The Rochester Manual: Practical Patient Care

The Rochester Manual:

Practical Patient Care

Medicine, Surgery, Pediatrics, OB-Gyn and Psychiatry

Editors: Karl A Illig, MD
and
Wendy Cowles Husser, MA, MPA

Introduction

A truly meaningful addition to a medical library is one that provides desired information by authors who are appreciative of the needs of a targeted audience. The audience that this work addresses includes medical students who course through compacted exposure to a wide variety of clinical arenas and are expected to gain an appreciation of the salient issues specific to each specialty and that these issues often transcend several disciplines. This work also provides a brief exposure to a broad variety of medical issues for reinforcement of knowledge gained in the past for those whose specialties have limited exposure to other fields. Residents, practitioners, and nurses all can benefit from reinforcement.

The authors—residents most closely aligned chronologically to students and their needs—are the most likely to be appreciative of the audience's desires and needs, the constraints of time, and the imperative of a succinct, readily understandable presentation of the most pertinent information.

This book addresses a need by a group of authors who recognize the elements required to satisfy that need and, as such, is truly meaningful.

SI Schwartz, MD

Distinguished Alumni Professor and Chair
Department of Surgery
University of Rochester Medical Center

Acknowledgements

Our first acknowledgment goes to the core of this book; to the students and medical professionals so often called on to make rapid decisions about patient care. This book was designed to fill a niche we believed was empty. Many textbooks exist in all fields of medicine that cover every detail of every disease; too often the clinical education of 3rd year medical students follows the same pattern of a flood of sometimes unconnected minutiae. Details are critical in medicine, but an initial, solid grasp of basic concepts should come first, creating the framework within which to assimilate the details as they come later.

Our second acknowledgment goes to the writers, senior residents and fellows at the University of Rochester who provide their own mental algorithms for conceptualizing the problem itself and for determining treatment options in a way that they wish had been available to them. Our book attempts to discuss the "big picture" in a readable way so that details can be assimilated, recalled, and understood.

Our third acknowledgment is directed at our reviewers, most of whom are at the University of Rochester, a few of whom are scattered around the United States. They criticized for accuracy and understanding, and pushed us to refine our material.

Finally, we are indebted to Beth Konieczny who cheerfully accepted our last minute directions and organized the flow of manuscripts and information among authors, editors, and publisher.

Karl A Illig

Dr. Illig was born in Rochester, NY, and despite four years of college at Harvard (majoring in springboard diving) and four years of medical school at Cornell in New York City (majoring in rugby), he knew there was "no place like home." His surgical residency at the University of Rochester, completed in 1995, included 2 years of research in trauma and general surgery. He is currently a fellow in vascular surgery with research projects underway on primary fibrinolysis and aortic and carotid surgery; clinical interests, other than vascular surgery, include trauma and education. He has 23 publications to his credit, and won the American College of Surgeons Committee on Trauma National Residents' Paper Competition in 1991. He loves golf, skiing, reading, scale modeling, and, most of all, his wife, Juliet, and son, Andrew.

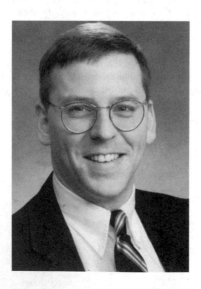

Wendy Cowles Husser

Ms. Husser has been an editor in the medical field for more than two decades. Her work includes 6 editions of *Principles of Surgery, Maingot's Abdominal Operations, The Year Book of Surgery,* and the *Handbook of Surgery, PreTest Self Assessment and Review, The Mapping of America;* she has lectured on writing for publishing. She earned her B.A. in English, and Masters in English Literature at the University of Rochester, and a Masters in Public Administration from the Maxwell School, Syracuse University. She has edited and produced hourly videos for national distribution on surgery and urology, and was the writer for one; she is coauthor on a paper on the liver, has edited hundreds of articles, several dozen chapters, and more than 240 editorials. She is currently working with European and American authors on an illustrated history of hernia, a history of surgery in America, the Centennial publication for the American Urological Foundation, and monographs covering a range of topics.

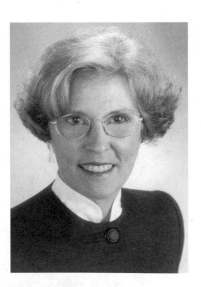

Dedication:

This book is dedicated to my wife,
Juliet, and son, Andrew,
whose support has been the one completely
irreplaceable thing in my life.

KAI

Author List[1]

Hassen Al-Amin, MD
Staff Fellow, Psychiatry
(Clinical Brain Disorders Branch, NIMH)

Sailija P Allanki, MD
Resident, Psychiatry

Paula Thomas Ardron, MD
Fellow, Pediatric Allergy and Immunology

Elise Becher, MD
Resident, Pediatrics

Bruce M Belin, MD
Resident, Surgery

Brent L Blackburn, MD
Resident, Pediatrics and Medicine

Dennis Blom, MD
Resident, Surgery

Peter N Bowers, MD
Fellow, Pediatric Cardiology

Ann-Marie Brooks, MD
Resident, Pediatrics

Diego Cahn-Hidalgo, MD
Resident, Medicine

Jae-Sung Cho, MD
Resident, Surgery

Marci J Chodroff, MD
Resident, Medicine

Rita A Clement, MD
Resident, Ob/Gyn

Paul D Danielson, MD
Resident, Surgery

Giuseppe Del Priore, MD
Assistant Professor, Gynecologic Oncology
(New York University)

Christina Deuber, MD
Resident, Pediatrics

John Downie, MD
Resident, Pediatrics

Dianne M Edgar, MD
Private Practice, OB/Gyn

Marc H Eigg, MD
Resident, Ob/Gyn

Carol Gagnon, MD
Resident, Pediatrics

Theresa M Gingras, MD
Resident, Pediatrics

Neal D Goldman, MD
Resident,Otorhinolaryngology

Andrew Goldstein, MD
Resident, Surgery

Jeffery A Goldstein, MD
Resident, Medicine

Joseph F Gomez, MD
Resident, Medicine

Carol Gondek, MD
Assistant Professor, Ob/Gyn
(University of Maryland Medical System)

Sheryl Gravelle-Camelo, MD
Private Practice, Pediatrics

Roy K Greenberg, MD
Resident, Surgery

Jennifer J Griggs, MD
Fellow, Hematology and Oncology

Mary Ellen Guido, MD
Fellow, Nephrology

Daniel F Gunther, MD
Resident, Pediatrics

Karen J Gurski, MD
Resident, Ob/Gyn

Jacqueline R Halliday, MD
Resident, Ob/Gyn

Frank Hamlett, MD
Fellow, Child Psychiatry

William G Harmon, MD
Resident, Pediatrics

Lindsey C Henson, MD, PhD
Assistant Professor, Anesthesiology

Steven M Horowitz, MD
Resident, Medicine

Khalid M Hubeishy, MD
Fellow, Emergency Psychiatry

Pasquale Iannoli, MD
Resident, Surgery

Karl A Illig, MD
Fellow, Vascular Surgery

(continued)

Author List *continued*

Wallace E Johnson, MD
Resident, Medicine

Michelle Sheri Jones, MD
Resident, Pediatrics

Jeffrey M Kaczorowski, MD
Resident, Pediatrics

David C Kaufman, MD
Clinical Assistant Professor, Surgery

Michael C Keefer, MD
Asst. Prof., Infectious Diseases

Kavita R Kolluri, MD
Resident, Medicine

F Eun-Hyung Lee, MD
Resident, Medicine

Andrew C Lee, MD
Assistant Professor, Anesthesiology

Men-Jean Lee, MD
Assistant Professor, Maternal-Fetal Medicine
(New York University)

Paul F Lehoullier, MD, PhD
Resident, Pediatrics

Nicole C Maronian, MD
Resident, Otorhinolaryngology

Kevin R McCormick, MD
Resident, Medicine

Ayesa N Mian, MD
Fellow, Pediatric Nephrology

Nicholas J Morrissey, MD
Resident, Surgery

Michael D Moxley, MD
Attending, Ob/Gyn
(St. Agnes Hospital, Baltimore, MD)

Wiley Nifong, MD
Resident, Surgery

Nicki Panoskaltsis, MD
Resident, Medicine

Timothy Pittinger, MD
Resident, Surgery

Anton P Porsteinsson, MD
Sr. Instructor, Psychiatry

A Andrew Rudman, MD
Resident, Medicine

Mustasim Rumi, MD
Resident, Surgery (Tufts University)

Margaret Salamon, MD
Instructor, Ob/Gyn (Northwestern University)

Timur P Sarac, MD
Resident, Surgery

Anna Seydel, MD
Resident, Surgery

Laura Jean Shipley, MD
Clinical Instructor, Pediatrics

Steven M Scofield, MD
Resident, Pediatrics and Medicine

Sharon Space, MD
Fellow, Pediatric Hematology/Oncology

Katharyne M Sullivan, MD
Fellow, Child Psychiatry

Calvert Warren, MD
Sr. Instructor, Psychiatry

Christopher L Wu, MD
Assistant Professor, Anesthesiology

1 Unless otherwise identified, all authors are at the University of Rochester

Reviewer List

Sincere appreciation to the following who provided
critical reviews for our chapters and supported the efforts
to produce our book.

James T Adams, MD
  Professor, Surgery

Michael J Apostolakos, MD
  Assistant Professor, Medicine

Curtis G Benesch, MD
  Senior Instructor, Neurology

Palmer Q Bessey, MD
  Professor, Surgery

Robert F Betts, MD
  Professor, Medicine - Infectious Diseases

Donald R Bordley, MD
  Associate Professor, Medicine

Oscar Bronsther, MD
  Associate Professor, Surgery

Marilyn R Brown, MD
  Associate Professor, Pediatrics-
  Gastroenterology/Nutrition

Mary T Caserta, MD
  Assistant Professor, Pediatrics -
  Infectious Diseases/Immunology

Edward B Clark, MD
  Professor, Pediatrics

Frances A Collichio, MD
  Assistant Professor, Cancer Center

Carl T D'Angio, MD
  Assistant Professor, Pediatrics-Neonatology

Robert W Emmens, MD
  Clinical Associate Professor, Pediatric Surgery

Andrea Kay Faulkner, MD
  Senior Instructor, Psychiatry-
  Child & Adolescent Services

Lynn C Garfunkel, MD
  Assistant Professor, Pediatrics

Francis Gigliotti, MD
  Associate Professor, Pediatrics-
  Infectious Diseases/Immunology

John Christopher Glantz, MD
  Assistant Professor, Obstetrics & Gynecology

Richard M Green, MD
Associate Professor, Surgery-Vascular Division

Ann E Zettelmaier Griepp, MD
Assistant Professor, Psychiatry

J Peter Harris, MD
Associate Professor, Pediatrics

George L Hicks, MD
Associate Professor, Surgery-Cardiothoracic Division

Kathleen M Hoeger, MD
Assistant Professor, Obstetrics & Gynecology

Cynthia R Howard, MD
Assistant Professor, General Pediatrics

David W Johnstone, MD
Assistant Professor, Surgery-Cardiothoracic Division

Albert P Jones Jr, MD
Clinical Associate Professor, Obstetrics & Gynecology

Nicholas Jospe, MD
Associate Professor, Pediatrics-Endocrinology

James W Kendig, MD
Associate Professor, Pediatrics-Neonatology

David N Korones, MD
Assistant Professor, Pediatrics-Hematology/Oncology

Richard E Kreipe, MD
Associate Professor, Pediatrics-Adolescent Medicine

David A Krusch, MD
Associate Professor, Surgery

Nancy E Lanphear, MD
Clinical Instructor, Pediatrics

Patrick C Lee, MD
Assistant Professor, Surgery

Jane L Liesveld, MD
Assistant Professor, Medicine

John R Looney, MD
Associate Professor, Medicine-Immunology

Thomas J McNanley MD
Assistant Professor, Obstetrics & Gynecology

Walid M Nassif, MD
Assistant Professor, Psychiatry-
Behavioral/Psychosocial Medicine

Lawrence F Nazarian, MD
Clinical Professor, Pediatrics
(continued)

Reviewer List *continued*

Table of Contents

Pediatrics
Jeffrey M Kaczorowski and
Laura Jean Shipley, Section Editors

OB/Gyn
   Men-Jean Lee and Giuseppe Del Priore, Section Editors

Psychiatry
Hassen Al-Amin and Anton P Porsteinsson,
Section Editors

Multidisciplinary

Roy K Greenberg
Section Editor

Multidisciplinary

1   Airway and Ventilator Management

The first priority in the treatment of any sick patient is the provision of an adequate airway. Because decompensation can be so rapid if the airway is lost, the evaluation and management of the patient with respiratory compromise can be exceedingly stressful. The two most important concepts to be comfortable with at this point are **when** and **how** to control the **airway** (the passage from the outside world to the alveoli), and how to manage a patient who requires **mechanical ventilation**.

Initial Assessment

The first steps in the evaluation of a patient with possible respiratory compromise are to relax, take a deep breath, and not panic. It is essential, especially for the inexperienced, to be able to interpret the situation and respond with control and logic.

Examine the patient for spontaneous respirations by listening to and watching the chest. Patients who can cough or talk are likely to be able to maintain their own airways in the short term. You may need to temporarily stop respiratory assistance (such as mask bagging) and observe for 10-15 seconds. The amount of work the patient appears to be doing to breathe should be noted, as should signs and symptoms of hypoxia such as cyanosis and altered mental status. The presence of stridor (harsh inspiratory sounds that arise from the upper airway) or retractions (extreme respiratory muscular effort) are signs of impending respiratory failure. Pulmonary crackles are usually indicative of interstitial fluid (pulmonary edema) or collapsed alveoli, ronchi are associated with increased intraluminal airway secretions, and wheezes suggest reactive airway disease or interstitial fluid overload.

The decision whether a patient needs help getting oxygen to the lungs is not always straightforward—clinical judgement and experience are necessary. Patients who are still breathing need help, in general, if they're working too hard (and, by extrapolation, won't be able to keep it up), have mechanical problems with their airway (such as those caused by trauma, anesthesia, or unconsciousness), or if high pressures must be delivered to the alveoli to improve oxygenation.

If Help is Needed

Once the decision is made that assistance is needed, action must be prompt and decisive. A major caveat when dealing with a patient with an impaired airway is that if the patient has suffered any blunt trauma, the cervical spine must always be assumed to be injured, and the patient **must not be moved**. First, **open the airway** using the **jaw thrust**, and clean debris (vomitus, foreign bodies) from the mouth by hand or with **suction**. The tongue is the most common obstruction in an unresponsive patient; the jaw thrust moves the tongue forward. An effective jaw thrust is done by placing one index finger behind each side of the patient's mandible at the angle of the jaw and applying considerable force (the most common error is not applying enough).

Once the airway is open, **ventilation** is the next step. If the patient is not breathing spontaneously or the airway is expected to be in jeopardy for more than a few minutes, more help is necessary. A **bag valve mask** (**BVM**) is a plastic mask that is connected by a series of one-way valves to an oxygen source that can be used to force oxygen into the lungs (and passively allow CO_2 to be expired). An airtight seal is required and is accomplished by pulling the jaw forward with a jaw thrust (not by pushing the mask into the face or the patient's tongue will obstruct the airway). An **oral airway** is a plastic splint placed in the mouth used to hold the tongue forward, and a **nasal airway** is a pliable tube that stents the airway from the nose to the base of the tongue. Both facilitate the use of the BVM, but oral airways are not well tolerated by patients who are awake. **Suction** remains critically important to have available at all times.

Intubation

One of the most difficult decisions and important clinical skills to acquire is that of knowing when to intubate a patient. There is no definitive algorithm, and no book can provide definitive answers. The decision is not based on a specific arterial blood gas (ABG) value, an inspiratory rate, or any other single clinical finding, but is a decision made on the basis of all available data, including the judgment about whether the problem is temporary or relatively permanent, the underlying disease process, and the patient's premorbid status. Respiratory distress usually occurs gradually. There is not always an exact time to intubate, but there is a period of time within which the decision is made.

Why intubate?

Why intubate? In other words, what advantage does an endotracheal tube provide? There are two major functions of the endotracheal tube. Most important is the ability, due to the inflatable cuff, to deliver air under pressure (**positive-pressure ventilation**). Mechanical "control" of the airway is another; the tube ensures the maintenance of a direct, open passageway from the outside world to the trachea.

Intubation

Once the decision has been made to intubate, the patient should be adequately prepared. Oxygen saturation should be monitored; **preoxygenation** by BVM to establish arterial saturation as complete as possible is important if time and the airway status permit. The patient should be positioned for intubation with unrestricted access to the head and neck, and **suction should be turned on** (not just "available"). The most commonly used technique is **oral intubation**. A laryngoscope (a straight or curved metal tongue blade with a light source) is used to visualize the vocal cords and pass the endotracheal tube under direct vision through them into the trachea. The laryngoscope stimulates gagging; oral intubation is thus much easier in unconscious patients. **Nasotracheal intubation** is useful in patients who have oral pathology, are somewhat awake, or cannot tolerate an orotracheal tube. Blind nasal intubation is particularly useful since it can be done in an awake, unsedated patient, without using a laryngoscope. It is done by advancing an endotracheal tube through the nose, relying on the presence of audible breath sounds to signal the correct position. Obviously blind nasotracheal intubation requires that the patient is able to breath; it is not an option in an apneic patient. This technique may be safer than orotracheal intubation if the status of the cervical spine is in question (since neck extension is not required). The greatest disadvantage of blind nasal intubation is the possibility of bleeding from injury to the vascular oronasopharyngeal mucosa which can make intubation more difficult.

Sedation, commonly using benzodiazepines, barbiturates, or other medications is frequently required for intubation. Full pharmacologic paralysis is sometimes required, but this technique should be attempted only by those who are very experienced in airway management (because if intubation is unsuccessful, the patient can no longer breath or protect his or her own airway). Finally, a **surgical cricothyroidotomy** is an option if intubation is unsuccessful or impossible (for example, after major maxillofacial trauma) and the airway is acutely compromised. The incision is made through the cricothyroid membrane just beneath the thyroid cartilage and is, in experienced hands, extremely rapid (seconds).

The Ventilator

Intubation implies that the problem is expected to last more than a few minutes or hours and, thus, that ventilation by hand will be impractical. A mechanical ventilator reliably provides oxygenation and ventilation for the duration of the patient's needs, and is used in essentially every intubated patient.

The concepts of oxygenation and ventilation are very important. **Oxygenation** is the delivery of oxygen to the alveoli and blood. There is a great deal of reserve; under normal conditions, air with high oxygen content can sit in the alveoli for many minutes while normal arterial oxygen content (PaO_2) is maintained. CO_2, however, is constantly delivered to the alveoli by the flow of blood, and must be continually removed by regular exchange of air, or **ventilation**. While they can interact, they are two separate concepts, and can be (and usually are) treated separately. In other words, disorders and treatment of each occurs independently of each other.

Oxygenation

Oxygenation is altered by adjusting the **fraction of inspired O_2 (FIO_2)** from 21%-100%. Too much oxygen is harmful because of alveolar damage due to free radical reactions. In general, FIO_2 should be at the lowest level possible that will maintain adequate oxygen delivery to the tissues (see Chapter 5, "Shock"). An FIO_2 of up to

Multidisciplinary
Airway and Ventilator Management
continued

50%-60% is safe for long periods; higher levels begin to be harmful by 48-72 hours or so. The other way to affect oxygenation is by increasing the actual pressure within the lungs by using **positive end-expiratory pressure (PEEP)**, discussed below.

Ventilation

Ventilation is provided by adjusting the **tidal volume** (volume of air delivered per breath) and **rate**, the product of which is the **minute ventilation**. The goal is to adjust the minute ventilation to attain the desired pH.

Ventilatory modes

Modern ventilators are computers, capable of performing a mechanical task (delivering air) in a number of different ways (called **modes**). In **assist-control (AC)** mode, each attempted breath by the patient triggers delivery of a set tidal volume. If no breaths are triggered, or the rate is low, a guaranteed back-up minute volume is delivered at the set tidal volume and rate. **Synchronized intermittent mandatory ventilation (SIMV)** is similar to AC, except that spontaneous breaths triggered by the patient lead to delivery of whatever tidal volume the patient can produce, not the full, set tidal volume. In a breathing patient, SIMV requires that the patient do more work, but AC and SIMV are identical in those who are apneic. **Pressure support (PS)** is a mode that increases flow to a set level of positive pressure during inhalation, reducing the work needed to breathe. The patient continues to be able to pull flow from the ventilator above the PS level until the flow rate decreases. There are no mandatory breaths; patients determine their own respiratory rate if no other mode is used.

CPAP (continuous positive airway pressure) and **PEEP (positive end-expiratory pressure)** are ventilator techniques that are similar and should be considered together. They both consist of raising the baseline pressure above the zero level, with the goal of recruiting alveoli, thereby improving oxygenation. PEEP is used during positive-pressure ventilation, and CPAP essentially provides a low level of assistance during spontaneous respiration roughly equal to the extra work needed to breath through the long, narrow endotracheal tube, and is thus commonly used to test the patient's ability to breathe without the ventilator.

Ventilator settings

When you place someone on the ventilator, you specify the **ventilator settings**. The best way to do this is to make an educated guess (erring on the conservative side) based on the patient's size and the clinical situation, then measure the arterial blood gas (ABG) after equilibration and make changes as needed. Generally, you specify the mode, the tidal volume (10-15cc/kg) and minimum rate (often 12-14 breaths per minute) to determine ventilation, the FIO_2 (start at 60% and wean as able) to determine oxygenation, and the level of PEEP and pressure support (typically 5mmHg each) to keep the alveoli open and reduce the work of breathing.

In order for the ventilator to operate, a triggering device must be chosen. The usual trigger is the negative pressure created by the patient. Obviously, both SIMV and AC modes will deliver at least the set minimum minute ventilation if the patient does not ever trigger the ventilator (if the patient is iatrogenically paralyzed, for example). The peak flow and inspiratory to expiratory (I:E) ratio determine the kinetics of ventilation. The peak flow is the rate of delivery of air (inspiration). If high, for example, inspiration is quick and the majority of each breath is expiration. This is closest to normal breathing.

Monitoring While on the Ventilator

Monitoring the adequacy of oxygenation and ventilation is of utmost importance. **Continuous pulse oxymetry** gives a measure of the oxygen saturation of hemoglobin (the acceptable range is typically 90%-100%), but provides no information about ventilation. To assess ventilation and accurately measure the PaO_2, the ABG is frequently used. Interpreting the ABG is quite straightforward. Three variables are of interest: the pH, the PaO_2, and the pCO_2.

The pH measures the acidity of the blood and is affected by both metabolic and respiratory factors (see Chapter 2, "Acid-Base Disorders"). **It is critically important to clearly understand the relationship between the other two variables and oxygenation and ventilation**. The PaO_2 measures oxygenation; if it is too high or too low, adjust the FIO_2 and/or PEEP. The pCO_2 measures ventilation; if too high or too low, adjust the tidal volume and/or respiratory rate. Oxygenation and ventilation, for our purposes, do not interact or affect one another! You can look at each as **separate** entities and adjust the ventilator settings **separately**.

Use your head while monitoring a patient on the ventilator. Pulse oxymetry is cheap and easy and can be used in a continuous fashion. Obviously, if the patient is unstable, frequent ABGs will be required, but when the patient is more stable, you can taper off.

Weaning and Extubation

**Weaning
parameters**

It is important to remember the reason you placed the patient on the ventilator in the first place. Four major points are considered when trying to discontinue mechanical ventilation: ventilation, oxygenation, secretions, and airway protection.

Ventilation is probably most important, because the problem that patients most often have is inability to move enough air back and forth to ventilate themselves. "**Weaning parameters**" are obtained while still intubated and predict successful extubation (defined as not having to put the tube back in). **Vital capacity** usually needs to be at least 10cc/kg, although the **minute volume** may better predict the ability to sustain ventilation over more than a breath or two. Patients should also be able to generate at least -30 cm H_2O (**negative inspiratory force**, **NIF**). The quotient of the respiratory rate to tidal volume (in liters) can be calculated; if less than 100, it is likely mechanical ventilation can be discontinued. Oxygenation must be adequate at levels of FIO_2 that can be delivered without the endotracheal tube (i.e., at low levels of PEEP). The presence of excessive airway secretions requires judgment. Some secretions are inevitable. If the patient is awake and the secretions are not purulent, it's probably OK. Finally, the ability of the patient to protect the airway must be assured. The presence of appropriate gag and cough reflexes usually indicates the ability to protect the airway; note that patients do not have to be awake and responsive in order to accomplish this task.

Weaning can begin if the patient is not acutely ill and there are no signs of active infection. Adequate nutrition and appropriate treatment of infection are the most important factors in successful weaning, and attempts at obtaining good sleep-wake cycles are also helpful. There are many different techniques that may be used. Slowly decreasing the level of ventilatory support (rate) or attempts at interval training with periods of work alternating with higher levels of support and rest are both useful. A nice method, especially for patients who are awake but very weak, is to reduce the rate drastically while providing a high level of pressure support (which is then gradually decreased).

Tracheostomy

If it appears unlikely that the patient can be weaned from mechanical ventilation within a reasonable time frame, a decision regarding potential **tracheostomy** must be entertained. A tracheostomy is a surgical hole in the trachea below the vocal cords. It provides access for suctioning, gets the tube out of the mouth and tape off the face, is secure, and is much more comfortable for the patient than is an endotracheal tube. In addition, the work of breathing is reduced markedly because the tube is so short. Finally, "extubation" is very simple: merely disconnect the tubing and watch the patient for a few minutes. These are major advantages; it is not at all uncommon for a patient who "cannot be weaned" to be free of the ventilator within a few days of tracheostomy. This does not mean the tracheostomy was unnecessary; rather, that it might have helped sooner!

There is no magic day that an endotracheal tube has been in too long and the patient needs a tracheostomy. Formerly, the risk of pressure necrosis of the trachea by the endotracheal tube's cuff was believed to be significant by 10-14 days, but modern, low-pressure cuffs have made this point less relevant. Patient comfort, reduction in maxillofacial infection, and improved pulmonary toilet are the primary issues. Generally, a tracheostomy is advised if intubation seems to be necessary beyond 2 weeks or so, but this decision is very variable and depends on how much progress patients are making (i.e., whether they will be extubated in the next few days). There is some data to suggest that very early tracheostomy (within a few days if prolonged ventilation is expected) improves outcome, but data are sparse. Special tracheostomy tubes allow some awake and cooperative patients the ability to talk even when on the ventilator.
(continued)

Multidisciplinary
Airway and Ventilator Management
continued

Oxygen Delivery

Finally, it's important to understand oxygen delivery systems for non-ventilated patients, such as nasal prongs, face masks, and venturi devices. Estimation of the inspired oxygen concentration (FIO_2) is the first step. 100% oxygen flows from the tank (or wall); the unknown factor is how much air (21% oxygen) is entrained from the surroundings. The FIO_2 depends on the patient's own ventilation. For example, in a patient with a minute volume of 6L/min (21% O_2) wearing nasal prongs set at a flow of 2L/min (100% O_2), most of the inspired oxygen will be from the 100% source. If the minute volume increases, however, relatively more room air (21%) will be entrained and the FIO_2 will decrease. Thus, the FIO_2 varies significantly depending on the patient's minute volume. Some oxygen delivery devices use reservoirs to store pure oxygen, such as the bag on a non-rebreather mask. Sometimes the reservoir is not so apparent: when using nasal prongs, the nose and nasopharynx act as an oxygen reservoir. Some devices are designed to deliver a set FIO_2, entraining varying amounts of the 100% oxygen from the source according to the air velocity and size of aperture provided. If a patient is intubated and on the ventilator, of course, they will receive exactly the FIO_2 you set.

Oxygen is a great drug: use it in every patient with airway or ventilation compromise. The old adage that many COPD patients require a hypoxic drive is rarely true; it's a lot easier to assist ventilation if you're wrong, than it is to reverse hypoxic injury. ∎

2   Acid-Base Disorders

Discussions of acid-base physiology can be approached from a clinical or biochemical perspective. The clinical approach helps clarify treatment but rarely provides much of an appreciation for the basic science behind it; the bio-chemical approach tends to be confusing and carries with it a strong hypnotic-sedative effect. It's a topic that is vital to understand, however, and an approach via the middle ground might be most educational.

Interpretation of Acid-base Status

The **arterial blood gas (ABG)** is obtained from a direct arterial puncture. The two most important values when dealing with acid-base status are the **pH** and partial pressure of carbon dioxide (**PCO_2**). The **HCO_3** is obtained from measurement of serum electrolytes (SMA-7). CO_2 is excreted solely by the lungs, while the kidneys are the major regulators of HCO_3.

When evaluating a patient suspected of having an acid-base disturbance, the first and easiest question to answer is, "What is the hydrogen ion concentration [H^+] in the blood?" Knowing the pH or the [H^+] is the first step in the evaluation of any acid base disturbance. The laboratory actually measures [H^+], not pH. The pH is a calculated value equal to the negative log of [H^+]—using pH rather than just referring to the actual [H^+] in the blood is a convention. If pH is low (less than 7.35) or [H^+] is high (more than 45nM/L), the patient has an **acidemia**. If the pH is high (more than 7.45) or the [H^+] is low (less than 35nM/L), the patient has an **alkalemia**. The "-emia" is determined by the measured pH, while an "-osis" is a pathologic process, and the patient may have more than one at a time.

After pH is determined, the next step is to determine the cause of the problem. It can be very easy or quite difficult to determine every factor involved, because both **metabolic** and **respiratory** disturbances contribute. In a simple acid-base disorder, there is only one problem—metabolic or respiratory. Complex acid-base disorders are caused by both; the final pH depends on the magnitude of each. *(continued)*

Multidisciplinary
Acid Based Disorders *continued*

A **simple acid-base disorder** is present when only one problem exists. The pH, HCO_3, and PCO_2 will determine the acid/base disturbance:

pH	PCO_2 /HCO_3	Nomenclature of Disorder
Low	High PCO_2	Respiratory acidosis
Low	Low HCO_3	Metabolic acidosis
High	Low PCO_2	Respiratory alkalosis
High	High HCO_3	Metabolic alkalosis

Simple disorders mean that one factor is abnormal, and the other is altered in the expected direction required to drive the blood back toward neutrality. The question of which is the primary problem and which is compensation must be answered by looking at the pH and clinical situation (see below). If HCO_3 is low and PCO_2 is high, for example, both of which **independently** suggest that acidosis is present, the patient must have a **complex** acid-base disturbance. The point is of course, that compensation acts to drive the pH back towards normal—PCO_2 should decrease to compensate for a decreased HCO_3 (primary metabolic acidosis), for example. If this relationship is not present, or, more subtly, if the direction is right but the magnitude is not, a complex disorder exists. Any combination of metabolic and respiratory disturbance can occur at the same time, except a respiratory acidosis and alkalosis (you can't breath fast and slow at the same time).

Compensation

What is **compensation**? If a patient develops an acidosis or alkalosis as the result of a respiratory or metabolic disturbance, the body has the ability to partially correct the problem. In the setting of a primary respiratory problem, the kidneys can respond by either secreting or reabsorbing bicarbonate (metabolic compensation). If the patient has a primary metabolic problem, the lung can compensate by "excreting" (hyperventilating) or, to a limited extent, retaining CO_2. It is no surprise that PCO_2 and HCO_3 are closely intertwined molecules. If a primary disorder alters the concentration of one of these measured parameters, the other is modified by the compensatory mechanisms. Therefore, to determine whether a single disorder with normal compensation is present instead of two separate disorders, you have to calculate the level to be expected if perfect compensation were present:

Primary Disorder	Expected Compensation
Metabolic acidosis	PCO_2 drops to equal (HCO_3 x 1.5) + 8
Metabolic alkalosis	PCO_2 increases to equal HCO_3 +15
Respiratory acidosis	HCO_3 increases 3 for each 10 increase in PCO_2
Respiratory alkalosis	HCO_3 drops 5 for each 10 decrease in PCO_2

If the measured value is above or below the expected calculated value, a secondary disturbance must be present.

There are two important caveats. First, compensation for acute respiratory problems is poor–in other words, compensation takes a little time. For example, the kidneys cannot reabsorb or excrete HCO_3 to a significant degree immediately (it takes a few hours to gear up). Second, respiratory compensation for a metabolic alkalosis is poor, because, to compensate, hypoventilation must take place. Of course, adequate oxygenation (see Chapter 1, "Airway and Ventilator Management") takes "priority" over pH in the body's scheme of things, so the CO_2 usually won't rise very much despite a severe metabolic alkalosis.

Anion Gap Disorders

The **anion gap** is the difference between **measured** major anions and cations on the SMA-7. Humans are electrically neutral. The idea that because an anion gap exists there must be more cations than anions (producing an electrical charge) is a misconception. The reality is that conventional laboratory tests (specifically the SMA-7) measure more cations than anions. In reality:

Unmeasured anions + Cl^- + HCO_3^- = Unmeasured cations + Na^+

(continued)

Cations like potassium, magnesium and calcium and
anions like albumin and phosphate can be measured but
are generally not part of the **anion gap equation**:

$$\text{Anion Gap} = Na^+ - (Cl^- + HCO_3^-)$$

There is always an anion gap of approximately 10meq/L
due to the normally unmeasured anions (there are more
unmeasured anions than unmeasured cations). The utility
of the anion gap is that it provides a way to estimate
whether a metabolic acidosis is accompanied by an
increase in unmeasured anions (**anion gap acidosis**). If
so, the calculated anion gap will increase because of the
presence of a new, unmeasured anion (not accounted for
in the equation). A convenient mnemonic to remember
the causes of anion-gap acidosis is the term MUD PILES:
methanol, uremia, diabetic ketoacidosis, paraldehyde, isoniazid or iron toxicity, lactic acidosis (probably the most
common), eating disorders (starvation), and salicylates.

A **triple disorder** can even be present, where concomitant metabolic and respiratory disturbances all coexist.
Trying to figure out this situation is one of the most difficult aspects in the interpretation of acid-base disturbances. The major question in the setting of an anion gap
acidosis is whether or not the decrease in HCO_3 is equivalent to the increase in the gap (in other words, is simple
compensation occurring)? If so, then the anions causing
the gap are the sole cause of the acidosis, but if not,
something else must be causing the altered HCO_3 (i.e., a
concomitant metabolic disturbance).

Clinical Acid-base Interpretation

Take a deep breath (lowering your PCO_2). Although the
concepts and number of terms to worry about are fairly
limited, the number of permutations quickly becomes
unmanageable. It is critically important to remember that
interpretation of the numerical values in isolation is
impossible in all but the simplest situations—the ABG
and SMA-7 must be interpreted in light of the current
clinical situation. Fortunately, certain situations and combinations of events are common.

Respiratory acidosis

Respiratory acidosis is caused by retention of CO_2. Any problems with breathing (such as acute respiratory failure or chronic obstructive pulmonary disease) will lead to respiratory acidosis, as will mechanical problems with ventilation (such as a low ventilator setting; see Chapter 1, "Airway and Ventilator Management" or pneumothorax; see Chapter 35, "Thoracic Surgery"). The kidneys compensate by reabsorbing HCO_3 to raise its concentration in the blood. Chronic retention is better tolerated and better compensated for (i.e., HCO_3 is higher and pH is near normal) than is acute (when HCO_3 may not be altered at all).

Respiratory alkalosis

Respiratory alkalosis is caused by hyperventilation and excess CO_2 excretion. This can be caused by hyperventilation due to agitation, pain, or brain injury, early sepsis, or specific problems like salicylate overdose. The kidneys compensate by excreting HCO_3 to lower its concentration in the blood. Chronic hyperventilation is rare, but leads to better compensation than does acute.

Metabolic acidosis

Non-anion gap metabolic acidosis is caused by loss of HCO_3, most commonly due to diarrhea or renal tubular acidosis. Urine electrolytes are very helpful in this situation. If HCO_3 stool losses are high, the kidneys should make ammonium as they secrete H^+ to compensate. In a fashion analogous to the serum anion gap, the difference between the urinary chloride and the sum of your sodium and potassium will give you an estimate of the amount of ammonium, the major unmeasured cation, in the urine:

$$\text{Urinary Anion Gap} = (Na^+ + K^+) - Cl^-$$

If the urine anion gap is negative (more chloride than cations, implying the presence of unmeasured cations such as ammonium) the kidneys are responding appropriately to an acidemia from another cause (such as diarrhea). If the urine anion gap is positive or zero (no ammonium production) the kidneys are not compensating appropriately and it is probable that an intrinsic renal problem (such as renal tubular acidosis) exists. In any metabolic acidosis the lungs compensate by "excreting" more CO_2 by hyperventilating.

Anion gap metabolic acidosis is caused by the presence of unmeasured anions as discussed above. One of the more common causes is lactic acid, produced by muscles

Multidisciplinary
Acid Based Disorders *continued*

and other tissues as the product of anaerobic metabolism. Most commonly this indicates tissue hypoxia due to impaired oxygen delivery and/or utilization, often due to sepsis. The cells shift to anaerobic metabolism and release lactic acid. Other common causes are poisoning (methanol, paraldehyde, and salicylates), uremia from renal failure, and diabetic ketoacidosis. Again, pulmonary compensation is by hyperventilation.

Metabolic alkalosis

Metabolic alkalosis is caused by too much HCO_3 or too little H^+. Its causes are a little less intuitively obvious, but there are two very common situations in hospitalized patients in which metabolic alkalosis is often present. Contraction alkalosis is caused by intravascular volume depletion, commonly as the result of iatrogenic diuresis. The kidneys respond by reabsorbing Na^+ in an effort to increase intravascular volume, and excrete H^+ to maintain electrical neutrality, thus raising the pH. The other common cause of H^+ loss is via removal of acidic gastric contents via vomiting or nasogastric suction. Dehydration is also often present in this situation, adding the effects of a contraction alkalosis. Again, the first "priority" of the kidneys is to preserve intravascular volume, and Na^+ is reabsorbed while H^+ is excreted. This produces the "paradoxical aciduria" seen with a contraction alkalosis.

Usually a mild metabolic alkalosis is well tolerated. The goal of treatment is to treat the underlying problem by replacing intravascular volume (with normal saline). Serum potassium must also be replaced so that the kidney can excrete potassium rather than H^+. If the alkalosis is due to high nasogastric output, reducing the acid output of the stomach (for example, by administering an H_2-blocker) will stop the problem at its source. If the alkalosis is very severe a patient can be given, under very controlled circumstances, a hydrochloric acid drip (although this technique is a little controversial). Respiratory compensation is poor, because hypoventilation (raising PCO_2) produces hypoxia and subjective distress and therefore does not occur to a useful degree. ■

It is in the recent decades only that "mainstream" medicine recognized the importance of nutritional therapy in ill patients. It has been estimated that half of all hospitalized patients suffer from some degree of nutritional impairment, and it is clear that nutritional deficits contribute substantially to morbidity and mortality.

Physiology

The function of nutrition is twofold: to provide energy (calories) in the form of adenosine triphospate (ATP), and to provide structural building blocks and reagents for the body's chemical reactions and cellular healing and turnover. Major molecules used by the body are divided into three categories: carbohydrates, lipids, and proteins. The body can convert any of these into any other fairly freely, with the exception that lipids cannot be efficiently converted to carbohydrates or proteins. Carbohydrates and lipids are the major energy source, yielding ATP via the Krebs cycle and electron transport chain, while proteins are normally used for structural and functional purposes (see Figure 3.1 on following page).

Carbohydrates (in the form of glycogen) are used for short-term energy storage (less than 24 hours), while lipids (fat cells) are the major long-term energy source. There is no "nonessential" form of protein in storage; each molecule used is taken away from a structural (e.g., muscle) or functional (e.g., albumin) role. The basic goal of nutritional support is to provide nonprotein fuel sources (carbohydrates and fats) so that protein can be used for synthesis and regeneration.

Nitrogen balance

An often confusing point is the interchangeability of nitrogen and protein in the clinical setting. Nitrogen is not present in lipids or in carbohydrates, only in proteins; thus, when proteins are broken down for energy, nitrogen is excreted in the urine. It is also technically easy to measure, and thus protein is usually discussed clinically as nitrogen. Each 6.25 grams of protein yields 1 gram of nitrogen, and vice versa. **Nitrogen balance** refers to the relationship between nitrogen

Multidisciplinary
Nutrition *continued*

Figure 3.1
Simplified diagram of the fate of the three major nutritional components. Adapted from Alberts B, Bray D, Lewis J, Raff M, Roberts K, and Watson JD. Molecular Biology of the Cell, 2nd edt. New York: Garland, 1989, with permission.

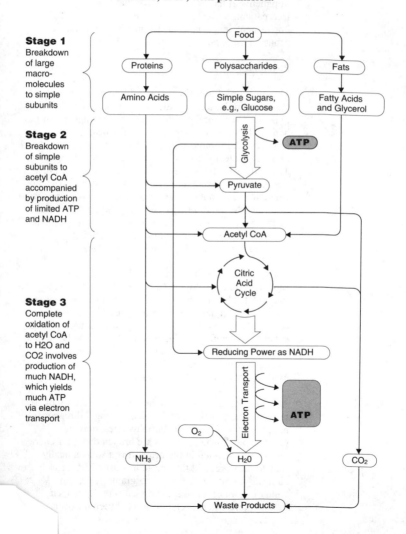

Stage 1
Breakdown of large macro-molecules to simple subunits

Stage 2
Breakdown of simple subunits to acetyl CoA accompanied by production of limited ATP and NADH

Stage 3
Complete oxidation of acetyl CoA to H2O and CO2 involves production of much NADH, which yields much ATP via electron transport

intake and nitrogen loss in urine, feces, and wounds (thus, ingested and excreted protein).

Pathophysiology

There are three situations where the body is using stored nutrients: **short-term fasting** (between meals), long-term **starvation**, and significant **stress** caused by sepsis, trauma, or other major insult.

Fasting

In the normal, **short-term** between-meals state, the body uses glucose as a fuel, primarily from circulating, recently ingested carbohydrates, and also from liver and muscle glycogen, regulated by insulin and glucagon. Proteins are used for synthesis, and excess calories are converted to stored fat.

Starvation

In **starvation**, a different situation exists. Only small amounts of stored carbohydrates are available, primarily in the form of liver glycogen, and these carbohydrates are quickly exhausted (within 12-48 hours). Fats are the primary source of long-term energy storage and are burned to produce ATP by most of the body. Some cells, notably neurons (the brain), and cells of the hematologic system (red and white cells), use glucose only. Since fats cannot efficiently be converted into glucose, protein is used for this purpose, at the expense of structure and function. This causes an increased urinary nitrogen excretion (signifying increased proteolysis). The administration of carbohydrates can decrease this protein breakdown, leading to reduced nitrogen excretion; this is the so-called "protein-sparing" effect. In prolonged starvation, however, the brain adapts to allow utilization of lipids (as ketone bodies), leading to reduced protein breakdown and urinary nitrogen excretion. Hematologic cells still must have glucose, though, so a certain amount of obligatory protein breakdown (and nitrogen excretion) continues. The net result is utilization of stored fat. If some carbohydrates are administered to reduce proteolysis, "fat loss" (dieting) results!

Stress

Major **stress** (major trauma, sepsis, and critical illness in general), however, results in fundamentally different events. As in starvation, there is early exhaustion of liver glycogen and increased proteolysis. For reasons that are not well understood, however, in stress the brain does **not** shift to the utilization of ketone bodies, but continues to require glucose. This glucose, again, mostly comes from protein, because conversion from fats is so inefficient. Furthermore, even if glucose is supplied, probably due to cytokines and hormones the body continues to break down protein and excrete nitrogen in the urine. The "protein-sparing" effect of glucose is **not** seen in major stress, and the early, high levels of protein breakdown and urinary nitrogen excretion persist. Unfortunately, since there is no storage form of protein, function is lost when proteolysis occurs. Muscle is a primary source of protein, and the diaphragm is a large muscle, contributing to the difficulties in weaning septic patients from the ventilator. Other significant sources of protein are immunoglobulins, other circulating proteins such as albumin, the liver, and the intestinal tract.

The major nutritional problem in septic or post-traumatic patients is that even if sufficient calories and glucose are given, obligatory protein breakdown occurs. There is no way to ameliorate this early negative nitrogen balance, and, in fact, such attempts may be harmful due to overfeeding. The only "cures," at present, are cure of the underlying problem or prolonged support of the patient during the proteolytic state until healing takes place.

Nutritional Assessment

There are essentially three ways of assessing a patient's nutritional status. The first, **subjective global assessment**, is simply observations made on the basis of the history, physical exam, simple laboratory tests, and clinical judgment. A practical (and only partially facetious) starting point is to assume that **every** patient, other than those with very simple problems, is (or will be) malnourished. Important clues to nutritional deficits are a history of recent weight loss (more important than static weight, even if "abnormal"), prolonged inability to eat (whether preexistent or anticipated), muscle wasting, decreased fat stores, or reduction in certain serum values (such as albumin, prealbumin, transferrin, or the absolute lymphocyte count) that have been shown to correlate with malnutrition. This method is probably the most clinically useful. The second method is to use a **formula** to estimate basal energy needs based on height, weight, and age (such as the Harris-Benedict equation), multiplying by a stress factor (ranging from 1.0 to as high as 2.0) for fevers, infection, trauma, or other ongoing problems, as appropriate. This is most often done by the nutritional support team when their assistance is needed; such formulas are quite straightforward. The final method is actually to calculate energy needs using a **metabolic cart** and indirect calorimetry (direct calorimetry would be messy and non-repeatable!), measuring O_2 consumption and CO_2 production as an indication of fuel metabolism, and is usually reserved for research or very difficult clinical situations.

Requirements

Calories

Calories are provided primarily as glucose and lipids, and needs are usually around 20-35kcals/kg/day. Severe stress can increase requirements to as much as 40 or more kcals/kg/day, and children, because growth is also needed, can require as much as 175kcals/kg/day. Each gram of lipid yields 9kcal of energy, protein yields 5kcal/gm, and carbohydrates yield 4kcal/gm. As discussed above, it is important to provide enough calories as glucose and lipids to let the body utilize protein for synthesis; thus the ratio of calories to protein should be about 120-150kcals per 1 gram of nitrogen. With significant stress, because obligate proteolysis persists, more protein must be given, resulting in a decrease in the ratio to 100:1 or so. Overfeeding of calories is of no benefit and may be actively harmful, increasing hepatic workload and possibly contributing to immunosuppression.

Carbohydrates

Carbohydrates are primarily given for caloric needs as discussed above. Typical needs are 150-400gm/day, which supply about 50%-70% of total calories. The body can only utilize about 5mg/kg/min. Too much carbohydrate is also harmful, resulting in hyperglycemia, increased conversion of glucose to lipid (burning ATP), fatty deposition within the liver, and production of too much CO_2. This may contribute to difficulties in weaning the patient from the ventilator, because glucose results in the production of more CO_2 per O_2 used (the respiratory quotient, RQ) than does lipid. Stressed patients handle glucose poorly for a variety of reasons, due in part to end-organ insulin resistance; hyperglycemia is common.

Lipids

Lipids are given to provide calories (about 30%), to provide linoleic acid, which cannot be synthesized, and to "spare" some protein breakdown by providing ketone bodies for the brain. General needs are about 2.5gm/kg/day. Fats in the form of omega-3 fatty acids ("fish oil") may be beneficial by reducing pro-inflammatory precursors, but too much fat may be somewhat immunosuppressive. Fats are especially helpful as caloric sources in the relatively glucose intolerant stressed patient.

Proteins

Proteins are ideally used only for synthesis and to provide essential amino acids (thus making mandatory the provision of adequate nonprotein calories), although some are unavoidably burned as fuel. Adults need about 0.8gm/kg/day, while children need more (up to 1.5gm/kg/day) to support growth. Branched-chain amino acids (Ile, Leu, Val) are metabolized purely by muscles and thus may be beneficial with liver dysfunction. Glutamine is the primary fuel for the enterocytes, plays a major role interorgan nitrogen transfer, and is preferentially metabolized in severe stress. It is currently available in enteral, but not parenteral, formulas. Although unstable in solution, increasing evidence suggests it should routinely be used, and strategies for its parenteral administration are evolving.

Vitamins, electrolytes, trace elements

Vitamins, **electrolytes**, and **trace elements** must also be provided. In general, stores of the fat-soluble vitamins are well preserved, while those of the water-soluble vitamins are more rapidly depleted. There is accumulating evidence that the administration of iron may be immunosuppressive in severe stress.

Delivery

Who needs nutritional support? Obviously, anyone who is or will be malnourished and cannot meet their own needs. The rule of thumb is that healthy patients who are unable to eat for 7-10 days (total pre- **and** postoperatively) should have supplemental nutrients provided. Patients who start out malnourished should receive supplemental nutrition sooner. A special case is whether a mildly malnourished patient, unable to eat or be supported with tube feedings, should receive preoperative parenteral nutrition. Contrary to conventional wisdom, the answer is usually **no**! It has been shown empirically that the majority of patients actually do worse in this situation. The reason is that the risks of parenteral nutrition (initial central access and infection) and high costs outweigh the very minimal benefits. Preoperative parenteral nutrition is beneficial only in the subgroup of extremely malnourished patients, and only if continued for a long period of time (more than a week). At the time of surgery, enteral access in the form of a jejunostomy or gastrostomy should be established.

Enteral feeding

Nutrition can be administered **enterally** (within the gut) or **parenterally** (hyperalimentation or total parenteral nutrition; TPN). **Always use the gut if able.** Theoretically, enteral feeding is more physiologic, because nutrients enter the portal system and liver rather than the systemic veins. Parenteral feeding clearly results in atrophy of the enterocytes and gut mucosa, possibly contributing to impaired barrier function. Enteral feeding is cheaper, easier, and associated with fewer complications. Empirical studies are surprisingly sparse, but accumulating evidence suggests improved overall outcome with enteral feeding, especially after trauma or burns.

Enteral feeding can be accomplished using a variety of techniques. Access to the stomach can be via the oral route (what we all do every day), by means of a nasogastric feeding tube, a percutaneously-placed endoscopic gastrostomy (PEG), or a surgically placed gastrostomy. Feeding into the stomach is most physiologic, and, because the stomach is a storage organ, can be administered as boluses (three times a day) of any tonicity. With gastric access, regurgitation and aspiration can be a problem, especially if a feeding tube passes through the lower esophageal sphincter, or if the patient is recumbent. This route is best used in patients with an absolutely normal GI tract who cannot eat (due to oropharyngeal cancer, other obstructive problems, endotracheal tubes, and so on).

Feeding into the small bowel (duodenum or jejunum) reduces the risk of aspiration by interposing another sphincter (the pylorus) between the food and the lungs. Access is more complicated, requiring a transpyloric nasoduodenal tube or surgically- or laparoscopically-placed jejunostomy; it is critical to anticipate this need at the time of laparotomy for major trauma or sepsis. The small bowel is much less affected by ileus or dysmotility problems than is the stomach, and such feedings are often well tolerated immediately after surgery or burns, and

Multidisciplinary
Nutrition *continued*

even in situations where prolonged ileus is expected to be present. Thus, this route is best used if the stomach is expected to work poorly (acute or major trauma, sepsis, or stress) or if the patient has failed intragastric feeds due to intolerance or aspiration. Nutrients must be administered as a constant infusion, because there is no reservoir function, and the nutrients usually need to be initially dilute until the small bowel adapts.

Multiple formulations for enteral nutrition are available depending on the clinical situation. Provision is based on calculated caloric and fluid requirements. Adequate protein, lipids, and other required nutrients are usually present in adequate amounts without special consideration.

Parenteral nutrition

Only if the gastrointestinal tract is unusable should **parenteral** nutrition be considered—a sick patient who "will not eat" should be given a feeding tube, not TPN. Situations where TPN is appropriate are short gut syndrome after resection, neonatal necrotizing enterocolitis or "immature gut," severe pancreatitis, mechanical bowel obstruction, or failure of all efforts at enteral feeding, for example. TPN refers to the provision of 100% of a person's nutritional needs intravenously. Because of high osmolality (often 25% dextrose), it must be given via a central vein, i.e., requires a "central line" (peripheral parenteral nutrition can be given via a peripheral catheter, but glucose delivery is limited to 10% dextrose, providing inadequate calories and calorie:protein ratios). TPN can be given at home, can support children through normal growth and development, and patients on TPN can conceive and bear normal children.

TPN is created daily in the pharmacy for each patient. Therefore, components must be calculated individually. In general, one starts with a standard amino acid mixture (typically 4.5%), adds carbohydrate and lipid emulsion to provide calories in accordance with the guidelines presented above, then adds electrolytes, minerals, vitamins, trace elements, and insulin as needed. Usually calculations are done at the initiation of feeding, often with the help of the nutritional support service, and modifications are made later according to the patient's response. ■

4   Response to Injury

Homeostasis refers to the state of normal metabolism—it describes the process by which metabolism and energy are regulated to maintain the organism in a state of physiologic status quo. When anything disrupts this steady-state situation, a **"stress response"** is said to occur, referring to the constellation of changes seen after tissue injury. This response is elicited by any major physiologic stress, such as injury or sepsis; even elective surgery elicits some response. In general, **the magnitude of the stress response is proportional to the magnitude of the physiologic insult**.

Why Does the Stress Response Exist?

There are many different ways to approach this topic. Traditionally, the broad variety of changes that take place are viewed chronologically in cross section, from early after the response is initiated to late in the patients' course (until they recover or die), or discussed according to individual organ systems (such as the hypothalamic-pituitary axis, the renin-angiotensin system, and so on). From this viewpoint the entire response is divided into an **early,** or **catabolic** phase, where, as the name implies, metabolism is altered to support processes immediately essential to short-term survival, usually at the expense of energy stores and the body's structural components, a **late,** or **early anabolic** phase, where metabolism shifts back toward preservation of structure and function necessary for long-term, normal function, and nutrient balance is positive, and a **recovery**, or **late anabolic** phase, where depleted stores themselves (such as fat) are repleted.

This chapter, in contrast, will explore the stress response from a **teleologic** viewpoint, attempting to answer the question of "why" the various pathways and hormones evolved to perhaps convey a better sense of the purpose of the stress response rather than just its components. Looking at it this way, the stress response evolved for several reasons: to protect delivery of nutrients to the cells by **protecting circulating volume**, to improve cellular energy levels by **increasing circulating substrate**, to heal injury by **protecting the body's physical integrity**, and to fight sepsis by **increasing immunocompetence**.

A fundamental point to remember is that these responses evolved when modern medicine wasn't around—either they worked quickly, or the organism died. Now that we have the ability to keep critically ill patients alive beyond this short-term period, it has become apparent (and is a recurring theme in this discussion) that almost every component of the stress response produces damage, as well.

Protection of Circulating Volume

Perhaps the variable the body "wants" to protect most is **circulating volume**. If the organism is injured, hemorrhage often results. Oxygen delivery to the cells is the fundamental reason that we're alive. More vital than the red cells themselves, however, is the actual physical fluid that carries them around and allows the heart to distend during diastole so that it can pump—in other words, volume itself, rather than red cell mass (or hematocrit), is the critical variable. The body tolerates half its normal red cell mass much better than it does half its normal circulating volume, for example.

Response to hypovolemia

Volume status (pressure) is sensed by stretch and pressure receptors in the aorta, atria, and carotid and renal arteries. Decreased blood pressure and afferent neurologic impulses from the site of injury result in release of multiple hormones. **Vasopressin (antidiuretic hormone, ADH)** is released by the posterior pituitary. This directly causes volume retention by stimulating renal reabsorption of sodium, and also causes vasoconstriction. **Renin** is released by the kidney, catalyzing the creation of angiotensin I that acts as a substrate for the formation of angiotensin II in the lung. **Angiotensin II** is the most powerful vasoconstrictor known, and also stimulates the release of aldosterone from the adrenal cortex. **Aldosterone**, like ADH, also increases renal resorption of sodium and water. The autonomic nervous system itself is activated (or tonic suppression is decreased), causing release of vasoconstrictive **catecholamines**, while **ACTH**, released by the anterior pituitary, augments adrenal release of aldosterone and catecholamines (and cortisol). An additional mechanism that comes into play in situations of hypovolemia is **stimulation of thirst**, a phenomenon that is commonly seen in the emergency room after major trauma. Finally, perfusion of the heart and brain are often preferentially protected by peripheral **vasoconstriction** (due to systemic catecholamines, local neurologically-mediated vasoconstriction, ADH, angiotensin II, and other factors). Although the body's efforts are primarily directed at preserving volume, red cell mass is not ignored. Anemia stimulates renal release of **erythropoetin** that more gradually stimulates the bone marrow to produce more red blood cells.

When these effects persist, however, harm results. By reducing global (and renal) cellular perfusion (see Chapter 5, "Shock"), irreversible damage may be done to the organism as a whole. The increased capillary and cellular permeability and relative water retention result in tissue edema ("third-spacing," see Chapter 27, "Postoperative Care"), and continued release of catecholamines increases myocardial work and oxygen consumption.

Provision of Circulating Substrate

The ultimate requirement of all cells is the formation of ATP to drive chemical reactions. To do this, the cells must receive oxygen and carbohydrates, lipids, or amino acids. With hypovolemia, this delivery is threatened, thus the mechanisms in the section above also act to provide continued substrate delivery.

Nutrition

Nutritional abnormalities in the stressed state are covered in detail in Chapter 3, "Nutrition." Normal metabolism consists of net synthesis (anabolism) when substrate and energy are abundant and net catabolism when they are not. Although protein, lipid, and carbohydrate all can be used to synthesize ATP, the brain and hematologic system have an obligate need for glucose. Storage is limited, however (about a day's worth). In uncomplicated starvation, after carbohydrate stores are depleted, proteins are initially broken down to provide precursors for gluconeogenesis. If uncomplicated starvation is prolonged, the body can shift toward greater utilization of lipids, "sparing" protein catabolism (dieting). After significant injury, sepsis, or other stress, however, this shift does not take place, and protein breakdown continues unabated even if

Multidisciplinary
Response to Injury *continued*

"adequate" nutrition is provided. Unfortunately, since all protein has some function, proteolysis results in loss of needed muscular, synthetic, or immune activity.

Acute-phase response

As well as for ATP production, amino acids derived from skeletal muscle proteolysis are also used for synthesis of new molecules called **acute-phase proteins**. Acute-phase proteins are a heterogeneous group of molecules with multiple different functions that have been found to be synthesized and released together during stress. Although traditionally lumped together, most have different functions (many tend to aid in improving the function of the immune system). Part of the response, too, is the relative inhibition of the synthesis of less acutely-essential proteins such as albumin and transferrin.

Other hormones

Stress-induced elevations in **catecholamines** (resulting from hypovolemia, direct neural impulses from the site of injury, and emotional responses), **cortisol** (stimulated by ACTH), **growth hormone** (from the pituitary), and **glucagon** (released by the pancreas) all signal the need to generate new substrates for energy production. Under the influence of these hormones, free fatty acids (from adipose tissue) and protein (from tissues) are mobilized. An insulin resistance occurs resulting in hyperglycemia (primarily due to the effects of cortisol and catecholamines).

Unfortunately, although useful in the short term (resulting in increased gluconeogenic precursors and mobilization of resources toward energy production rather than growth and synthesis), these effects create new problems. Useful protein is broken down (such as diaphragm muscle and immunoglobulins), hyperglycemia persists (increasing hepatic workload and complicating the management of these patients), and the body's resources are quickly exhausted.

Protection of Bodily Integrity

Often throughout the evolution of these reactions the organism was physically injured. Healing damaged tissue, therefore, became another priority. Initial **vasoconstriction** at the site of injury (to aid in hemostasis) followed by **increased permeability** and **vasodilation** (to improve delivery of useful mediators) are the first such effects seen. There is a physiologic leukocytosis resulting from acute vascular demargination, and an **increased delivery of cellular mediators** of healing such as macrophages, neutrophils, and fibroblasts (see Chapter 29, "Wounds") along with stimulation of chemotaxis. In general, resources are mobilized to allow the organism to physically remove itself from danger (catecholamines increase heart rate and cardiac output, dilate pupils, for example) and to improve wound healing.

Again, however, many of the events occurring elsewhere in the body after injury are detrimental to local injury repair. Cortisol inhibits inflammation (thus healing), and the protein breakdown needed for ATP production occurs at the expense of synthesis of molecules needed for repair.

Protection against Sepsis

A fundamental pathway detailed over the past decade or so describes the response to Gram-negative infection. Gram-negative bacteria release **endotoxin** that causes the release of **tumor necrosis factor** (**TNF**) from macrophages and perhaps endothelial cells. TNF seems to be a primary mediator of the "septic response," and causes fever, vasodilatation and increased capillary permeability, chemotaxis, and, in higher doses, tissue injury and death. **Interleukin-1** (**IL-1**), also a macrophage product, is similar to TNF in function. IL-1 also stimulates T-cell activation (see Chapter 10, "Immunology"). The **fever** caused by both these molecules is a hallmark of the inflammatory response, and may function to make the environment less favorable to bacteria. **IL-6** is probably the molecule that signals the liver to start synthesis of the acute-phase proteins. These **cytokines** all act over very short distances (as opposed to hormonal function), making detection very difficult, although in very high amounts (such as occurring after maximal insult) they may have systemic effects, as well. A common finding after stress of any magnitude is **leukocytosis**. This effect results from "mobilization" (**demargination**) of white cells sequestered along the walls of blood vessels, and again serves (in a teleologic sense) to improve immune function. Production itself (by the marrow) is also increased. It is important to remember that fever and leukocytosis are properties of inflammation and the stress response, from whatever source, and do not automatically denote infection.

Interestingly, many of the changes seen in cancer cachexia parallel (in a subdued fashion) some of the effects of these mediators; cancer cachexia could be merely the "side effect" of the molecules released by the body (such as TNF) to fight the tumor.

The Stress Response Unchecked

With millions of years to evolve, you'd think that the system protecting the body during severe stress or injury would work pretty well. Unfortunately (in this context), modern medicine has made it possible to live much longer than the system was ever able to evolve for. Before modern medicine, you would either die right away or rapidly improve. The stress response was not meant to be of any chronic use. It is clear that all these responses create some problems as they do their work. Certainly in the short term, their beneficial effects far exceed their adverse effects. In the long term, however, the reverse might be true.

The stress response unchecked

For years it has been recognized that there is a group of patients who appear "septic," yet have no identifiable infectious focus. There are two philosophic viewpoints to explain this. The first is that there are ongoing, undiscovered, or untreated insults that result in persistent activation of the stress response. For example, the initial injury (such as a fractured femur) has been fixed, but a pneumonia then occurs. When that is controlled, the worsening immunosuppression allows a new problem to arise, and so on. The second viewpoint suggests that the source has been truly eradicated, but the whole stress response has become autonomous, and that the cycle has become self-perpetuating. In other words, the patient is now suffering from unchecked activation of their own mediators ("mediator-itis"). The concept that the stress response can become autonomous is somewhat fatalistic, but does imply that there is a point in the course of some very ill patients where specific blockade of a component or components of the cycle can be of benefit. Certainly this hypothetical point would be late: because it performs such a vital role early after the insult, the elimination of the stress response too early would result in the patient never making it through the illness at all.

SIRS

A new term is increasingly used: **systemic inflammatory response syndrome (SIRS)**, denoting the fact that it is very often the inflammatory response itself, rather than just infection or injury, that is the basis for the patient's illness. **Sepsis** thus denotes true systemic infection, and implies specific treatment is possible. Most organs have a stereotypical clinical and pathologic response to injury that is similar with a variety of insults. The lung is the prime example. Inhalation injury, hypotension, or endotoxin can all injure the pulmonary endothelium. No matter the insult, however, the reaction is the same, producing what we call **adult respiratory distress syndrome (ARDS)**.

Thus, a patient with SIRS may have had an initial insult that has been adequately eradicated and treated. The patient might still have ARDS and abnormally increased capillary permeability due to continued macrophage activation and cytokine release, continued fluid retention due to inappropriate ADH secretion, tachycardia due to continued catecholamine release, immune deficiencies due to high levels of cortisol, glucose, and proteolysis needed for energy formation, continued hyperglycemia, and worsening skeletal muscle weakness due to protein breakdown. In the normal situation, these responses will abate, and the patient will recover. If they do not, a diligent search must be made for undiagnosed and untreated, ongoing stimuli. No matter what you believe in, it is incumbent on the physician caring for any critically ill patient to continue to search for new or undiscovered problems, and to continue to maximally support patients (while meaningful recovery is possible) until they recover. ∎

5   **Shock**

Shock is the clinical syndrome of inadequate tissue perfusion or oxygenation, regardless of etiology. One of the most common (and frustrating) mistakes made in the care of critically ill patients is to choose a specific parameter to follow (such as blood pressure), while ignoring the overall clinical situation. The most basic requirement for health is the delivery of adequate oxygen to and subsequent utilization by the cells of the body. Utilization depends on cellular, mitochondrial, and molecular "health," and, in many cases, is beyond our control. Therefore, the basic variable we can alter is oxygen delivery. It cannot be overemphasized that **adequate oxygen delivery**, rather than blood pressure, cardiac output, or urine output, is the most basic need of any patient.

Tissue perfusion (oxygen delivery) is dependent on both the **oxygen content** of the blood and the mechanical **cardiac output**. This chapter will address shock as a clinical entity and focus on arterial oxygen content, while the next (Chapter 6, "Basic Hemodynamics and Invasive Monitoring") will focus on cardiac output and the Swan-Ganz catheter.

Shock

Shock exists at a cellular level. We often cannot detect its presence until the body's macroscopic compensatory mechanisms come into play. The skin can be cool and clammy, reflecting decreased cutaneous perfusion, and there may be confusion, reflecting decreased cerebral perfusion. With decreasing renal perfusion, **urine output falls**. The heart will compensate for reduced intravascular volume by becoming **tachycardic**. A widened pulse pressure is often seen. More invasive monitoring reveals decreased cardiac output, increased oxygen extraction by the tissues, and lactic acidosis, reflecting a shift to anaerobic metabolism. Finally, when compensatory mechanisms fail, **hypotension** results. None of these parameters defines shock, but all are helpful in suggesting its presence.

There are four "classic" types of shock: hypovolemic, septic, cardiogenic, and neurogenic; some would add anaphylactic and obstructive shock to the list. These classic divisions can overlap and coexist in the actual clinical setting, but all six shock states are governed by many of the same physiologic principles.

Hypovolemic Shock

Hypovolemic shock exists when the intravascular volume decreases sufficiently to compromise cardiac output and tissue perfusion. The most common cause of hypovolemia is hemorrhage; non-traumatic hypovolemia may be the result of "third-spacing" due to surgery, ileus, or sepsis (see Chapter 6, "Basic Hemodynamics and Invasive Monitoring", and Chapter 27, "Postoperative Care"), persistent emesis or diarrhea, high ostomy output, fever, or iatrogenic dehydration with diuretics. Intravenous fluid replacement is the necessary treatment. Restoring the intravascular volume remedies tissue and renal hypoperfusion and the associated acidosis and oliguria, respectively. A critical error is to focus on the establishment of urine output, administer a diuretic, and forget that urine output is a sign, not the goal *per se*. Diuresis will only worsen the underlying hypovolemia. The underlying dehydration must be addressed—urine output will increase on its own when the kidneys are adequately perfused. Fluid selection for resuscitation is dictated by the clinical situation—the theory is to replace lost fluid in amount and composition. In general, isotonic lactated Ringer's solution is the optimal solution to replace volume, because it very closely mimics serum (see Chapter 7, "Basic Fluid and Electrolytes," and Chapter 27, "Postoperative Care"), while packed red blood cells are reserved for clinically significant anemia.

Fluid replacement will succeed as long as the patient maintains perfusion to the vital organs (brain and heart, and kidneys) via autoregulation. If the shock state is allowed to persist for a period of time without adequate treatment, compensatory mechanisms will ultimately fail and the patient will no longer be able to support blood pressure and perfusion and oxygen delivery to the vital organs. This is decompensated shock; after this point, the organ system or patient will likely not be salvageable despite aggressive resuscitation.
(continued)

Multidisciplinary
Shock *continued*

Septic Shock

Septic shock, including its definition, mechanism, and treatment, is currently a topic of much interest among critical care experts. Sepsis is a shock state that results from a systemic inflammatory response to a variety of insults, most notably endotoxin. Much of the actual septic picture may well be mediated by the body's own natural molecules (such as tumor necrosis factor, the interleukins, bradykinin, serotonin, histamine, nitric oxide, and other vasoactive molecules) released appropriately (at least, at first) in response to an insult. Although it might serve as an inciting event, active infection is not necessary for sepsis, and a septic focus often cannot be identified. As a result, antibiotic therapy alone has had little effect on the overall mortality from sepsis, and many clinicians now prefer the term "**systemic inflammatory response syndrome**" (**SIRS**; see also Chapter 4, "Response to Injury").

Sepsis not only causes hemodynamic aberrations, but also leads to cellular dysfunction by interfering with metabolism and oxygen utilization. Early septic shock is referred to as the hyperdynamic or "warm" phase of sepsis and is characterized by increased cardiac output, relative hypotension, and decreased systemic vascular resistance. Again, focus on the big picture (tissue perfusion) and resist the temptation to administer alpha agonists ("pressors") to treat falling blood pressure and low systemic vascular resistance. Patients in the early phase of septic shock do much better with large volumes of intravascular fluid replacement. Pressors, while increasing blood pressure, may actually worsen cellular oxygen delivery by peripheral vasoconstriction and worsen the shock. Much of the intravascular volume delivered, however, is lost to "third-spacing" (see Chapter 27, "Postoperative Care"), producing marked total body edema; much of the decrease in systemic resistance is due to **capillary leak** and thus not necessarily treatable with vasoconstrictors. The hypodynamic or "cold" phase occurs later and is marked by falling cardiac index; this phase often requires the last-ditch use of pressors in addition to volume replacement to maintain adequate perfusion to the heart and brain. Salvage rates fall dramatically as the septic process deteriorates from the hyperdynamic to the hypodynamic stage.

Cardiogenic Shock

Cardiogenic shock describes the low flow state secondary to low cardiac output associated with a primary cardiac problem, described clinically as "pump failure." It can be the result of poor ventricular function following myocardial infarction or ongoing myocardial ischemia, structural abnormalities such as valvular disruption, rupture of ventricular aneurysm, tamponade, or dysrhythmia. Patients in cardiogenic shock present with typical signs of hypoperfusion (hypotension, pallor, oliguria), but are generally euvolemic. Pulmonary artery pressures tend to be elevated secondary to poor cardiac output, with subsequent pulmonary edema. Inotropic agents such as dobutamine or dopamine are useful while primary mechanisms for pump failure are found and corrected.
Echocardiography is useful in evaluating cardiac performance noninvasively and in investigating anatomic causes for pump failure. It is this population of patients that benefits most from the intra-aortic balloon pump (which augments diastolic coronary artery perfusion and reduces systolic afterload).

Neurogenic Shock

A **loss of sympathetic tone** to the cardiovascular system occurs after disruption of the spinal cord, typically due to trauma. Vasodilatation, paradoxical bradycardia, and inability to autoregulate blood pressure follows. These patients are typically euvolemic at the time of injury. Unless terminal, shock is rarely the result of isolated head injury; other sources must be sought in the hypotensive multiply-injured patient.

The spinal cord injury and subsequent vasodilatation result in a low systemic vascular resistance inappropriate for the normal volume status. While fluid resuscitation is useful in the short term, alpha agonists are often needed to counter the inappropriate vasodilatation.

Anaphylactic Shock

Anaphylaxis is an **immediate hypersensitivity reaction** mediated by massive IgE release after exposure of a sensitized individual to a specific antigen, usually in the form of medication, food, or animal venom. Anaphylaxis is characterized by urticaria, pruritus, bronchospasm, and cardiovascular collapse; mast cell degranulation is the primary source of the mediating vasoactive amines. This form of shock is unique because both oxygenation and perfusion are acutely impeded. Treatment is airway control, oxygenation, and support of the blood pressure. These patients benefit from epinephrine and diphenhydramine (Benadryl): the non-selective beta activity of epinephrine relieves bronchospasm, and improves cardiac output, and Benadryl serves to stabilize mast cell membranes, alleviate pruritis, and control urticaria. Steroids sometimes play a role in acute anaphylactic reactions to control airway edema and "stabilize" the immune and inflammatory systems.

Obstructive Shock

Finally, shock can result from **simple mechanical obstruction** of cardiac output, such as that seen with caval obstruction due to the mediastinal shift of a tension pneumothorax or a pulmonary embolus. The pathophysiology is variable and depends on the site of obstruction. Aggressive fluid replacement will buy time to correct the underlying problem.

Pathophysiology

Oxygen delivery is proportional to the oxygen content of the blood times the cardiac output, or:

Oxygen delivery = Arterial Oxygen Content (CaO_2)
x Cardiac Output (CO).

Oxygen content (CaO_2) is calculated as:

Oxygen content = O_2 carried by RBCs + O_2 dissolved
in the blood

or

$$CaO_2 = (Hb \times SaO_2 \times 1.39) + (0.0031 \times PaO_2)$$

where Hb is hemoglobin concentration, SaO_2 is arterial oxygen saturation, and PaO_2 is partial pressure of arterial O_2.

Recall that O_2 exists in both the bound and unbound form. The bound form is represented by the first term, with 1.39 (oxygen carrying capacity) representing the amount of O_2 (mL) bound to 1 gram of human hemoglobin **under normal conditions**. The unbound or dissolved portion is represented by the second term, with 0.0031 representing the solubility factor of O_2 in plasma. Since the second term is always a very small number, it is clinically insignificant and the equation simplifies to:

$$CaO_2 = Hb \text{ x } SaO_2 \text{ x } 1.39$$

To affect oxygen delivery, arterial oxygen content and cardiac output must be controlled. Cardiac output is dependent on stroke volume and heart rate, addressed in the next chapter ("Basic Hemodynamics"). Arterial oxygen content, as shown above, is dependent on **hemoglobin concentration**, **arterial oxygen saturation**, and the **oxygen carrying capacity**.

Hemoglobin Concentration

Hemoglobin concentration is maximized by transfusion. Blood volume and blood's oxygen-carrying capacity are two different things. For example, chronic anemia affects oxygen carrying capacity but not intravascular volume, while acute blood loss compromises both. Unfortunately, as the hemoglobin concentration is increased, blood viscosity is also. There is a point where raising the hematocrit is no longer helpful because viscosity is increased and microvascular perfusion (very difficult to measure) is impaired. Further, there are the myriad adverse effects of transfusion to consider. It appears that a hematocrit of 30% (much lower than "normal") is optimal.

Arterial Oxygen Saturation

It is imperative that adequate **partial pressures of oxygen** are maintained. "Adequate" saturation is generally 90% or greater, especially in the face of impaired cardiac function or decreased hemoglobin concentrations. Optimal saturation might require intubation, mechanical ventilation, and/or supplemental oxygen. Typically, one should optimize hemoglobin and saturation before modifying other parameters (i.e., stroke volume or heart rate). *(continued)*

Oxygen Carrying Capacity

The numerical term describing **oxygen carrying capacity**
(1.39) in the simplified equation is not a constant, but can
be affected by temperature, pH, and pCO_2. The relationship between the partial pressure of oxygen and the
hemoglobin saturation is described by the oxyhemoglobin
dissociation curve. Acidosis tends to shift the curve to the
right, thereby facilitating oxygen unloading for a given
partial pressure in relatively ischemic/anaerobic tissues.
Markedly elevated pH (alkalemia) can cause paradoxically poor unloading of oxygen where it is most needed
(left shifted curve). Similarly, hypercarbic states promote
oxygen delivery for the same reasons. This is the funda-

Figure 5.1
**Normal oxygen-hemoglobin dissociation curve (at
37°C and pH of 7.40). Note that (on the average) the
partial pressure at which hemoglobin is 50% saturated, the P_{50}, corresponds to an oxygen tension of
27mmHg—quite low. A saturation of 97% corresponds
to a partial pressure of 100mmHg.**

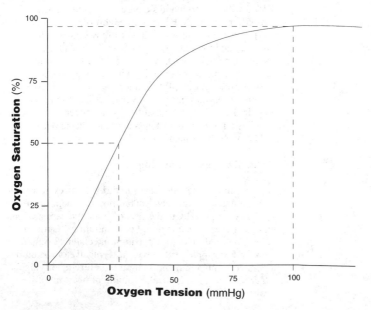

mental principle behind the concept of "permissive hyper-capnea"—allowing the patient to have higher arterial pCO_2 to improve oxygen delivery.

Temperature control in critically ill patients or trauma victims with environmental injury (severe hypothermia) is a vexing issue. Besides direct cardiovascular effects, temperature affects oxygen carrying capacity. As temperature decreases, the affinity of hemoglobin for oxygen increases (left-shifted curve) resulting in impairment of tissue unloading. As a result, it is vital to maintain relative normothermia. Common techniques include warming devices, warmed intravenous fluids, increased ambient temperature, and warm peritoneal, gastric, and thoracic lavage.

Transfusion of blood depleted in 2, 3-diphosphoglycerate (DPG) results in a left-shifted oxyhemoglobin dissociation curve leading to a higher hemoglobin affinity for oxygen and subsequent decreased unloading of oxygen. In general, transfused red blood cells should be assumed to be deficient in DPG, and DPG levels do not return to normal levels until 24-48 hours after transfusion. ■

6 Basic Hemodynamics and Invasive Monitoring

As discussed in the previous chapter, the ultimate goal in any patient is the delivery of adequate oxygen to the cells of the various organ systems, because cells depend on oxygen to maintain aerobic metabolism. Oxygen delivery can be broken down into two factors: oxygen content and blood flow (cardiac output):

$$\text{Oxygen delivery} = \text{Arterial Oxygen Content } (CaO_2) \times \text{Cardiac Output (CO)}$$

Oxygen content was discussed in the previous chapter ("Shock").

Cardiac output (CO)

Cardiac output is defined as the volume of blood pumped by the heart per unit time. This is equal to the **heart rate** (**HR**) times the **stroke volume** (**SV**), or:

$$\text{CO (liters/minute)} = \text{HR (beats/minute)} \times \text{SV (liters/beat)}$$

Each of these variables can be modified. **Heart rate** can be controlled chemically or electrically (see Chapter 13, "Basic ACLS"). A faster heart rate does not necessarily mean a greater cardiac output; if the ability of the heart to fill during diastole (preload) is compromised, stroke volume is decreased. **Stroke volume** is determined by **preload**, **afterload**, and **contractility**. **Preload** is the end-diastolic myocardial fiber length, which clinically is essentially the volume status of the patient. **Afterload** is the resistance against which the left ventricle has to beat, and **contractility** is the force with which the heart contracts for a given preload or end-diastolic volume (analogous to the concept of compliance, contractility refers to the relationship between two variables and is not an intrinsic number). Contractility is expressed as the position of the **Starling curve**, and in clinical practice is usually subjectively assessed.

CO determinants

The formula above makes things quite simple: any fall in cardiac output **must** be due to a change in one or a combination of the four factors above—**heart rate, preload,**

afterload, or **contractility**. There is nothing else to remember. This concept is critically important, and when faced with a sick patient, thinking about each factor individually will clarify your thinking and simplify the issue dramatically.

Clinically, diminishing cardiac output is heralded by a well-defined sequence of signs and symptoms. First, **urine output falls** as renal perfusion drops. This is a compensatory mechanism in an attempt to maximize blood volume, thus maximizing preload. Second, **heart rate increases**, again in an effort to compensate by increasing cardiac output. Finally, **blood pressure falls** as compensatory mechanisms fail.

Invasive Monitoring

Ideally quantitative data supplement clinical findings. Because this involves invasive monitoring devices that are not without risk, this correlation is reserved for patients that present an ambiguous picture or when one is attempting to modify the specific components of the above relationships in a sick patient.

CVP

Obviously, the history, physical examination, and simple clinical parameters such as the vital signs, urine output, and radiologic and laboratory data are the first step in any sick patient. If questions persist, a central venous catheter can be inserted to measure the **central venous pressure**. This, however, gives limited information, essentially the "right-sided" preload only. If the situation is unclear, more specialized monitoring in an intensive care setting is needed.

Swan-Ganz catheter

One of the most useful monitoring devices in a sick patient is the **Swan-Ganz catheter**. This is a long, multi-lumen catheter with an inflatable balloon at the end. It is placed into the **venous** system via a central vein and "floated" into position, allowing it to follow the flow of blood by inflating the balloon. A pressure transducer conveys characteristic wave forms as the catheter passes through the various cardiac chambers (right atrium and ventricle) into the pulmonary artery. When the catheter is in a large branch of the pulmonary artery, the balloon occludes the narrowing vessel. At this point, with the balloon occluding flow, resistance through the pulmonary capillary bed thus ceases and the measured pressure represents the static pressure distal to the balloon. Consequently, the wave form becomes flat. This is commonly called the **pulmonary capillary wedge pressure (PCWP)**. Because there is no resistance and no intervening valves, the PCWP is (with certain limitations) the same as the left atrial pressure—and because, during diastole the mitral valve is open, it reflects the left ventricular end-diastolic pressure, or **left-sided preload**. This concept is critically important—the advantage of the Swan-Ganz catheter is that it allows you to measure "left-sided," intracardiac pressures from the relatively non-invasive right side of the heart. With the catheter tip in the right position, leaving the balloon deflated measures the pulmonary artery pressure, and inflating it (PCWP) essentially measures the left atrial and left ventricular diastolic pressure.

CO & CI

The second useful function of the Swan-Ganz catheter is its ability to measure certain derived values. Most importantly, the cardiac output can be calculated using thermodilution. By injecting a known quantity of saline at a known temperature through a port a known distance proximal to a thermistor, the computer can calculate the amount of blood diluting the injectate, and, based on the temperature gradient, derive an approximation of blood flow per unit time, which is the **cardiac output**. The cardiac output is usually indexed to patient size by dividing it by the body surface area to yield the **cardiac index**.

SVR

Additionally, by knowing the cardiac output and various pressures, we can now calculate the afterload, or the resistance against which the heart pumps. The easiest way to derive this is to revert back to basic physics and Ohm's Law:

V (potential) = I (flow) x R (resistance)

Translating this into clinical terms, potential energy is the pressure gradient, or the difference between the mean arterial pressure (MAP) and central venous pressure (CVP). Flow is equivalent to the cardiac output (CO), and resistance is the systemic vascular resistance (SVR), or afterload, which is the variable of interest. In other words:

$$\text{Resistance} = \text{Potential} / \text{Flow}$$

or

$$\text{SVR} = \text{Pressure Gradient} / \text{CO}$$

Clinically we must multiply this value by a constant to translate it into usable units:

Contractility

$$\text{SVR} = [(\text{MAP-CVP}) / \text{CO}] \times 80$$

Using the Swan-Ganz catheter, we can measure cardiac output, estimate right- and left-sided preload independently, and derive the systemic vascular resistance. Contractility, as discussed above, is a relationship between two variables (analogous to compliance) and thus is not a value that can be directly measured. It refers to the contractile force developed for a given fiber length (or preload/end-diastolic pressure) and is reflective of the health of the myocytes themselves. One can measure cardiac output at different preloads before and after an intervention, thus constructing two different Starling curves, but this is too time-consuming to be of consistent clinical value. In practice, judgments are made as to the contractility based on the clinical situation and the other values.

Oxygen consumption

A final measurement that is becoming very useful is **venous oximetry**. The tip of the Swan-Ganz catheter is in the pulmonary artery, which contains mixed venous blood just prior to oxygenation in the pulmonary capillaries. Using an oximetric probe, one can calculate the venous oxygen content using the same formula demonstrated above. The difference between the arterial and venous oxygen content represents the **oxygen consumption** of the body as a whole. The oxygen consumption, measured as arteriovenous oxygen **difference**, increases with increasing oxygen extraction by the tissues or with reduced oxygen delivery, reflected as a **falling** mixed venous oxygen saturation. This serves as an early warning system that cardiac output may be decreasing. Conversely, if the mixed venous saturation is **rising**, the tissues are not extracting enough oxygen. This can be secondary to a metabolic derangement or a delivery problem (such as shunting). Venous oximetry is very helpful because is provides us with a good moment to moment assessment of cardiac output as well as the ability to calculate oxygen consumption.

(continued)

Multidisciplinary
Basic Hemodynamics and
Invasive Monitoring *continued*

Clinical Correlation

In the most common, non-ICU inpatient clinical situation, the presence of shock may not be so clear-cut. In practice, the most common scenario is that you are called to see a patient with reduced urine output, tachycardia, or hypotension, in order of severity. The first step, philosophically, is to determine whether the patient's problems are the result of **too little fluid** (septic, neurogenic, or hypovolemic shock) or (relatively) **too much fluid** (cardiogenic shock), as the treatment for the first is volume, and the second, inotropic support (see Chapter 5, "Shock"). Thus, if you are faced with a sick patient not in obvious congestive heart failure and you don't know what's going on, give fluids! At worst, you will buy time to figure things out, and most of the time you will already be treating the problem.

First, give fluids. You are treating the most common pathophysiologic cause (hypovolemia) as discussed above. Obviously you should be cautious when faced with an elderly patient with distended neck veins and crushing chest pain, and you should exclude renal disease (or catheter malfunction) when dealing with oliguria, but, in general, you will do much more good than harm by administering fluids.

Second, if there is no response, **measure right-sided or central venous filling pressure with a central line**. This should make the critical distinction between the forms of shock with predominant hypovolemic components (hypovolemic, septic, and neurogenic, which result in a low CVP), the presence of which should lead to further fluid resuscitation, and that with potential relative hypervolemia (cardiogenic, which leads to a high CVP) the presence of which should suggest that inotropic support is needed.

Third, if there is **still no response or the situation is unclear**, the next step is to **insert a Swan-Ganz catheter**. This allows you to measure left-sided cardiac function, to measure cardiac output directly, to estimate contractility better, to judge tissue oxygen utilization, and to calculate systemic vascular resistance (afterload). ■

One of the most basic elements of patient care is fluid and electrolyte management. The anatomy of body fluids and the physiologic principles that maintain normal fluid and electrolyte balance must be understood so that derangements can be identified and treated.

Distribution of Body Fluids

Approximately 60% of a person's body weight is water (**total body water, TBW**). Fat is relatively free of water —lean individuals have a greater proportion of water to body weight than do the obese. Body water is divided into two functional compartments. Most water is **intracellular**, making up approximately 40% of an individual's body weight (two-thirds of TBW), and the rest is **extracellular**, accounting for about 20% (one-third of TBW). The extracellular compartment is further divided into **interstitial** and **intravascular** components, constituting 15% and 5%, respectively, of body weight. A 70kg person, therefore, has about 42 liters of total body water, 28 liters of which are intracellular, 10.5 liters interstitial, and 3.5 liters intravascular fluid. Under abnormal conditions, "**third-space**" fluids may also exist (see Chapter 27, "Postoperative Care"). The "third space" is always pathologic, by definition, and refers to fluids from the intravascular and intracellular spaces that have accumulated in various tissues as the result of the altered hormonal milieu and cellular membrane changes seen with critical illness. This fluid still exists, but is not exchangeable or in equilibrium with the remainder of the body's fluid. When the underlying problem is corrected, a diuresis occurs as the fluid moves back into the intravascular space and is excreted by the kidneys. Third-spacing is manifest by tissue and bowel wall edema and abnormal collections such as ascites and effusions, and explains why a critically ill patient can be "intravascularly hypovolemic" and "total body fluid overloaded" at the same time.

Composition   Composition of the fluid in the separate spaces differs. The principal intracellular cations are **potassium** and **magnesium**, while the principal anions are **proteins** and **phosphates**. The major extracellular cation is **sodium**, while **chloride** and **bicarbonate** are the primary extracellular anions. The total electrical charge in each compartment is neutral. Protein is present in every compartment, although there is a relatively small amount of protein in the interstitial space compared with the intravascular space.

Fluid Regulation

There are two opposing forces involved in fluid shifts: hydrostatic and colloid oncotic pressure. **Hydrostatic pressure** is the force exerted by the volume of fluid in a confined space; high hydrostatic pressure pushes fluid away. Water moves to equalize the osmolality of solutions on separate sides of a semipermeable membrane—**colloid oncotic pressure** is the "pull" exerted on water by the nonpermeable molecules in a system; high colloid oncotic pressure "pulls" fluid towards itself. These forces depend on a functional semipermeable membrane between two spaces with differing composition:

Figure 7.1
Directions of forces causing movement of fluids across a semipermeable membrane.

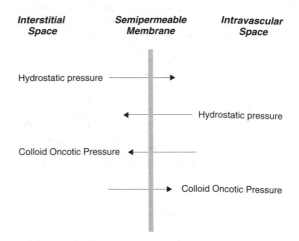

| Interstitial Space | Semipermeable Membrane | Intravascular Space |

Hydrostatic pressure ———▶

◀——— Hydrostatic pressure

Colloid Oncotic Pressure ◀———

———▶ Colloid Oncotic Pressure

Clinical examples are common. Increased intravascular hydrostatic pressure caused by venous hypertension secondary to congestive heart failure forces fluid into the interstitial space, causing edema. In a similar fashion, liver failure causing hypoproteinemia produces a low intravascular colloid oncotic pressure; water will preferentially move out of the vessels into the tissues, again producing edema.

Regulation of osmolality

Intake, output, production, and distribution of proteins and ions are governed by multiple systems. **Osmolality** is proportionate to the total number of dissolved particles per kilogram of solvent. Receptors in the brain sense changes in osmolality and control the secretion of **antidiuretic hormone** (**ADH**) which modifies the permeability of the renal tubules. A rise in plasma osmolality leads to increased secretion of ADH which causes resorption of water by the kidneys, and a fall leads to reduced levels of ADH and reduced renal water reabsorption.

Normal osmolality is 285-295mosm/kg H_2O; abnormal plasma osmolality is often due to an abnormal fluid balance. Osmolality can be measured directly by the lab or approximated from serum ion concentrations:

$$\text{Plasma osmolality} = (\text{Na} \times 2) + (\text{glucose}/18) + (\text{BUN}/2.8)$$

This calculated value may be inaccurate if unmeasured ions, such as lactate or mannitol, are present. Sodium is the prime osmotically active extracellular molecule and thus contributes most to the equation above.

Maintenance Fluids

The basic objective of "fluid and electrolyte therapy" is to maintain normal body fluid load, distribution, osmolality, and ionic concentrations. The easiest way to calculate **maintenance fluids** is to measure normal fluid and electrolyte **losses**, and thus figure out what is needed to maintain status quo (see also Chapter 27, "Postoperative Care").

Fluids

For simplicity's sake, fluid losses can be grouped into two categories: urine and everything else. **Urine** accounts for most of the daily fluid loss under normal circumstances;

the average adult produces **0.5-1.0 cc/kg/hr** of urine. A 70kg person will therefore produce about 40-60cc/hr, or 1200cc/day. "**Everything else**" includes water lost as sweat and in exhaled air (**insensible**, because these losses are hard to measure), water lost in the stool, and water lost as "water of hydration" needed to hydrolyze protein bonds, totaling approximately 800cc/day. Daily losses under normal, nonstressed conditions thus roughly approximate **2 liters**. Replacement then requires the same amount, which works out to be about **85cc/hour**. Loss can also be calculated based on body surface area and weight; this is especially useful when dealing with fluid administration in children (see Chapter 45, "Infant Fluids, Electrolytes, and Nutrition").

Electrolytes

The next step is to determine the electrolytes lost and replacement needed. The most important are sodium and potassium; other electrolytes are lost but are less vital to the regulation of body fluid. Average daily sodium loss is 2meq/kg, and that of potassium is about 0.5meq/kg. Therefore, a 70kg person will lose 140meq/day of sodium and 35meq/day of potassium. What IV fluids are needed?

	Na^+	K^+	Cl^-	HCO_3	Osm
Serum	140	4	100	26	300
Normal Saline (NS, 0.9%)	154	154	0	0	308
1/2 NS (0.45%)	77	77	0	0	154
Lactated Ringer's (LR)	130	4	109	(28)	275 (Ca = 3)

A 70kg person needs 140meq of sodium in 2 liters of fluid per day. Two liters of 1/2 NS will provide 154meq of sodium; if 20meq of potassium is added to each liter (totaling 40meq), we have come close to exactly replacing the daily loss of water, sodium and potassium. Although full caloric support cannot be provided with IV fluids in a peripheral vein (see Chapter 3, "Nutrition"), the addition of 100gm/day of dextrose (5% dextrose; 5g/dL) will help. Putting this all together will yield **D_5 1/2NS** with **20meq KCl/L** at **85cc/hr**—this should look familiar!

Although the concepts above are useful in understanding why we give what we give, they provide only the starting point. As in all medicine, nothing is ever as idealized as it seems. In practice, you start with an educated guess and modify subsequent therapy according to response. This means that the fluid and electrolyte status of patients receiving any fluid should be monitored, and changes should be made based on the evolving clinical picture.

Volume

Hypovolemia may be the most common disorder of fluid and electrolyte physiology. Blood loss, vomiting, diarrhea, nasogastric suctioning, inadequate intake, and third spacing due to sepsis or injury are the most common causes of hypovolemia. Fluid shifts occur rapidly between compartments, but enough fluid must be contained in the intravascular space for the heart to adequately fill during diastole.

Replacement strategies

In hypovolemia resulting from "surgical" problems such as hemorrhage or third spacing, losses are often **isotonic**. Therefore, the best replacement strategy is to use isotonic solutions. Although whole blood is essentially perfectly isotonic, the issues of disease transmission, availability, and allergic reactions preclude its routine use for simple hypovolemia. Instead, **lactated Ringer's solution**, a crystalloid specifically formulated for isotonic replacement, is used. Conversely, in many instances where hypovolemia results from "medical" causes such as dehydration due to illness, replacement with solutions higher in sodium and lower in potassium is best —**normal saline**.

Certain other common situations empirically require certain fluids. For example, fluid lost from the upper gastrointestinal tract (e.g., with nasogastric suction) typically contains high levels of sodium and chloride, as well as acid, and optimal replacement is with the mildly acidic normal saline. Bile and pancreatic secretions both contain bicarbonate, and losses from diarrhea also tend to be isotonic and basic. In both these situations the mildly basic lactated Ringer's solution most closely approximates the solutions and electrolytes lost.

Signs and symptoms

In an otherwise normal patient with progressive hypovolemia, a characteristic sequence of signs and symptoms develops (see Chapter 6, "Basic Hemodynamics and Invasive Monitoring"). First, **urine output drops** as the kidneys attempt to compensate by increasing sodium and water reabsorption. Next, **heart rate increases** as the heart compensates by increasing rate to maintain cardiac output in the face of reduced stroke volume. Finally, **blood pressure falls** as compensation fails. The goal of taking care of these patients is to recognize developing hypovolemia and to treat it with volume replacement before this final stage is reached. **Do not treat oliguria with diuretics** until you are **sure** that compensation for hypovolemia is not the cause!

While symptoms and signs in an "otherwise normal patient" are obvious, often in "real life" it is difficult to determine volume status. Has the urine output dropped because of hypovolemia or low cardiac output ("prerenal" oliguria, denoting decreased renal perfusion) or from renal failure itself ("renal" oliguria)? Along with checking the BUN and creatinine, an easy and more reliable method to quickly identify renal oliguria is to compare urine and serum electrolytes and osmolarity. **Fractional excretion of sodium** can be calculated as follows:

$$FE_{Na} = [(\text{urine Na/urine Cr}) \times (\text{serum Cr/serum Na})] \times 100$$

A FE_{Na} less than 1 suggests the presence of a prerenal state due to poor perfusion from whatever cause, while that greater than 1 suggests that an intrinsic renal problem is present.

Crystalloid and colloids

You are almost guaranteed to hear the terms crystalloid and colloid your first day in an ICU or on the surgical service. **Crystalloid** refers to any solution based on water containing only small, common ions, while **colloid** refers to solutions containing large, osmotically active molecules. LR and NS are crystalloids, while albumin and hetastarch (Hespan) are colloids. Packed red blood cells and fresh frozen plasma are technically colloids, but are usually referred to separately as **blood products**. Colloids, **in theory**, produce a greater intravascular volume increase for a given volume infused because their oncotic pressure causes extravascular interstitial water to move into the intravascular space. While the same physiologic effect can be accomplished with a smaller volume of colloid than crystalloid, in practice this is not clinically relevant. In fact, in disease states the osmotically active particles in colloid solutions will move quickly out through the "leaky" capillaries, prolonging tissue edema. Literally decades of research has established that patients do equally well when given crystalloid or colloid. Because of its much lower cost and essentially zero risk of allergic reactions and disease transmission, crystalloid is thus preferred in most situations where volume is needed.

Hypervolemia

Hypervolemia occurs in essentially two situations: iatrogenic volume overload and renal failure. A third situation, congestive heart failure (CHF), is a form of **relative** hypervolemia, where, although volume status may be normal, the diseased heart's ability to pump is overwhelmed, causing fluid to build up in the lungs and periphery. Hypervolemia in the setting of normal renal function is treated easily with diuretics; furosemide (Lasix) has the added benefit of causing pulmonary vasodilatation, accounting for the otherwise paradoxical observation that it relieves the respiratory distress seen in CHF before diuresis has occurred. The relative hypervolemia of CHF can, of course, also be treated by increasing the heart's ability to pump with inotropic agents (see Chapter 6, "Basic Hemodynamics"). If the kidneys are not working, dialysis, which removes fluids and allows regulation of electrolyte levels, or ultrafiltration, which removes fluids only, are the only options.

One very common special case deserves re-emphasis. The total-body edema seen in critically ill patients who are third spacing is **not** hypervolemia. **Intravascular** volume is the critical variable; most often, despite **total body fluid overload** (edema), such patients have **intravascular hypovolemia**. Therefore, their oliguria should **not** be treated with diuretics unless you are sure that their **intravascular** volume is elevated.

Sodium

Hyponatremia

Hyponatremia is most conveniently approached according to whether the patient is hyper-, hypo-, or euvolemic. The most common form, **dilutional** or **hypervolemic hyponatremia**, is caused by the presence of excess free water; this is commonly seen during sepsis or critical illness when antidiuretic hormone (ADH) and aldosterone levels are increased (see Chapter 4, "Response to Injury"). Mild hyponatremia is initially treated by free water restriction. **Hypovolemic hyponatremia** is com-

Multidisciplinary
Basic Fluids and Electrolytes *continued*

monly the result of situations where both water and sodium are lost, such as excessive diuretic use or nasogastric suction, and is thus best treated by replacement of volume and sodium. **Euvolemic hyponatremia** most often is seen in the syndrome of inappropriate ADH secretion (SIADH), which produces a low serum sodium, elevated urine sodium, and normal to high urine osmolarity. The treatment of choice here also is free water restriction. **Pseudohyponatremia** is a laboratory artifact typically seen with severe hyperglycemia, where glucose molecules cause influx of water that dilutes and artificially decreases the sodium concentration. The measured serum sodium level should be adjusted upwards 1.6meq/L for every 100mg/dL increase in glucose over normal (100mg/dL).

The body tolerates fluctuations in sodium relatively well; like anything else, slow changes are better tolerated than are fast. Regardless of cause, clinical manifestations (primarily neurologic) are rare until the sodium level drops below 120meq/L. At this level replacement with hypertonic solutions should be considered; replacement must be cautious and slow to avoid neurologic injury.

Hypernatremia

Hypernatremia is usually the result of volume depletion from inadequate intake, diabetes insipidus, or diuretic use; volume is replaced by hypotonic crystalloid solutions.

Potassium

Hypokalemia

Potassium is an important molecule, for three reasons: its extracellular concentration is low, making small preterbations proportionately more significant, it's easily excreted by the kidney, and the heart and neurons are exquisitely sensitive to abnormal levels. Volume loss (typically from gastrointestinal loss or diuretic use) with inadequate replacement is the most common cause of **hypokalemia**. Symptoms are typically the result of cardiac arrhythmias, ileus, or neurologic abnormalities. When possible, potassium should be replaced enterally, although intravenous replacement is safe if care is exercised. In general, 10meq will increase the serum level 0.05-0.1meq/L. Serum levels should be followed very closely.

Hyperkalemia

Hyperkalemia is most commonly caused by renal failure; patients with severe trauma, major burns, prolonged extremity ischemia, or crush injuries (all resulting in widespread cellular lysis) may also become hyperkalemic as intracellular potassium stores are released; hyperkalemia is rare if the kidneys are working normally. Untreated hyperkalemia can be rapidly fatal because of its cardiotoxic effects. Arrhythmias, peaked T-waves, and widened QRS complexes are typically seen at levels of 5.5meq/dL and greater. A very common cause of elevated potassium levels is hemolysis of the sample prior to measurement; the test should be repeated if the clinical situation does not seem to fit.

The goal of treatment is to lower the extracellular potassium concentration, which can be accomplished by either promoting cellular uptake or actually removing the potassium from the body. Raising serum pH with **bicarbonate** will cause potassium to move into the cells in exchange for protons; **insulin** does the same. **Dextrose** must be given concurrently to avoid hyperglycemia. Definitive correction, however, requires actual removal of potassium. **Potassium exchange resins** (sodium polystyrene sulfonate, Kayexalate) can be given orally or rectally. **Dialysis**, used as a last resort, is quite effective. Administration of **calcium** stabilizes the myocardium and reduces the risk of an arrhythmia, but has no effect on the potassium level per se.

Magnesium

Magnesium's importance has been recognized only in the past decade or so. It acts mainly as an enzyme cofactor; acute changes in its serum concentration affect mainly cardiac and skeletal muscle. Symptoms of **hypomagnesemia** include arrhythmias, muscle fasciculations, and weakness. The kidney is very effective at magnesium conservation; consequently hypomagnesemia is usually the result of a combination of poor oral intake, excessive GI loss, and inadequate IV replacement. Magnesium is easily replaced either intravenously or orally. **Hypermagnesemia** is rare, potentially occurring with renal failure, and is usually not symptomatic. *(continued)*

**Multidisciplinary
Basic Fluids and Electrolytes** *continued*

Calcium

Hypocalcemia

Hypocalcemia is relatively common, especially in the setting of malnutrition, vitamin D deficiency, hypoparathyroidism, pancreatitis, renal failure, or recent surgery. Interpretation of calcium levels is notoriously tricky. The laboratory reports **total serum calcium**, not the physiologically active **ionized calcium**. About half of the blood's calcium is bound to albumin, and hypoalbuminemia will lead to a low reported calcium level despite an adequate amount of active, ionized calcium. A "correction" formula can be used to adjust for this:

$$\text{Corrected Ca} = 0.8 \times (4.0\text{-measured albumin}) + \text{reported serum Ca}$$

Note that the reported, total serum calcium is an accurate number—the lab hasn't made a mistake. What you are doing by "correcting" the value is creating an artificial number to make comparison with the normal value easier. The "corrected," artificial value correlates better with physiologic effects in the setting of hypoalbuminemia. An ionized calcium level can also be ordered, but is often difficult to interpret.

Symptoms of hypocalcemia include peripheral and perioral paresthesias, muscle weakness or twitching, tetany, and, rarely, seizures. **Chvostek's sign** is facial twitching elicited by tapping on the facial nerve in the cheek, while **Trousseau's sign** is carpopedal spasm after brief upper extremity ischemia produced by inflating a brachial blood pressure cuff to greater than systolic pressure for 3-5 minutes. Characteristic EKG changes are prolonged ST segments and Q-T intervals. Hypocalcemia ("symptomatic or seven" is one guideline) is best treated with intravenous calcium gluconate or chloride; calcium can also be given orally (calcium carbonate, Os-Cal, or Tums, for example).

Hypercalcemia

The most common causes of **hypercalcemia** are **hyperparathyroidism** in the general population, and **malignancy**, usually with bony metastases, in hospitalized patients; thiazide diuretic use, sarcoidosis, and parathyroid hormone-producing malignancy are three less common causes. Hypercalcemia caused by hyperparathyroidism is usually mild and asymptomatic and is often discovered by routine laboratory screening. Symptoms, when they occur, are often not noticed but are fairly classic in retrospect, consisting of kidney stones, abdominal pain, bony pain, and psychiatric disturbances ("stones, abdominal groans, painful bones, and psychic overtones..."). Asymptomatic patients with moderate hypercalcemia should undergo workup, and hyperparathyroidism, if present, should probably be treated by parathyroidectomy, although opinions vary about those with only minimally elevated calcium levels. Serious (serum level greater than 13mg/dL) or symptomatic (delirium, polydipsia, polyuria, nausea, and vomiting) hypercalcemia is most often associated with metastatic cancer and usually requires treatment with diuresis and hydration. ■

8 Hemostasis, Thrombosis and Transfusion

Intricate biologic relationships exist between blood and the vessel wall, allowing blood to remain a liquid and flow easily under normal conditions, yet maintaining a mechanism whereby it can be rapidly converted to a solid clot. When abnormalities in these relationships occur, significant morbidity is often the result.

Hemostasis

Tissues are highly thrombogenic. The vascular system has a natural barrier that exists between flowing blood and these tissues: the **endothelium**. Vascular endothelium is highly active and plays many roles, the most important of which are prevention of thrombosis and mediation of vascular repair. Intact endothelium is highly thromboresistant, and the fundamental event underlying essentially all episodes of clot formation is **endothelial damage** with exposure of blood to the subendothelial tissues. The process of clotting occurs in two steps: **primary** and **secondary hemostasis**. After hemostasis, **thrombolysis** acts to prevent the process from continuing out of control.

Primary hemostasis

Primary hemostasis refers to the initial, cellular clotting response. When endothelium is damaged, the collagen-laden subendothelium is exposed. The very first reaction to injury is **vasoconstriction**, occurring within seconds. Very quickly, **platelets adhere** to the damaged vessel wall with the help of von Willebrand factor (vWF) that binds to the exposed collagen and the platelet, linking them together. The adherent, newly activated platelets change shape, degranulate, and release chemotactic signals leading to **platelet aggregation**. This step requires fibrin from secondary hemostasis to bind the platelets together. Platelet thromboxane, inhibited by aspirin, is a potent vasoconstrictor and platelet aggregator. At this point the conglomeration of blood components is called a platelet plug, the product of primary hemostasis.

Secondary hemostasis

Secondary hemostasis is the molecular half of thrombosis, with activation of fibrin being the final common pathway. Clotting occurs via the intrinsic (interaction of factor XII and platelets) and extrinsic (activation of factor VII by subendothelial thromboplastin) pathways. The extrinsic pathway creates a large amount of fibrin within seconds, while the intrinsic pathway is slower. Both pathways activate their respective arms of the coagulation cascade, which converge in the formation of **thrombin** (factor IIa), a potent platelet aggregator that forms **fibrin** (factor Ia) from fibrinogen. The fibrin consolidates the platelet plug with a mesh-like network, and activates platelet receptors to cause clot retraction. Calcium is necessary for most reactions of secondary hemostasis to occur. An important later step is vasodilatation due to histamine release by the platelets, which acts to increase the delivery of inflammatory cells to the wound.

Thrombolysis

Thrombolysis is the process whereby clot formation is kept in check to prevent the thrombus from extending throughout the body. There are several major mechanisms by which this is accomplished. First, the proteolytic enzymes that are produced to activate the coagulation cascade also function to degrade cascade cofactors, thus limiting their local supply. Plasminogen, synthesized by the liver, is activated by factors such as tissue plasminogen activator (tPA) released by the intact endothelium adjacent to the clot. The resulting **plasmin** acts to dissolve fibrin where it overlaps normal endothelium. Additionally, the continued flow of blood serves to wash away thrombotic substances. Final endothelial repair and growth is due primarily to the release of platelet growth factors.

To clot normally, one needs exposed subendothelium (endothelial damage), functional platelets in conjunction with von Willebrand factor, intact coagulation cascade proteins in conjunction with calcium, and a normal fibrinolytic system.

Hemostatic Disorders

Disorders leading to excessive bleeding can be hereditary or acquired. The most common **hereditary** hemostatic defect is Hemophilia A, which results from a markedly diminished factor VIII level (see Chapter 17, "Hematology"). Bleeding occurs in these patients spontaneously and with mild trauma. Treatment consists of transfusion of factor VIII concentrate if severe, cryoprecipitate (less risk of disease transmission) if mild. Hemophilia B (Christmas Disease), results from a deficiency in factor IX, and is treated with factor IX concentrate. von Willebrand's disease, where patients lack von Willebrand's factor, leads to platelet dysfunction because platelet adherence is abnormal; this is treated with cryoprecipitate.

Platelet disorders

Acquired disorders are more common. Acquired platelet disorders are usually secondary to either drugs or to altered organ function. **Qualitative** platelet defects (normal number but impaired function), for example, can be due to aspirin use, which irreversibly inhibits platelet thromboxane formation, or to uremia, which affects the interaction between platelets, factor VIII, and von Willebrand factor. **Quantitative** disorders (reduced number of normally functioning platelets) are commonly due to hemorrhage, hypersplenism, or bone marrow failure. Because platelets are necessary for primary hemostasis, the **bleeding time** will be the primary laboratory abnormality in any platelet disorder, while the platelet count will be reduced only in quantitative disorders.

Factor disorders

Disorders of **coagulation factors** are most commonly seen in patients with liver disease (the liver produces all of the clotting factors except VIII), or in patients taking warfarin (Coumadin, which inhibits production of the vitamin K dependent factors-II, VII, IX, X). These will produce abnormalities in the **prothrombin (PT)** or **partial thromboplastin (PTT) times**, which measure the extrinsic and intrinsic pathways, respectively.

DIC

The most commonly seen **fibrinolytic disorder** is a combined thrombotic and hemorrhagic disorder: **disseminated intravascular coagulation (DIC)**. This usually results from a stimulus (such as sepsis) causing continuous clot formation and breakdown. This results in a "consumptive coagulopathy," leading to a diminished platelet count, prolonged coagulation times and decreased fibrinogen levels, with increases in the breakdown products of fibrin (fibrin split products).

Thrombotic Disorders

Virchow's triad refers to the three factors that predispose to thrombosis: stasis, endothelial injury, and hypercoagulable states. Hypercoagulable states can be hereditary, such as Protein C, S or anti-thrombin III deficiencies, or

acquired, as seen in patients with malignancies or polycythemia vera. Endothelial injury, discussed above,
results from trauma, abnormal blood flow patterns, repetitive stress, or, most importantly, atherosclerosis, lipids,
and smoking. Stasis occurs with inactivity, most importantly due to prolonged sitting or iatrogenically-imposed
paralysis during surgery, or in the atria of the heart in the
setting of atrial fibrillation. Patients can present with clots
in the venous or arterial systems. In general, acquired disorders secondary to atherosclerosis and smoking are
extremely common; hereditary disorders are rare but
often lethal.

Evaluation and Workup

Among the most abused laboratory studies are those
monitoring the coagulation system. In general, coagulation studies are insensitive and are not needed unless
there is a primary hematologic problem, a history suggestive of abnormal bleeding, or the patient will undergo
surgery when systemic heparinization is planned (cardiac,
vascular) or when any bleeding would be catastrophic
(neurosurgery).

In the evaluation of any patient, especially those with suspected hematologic problems, a careful history including
evidence of previous bleeding or clotting disorders and
relevant medications (including aspirin), as well as any
relevant family history, is required. A careful exam is also
important, including evaluation of the pulses and the
identification of any extremity edema. If appropriate, as
discussed above, baseline laboratory tests are obtained.

PT and PTT

The **prothrombin time** (**PT**) is an assessment of the
extrinsic pathway, and is now commonly and more accurately expressed as an **international normalized ratio**
(**INR**) which is a ratio of the PT to a control value modified by a reagent factor. The **activated partial thromboplastin time** (**PTT**) similarly is an assessment of the
intrinsic pathway. The **platelet count** is used to detect a
thrombocytopenia or thrombocytosis (quantitative platelet
disorder), and the **bleeding time** is used to detect a qualitative platelet disorder (adequate number of poorly functioning platelets). Further, more sophisticated tests are
performed as directed by problems pinpointed above.
(continued)

Multidisciplinary
Hemostasis, Thrombosis and Transfusion
continued

Transfusion and Hemorrhage

PRBCs

Although a variety of blood products is available, in routine clinical practice there are only 3 or 4 components commonly used.

Packed red blood cells (PRBCs) have a hematocrit of about 70%, and transfusion of one unit will raise the patient's hematocrit by about 3%. Blood transfusions obviously carry some risk. Transmission of the HIV virus is quite uncommon today (the risk was estimated to be about one in 100,000 units transfused in the early 90s), but risk of transmitting Hepatitis B and C is still significant. Transfusion reactions can occur, and are classified as **febrile**, resulting from patient antibodies to cellular or molecular components of the transfused blood, or, less commonly, **hemolytic**, resulting from ABO or other antigen incompatibility. Further, a transfusion itself is inherently immunosuppressive. Thus, blood should be reserved for situations where the benefit exceeds the risk. Usually this means that PRBC's should be reserved for repletion of oxygen-carrying capacity (red cell mass, hematocrit), and not used for volume replacement. These "side effects" of blood transfusion, moreover, have essentially eliminated the use of whole blood.

FFP

During storage, coagulation factors and platelets are depleted. **Fresh frozen plasma (FFP)** contains blood proteins including most coagulation factors (excluding factor VIII). A common practice is to transfuse 2 units of FFP and 4-6 units of **platelets** for every 10 or so units of red cells transfused to avoid dilutional coagulopathy and thrombocytopenia. Both agents can transmit disease and produce transfusion reactions, however, and there is much evidence that in situations other than massive transfusion (replacement of several blood volumes) their use should be restricted to situations where specific, clinically relevant deficiencies exist. Finally, **cryoprecipitate** is rich in factor VIII and von Willebrand's factor, and is thus useful in the treatment of von Willebrand's disease, mild Hemophilia A, DIC, and uremia.

A patient who is actively bleeding is a special problem. Assuming, for our purposes, that the airway and breathing are controlled, ensuring an adequate circulating volume and control of hemorrhage are the first steps. In the short term, replacement of fluid mass is most critical to supply preload to the heart. Actual oxygen-carrying capacity is surprisingly well preserved. Thus, **volume** replacement is initiated with isotonic crystalloid such as normal saline (NS) or lactated Ringer's solution (LR, closest to plasma). Multiple, large-bore (18 or 16g) IVs are necessary, because the rapidity of volume replacement is often critical. When actual **oxygen-carrying capacity** is significantly affected, as assessed by hematocrit or clinical judgment, PRBCs are infused, and specific blood products are used to treat specific coagulopathies. The hematocrit, because it is a percentage, will be normal immediately after acute blood loss, but patients tolerate a low hematocrit quite well, with improved microvascular perfusion due to lowered viscosity with significant anemia being the trade-off.

Often, the source and cause of blood loss are obvious. With any bleeding patient, especially those with no obvious reason to bleed, a coagulopathy (pathologic or iatrogenic) should be sought and treated, if present. Abnormalities of the intrinsic pathway, often due to heparin (elevated PTT), can be counteracted by protamine. Abnormalities of the extrinsic pathway, often due to Coumadin administration or liver failure (elevated PT), can be reversed quickly by FFP (directly repleting proteins) or more slowly by Vitamin K (to stimulate synthesis). Vitamin K is less effective if the liver's synthetic function is impaired. The same principles are used when evaluating a patient who is receiving anticoagulants prior to an operation.

Deep Venous Thrombosis (DVT)

A lower extremity DVT, or clot in the venous system of the leg, is among the most common hematologic disorders seen. The "typical" patient presents with a swollen leg after some predisposing factor such as an operation, a long, sedentary car ride, or a malignancy. Unfortunately, this classic presentation is unusual. Many patients with a swollen leg have no clot, and a significant number of patients who die as the result of pulmonary embolization have no antecedent symptoms. It has been estimated that the diagnosis of a DVT is accurate clinically only about half the time. Luckily, a good screening test is available: **duplex ultrasound** (see Chapter 37, "Vascular Surgery"). It is noninvasive, and, in experienced hands, quite accurate. A clot is detected by direct visualization or by the lack of flow or compressibility in the vein. Although it is invasive, painful and involves the use of contrast, the gold standard probably remains the **phlebogram** because it gives a direct picture of the vessels.

Complications

Clots in the veins of the leg require treatment for prevention of **pulmonary embolus (PE)** and **post-phlebitic** or **chronic venous stasis syndrome**. Venous return itself is almost always enough preserved (via collaterals) to support adequate perfusion to the leg. In general, any clot in the femoral or iliac vessels requires therapy, but the situation is less clear with those limited to the calf. Isolated calf vein thrombosis per se has a lower incidence of embolic events, but can progress to femoral thrombosis if not treated.

Treatment

Treatment involves two major principles: prevention of PE while the clot is unstable, and prevention of local propagation. The first objective is addressed through bed rest for 4-7 days while the clot adheres to the endothelium. Elevation of the extremity will help with edema resolution. Prevention of local propagation is accomplished with anticoagulation. Anticoagulation with heparin or Coumadin does not lyse the clot, but it does prevent propagation while the body itself takes care of thrombolysis. Actual thrombolytics and surgical thrombectomy have not been shown to reliably reduce the incidence of late post-phlebitic changes, and in general are seldom used in simple DVT.

Heparinization

Baseline laboratory values are obtained, and the patient is started on a heparin drip after an initial bolus. **Heparin** is used initially because its onset is immediate. It acts by potentiating the actions of anti-thrombin III that prevents thrombin from activating the platelets and converting fibrinogen to fibrin. Because heparin binds to other proteins its pharmacokinetics vary, and thus, the patient's coagulation parameters must be followed closely until a steady state is reached. The PTT is used to monitor heparin therapy, and is usually considered therapeutic if it is between 1.5-2.5 times normal (50-85 seconds or so). One impor-

tant "side effect" of heparin is acquired thrombocytopenia, due to anti-platelet antibody formation. Platelet
counts should be measured daily in any patient receiving
heparin in any form, and all sources (including flushes)
must be stopped if the syndrome occurs.

Oral anticoagulation

Because patients cannot receive a continuous IV infusion
for the rest of their lives, oral anticoagulation is begun
with warfarin (Coumadin). Coumadin is a vitamin K
antagonist and consequently diminishes the levels of the
vitamin K dependent coagulation factors (II, VII, IX, and
X). Coumadin is given orally and is therefore the drug of
choice for long term anticoagulation, and its effect is
monitored by the PT or INR. Proteins C and S, which are
anticoagulants, are also vitamin K-dependent and thus are
also diminished with Coumadin therapy. Because of their
short half-lives, levels decrease faster than the clotting
factors, and patients may be transiently hypercoagulable
immediately after the initiation of Coumadin therapy. This
is why Coumadin is not started until the patient is thera-
peutically anticoagulated with heparin. The development
of a steady-state therapeutic effect often takes 4-7 days.
By this time the clot is adherent and the patient may be
discharged.

Caval interruption

If contraindications to anti-coagulation are present (recent
neurosurgery, "failure" of anticoagulation, ongoing bleeding) interruption of the inferior vena cava with a percutaneously or surgically placed filter is an option. While the
underlying problem (clot in the leg) is not addressed, the
major, potentially fatal problem (pulmonary embolus) is
almost perfectly prevented. ■

Multidisciplinary

Endocrinology

The endocrine system is composed of the **pancreas** and **pituitary**, **adrenal**, **thyroid**, and **parathyroid glands**. These glands release hormones that regulate the activity of organs throughout the body. Hormones are substances released into the blood that act at a distance, and, as such, are fundamental to the coordination of the organ systems.

Pancreas

The **islets of Langerhans** are small nests of cells within the pancreas responsible for hormone production. They are composed of four cell types. **Alpha cells** secrete **glucagon**, which raises blood glucose levels primarily by causing the breakdown of glycogen. **Beta cells** secrete **insulin**, which lowers blood glucose levels by promoting glucose entry into cells. Insulin also promotes protein synthesis, lipogenesis, and glycogen storage and thus has profound, global, anabolic effects, while glucagon, in general, has the opposite function. **Delta cells** secrete **somatostatin**, a peptide that functions to inhibit pancreatic and gastrointestinal hormone release, and **F cells** produce pancreatic polypeptide, an inhibitor of endocrine function.

Diabetes

Diabetes mellitus is manifest by hyperglycemia, and is discussed in more depth in Chapter 53, "Pediatric Endocrinology." Symptoms include osmotic polyuria, resultant polydipsia, and polyphagia, and glucosuria is present if the blood glucose level exceeds the threshold for tubular reabsorption (250mg/dL or so). Diabetes is the result of inadequate insulin, either because of an absolute deficiency or because of resistance at the receptor level. Type I (usually juvenile-onset) diabetes is caused by deficient insulin production due to beta cell destruction; these patients always require insulin, and are prone to develop diabetic ketoacidosis. Type II (usually adult-onset) diabetes is caused by resistance of peripheral cells to insulin and is usually associated with prolonged obesity. Type II diabetes can usually be managed by diet and weight modification alone, but may require the use of oral hypoglycemics or even insulin, if very severe. These patients can develop non-ketotic, hyperosmolar coma, caused by the hypovolemia due to the osmotic effects of severe hyperglycemia (as high as 2000mg/dL) and glucosuria.

Hypoglycemia

Hypoglycemia is defined as a plasma glucose level less than 65mg/dL; symptoms are most dependent on the rate of decline and duration of hypoglycemia. Initial signs and symptoms are due to reflex **adrenergic hyperactivity** and consist of tachycardia, tachypnea, palpitations, diaphoresis, anxiety, weakness, tremors, hunger, and nausea. If hypoglycemia persists, evidence of **cortical dysfunction** such as disorientation, hallucinations, strange behavior, frontal release signs, and seizure activity arise. The final or **medullary** stage of hypoglycemia includes a decreased respiratory rate, bradycardia, pupillary dilatation, coma, and death. Hypoglycemia is caused by excess insulin, which, in turn, is most often due to an insulin overdose in a diabetic patient or to an insulin-producing tumor. Excess use of sulfonylurea drugs, beta-blockers, and alcohol can also produce hypoglycemia. Treatment is glucose replacement; workup is required if the condition persists or recurs.

Pituitary

The pituitary gland is the control center for most of the rest of the endocrine system. It is composed of the functionally separate **anterior (adenohypophysis)** and **posterior (neurohypophysis)** pituitary glands, and is connected to the hypothalamus by a stalk. The anterior pituitary has hormone-producing cells that respond to **releasing hormones** secreted by the hypothalamus, conveyed by a portal venous system, while the posterior pituitary has no discrete cell bodies, but consists of the termination of nerve fibers passing down the stalk from the hypothalamus.

The anterior pituitary produces five major hormones, each "released" by the respective hypothalamic releasing hormone. **Thyroid stimulating hormone (TSH)** stimulates the thyroid to grow and produce thyroxine, **adrenocortotropic hormone (ACTH)** stimulates the adrenal cortex to produce mineralo- and glucocorticoids, **growth hormone (GH)** stimulates growth in children and is a general anabolic hormone in adults, and **leutenizing hormone (LH)** and **follicle-stimulating hormone (FSH)**, act to regulate the ovulatory cycle. The nerve fibers to the

Multidisciplinary
Endocrinology *continued*

posterior pituitary convey the hormones **vasopressin (antidiuretic hormone; ADH)** and **oxytocin**, which are stored for release at timed intervals. ADH increases renal water reabsorption, while oxytocin assists in breast feeding.

Disorders of the pituitary gland cause symptoms either by compression of the optic chiasm (producing a homonymous, bitemporal hemianopsia) or by excessive or deficient release of one or more hormones. Pituitary tumors are usually benign **microadenomas**, usually of one cell type, usually releasing one hormone. **Prolactinoma** is the most common microadenoma, causing impotence and decreased libido in men, and galactorrhea and amenorrhea in women. Treatment is operative removal of the adenoma.

Acromegaly is caused by overproduction of GH in the adult (gigantism results in a child whose growth plates have not yet fused). Acromegaly causes characteristic physical features such as mandibular enlargement, frontal bossing, and growth of the hands, feet, and tongue. Diabetes can occur due to glucose intolerance caused by excess GH. Onset is usually insidious, and treatment consists of a combination of surgery, radiation therapy, and somatostatin.

Pituitary insufficiency can be of two types: **panhypopituitarism** or **selective hypopituitarism**. Panhypopituitarism can result from a number of problems, including tumor, trauma, postpartum pituitary necrosis, and operative removal of the gland. Symptoms are caused by hormone deficiency; the most troublesome being ACTH. Treatment consists of hormone replacement. Selective hypopituitarism is most commonly caused by chronic, exogenous steroid administration, leading to suppression of pituitary ACTH production.

There are two common disorders of the posterior pituitary. The **syndrome of inappropriate antidiuretic hormone (SIADH)** refers to the situation where ADH is produced in the absence of a hyperosmolar state. SIADH causes inappropriate renal water reabsorption leading to hypo-osmolality and hyponatremia, and can be caused by head trauma, tuberculosis, infection, and some drugs. SIADH is usually self-limited and is treated with volume restriction. The converse of SIADH is **diabetes insipidus (DI)** caused by ADH insufficiency, often after head trauma. Urine is inappropriately dilute; diagnosis is confirmed by the presence of dilute urine in the presence of high serum osmolality. DI can be central (lack of ADH secretion) or nephrogenic (distal tubular cells unresponsive to ADH), differentiation of the two can be accomplished by noting the response to exogenous ADH administration.

Adrenal Gland

The adrenal gland is made up of two embryologically unrelated parts, the **cortex** and the **medulla**. The cortex produces three classes of steroid hormones: glucocorticoids, which regulate carbohydrate, protein, and lipid metabolism, mineralocorticoids, which regulate fluid and electrolyte balance, and the sex steroids. The medulla produces catecholamines. In response to **corticotropin releasing factor** from the hypothalamus, the anterior pituitary gland releases **ACTH** which stimulates the adrenal gland to produce and release glucocorticoids (and, to a lesser extent, mineralocorticoids). Cortisol levels fluctuate rapidly making simple, one-time measurement of levels unreliable as a measure of adrenal function.

Adrenal insufficiency

Primary adrenocortical insufficiency refers to dysfunction at the level of the adrenal gland itself, usually from destruction of functioning tissue. The most common causes include autoimmune destruction, adrenal hemorrhage or infarction, and tuberculosis. Congenital enzyme deficiencies also occur, but are less common. **Chronic primary adrenocortical insufficiency** (**Addison's disease**) often produces skin pigmentation due to high levels of melanocyte-stimulating fragments of the ACTH precursor molecule (produced in high amounts due to the loss of negative feedback). **Secondary adrenocortical insufficiency** results from a dysfunction at the level of the hypothalamus or pituitary gland with resultant ACTH deficiency. Iatrogenic suppression of the hypothalamic-pituitary-adrenal axis by exogenously administered glucocorticoids is probably the most common cause. **Acute adrenocortical insufficiency** (**Addisonian crisis**) usually occurs after an acute stressor such as infection or trauma in the setting of chronic adrenal deficiency or iatrogenic

Multidisciplinary
Endocrinology *continued*

suppression. Signs and symptoms are nonspecific, and include fever or hypothermia, hypotension, abdominal pain, nausea, vomiting, mental status changes, and weakness; diagnosis is very difficult, in part because these patients are often critically ill to begin with. **A patient who has received steroids for two or more weeks within the past two years and who has an unexplained problem should be assumed to have adrenal insufficiency until proved otherwise.** If suspicion is high, exogenous steroids can be given before laboratory confirmation is obtained. In nonemergent situations, serum cortisol levels can be obtained after the adrenal gland is stimulated by ACTH.

Cushing's syndrome

Overproduction of cortisol is called **Cushing's syndrome**. **Cushing's disease** is the special case of Cushing's syndrome caused by an ACTH-producing pituitary microadenoma with resultant bilateral adrenal hyperplasia. Cushing's syndrome can also be caused by a primary problem with the adrenal gland (adenoma or tumor) or an ectopic source of ACTH (such as a small-cell lung tumor). Cushing's syndrome presents with a characteristic constellation of physical findings, including truncal obesity, round, "moon-like" face, a so-called "buffalo hump," and abdominal striae.

Hyperaldosteronism

The combination of hypokalemia and hypertension suggests **hyperaldosteronism**, also known as **Conn's syndrome**. An adrenocortical adenoma or diffuse hyperplasia can lead to the overproduction of aldosterone, which causes potassium excretion, sodium and volume retention, and resultant hypertension; as opposed to primary renovascular hypertension, plasma renin levels will be low.

Pheochromocytoma

The most important neoplasm of the adrenal medulla is **pheochromocytoma**, a catecholamine-producing tumor that can arise anywhere neuroendocrine tissue is present. Ten percent are malignant, 10% familial, 10% bilateral, and 10% extra-adrenal or multiple. Epinephrine, and, occasionally, norepinephrine are secreted in episodic fashion, leading to the characteristic paroxysms of tachycardia, hypertension, and headache; occasionally an episode of "malignant" hypertension on induction of anesthesia for an unrelated operation will be the presenting "symptom." Operative removal is required; to do so safely, alpha followed by beta blockade ("a before b") and volume loading for several weeks is needed, and early control of the adrenal vein at the time of operation is helpful.

Incidental adrenal masses are noted occasionally on CT or MRI studies ordered for other reasons. A hormonally inactive mass smaller than 6cm is extremely unlikely to be malignant and should be observed.

Thyroid

Two cell types are present within the thyroid. In response to pituitary TSH, **follicular cells** metabolize iodine to produce, store, and release **T3 and T4 (triiodyronine and thyroxine**, respectively), which help regulate cellular metabolism. In response to elevated serum calcium levels, **parafollicular cells (C-cells)** secrete **calcitonin** which inhibits osteoclast activity. The physiologic relevance of calcitonin in humans is unclear; total thyroidectomy seems not to alter calcium homeostasis at all. The terms hyper- and hypothyroidism refer respectively, thus, to over- and underactivity of thyroxine.

Hyper-thyroidism

Hyperthyroidism causes an increased metabolic rate, leading to weight loss, heat intolerance, palpitations, and tachycardia, and can be due to excess TSH or primary overactivity of the thyroid itself. The most common causes of hyperthyroidism are Grave's disease, thyroiditis, and diffuse toxic goiter. **Grave's disease** occurs predominantly in young women, presents with exophthalmos, and seems to be caused by an antibody that stimulates the TSH receptor. Hyperthyroidism in the setting of a negative Grave's workup is usually due to thyroiditis or a neoplasm (rare).

Hypo-thyroidism

Hypothyroidism usually produces cold intolerance, lethargy, weight gain, and depression, and occasionally periorbital edema and a nonpitting puffiness (myxedema) throughout the body. **Hashimoto's thyroiditis** is the most common cause of hypothyroidism, and is caused by antibodies directed against thyroglobulin and thyroid peroxidase; there is some evidence that an increased risk of carcinoma occurs in these patients. **Iatrogenic** elimination of thyroid tissue by operative excision, radiation, or radioac

Multidisciplinary
Endocrinology *continued*

tive iodine administration also causes hypothyroidism. Patients with hypothyroidism from any cause are easily treated with exogenous thyroxine (Synthroid).

Thyroid nodules

Thyroid nodules are relatively common (present in 4% of the population) and thus are frequently discovered on routine exam. Prior radiation exposure or the presence of pain or hoarseness are suggestive of malignancy. Several algorithms can be followed for workup of such nodules, with the overall objective to distinguish benign from malignant tissue. Thyroid function tests are not terribly useful, because global function is usually normal, but isotope scintography ("thyroid scanning") is: most malignant tumors are "cold." Most solitary nodules eventually require fine needle aspiration cytology; interpretation depends on the tissue type present. In general, differentiation of purely papillary masses into benign and malignant types is fairly reliable, but the same is not true for follicular masses – malignancy, in this case, can only be determined with certainty by permanent section. Thus, "papillary adenoma" usually reliably denotes absence of malignancy, but any follicular tissue essentially mandates formal operative resection.

Thyroid Ca

Thyroid carcinoma, the most common endocrine malignancy, is twice as common in women. Papillary, follicular, anaplastic, and medullary carcinomas, as well as lymphomas, arise from the cells within the thyroid gland. **Papillary carcinoma** is most common (60%-70%), is relatively nonaggressive, and is rarely a cause of mortality; the presence of psommoma bodies are its histologic hallmark. Operative resection is required, although there is considerable controversy over whether the entire gland or just the lobe containing the palpable tumor should be removed. Although the incidence of undetected, microscopic foci in the opposite lobe is high, these foci, as well as lymph nodes containing metastatic foci of tumor do **not** worsen prognosis if left in place. **Follicular carcinoma** is less common, but has a higher rate of spread to lymph nodes. **Medullary carcinomas** arise from the parafollicular cells, and represent only about 3% of all thyroid cancers; about 20% of medullary carcinomas are, in part, genetically transmitted. **Anaplastic carcinoma** is the most aggressive of the thyroid carcinomas and carries a dismal prognosis.

Parathyroid

Hyper-parathyroidism

The paired **parathyroid glands** are usually located on the posterior surface of the thyroid. During development, they migrate caudally. The superior parathyroids, originating from the 4th pharyngeal pouch, migrate in association with the thyroid gland, while the inferior parathyroids, arising from the 3rd pouch, migrate with the thymus. The final locations of the inferior glands are much more variable than are those of the superior glands.

In response to serum calcium levels, the parathyroid glands synthesize and secrete **parathyroid hormone (PTH)**, which helps to regulate (increase) the concentration of serum calcium; the parathyroids are independent of pituitary control. **Hyperparathyroidism** is the most common cause of hypercalcemia in non-hospitalized patients (see Chapter 7, "Basic Fluids and Electrolytes"), and hyperparathyroidism is usually discovered on routine laboratory screening of asymptomatic patients. PTH levels are usually elevated. **Primary hyperparathyroidism** is due to an overproduction of PTH by the gland itself, leading to elevated PTH and calcium levels. Most are due to an adenoma, and the rest, to diffuse hyperplasia; cancer is exceedingly rare. Treatment involves operative exploration; intraoperative decision making is made more interesting by the fact that both asymmetric hyperplasia and multiple adenomas occur. Radiologic studies are **not** usually helpful or cost-effective unless the patient has had a previously unsuccessful parathyroid exploration.

Secondary hyperparathyroidism is caused by chronic renal failure. Diminished glomerular filtration leads to retention of phosphate and excretion of calcium; the parathyroids compensate by increasing secretion of PTH. Medical management includes dialysis and calcium and vitamin D supplementation. With continued parathyroid stimulation by renal failure, the glands become autonomous. Patients who regain normal renal function after a renal transplant should regain near-normal renal function and calcium levels; if the parathyroids continue to secrete PTH, **tertiary hyperparathyroidism** is said to be present. Operation may be required to avoid excessive bone reabsorption and soft tissue calcification. ■

10   Immunology

Immunology is the study of the organism's defense against and response to pathogens. The immune system can respond in a **nonspecific** way to infection, injury, and even malignancy, and, by the process of **acquired immunity**, in a **specific** way against individual pathogens. Nonspecific immunity involves skin, mucosal, and secretory barriers to invasion, natural killer cells, polymorphonuclear leukocytes (PMNs), and macrophages, while acquired immunity is primarily a function of the lymphocytes and immunoglobulins. Fundamental to a healthy immune system is an organism's capability of differentiating "**self**" from "**non-self**."

"Self" and "Non-Self"

Cellular recognition is dependent on membrane-expressed proteins called **human leukocyte antigens** (**HLA**, after the cells on which they were initially discovered). The DNA that codes for these is called the **major histocompatability complex** (**MHC**) on a section of chromosome 6. In other words, the **MHC** is the DNA that codes for the **HLA** proteins (don't get confused!). Two separate classes of MHC-derived proteins are produced: class I proteins (HLA-A, -B, and -C) are expressed on the surface of virtually all nucleated cells, while class II proteins (HLA-D, -DR, -DQ, and -DW/DR) are expressed primarily by **B lymphocytes** and **antigen-presenting cells** (**APC**, macrophages, and dendritic cells). Foreign proteins are taken up non-specifically by APCs; the phagocytized, fragmented proteins, serving as antigens, are then expressed on the cell surface of the APC in conjunction with the cell's class II proteins. This form of presentation (foreign antigen plus class II HLA on the surface of an APC) activates the rest of the immune system to specifically recognize the original foreign protein as "non-self."

The immune response can be broadly divided into two arms, **humoral** and **cellular**. The humoral arm is mediated by proteins that bind to and help destroy foreign antigens, while the cellular arm is mediated by specific cell-to-cell interactions. An **antigen** is a molecule that can be recognized as foreign by the effectors of the immune system. Antigens are recognized by **immunoglobulins**

(**Ig**) produced by B-lymphocytes or by the T-cell antigen receptor (TAR). Igs recognize and bind to soluble antigens while T-cells recognize antigen processed by APCs. Antigens can be large or small; the specific portion of the antigen that is recognized as foreign and is responsible for activation of the immune system (and bound by the Ig) is called the **epitope**.

Humoral Response

B-lymphocytes are the major cellular effectors of the humoral response. Individual B-cells, normally quiescent, can be programmed to make a specific antibody directed against an epitope. On exposure to the antigen, a B-cell will be stimulated to **clonally expand**, differentiate into antibody-producing **plasma cells**, and increase the production of antibodies specifically directed against that (and only that) antigen.

Antibodies

Antibodies are not created specifically to recognize certain antigens. Instead, a huge variety of antibodies exists from birth, and statistically one (really many, in varying degrees of specificity) will always recognize any possible configuration of molecules that make up any antigen. Once the antigen is recognized and the appropriate B-cell activated, those B-cell(s) bearing the antibody(s) are stimulated to clonally expand. If the same (or similar) antigen returns, the secondary (**amnestic**) response is much faster and of much greater magnitude, because multiple copies already exist of the specific Ig and specifically activated B-cells.

Antibodies are Y-shaped polypeptides, and are composed of two identical heavy chains and two identical light chains attached by disulfide bonds. Variable and hypervariable regions of the antibody (on the two upper ends of the "Y") determine its antigenic specificity, while the constant region (the bottom or stem of the "Y") allows the molecule to bind to the cell surface receptors of effector cells as well as with other components of the immune system such as complement proteins (see below).

Isotypes

There are five different antibody types (**isotypes**). **IgM**, a pentamer, is the largest of the immunoglobulins; IgM is the principal antibody produced **early** in the response to antigen (while IgG production is gearing up) and is pre-

Multidisciplinary
Immunology *continued*

sent on the surface of quiescent B-cells. **IgG** is the most common serum immunoglobulin. IgM and IgG activate complement, and IgG is recognized by receptors on phagocytic cells. **IgA**, which is found primarily in solution in mucosal secretions, acts as a first line of defense against invading pathogens. **IgD** coats the B-cells and may serve as a receptor, causing B-cell activation, while **IgE**, the principle effector of allergic reactions, when bound with antigen, binds to mast cells and basophils causing degranulation and release of active substances (such as histamine). IgG, IgA, and IgE are produced during the secondary response as IgM-producing B-cell clones specific for an anitgen are activated and induced to switch.

Cellular Response

The principal mediators of the cellular arm of the immune system are the **T-lymphocytes**. T-cells have heterodimeric antigen-specific receptors on their surface as well as additional associated transmembrane proteins that form a complex (**T-cell antigen receptor**, **TAR**). This complex includes **CD3**, a determinant expressed on all mature T-cells. T-lymphocytes are classified according to the other CD receptor expressed; the two major groups are **helper/inducer** (**CD4**) and **cytotoxic/suppressor** (**CD8**) T-cells. Helper T-cells assist B-cells in mounting an antibody response and stimulate proliferation and differentiation of other cellular elements of the immune system and cytotoxic T-cells recognize and directly lyse foreign or malignant cells.

Circulating **monocytes** and their noncirculating equivalents, **macrophages**, were originally recognized by their ability to phagocytose foreign cells or particles. Monocytes originate in the bone marrow, are released into the blood for 24 hours or so, then enter specific tissues (where they are then called macrophages). Macrophages, which do not possess antigen-specific receptors, have multiple, often nonspecific roles. **Phagocytosis** can be made much more efficient by the presence of **opsonins**, molecules (often the constant region of an immunoglobulin or products of the complement cascade) bound to the surface of the antigen that enhance recognition (and consequent destruction) of the antigen by phagocytes. Macrophages, as **APCs**, **process antigens** and present them to T-lymphocytes, as discussed above. A very important function of macrophages is the production of **cytokines**, including **interleukin (IL)-1** and **tumor necrosis factor (TNF)**. Macrophages are critically important to the immune response; because no person has ever been found without them, their congenital absence is assumed to be incompatible with life.

Natural killer (NK) cells function as fairly nonspecific killers of invading organisms; they can be "turbocharged" by cytokines (a generic term for molecules that affect immunoreactivity including TNF, the interleukins, and the interferons) and are then called **lymphokine activated killer (LAK)** cells (under investigation as tumoricidal agents).

Complement

The **complement system** is a group of serum proteins that can be activated to opsonize and lyse pathogenic antigens and cells. There are two pathways for complement activation. In the **classical** pathway, complement is activated by antigen-antibody complexes, while in the **alternative** pathway the antigen itself (i.e., viral capsule or bacterial endotoxin) stimulates the cascade. Activation by either produces an amplifying cascade leading to the creation of **membrane attack complexes (MAC)** that destroy membranes of foreign cells, activated molecules that act as **opsonins**, and activated molecules that act as **chemotactic agents** for PMNs and macrophages.

Cytokines

The term "**cytokine**" (**lymphokine**, if produced by a lymphocyte) is given to various proteins produced by cells of the immune system that are involved in the regulation of the immune response. Cytokines, generally small molecules that bind to cell surface receptors, often function as local mediators, but they may cause systemic effects, especially if present in supraphysiologic amounts. The most important cytokines thus far identified are the interferons, interleukins and tumor necrosis factor.

Interferons

There are three important **interferons (IFN)**. IFN-alpha and -beta are concerned principally with the host response to viral infection. Their production is induced by viral infection, and they induce non-specific resistance to viral infection in neighboring, uninfected cells. IFN-gamma activates macrophages and NK cells and induces the expression of MHC products on a variety of cells, thereby enhancing antigen presentation.

Interleukins

The **interleukins** are a family of cytokines that seem to act as communication molecules between cells of the immune system. **Interleukin (IL) -1** is produced mainly by activated macrophages in response to antigen or injury, and activates helper (CD-4) T-cells. IL-1 also has systemic effects such as fever induction, hypotension, leukocyte adherence to endothelium, and cortisol release. Activated helper T-cells produce **IL-2** in response to stimulation by IL-1 and antigen. IL-2 enhances T-cell activation and induces proliferation of the T-cell and the IL-2 receptor in a self-augmenting cycle; this interaction is critical to the process of cell-mediated immunity and to

Figure 10.1
Simplified macrophage—helper T-lymphocyte interaction. In response to a stimulant such as endotoxin, the macrophage produces IL-1, which stimulates the production of IL-2 by the T-cell. IL-2 stimulates production of more IL-2 and expression of the IL-2 receptor. Steroids inhibit macrophages and IL-1 production, and Cyclosporine A and FK-506 inhibit IL-2 production. Azothioprine, antilymphocyte globulin, and OKT3 all act to inhibit the T-lymphocyte in various ways (see Chapter 39, "Transplantation").

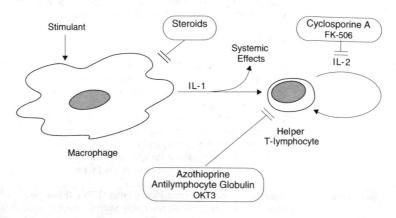

understand the mechanism of action of the drugs used for prevention of rejection after an organ transplant (see Chapter 39, "Transplantation").

IL-4, produced by helper T-cells, is a principal B-cell stimulating and differentiating factor which is critical for the production of IgE. IL-5 plays a minor role in B-cell activation but is important for IgA isotype switching and for eosinophil production. IL-6 was originally described for its role in B-cell activation, but is now known to be the principal stimulus for the hepatic **acute phase response** (see Chapter 4, "Response to Injury").

TNF

Tumor necrosis factor (**TNF**), once called **cachexin** (because of its initial discovery as the molecule mediating parasite- and tumor-associated cachexia) is produced by activated macrophages. It is produced in response to endotoxemia, and may represent the "final common pathway" for endotoxin-associated sepsis, cancer cachexia, and the **systemic inflammatory response syndrome** (**SIRS**). It causes many systemic effects including fever, vasodilatation, and hypotension, and may cause tumor necrosis under certain conditions (but its net benefit as an anti-tumor agent has been minimal). TNF and IL-1 are early mediators of many of the effects of acute injury (see Chapter 4, "Response to Injury").

Organs of the Immune System

Lymph nodes are found throughout the body in chains along major vessels and draining specific organs. Lymphatic fluid drained from tissues is "surveyed" by the T- and B-cells in the nodes, which are stimulated to divide in response to antigen. As a result, a lymph node draining an infected area (the infection can be subclinical) will often increase in size and/or become red and painful. Non-encapsulated **lymphoid tissue**, which has the same function as the lymph nodes, is scattered throughout the body in locations near the "outside world" such as the oropharynx (tonsils), bronchi, and gastrointestinal tract (Peyers patches) where antigen exposure is high.

The **bone marrow** is the site where progenitor cells of the immune system are produced and where a certain part of their early development takes place; the **thymus** is the

Multidisciplinary
Immunology *continued*

location where T-lymphocytes are "taught" to respond to their specific antigens and leave "self" antigens alone. The **spleen** contains large collections of B- and T-cells surrounding porous sinusoids and venules. Blood passing through is likewise "surveyed" for micro-organisms (and senescent red blood cells), and lymphocytes respond appropriately when antigen is identified. The spleen is particularly important in the response to encapsulated bacteria; patients who require splenectomy for trauma are at later risk for **overwhelming post-splenectomy sepsis** (**OPSS**) after infection with these organisms.

The Coordinated Immune Response

Now is the time to put it all together. How does all this interact in "real-life?"

Viral infection

In a **viral infection**, the initial event in the specific immune response is recognition of the invading organism by T- and B-cells after processing and presentation as "non-self" by antigen-presenting cells. B-cells whose surface antibodies recognize the viral antigen are thereby stimulated to divide and produce more of that antibody, roughly in proportion to the specificity of recognition to the various epitopes and antigens. Similarly, helper (CD4) T-cells that recognize the virus in the context of HLA class II antigens produce cytokines that further stimulate antigen-specific B-cells. Most of the antibody initially produced is IgM, but later, as IgG production increases, this becomes the major isotype. The antibody neutralizes the virus particle (prevents it from binding to cells in preparation for infection) and opsonizes it for phagocytosis and destruction by macrophages. Virus-specific cytotoxic (CD8) T-cells are also induced and are often critical for clearing the viral infection by lysing and destroying infected host cells after recognizing viral peptides (plus HLA class II antigens) on their surfaces.

Bacterial infection

A **bacterial infection** elicits a similar but slightly more elaborate response. Once again, antibody-bearing B-cells recognize bacterial antigen. The specific B-cells, with help from helper T-cells, proliferate and produce specific antibody. The opsonized bacteria are engulfed by neutrophils and macrophages, and killed by exposure to enzymes and reactive oxygen products (the **respiratory burst**). The complement system is also activated by antibodies bound to antigen; the MAC lyses many bacteria, and products of the cascade produce further opsonization and PMN and macrophage chemotaxis. Cytokines released by the activated cells cause systemic effects such as fever, which may act to make the environment inhospitable for bacterial replication. The inflammatory response attempts to localize the infection and destroy the organisms; lymphocytes in the draining lymph nodes further fight spread of the antigens.

Abnormalities of the Immune System

Hypersensitivity is an exaggerated response to an antigen. **Type I hypersensitivity** (**anaphylaxis**) is caused by IgE (bound to the offending antigen) binding to and activating mast cells and basophils. These cells release granules containing histamine and other vasoactive substances; if rapid and/or massive, vascular collapse and hypotensive shock (due to systemic vasodilatation) as well as bronchoconstriction can result. Epinephrine can be lifesaving in this situation. **Type II hypersensitivity** (**direct cytotoxic response**) is an IgG- or IgM-mediated "self-cytotoxicity" manifest clinically as acute transfusion reactions, autoimmune hemolytic anemia, and hyperacute graft rejection, while **type III hypersensitivity** (**Arthus reaction** or **serum sickness** and other **immune-complex diseases**) occurs when antigen-antibody complexes become deposited in end-organ capillaries and larger blood vessel walls, activating complement and producing an acute localized (or systemic) inflammatory response. Finally, **type IV** (**delayed**) hypersensitivity occurs when T-cells recognize an antigen, proliferate, and release cytokines, activating macrophages and producing a local inflammatory reaction. This is the basis for testing for skin sensitivity (such as the PPD test for tuberculosis bacilli) to certain antigens.

Congenital defects

Congenital immunologic defects are, fortunately, uncommon. In **chronic granulomatous disease**, PMNs have a reduced or absent ability to produce reactive oxygen metabolites as part of the "respiratory burst" used to kill organisms, making the individual susceptible to repeated infections by catalase-producing bacteria. These bacteria are phagocytosed but not killed, and granulomas develop. In **Chediak-Higashi disease** bacterial killing by leukocytes is impaired, and patients suffer from recurrent infection by pyogenic bacteria. **Bruton's agammaglobu-linemia** is an X-linked genetic defect resulting in poor immunoglobulin production. Affected individuals frequently suffer from recurrent bacterial infections; these patients have normal cell-mediated immunity and defense against viral infections. **Transient hypogammaglobu-linemia of infancy** is characterized by decreased levels of IgG. Affected infants suffer from recurrent upper respiratory infections until approximately 4, when the immune system "grows up." **DiGeorge syndrome** results from failure of the thymus to develop normally. Cell-mediated immunity, which depends on T-cell "education" in the thymus, is impaired, and patients often suffer from overwhelming viral infection; humoral immunity (which also depends on helper T-cell function) is also impaired. **Wiskott-Aldrich Syndrome** and **ataxia-telangiectasia** are rare syndromes that have as part of their presentation a defect in cell-mediated immunity. Interestingly, these patients are at increased risk for hematologic malignancies, suggesting a role for cell-mediated immunity in surveillance and suppression of malignancy.

Acquired defects

Perhaps the most important forms of immunodeficiency are **acquired**. The **human immunodeficiency virus (HIV)** infects and eventually kills helper T-cells, and is more fully covered in Chapter 19, "HIV and AIDS." More common are causes we see every day but often fail to consider. In any **nutritionally depleted** patient there is likely to be some degree of immunodeficiency. Because the immune response depends to a large extent on protein synthesis (immunoglobulins, complement, and so on), malnutrition, which causes protein breakdown (see Chapter 3, "Nutrition"), will almost always produce some degree of impairment of the immune system.

Malignancy can cause immunosuppression. Hematologic malignancies can cause decreased production of normal, immunocompetent bone marrow-derived cells, and any cancer can cause nutritional depletion (cancer cachexia), possibly due to the reactive production of TNF by the body's own cells. ■

11   Oncology

Few diagnoses are as frightening as that of **cancer**. Not all cancers behave the same way, however, and even the discovery of widely metastatic disease does not necessarily portend imminent death. Appropriate care for a patient with cancer requires the expertise of many different physicians and health care workers, including internists, surgeons, medical and radiation oncologists, pathologists, radiologists, nurses, social workers, and volunteers (often cancer patients themselves). Because the care of a patient with cancer involves so many disciplines, communication between the various specialists is extremely important.

Recent advances in cancer include the development of new drugs with greater anti-tumor activity, novel approaches to the delivery of standard anti-tumor agents, changes in the way surgery, radiation, and chemotherapy are used and combined, the use of biologic response modifiers, discoveries in molecular biology, and new approaches to pain management and the care of terminally-ill patients. Perhaps the most important advances to come are better strategies to prevent cancer.

General Concepts

Most cancers (85%) are related to tobacco use or dietary factors. Tobacco is associated with cancers of the lung (the number one killer in both men and women), mouth, pharynx, larynx, esophagus, bladder, and pancreas. Alcohol contributes to cancers of the mouth, pharynx, larynx, esophagus, and liver, while diets high in fat and total calories are associated with cancers of the breast, colon, endometrium, and prostate. High fiber diets, in contrast, appear to reduce the risk of colon cancer. Environment carcinogens such as radiation and asbestos contribute to only 5% of cancers; the best cancer prevention strategy, therefore, is to eliminate the use of tobacco and to improve dietary habits.

Oncogenesis

The identification of oncogenes and tumor suppressor genes has improved understanding of the events leading to the abnormal proliferation of the cancer cell (**oncogenesis**). **Oncogenes** are DNA sequences present in normal cells that generally code for growth factors and receptors responsible for controlling the various stages of the cell cycle; minor abnormalities in the sequence of inappropriate activation can cause uncontrolled growth and malignant transformation. Because oncogenes act in a dominant fashion, only one abnormal allele is required to produce abnormalities of the cell cycle. **Tumor suppressor genes**, also usually present in normal cells, act to prevent tumor cell growth and proliferation; even one normal allele protects the host. Mutations in both oncogenes and tumor suppressor genes can lead to cancer. Multiple abnormalities in the control of cell proliferation over the lifetime of the host are required for the development of cancer; one-to-one correlations between specific oncogenes and corresponding tumors have not yet been discovered.

Screening

Screening is the detection of a problem in an asymptomatic patient. **Cancer screening** is a hotly debated, broad, politically-charged, and controversial topic, and different physician, patient, and political groups advocate or reject different screening methods with varying amounts of data to support their relative positions. In order for a screening test to be useful, several features must apply to the disease and screening test in question. The disease should be a major public health problem and should have a recognizable, asymptomatic phase. The screening test should be sensitive, specific, and reasonably predictive. Potential for cure should be improved by detection at an early stage, and treatment of patients should improve overall outcome. Finally, the screening method should be safe, i.e., **overall** morbidity and mortality should be reduced. In addition, from a purely economic standpoint, it should result in lower overall cost. Breast, cervical, and colon cancers are the only cancers for which screening has been shown to meet these criteria. Prostate cancer can be detected early in asymptomatic patients, but it has not yet been proved that early detection leads to improved overall survival, and routine chest x-rays (CXR) in smokers have likewise not been proved beneficial. Screening tests in high-risk patients are expected to have higher yield, and thus are generally performed earlier and/or more frequently.

Recommended screening strategies include **mammography** every 1-2 years for women between 40-49, with annual mammography after age 50; a baseline mammogram is performed between the ages of 35-39. Screening for cervical cancer by means of the **Papanicolaou (Pap) smear** (see Chapter 66, "Gynecologic Malignancies") is highly effective, and has almost eliminated cervical cancer among compliant women. Annual **stool testing for occult blood** and **sigmoidoscopy** every 3-5 years after age 50 is recommended to screen for colon cancer (see Chapter 32, "Colon and Rectum").

The words used to describe cancers are often, but not always, helpful in defining tumor behavior. For example, the term "aggressive" is used to describe a rapidly growing, early metastasizing tumor, while "indolent" means the opposite. Aggressive tumors can be highly treatable, however, and indolent tumors can be extremely refractory to treatment. Tumor behavior can also change over the lifetime of the patient; it is not uncommon for a slowly growing tumor to transform to a more aggressive type, manifest by the sudden development of widespread metastases or rapid growth at the primary site, and initially responsive cancers can develop resistance to chemotherapeutic drugs or radiation.

Metastatic cancer

Cancers can progress by both local invasion and by metastatic spread; a series of elaborate events must occur in order for a given tumor to **metastasize** (not all tumors have the same metastatic potential). After initiation of growth, tumors must develop their own blood supply in order to enlarge beyond 1-2cm or so, usually by the elaboration of angiogenesis factors. Malignant cells then break free from the primary and enter the circulation, facilitated by the production of enzymes that degrade the basement membrane and connective tissue and allow penetration. After entering the lymphatic system or bloodstream, cells must escape the body's own, highly efficient nonspecific scavenger and tumor surveillance systems. The few cells that remain at this point attach to subendothelium or capillary basement membrane by means of surface adhesion molecules. Proliferation and growth of the metastatic cells, with invasion at the site of metastasis, can then occur. In relation to the number of cells that detach from the primary, metastasis is actually a very rare event.

Either primary or metastatic tumors can kill the patient by local compression of vital organs, by organ failure due to replacement by tumor, by producing metabolic derangements such as hypoxia, acidosis, or hypercalcemia, and by causing the syndrome of **cancer cachexia**; most cancer deaths are due to metastatic spread. Cancer therapy itself also causes significant morbidity; most often, it is not possible to pinpoint the exact cause of death.

Principles of Cancer Diagnosis

Although the nonspecific symptoms of cancer such as weight loss are familiar to most people, symptoms and signs of each tumor will differ, and evaluation of each patient depends on the specific complaints and physical findings. A **tissue diagnosis** is almost always necessary for optimal workup, staging, treatment planning, and determination of prognosis. **Cytology** refers to the examination of individual cells, while **histology** is the examination of anatomically-complete tissue. Cytology can be very accurate for certain tumors (e.g., cervical), but usually a histologic sample is more accurate, because tumors are best characterized by their interaction with surrounding cells and "organs" such as blood vessels. The tumor focus most easily accessible with the lowest possible procedural risk should be used to obtain the sample. In addition to palpable masses or masses found on radiographic studies, palpable lymph nodes, peritoneal and pleural fluid, sputum, and bone marrow are useful (small inguinal lymph nodes are notoriously negative – "reactive hyperplasia only"). Serum tumor markers add useful information, although have not yet been shown to be valuable as screening tests. Always review the pathologic specimen with your own eyes (with a pathologist, if necessary), and have a general sense of the reliability of your laboratory.

Treatment before tissue diagnosis is rarely justified and generally is considered only in emergency situations, when delay would endanger the patient, or when suspicion is high and diagnosis may be difficult and/or risky .

Staging

Cancer staging is done to define the extent of disease, a necessary step in determining treatment and prognosis. Staging can be **clinical**, based on history, physical, laboratory, and radiologic data, or **pathologic (surgical)**, based on definitive histology. Both are useful, and which is more "accurate" depends on the criteria used to define treatment and prognosis for various therapies.

Cancer staging systems vary for each type of tumor. Several generalizations apply. **Stage 1** generally refers to small tumors confined within the anatomic boundaries of the affected tissue or organ; lymph nodes are usually not involved. **Stage 2** usually denotes a larger tumor, deeper invasion of the tumor, or regional lymph node involvement. **Stage 3** generally denotes extensive local invasion or a significant degree of lymph node involvement, and **stage 4** almost always denotes metastatic disease. Most tumors are now being staged with variations of the American Cancer Society's **TNM system**, with the status of the **tumor (T)**, **lymph nodes (N)**, and **metastases (M)** scored, and the results combined to yield the overall stage.

Along with staging of the cancer itself, an assessment of the patient's **performance status** is also important. Patients who are able to carry out activities of daily living with minimal burden imposed by the cancer are assigned a more favorable performance status than those who are dependent on others or significantly debilitated. In general, patients with a better performance status derive greater benefit from chemotherapy; many therapeutic trials include only patients who remain functional.

Principles of Cancer Treatment

Cancer can be treated by means of **surgery**, **radiation therapy**, **chemotherapy**, or **biologic therapy**. Surgery and radiation therapy are **local** treatments, while chemo- and biologic therapy are **systemic** treatments.

Surgical therapy

Operation for cancer is performed both for staging and to remove as much tumor as possible. Operation can be performed for **cure**, that is, resection undertaken with the goal of removing all cancer-bearing cells, or for **palliation**. Even if the tumor cannot be entirely removed from the body, in many instances the benefit of removing some tumor far outweighs the risks and discomfort of the operation itself (removing an obstructing bowel tumor even when known metastatic disease is present). In some cases removal of as much disease as possible (**debulking**) allows better chance of cure with adjuvant therapy, even if some tumor remains at the time of surgery (ovarian cancer). In some situations, resection of a single or several metastatic lesions is likely to prolong survival (isolated hepatic metastasis from colon cancer). Finally, several nonresective but essential procedures are needed by many cancer patients, most often for long-term venous access.

Radiotherapy

Radiation causes cell death by producing short-lived free radicals that injure the cells' DNA; radiation also interferes with cellular growth factors and cell-cycle regulation. For maximal free-radical formation, molecular oxygen is required; local hypoxia thus reduces the efficacy of radiation. Radiation is **not** specific for cancerous cells, rather, specific for **rapidly growing** cells. Thus, populations such as intestinal endothelium are also damaged, and the beam must be very carefully directed to exclude as much normal tissue as possible.

Approximately 50% of patients with cancer require radiation therapy at some point during their treatment course. Radiation therapy can be used as either the lone therapeutic modality or in combination with other treatment. Radiation therapy is most commonly used **after operation** for cancers of the head and neck, lung, breast, bladder, rectum, soft tissues, and bone, **in conjunction with chemotherapy** for lymphomas, lung cancer, and childhood malignancies, and for **palliation** of pain from metastases to bone, intracranial hypertension from brain lesions, obstruction from compression of vital organs, or fracture of weight-bearing bones from pathologic metastatic lesions. Radiation therapy is also given **before operation** to "downstage" the tumor and improve respectability for certain cancers. **Brachytherapy** is radiation delivered locally by instillation of a radiation source close to the site of the tumor, and has been used successfully in the treatment of cancers of the oral cavity, uterine cervix, prostate, lung, and brain.

The most important part of radiation therapy is treatment planning. The targeted tumor volume, choice of the treatment unit, design of the pattern of dose delivery, and the dose and time of the treatments must all be chosen before therapy begins. Careful consideration is given to all tissues in the treatment field in order to minimize toxicity. Certain tissues are extremely sensitive to radiation; the risk of damage eliminates the use of radiation in some parts of the body.

Chemotherapy

Chemotherapy, as opposed to surgery and radiation therapy, is a **systemic** treatment. Chemotherapy is given to patients who have cancer that is incurable by surgery and radiation alone. **Adjuvant** (postsurgical) **chemotherapy** is given to patients with a high risk of relapse after operation; classic examples of the use of adjuvant chemotherapy are breast cancer after mastectomy, colon cancer after tumor resection, ovarian cancer after debulking, and osteosarcoma. Chemotherapy is started as soon as the patient recovers from surgery and is given in maximally-tolerated doses for periods ranging from 4-12 months, depending on the type of cancer. **Neoadjuvant chemotherapy** is given **before** surgery with the goal of improving respectability and long-term survival; chemotherapy given before surgery can also provide information as to the responsiveness of the tumor to commonly used chemotherapeutic agents. Osteosarcomas, bladder cancer, anal cancer, esophageal cancer, and locally advanced breast cancer have all been effectively treated with neoadjuvant therapy. Some tumors are treated for attempted cure with chemotherapy alone, including Hodgkin's lymphoma, testicular carcinoma, and choriocarcinoma. Chemotherapy is most commonly used for **treatment of advanced disease**, either nonresectable local disease or metastases; the goal is improved survival and/or palliation of symptoms.

Most chemotherapeutic drugs damage cells by inhibiting the synthesis of DNA, damaging DNA already synthesized, or interfering with DNA repair; other targets of chemotherapy are RNA and microtubules. Again, chemotherapy is not specific to cancerous cells, but kills any rapidly growing cell (such as hair follicles and intestinal endothelium). Most cancers are treated with a combination of drugs with different actions (**combination chemotherapy**) in order to circumvent drug resistance and avoid or minimize overlapping toxicity. In general, maximally-tolerated doses are used, but most drugs have specific side effects that limit their use (the recent use of growth factors to "rescue" the bone marrow has allowed administration of greater doses of myelosuppressive drugs). Although nausea, diarrhea, mucositis, and hair loss are troublesome, they are usually tolerable and reversible. Renal, hepatic, nervous system, pulmonary, and cardiac toxicities, on the other hand, may be irreversible, and, if present, mandate dose

reduction. Most of these side effects are related to the
cumulative dose over time.

**Biologic
therapy**

Biologic or **immunotherapy** refers to techniques of augmenting the host's own anti-tumor immunologic defenses
by the administration of such immunologically active substances as interferons and interleukins, as well as to the
use of experimental therapies such as lymphokine activated killer (LAK) cells, tumor infiltrating lymphocytes
(TIL), monoclonal antibodies, and tumor vaccines (see
Chapter 10, "Immunology"). Most of these approaches
are in the early stages of development and do not represent standard care. Interferons are routinely used for the
treatment of chronic myeloid leukemia, renal cell carcinoma, and melanoma, while interleukin-2 is used in the
treatment of renal cell carcinoma and melanoma.

Supportive Care of the Cancer Patient

The emotional stress that cancer imposes on the patient,
family, and friends is tremendous. In addition to facing
the real possibility of death, patients fear that they will be
in pain, that they will be alone, and that they will die
away from their familiar environment. Often the most
helpful action for a patient with cancer, particularly
immediately after the diagnosis is determined, is to take
no action at all. Reassurance, compassion, and listening
are tremendously comforting. Nurses, social workers,
pastoral workers, and cancer volunteers are invaluable in
supporting the patient in this situation. Patients may have
difficulties bringing up concerns about financial matters,
sexuality, end-of-life issues, and self-image; discussion
and answers can be facilitated if the physician approaches
such subjects first. A phenomenon to remember is that a
patient will hear little of what you have to say after you
tell them they have cancer; be prepared to go over the
entire discussion again at another sitting.

Pain control

**In the vast majority of patients with cancer, adequate
pain control can be achieved quickly and consistently.**
There are, however, numerous obstacles to adequate pain
management in patients with cancer. Differing expectations between care providers and patients, poor communication, fear of "addiction" (by both the patient and physician), hesitancy on the part of the care providers to use
increasing doses of pain medications, adverse effects, and

cost are just a few of the factors interfering with pain control. A careful history is crucial to determine type and severity of pain, alleviating and exacerbating qualities, and the efficacy of the current pain management regimen. **Somatic** or **cutaneous pain**, usually well-localized, is due to activation of nociceptors in the skin and deep tissues, and responds to conventional non-steroidal anti-inflammatory agents or narcotic analgesics. **Visceral pain** is due to distension or irritation of deep, autonomically-innervated structures (see Chapter 25, "Abdominal Pain") and is usually dull or colicky; visceral pain responds to treatment with narcotic analgesics and antinausea medications. **Neuropathic pain**, the result of neural compression, infiltration, or injury, is described as excruciating, "burning," or "sharp," and is often associated with skeletal muscle pain and autonomic responses. Neuropathic pain often responds to tricyclic antidepressants and anti-convulsants. Side effects should be treated aggressively to avoid constipation, gastrointestinal bleeding, and dehydration caused by nausea. Nausea and sedation are often transient and may improve with development of tolerance (see also Chapter 12, "Anesthesiology and Pain Management").

Palliative Care

In addition to pain management, patients dying from cancer need close attention to problems affecting comfort such as nausea, constipation, anorexia, bowel obstruction, dyspnea, restlessness, and skin care. **Hospice care** provides comfort measures to patients dying of cancer. Because medical training most often teaches us to "do something," many physicians have difficulty adjusting to the idea of not aggressively "working up" new and chronic problems. Preserving the comfort of the dying patient is an active process that requires expertise and skill on the part of physicians and the entire team caring for the patient.

Many services exist for patients who have family and friends to help in their care at home. Most patients, as long as they have a reliable support person, can spend most (if not all) of their last days at home. Patients can be admitted to inpatient hospice units for improvement in pain control or for a respite for the patient's family and friends. ■

12   Anesthesiology and Pain Management

Anesthesiologists traditionally were involved in the intraoperative care of patients only, having little other contact outside the operating room. Modern anesthesiologists have branched out, however, and created a field that involves patient care during the entire perioperative period, including preoperative evaluation and preparation of patients for surgery, intraoperative care, and postoperative management of pain and other pathologic conditions. Intensive care medicine and the management of chronic pain are also significant components of modern anesthesiology.

Preoperative Preparation

Inpatients are prepared for surgery in the hospital, where they are seen by the surgeon, anesthesiologist, and any other consulting physicians necessary. Laboratory tests, preoperative teaching, and any other preparatory procedures are all done after admission (see Chapter 26, "Preoperative Care"). A large percentage of procedures, however, are now done on an outpatient or **ambulatory** basis. These patients require thorough preoperative preparation **before** they arrive at the hospital to ensure that they are ready for the OR and to avoid last-minute cancellations. Anesthesiologists are becoming increasingly involved in this preoperative evaluation and preparation and are now beginning to manage specific **preoperative clinics** for this purpose.

Preoperative evaluation

The first step in preparing a patient for the OR is a thorough **history** and **physical exam**. Based on the history, physical, and proposed operation, the anesthesiologist may order **preoperative tests**. Tests should be ordered only to gain information or answer questions that will significantly impact the patient's intraoperative or postoperative course; routine "shotgun" testing has not been shown to be of any benefit. The anesthesiologist also helps ensure that patients' **preoperative medical conditions** are under optimal control. Chronic conditions are reviewed with the patient and their primary physician to confirm that no further medical management is necessary. It is not expected that every patient will be "cured" before coming to the operating room, but their medical problems should be addressed and treated.

The **preoperative visit** also offers the opportunity to answer patients' questions and relieve anxiety; a thoughtful preoperative visit is at least as calming to a patient as is pharmacologic premedication. The preoperative visit is particularly useful in discussing the anesthetic plan and perioperative course of events with parents of small children.

Intraoperative Management

The anesthesiologist's responsibilities in the operating room include the provision of anesthesia or sedation, physiologic monitoring, and management of the patient's normal and abnormal physiology. In addition, the anesthesiologist manages perioperative intravenous fluids and blood and blood product transfusions.

Monitoring

Before the patient is anesthetized, **physiologic monitors** are applied. A noninvasive blood pressure monitor, EKG leads, pulse oximeter, and precordial or esophageal stethoscope are required for every patient. **Capnography** (measurement of expired CO_2) is used during general anesthesia. Additional monitoring devices, including an intraarterial blood pressure monitor, central venous or pulmonary artery catheter, transesophageal echocardiogram, nerve stimulator, or Foley catheter, are also used depending on the patient's preexisting medical condition, the anesthetic technique, and the extent of surgery planned.

Noninvasive blood pressure monitors are usually automated to free up the anesthesiologist to perform other tasks. Such monitors work by detecting arterial pressure changes within the cuff; mean arterial pressure is directly measured and systolic and diastolic pressures calculated. **Electrocardiography** is essential to monitor heart rate and rhythm; computerized analysis of the ST segments is now used routinely to provide early evidence of myocardial ischemia in "real time." The **pulse oximeter** measures oxygen content of the blood. Red and infrared light are transmitted through a tissue bed; oxygenated and deoxygenated hemoglobin absorb different amounts of these wavelengths, and the ratio of absorbances is used to calculate oxygen saturation.

Induction

During **general anesthesia**, the patient is rendered unconscious. General anesthesia involves three phases: induction, maintenance, and emergence. During **induction**, the patient is taken from a conscious to an unconscious state. Induction can be accomplished using intravenous (preferred in adults) or inhaled anesthetics (usually used in infants and children); IV induction agents commonly used include the barbiturates (thiopental, methohexital), propofol, etomidate, and ketamine. The anesthesiologist chooses the appropriate drug for each patient based on the patient's medical conditions and the drug's pharmacokinetic and pharmacodynamic properties. The endotracheal tube, if used, is usually inserted just after induction.

Maintenance

During the **maintenance phase** of general anesthesia between induction and emergence, a "steady state" of anesthesia is maintained using inhaled or intravenous anesthetics (or a combination of the two). Common inhaled agents include nitrous oxide, isoflurane, halothane, sevoflurane and desflurane; each has unique properties that are considered when a choice is made. Intravenous agents used for maintenance include a variety of opioids (Demerol, morphine, fentanyl, sufentanil, alfentanil), propofol, ketamine, or barbiturates; each can be given as a bolus injection or as a continuous infusion. Muscle relaxants are sometimes used during the maintenance phase to ensure relaxation, especially during abdominal operations.

Emergence

During **emergence** from general anesthesia the patient "wakes up," emerging from the unconscious to the conscious state. Maintenance of a patent airway and hemodynamic stability as the patient surfaces from general anesthesia are the most important considerations at this point. Timing of specific drug pharmacokinetic activity or pharmacologic reversal of previously administered drugs is crucial and often makes the difference between a smooth or stormy awakening.

Airway

When a patient is given a general anesthetic, **management of the airway** is a vital job of the anesthesiologist. The anesthesiologist performs a careful evaluation of the airway and develops a plan for management. This plan includes whether or not to use pharmacologic agents, preoxygenation (always), and the choice of which tools are to be used to ventilate the patient: patient positioning, ambubag/circle system, mask, oral and nasal airways, laryngeal mask, and endotracheal tubes are all options (see also Chapter 1, "Airway and Ventilator Management"). Airway manipulation is usually performed after the patient is anesthetized and paralyzed during induction, although intubation can be performed with the patient awake. A "**difficult airway**," by definition, poses a particularly challenging problem. If recognized prior to anesthetic administration, it can be handled in a planned, organized, and controlled fashion, but a difficult airway that is not discovered until after induction can result in a potentially fatal situation. **Airway evaluation** involves noting the degree of mouth opening and cervical spine mobility, visualization of the pharyngeal structures, measurement of the thyromental distance, and observation of any airway pathology.

Major conduction anesthesia

An alternative to general anesthesia is **major conduction anesthesia** (spinal or epidural anesthesia), which can be used alone, with sedation, or in conjunction with general anesthesia. **Spinal anesthesia** involves injecting concentrated local anesthetic into the subarachnoid space in order to provide a quick and complete blockade of the spinal nerves, while **epidural anesthesia** involves injecting dilute local anesthetic into the epidural space as a bolus or continuous infusion. Spinal anesthesia produces a total motor and sensory block, while epidural anesthesia produces a disproportionate sensory block; epidural techniques are relatively easier to apply in a continuous fashion. Major conduction blockade with either technique carries with it two types of **complications**: those produced during placement of the needle, and those resulting from blockade of the sympathetic nervous system. Bleeding, infection, epidural hematoma, nerve injury, and intraarterial injection are rare complications of injecting local anesthetic into the subarachnoid or epidural space. Sympathetic nervous system blockade always occurs, and if the level of the block is high enough (T_1-T_4), widespread vasodilation and bradycardia can occur. Depending on the degree of preoperative hydration and presence of preexisting cardiac disease, this can significantly decrease cardiac output and blood pressure. Major

Multidisciplinary
Anesthesiology and Pain Management
continued

conduction anesthesia requires the same monitoring and vigilance as does general anesthesia – even for minor procedures, patient outcome is not significantly different whether general or major conduction anesthesia is used. Local or regional **nerve blocks** can also be used for surgical anesthesia and the treatment of acute and chronic pain.

MAC

Even if local anesthetics are injected into the surgical site by the surgeon, **monitored anesthesia care** (**MAC**), the provision of sedation and continuous monitoring throughout the perioperative period, often makes the operation much easier. Sedation can range from minimal to a "near-general anesthesia" state. The anesthesiologist is "responsible" for sedation and monitoring, the surgeon, for local anesthesia and the procedure itself.

Postoperative Care

After the patient emerges from anesthesia, the anesthesiologist must ensure that the residual, life-threatening effects of the drugs used (i.e., general anesthetics, muscle relaxants, and opioids) have worn off. Adequacy of oxygenation and ventilation should be assured, and vital signs are followed closely in the post-anesthesia care unit (PACU or recovery room). Pain is treated, and medical conditions that existed preoperatively or those (such as hypothermia, dysrhythmias, or fluid imbalances) acquired intraoperatively are treated and corrected, if possible. When the patient's condition is stable, they can go to a regular hospital bed or be prepared for discharge home, if applicable.

Outside the Operating Room

Anesthesiologists assist with patient care throughout the hospital. Probably the busiest place anesthesiologists work outside the OR is the **obstetric suite**, where they are intimately involved in anesthesia and analgesia for labor and delivery, particularly by providing epidural analgesia for laboring mothers and anesthesia for Caesarean sections. The physiologic changes associated with pregnancy and pathologic conditions specific to the pregnant state create particular challenges. Regional anesthesia is preferred in the obstetric arena because most pregnant patients want to be awake for delivery and because they have a higher incidence of difficult airways, gastroesophageal reflux, and aspiration. The **radiology** and **gastroenterology suites**, **pediatrics ward**, and **burn/trauma units** are sites outside the operating room where anesthesiologists provide sedation, monitored care, or full general anesthesia. The provision of brief general anesthesia for **electroconvulsive therapy** takes place in the operating room or in a psychiatric treatment room.

In most hospitals, anesthesiologists are involved in **emergent airway management** during code situations or trauma (see Chapter 1, "Airway and Ventilator Management"). It is particularly important not to get into a "cannot intubate, cannot ventilate" situation; if a patient appears to have a difficult airway, securing the airway **before** rendering the patient unconscious and apneic is vital. Anesthesiologists are also involved in the management of patients requiring **intensive care**, along with internal medicine and surgical ICU specialists.

Acute and Chronic Pain

Because of expertise in regional anesthetic techniques and knowledge of the pharmacokinetics and dynamics of analgesic medications, anesthesiologists have taken a leadership role in the development of pain management as a specialty. **Pain management** is a relatively new field that attempts to overcome problems in the traditional approach to managing pain. Approximately 50% of surgical and medical patients, including children, report moderate or severe pain at some time during their hospital stay. Why is **inadequate pain control** such a widespread problem? Several reasons exist. Pain management is often not seen as a priority, and is delegated to the most inexperienced staff member (e.g., the intern). Unfounded fears of addiction and side effects (especially respiratory depression) often result in underdosage of medications. The task of adequately measuring pain is difficult and subjective, and there is wide variability in requirements for pain medication.

Pain Physiology   Pain is defined as an unpleasant sensory and emotional experience associated with actual or potential tissue damage, and is the final product of a combination of electrophysiologic events at the level of the neuron (collectively labeled as **nociception**) and the subjective and emotional

Multidisciplinary Anesthesiology and Pain Management

continued

experiences of the individual. Pain is created by several physiologic processes including **transduction**, where noxious stimuli are translated into electrical activity at the nerve endings, **transmission**, when impulses carrying nociceptive information are propagated to the central nervous system, **modulation**, whereby exogenous (narcotics) and endogenous (endorphins) analgesic agents modify nociceptive transmission, and **perception**, as transduction, transmission, and modulation all interact with the subjective experiences and emotional state of the individual to produce the final sensation. Unlike conditions for which diagnostic tests are readily available, there is no objective "test" to determine a patient's level of pain. Pain is usually quantified by **self-report rating scales** that seem to be reliable and reproducible over time.

Details about the pain should be elicited, including location, intensity, frequency and pattern (continuous or intermittent), quality, and aggravating and alleviating factors. Physical exam focuses on the pain and the physiologic responses to it; in most cases, for example, acute, postoperative pain results in increased sympathetic outflow causing tachycardia, hypertension, and tachypnea. Inspection can reveal an obvious cause of the pain such as a wound infection or ischemic tissue. Palpation of the site and surrounding areas should be the last maneuver performed; reproducibility and localization of the pain are two important pieces of data obtainable from palpation.

PCA

Treatment of **acute postoperative pain** is the most common pain control issue encountered in the hospital. Traditional scheduled parenteral opioid administration (i.e., Demerol 75mg IM q 3 hours) commonly results in insufficient analgesia or excessive side effects because of wide interpatient variability, delays in administration, and underestimation of dosage required. **Patient controlled analgesia** (**PCA**) allows constant intravenous or epidural delivery of an analgesic drug (usually an opioid), and allows the patient to control the amount of drug administered via a push-button control. If the patient does not feel pain or is overmedicated and sleepy, the push-button is not pressed and no medication is delivered, thus theoretically preventing overdosage. Decreased cumulative drug dose and greater patient satisfaction have been repeatedly demonstrated using PCA.

Tolerance and addiction

There is an unfounded belief that psychologic addiction (see Chapter 80, "Substance Abuse") can ensue when opioids are administered for the treatment of pain. In fact, less than 0.02% of patients with no prior history of substance abuse develop problems with opioid drugs after therapeutic opioid administration. **Tolerance** (increasing doses are required to produce the same effect) is a **pharmacologic** property of opioids and should be expected, while **physical dependence** is a **physiologic** property characterized by a withdrawal syndrome on abrupt discontinuation of the drug. Neither tolerance nor physical dependence is synonymous with **addiction**, which is a **psychic** state characterized by compulsive behavior to obtain the drug to experience its psychic effects.

Because of the recognition of the importance of pain control in patient care, the US Department of Health and Human Services has published a set of clinical practice guidelines titled "Acute Pain Management: Operative or Medical Procedures and Trauma", available at no charge to health professionals through the Agency for Health Care Policy and Research Clearinghouse at 1-800-358-9295. ∎

Medicine

Jennifer J Griggs
Section Editor

13   Basic ACLS (or, 'Where do I Stand During a Code?')

In-hospital "codes," the attempted resuscitation of dying patients, provide some of the most challenging situations for physicians. Despite what is suggested on television or in the movies, codes consist of much more than placing defibrillator paddles on a patient's chest and shouting "clear!" Codes are complex situations requiring preparation, organization, and clear thinking; it is the presence or absence of teamwork that often determines outcome.

The American Heart Association publishes a set of protocols for resuscitation and stabilization of patients with acutely abnormal cardiac function. Most recently updated in 1994, **advanced cardiac life support (ACLS)** is widely used to resuscitate patients with cardiac problems that occur while hospitalized, and is formally taught to essentially every internist and primary care physician early in their training. **This chapter is directed at the student or health care provider who has not yet taken the formal ACLS course**.

There is no Substitute for Memory

Even the most well-run code situations can be extremely chaotic. While debate and discussion often occur, a code is not the time to have to look things up, thus, **the specific ACLS protocols need to be committed to memory**. Once the steps of therapy are memorized, the fast-paced and often subtle changes in the patient's status can be anticipated and responded to more efficiently.

Keep a Cool Head

An old aphorism says, "in a code situation, **the first pulse to take is your own**." While there is a certain safety in numbers, it may happen that you are one of the first to arrive on the scene. There are several things that can be done by a student in the first few moments that make a huge difference down the line. First, confirm the vital signs. Is there a pulse? Are there spontaneous respirations? A measurable blood pressure? Next, place a back board under the patient, and start CPR if there is no cardiac activity (see below for a discussion of the issue of airway vs. CPR).

If there is someone already tending to the patient, make sure the crash cart and defibrillator are brought into the room. Locate the chart, determine the patient's diagnosis and primary physician, and find the latest progress note and medication list. Patients are often strangers to the code team; discovering what has been going on during the hospitalization is often very helpful in deciphering the situation.

Who's Running the Show?

There may quickly be many people tending to the patient. **Every code or emergency situation must have one and only one leader**. The leader of the code team, usually a senior resident, should make it clear who is in charge of the situation. If present, often the senior resident with primary responsibility for the patient, even if not on the code team, will be in charge, especially if the patient is on a non-medical service, but this responsibility may frequently be ceded to the code team depending on the specific situation, cause of the arrest, and training of those involved. Rapid communication and a quick decision are vital.

Location is Everything

While there is just so much space that can be taken up by physicians, nurses, respiratory therapists, and equipment, learning during a code, the student's priority, is greatly enhanced if within arm's length of the patient. Obviously, if performing a specific task, your place at the bedside is unquestioned.

For a student, excellent ways to help the victim as well as appreciate the events is to perform chest compressions or ventilate the patient, usually with the help of the respiratory therapist. If you are not helping, find an area where you can watch the cardiac monitor without obstructing the view of those running the code.

Although the room can become crowded very quickly, **there is no substitute for witnessing an actual code sit-**

uation. A professional attitude and awareness of the fast-paced action will allow you to remain close enough to learn from the situation.

Code "Etiquette"

In addition to performing chest compressions and ventilating the patient, there are many other ways to assist. Often the physician-in-charge will ask for a specific task. While some jobs (e.g., obtaining central access) may be inappropriate for a beginning student, most are well within your level of training. Obtaining an arterial blood gas or venous blood sample, placing an IV, or monitoring vital signs are some of the things you can do to stay helpful and involved.

This is certainly the time and place for a moderate degree of aggressiveness, especially if you want hands-on experience, although if in doubt, back off. **Patient care and outcome always take priority**, and it should be no blow to your confidence or esteem if your participation is declined. **This is not the time for turf battles** (at your or any other level); never try to perform any job that makes you feel uncomfortable or for which you have not been appropriately trained.

A Word About Electricity

Cardioversion is the application of current to the heart of a patient with an arrhythmia in an attempt to cause global myocardial depolarization and allow normal pacemakers to take over. Cardioversion can be **synchronized** to the EKG, which is safer because it avoids precipitating ventricular fibrillation due to application of energy during the T-wave, or **asynchronized**; cardioversion in a patient with a ventricular arrhythmia or asystole is, by definition, asynchronized. **Defibrillation** is the term usually used to denote asynchronous cardioversion in a patient with a malignant ventricular arrhythmia, although it does not differ, in theory, from cardioversion. Although both techniques are best approached by starting with a low level of current and moving upward until an effect is seen, defibrillation is usually performed with a higher level initially because there is less time to "waste." Much of the current during cardioversion is expended in the tissues of the chest wall; if the heart is exposed (by a thoracotomy or in the operating room), much less power is needed.

The application of synchronized cardioversion can be very confusing to the neophyte, because the paddles will not "fire" when the button is depressed. Pressure on the chest with the buttons pressed must be maintained for a second or two in this situation to allow the machine to "find" a suitable point in the cardiac cycle to fire.

Basic Principles and Protocols

The following are **highly simplified** protocols for resuscitation of patients with cardiac problems. Several points should be noted. First, **these are not meant to take the place of the full ACLS protocols, but are meant to provide a conceptual framework for understanding treatment**. Second, although the overall concepts are universally applicable, they apply only to patients with cardiac problems, not to patients with traumatic injuries (see Chapter 28, "Trauma"). Third, traditional teaching is that supply of oxygen to the lungs always takes first priority – providing blood to the tissues does no good if it doesn't have any oxygen in it. This means that providing oxygen and an artificial airway, if necessary (see Chapter 1, "Airway and Ventilator Management") take priority over chest compressions **if only one person is available to do both tasks**. Usually, however, especially in the hospital setting, both can be done simultaneously. There is some evidence that high-flow oxygen alone can temporarily sustain tissue oxygen delivery during CPR; thus, the most realistic strategy for a **lone, inexperienced rescuer** is to call for help, open the airway, administer high-flow oxygen, and start CPR; the ongoing priority, while awaiting help, is to continue chest compressions. Fourth, if no pulse is present (and oxygen is being delivered to the lungs), CPR should begin immediately in an attempt to get some blood to the tissues. Because certain arrhythmias have a very short "window of opportunity" within which they can be successfully defibrillated, determination of the specific arrhythmia may be critical. A student (not performing CPR) can rapidly attach the chest leads of the defibrillator, pending arrival of the code team, and thus be of significant help.

(continued)

Medicine
Basic ACLS *continued*

The initial distinction in any acutely ill patient is whether or not they have a pulse or blood pressure. Although patients without cardiac activity will be unconscious because their brain is not receiving oxygen, **unconsciousness can be caused by multiple factors and is not an indication that the patient needs CPR:**

Figure 13.1
Initial triage of dysrhythmias, unconsciousness, and other potential cardiac problems.

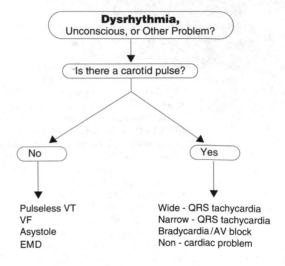

A more complete discussion of the pathophysiology of the various arrhythmias presented below follows in Chapter 14, "Cardiac Dysrhythmias."

Ventricular Fibrillation (VF) and Pulseless Ventricular Tachycardia (VT)

These arrhythmias do not perfuse the brain, coronary arteries, or remainder of the body, thus, they are not compatible with life and are therefore extreme emergencies.

Action must be prompt for survival. By definition, there is no palpable pulse or blood pressure; the patient will be unresponsive:

Figure 13.2
Simplified protocol for management of ventricular fibrillation and pulseless (i.e., no cardiac output) ventricular tachycardia.

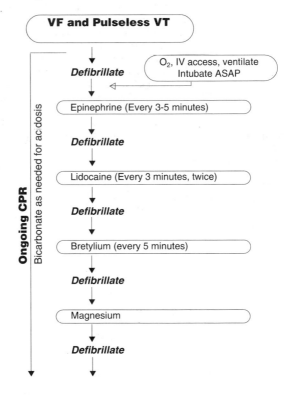

Survival from VF or VT demands rapid, early electrical countershock. As soon as a monitor-defibrillator is available, CPR should be interrupted so that "quick look" paddles can be applied to the chest to determine the rhythm. If VF or VT is confirmed, immediate defibrillation with 200 Joules is recommended. You will hear the order to "check for a pulse" after each defibrillation.
If you are within arm's length of the carotid, radial or femoral artery, palpate and report your findings. If you feel a pulse, the heart is beating and the tissues are being perfused.
(continued)

Medicine
Basic ACLS *continued*

Asystole

Again, this "arrhythmia" results in absent perfusion, and intervention must be immediate. Again, the patient will be unconscious without obtainable pulse or blood pressure. Prognosis for patients with aystole is poor. The patient often has end-stage cardiac function or has had a prolonged arrest with prolonged cerebral hypoxia. Because of the poor prognosis and the possibility that VF can masquerade as asystole, the diagnosis should be confirmed in at least two leads.

Figure 13.3
Simplified protocol for management of asystole and electromechanical dissociation.

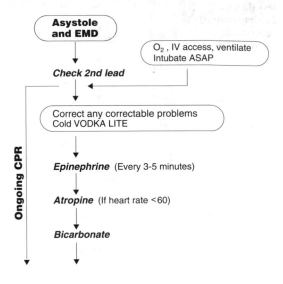

Electromechanical Dissociation (EMD)

EMD is the condition where the heart has electrical activity on the monitor but does not "beat" in a mechanical sense. No perfusion is taking place; blood pressure and pulse will be absent, and the patient unconscious. **EMD can be caused by curable problems such as a tension pneumothorax or cardiac tamponade** (see Chapters 28, "Trauma." and 5, "Shock").

Prognosis for patients with EMD is very poor unless an underlying cause can be identified and corrected. A good way to remember the most common causes is with the mnemonic Cold VODKA LITE. Cold refers to **hypothermia**. VODKA stands for **volume (hypovolemia)**, **oxygen (hypoxia)**, **drugs**, **potassium (hyperkalemia)**, and **acidosis**, and LITE for **lung (tension pneumothorax)**, **(myocardial) infarction**, **(cardiac) tamponade**, and **(pulmonary) embolism**.

Many arrhythmias do not cause cardiac arrest (see Figure 13.1). The patient can be conscious or unconscious, depending on the degree of cerebral perfusion and other medical conditions. Symptomatology can range from none – the arrhythmia is apparent only on a monitor; the absence of symptoms implying that the brain, heart, and peripheral tissues are receiving enough oxygen **for the time being** – to severe (hypotension, palpitations, sweating, chest pain, a feeling of impending doom).

Wide Complex Tachycardia with Pulse

These patients present with a range of signs and symptoms, as discussed above. If there is any doubt, **a wide complex tachycardia should be considered VT until proven otherwise**, because VT, even with a pulse, can convert to a life-threatening, pulseless arrhythmia in seconds:

Figure 13.4
Simplified protocol for management of wide-complex tachycardia with a pulse (i.e., with cardiac output).

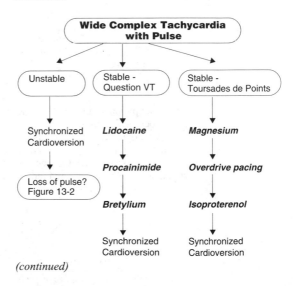

(continued)

Medicine
Basic ACLS *continued*

Cardioversion is the treatment of choice in an unstable patient. If the patient is less severely ill, time may be taken to administer sedation and to synchronize the cardioversion.

Bradycardia

Bradycardia can present with a wide range of symptoms. Again, the urgency of intervention depends on the degree of cerebral and coronary ischemia believed present:

Figure13.5
Simplified protocol for bradycardia.

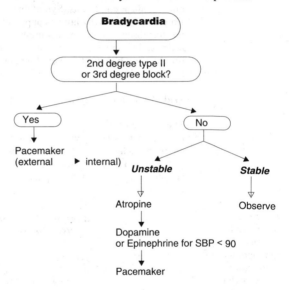

Unless the patient is in type II second degree or complete heart block, treatment is needed only if symptoms (e.g., chest pain, dyspnea, lightheadedness, hypotension, or ventricular ectopy) are present. Never use atropine in doses lower than 0.5mg at a time because such treatment can paradoxically exacerbate bradycardia.

Supraventricular Tachycardia (SVT)

Again, presentation is highly variable. SVT and its variants (including atrial fibrillation) are fairly common in hospitalized patients, and most episodes do not require a formal "code":

Figure 13.6 **Simplified protocol for narrow-complex tachycardia with a pulse.**

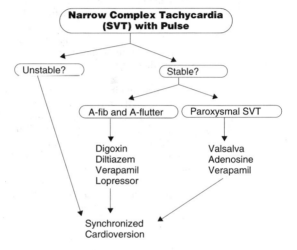

SVT requires emergency treatment when it causes cardiovascular dysfunction (e.g., hypotension) or when the tachycardia is likely to impair already tenuous myocardial blood flow (e.g., after an acute myocardial infarction). Synchronized cardioversion is the treatment of choice in unstable patients. In stable patients with SVT, vagal stimulation by means of a Valsalva maneuver can be helpful in differentiating between the various types of supraventricular tachyarrhythmias and can cause "spontaneous" conversion to sinus rhythm. Carotid massage is dangerous because of the relatively high incidence of carotid atherosclerosis; absence of a bruit is **not** an indication that disease is not present. ∎

Medicine

Cardiac Dysrhythmias

Dysrhythmia is a better term than is **arrhythmia**, which implies the complete absence of a rhythm, although both are used interchangeably. A **tachyarrhythmia** is a dysrhythmia faster than 100 beats per minute, and a **bradyarrhythmia**, one slower than 60. The history, physical examination, and electrocardiogram (ECG or EKG, used interchangeably) are the fundamental components needed for the recognition, diagnosis, and treatment of an abnormal cardiac rhythm.

A dysrhythmia is **not** synonymous with a myocardial infarction (MI). A dysrhythmia can be secondary to myocardial ischemia or an MI, but can also be caused by an electrical abnormality, mechanical stretching, electrolyte abnormalities, non-ischemic cardiac problems, or significant physiologic stress. In many cases, the cause is not known. A dysrhythmia can cause an MI, also, by increasing myocardial oxygen demand while decreasing supply. Diminished cardiac output and myocardial "stress" are the two principle reasons for treating dysrhythmias.

History

There are several important complaints to elicit when evaluating a patient with a possible dysrhythmia. **Palpitations** are one of the more common presenting symptoms. Questions designed to elicit the patient's definition of palpitations are a good way to begin. Does "palpitations" mean "my heart is beating fast" or "my heart is beating hard (pounding)?" Duration and frequency of palpitations are both crucial, as are any associated symptoms.

Both **lightheadedness** and **syncope** are caused by lack of oxygen to the brain; cardiac dysrhythmias are the underlying problem in almost a quarter of older patients who present with syncope. Dizziness or lightheadedness are usually caused by a tachyarrhythmia, whether regular or irregular. **Chest pain** in this setting is almost always due to myocardial ischemia (see Chapter 15, "Ischemic Heart Disease and Chest Pain"). **Shortness of breath** can be caused by high oxygen demand or impaired pulmonary oxygenation due to pulmonary edema. Because coronary perfusion and myocardial oxygenation occur during diastole, and increasing the heart rate decreases the time spent in diastole, tachyarrhythmias (and tachycardia in general) reduce myocardial oxygen supply as well as increase demand. **Congestive heart failure (CHF)** can be the cause or the effect of a dysrhythmia, especially in older patients or those with left ventricular failure.

Physical Exam

The **regularity** of the pulse and the **heart rate** are two critical elements of the physical examination; rate provides the most information. Cardiac dysrhythmias often have constant and characteristic rates, and whether a dysrhythmia is regular or irregular effectively eliminates many of the diagnostic possibilities right away.

Blood pressure should be specifically checked early in the evaluation; hemodynamic stability, reflecting the ability of the rhythm to perfuse both the body and the myocardium, is crucial in determining treatment. The presence and character of the first and second heart sounds, extra heart sounds, and murmurs are obviously important. Crackles, rales, or wheezes all suggest CHF, but the pulmonary exam is often normal in the presence of a dysrhythmia.

The Monitor and EKG

The ability to accurately interpret an EKG is fundamental to almost every field of medicine; each student, whether headed for medicine, surgery, pediatrics, or any other field, needs to be comfortable with this skill. Dubin's "Rapid Interpretation of EKG's" is the "bible" of EKG interpretation and should be read and studied. Both the cardiac monitor and 12-lead EKG provide the ability to graphically display the electrical rhythm over time, either on the screen or on paper. Analysis, covered fully in Dubin's, must be methodical; the most important factors in the analysis of a dysrhythmia are the rate, rhythm, PR and QRS intervals, and wave morphology. A Valsalva maneuver or certain drugs can slow a tachyarrhythmia in order to better define it. **Electrophysiology** is the subspecialty of cardiology that deals with the electrical system of the heart. Through cardiac catheterization the myocardium can be electrically stimulated at several points within the atria and ventricles to elicit electrical abnormalities, and the origin and morphology of and ability to elicit or suppress the abnormal rhythm can be tested. These studies can be used for both diagnosis and treatment.

Source

Of cardinal importance is whether the dysrhythmia arises from the atria (**supraventricular**) or ventricles (**ventricular** or **idioventricular**). The former are usually fast, produce narrow-complex QRSs, and preserve cardiac output, while the latter are often (but not always) slow, are manifest as widened QRSs, and are associated with loss of cardiac output, hence perfusion to the brain, heart, and other vital organs.

Atrial Fibrillation:

Atrial fibrillation, occasionally referred to as "delirium cordis" or total irregular pulse, is probably the most common dysrhythmia – certainly the most common seen by non-cardiologists. The exact mechanism is unknown, but, in general, the atria are in constant, uncoordinated electrical activity, or "fibrillation." The atria appear to be quivering when directly visualized, and never effectively contract. No P waves are present. The contribution of the atria to cardiac output, the "atrial kick," is variable but usually minimal; it is the **ventricular response** that determines symptoms and outcome. Ventricular response is variable, and depends on how many atrial impulses get to the conducting fibers.

A common cause of atrial fibrillation is atrial distention, which can be caused by valvular disease (classically mitral regurgitation or stenosis) or fluid overload. Atrial fibrillation can also be caused by coronary artery disease, hyperthyroidism, and hypertension, and commonly occurs in the postoperative state in elderly or otherwise susceptible individuals. Atrial fibrillation can be temporary or permanent, but, in comparison to atrial flutter, atrial fibrillation is more likely to be a chronic problem.

Figure 14.1
Atrial fibrillation. Note the lack of defined P-waves, "irregularly-irregular" ventricular rate, and QRS complexes of varying amplitude.

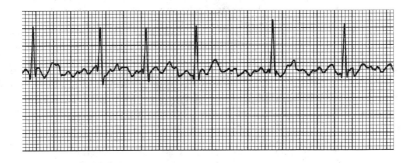

| Diagnosis | The hallmark of atrial fibrillation is an **"irregularly irregular"** heartbeat (i.e., ventricular response), as the interval between ventricular complexes changes from beat-to-beat. The ventricular response rate ranges from normal to 200, most commonly being between 100 and 160 in acute fibrillation. Patients are usually hemodynamically stable but may complain of palpitations, chest pain, or a general feeling of uneasiness – "something is wrong." |

| Problems | Atrial fibrillation causes two major problems. First, the atria can become large and "floppy," and this, combined with the relative akinesis of the atrial walls, increases the risk of **atrial thrombi**. These thrombi can break loose and cause arterial **embolization** to the cerebral, mesenteric, or peripheral vessels. The greatest risk of embolization occurs when longstanding fibrillation converts (spontaneously or therapeutically) to sinus rhythm; the accumulated clot suddenly is subjected to a contracting atrium and can then break free. The second problem is that of decreased cardiac output. The atria contribute varying amounts of "kick" to the overall cardiac output, and whether or not cardiac output is affected is variable. In general, it is the ventricular response that determines acute symptomatology; rates less than 150 are usually well tolerated. |

| Treatment | There are three issues involved in the treatment of atrial fibrillation: rate control, conversion to sinus rhythm, and |

treatment of sequelae. In general, the **rate** should be brought to less than 150 beats per minute in the acute situation to optimize short-term perfusion, and to less than 100 chronically to optimize long-term myocardial health. The higher the rate, the more symptomatic the patient, and the lower the blood pressure, the faster the rate needs to be controlled. An asymptomatic patient can be treated initially with digoxin, which is effective, but slow. Digoxin slows AV conduction – although fibrillation persists, the ventricular response is slowed and cardiac output is improved. Calcium channel blockers such as diltiazem or verapamil are fast and effective when given intravenously and are thus useful if the patient is unstable. There is a risk of myocardial depression, however, so calcium, which will act as an "antidote," should be available. Beta-blockers can also be used to slow AV conduction and thus "control" the ventricular rate. Synchronized cardioversion (see Chapter 13, "Basic ACLS") is the fastest but most invasive option for significantly unstable rhythms. An essential part of the evaluation of a patient with new or worsened atrial fibrillation is checking potassium, magnesium, and oxygen levels, all of which when abnormal can cause fibrillation.

Cardioversion to sinus rhythm is the second issue. Conversion is required if the patient requires their atrial "kick," i.e., cardiac output is depressed even with a normal ventricular rate. Digoxin does not cause conversion; it merely slows the AV response (conversion often occurs spontaneously, however, in cases of acute atrial fibrillation treated with digoxin). The calcium channel blockers can promote conversion, as can, of course, **electrical cardioversion**.

If the patient remains in atrial fibrillation, **prevention of embolization** becomes important. Coumadin is used to inhibit clot formation in patients who have long-standing atrial fibrillation, and in patients with known thrombi who have embolized. Patients undergoing elective cardioversion for chronic atrial fibrillation are often prophylactically anticoagulated before cardioversion, although it should be recognized that this does nothing to treat the clots already present. Generally, patients should be anticoagulated with heparin or Coumadin if they remain in atrial fibrillation for more than 48 hours. Of course, the benefit of preventing intracardiac thrombi must be weighed against the risk of hemorrhage.

Atrial Flutter

Although the mechanism is not known, **atrial flutter** can occur with or without structural heart disease. It occurs in either a paroxysmal or persistent fashion, and is more common in children, possibly because a child's heart does not have the muscle mass to sustain atrial fibrillation or other atrial dysrhythmias. The incidence of atrial flutter in adults is low and has been reported to be only 5% of that of atrial fibrillation.

Diagnosis As opposed to atrial fibrillation, the rhythm in atrial flutter is often regular. The EKG is very characteristic, revealing regular, "**sawtooth**" P waves, best seen in the inferior leads (II, III, AVF) and V1. As is the case with fibrillation, the critical determinant of cardiac output is the ventricular response, commonly described as the ratio of P waves to QRS complexes (2:1, 3:1, and so on). The atrial rate ranges from 250 to 450 beats per minute; the ventricular response anywhere from 2:1 to 8:1. An atrial rate of 300 with a ventricular response of 150 (2:1 conduction) is so classic that a regular, narrow-complex tachycardia at a rate of 150 beats per minute should be considered atrial flutter until proved otherwise.

Figure 14.2
Atrial flutter with a 4:1 ventricular response rate: atrial rate is 300 (remember, the P-wave buried in the QRS complex counts), ventricular, 75. Note the "sawtooth" P-waves and regular R-R interval.

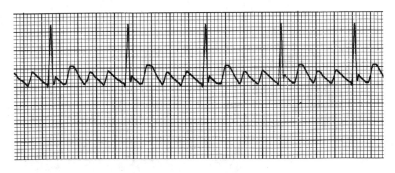

(continued)

The treatment of atrial flutter is similar to that of atrial fibrillation and depends on the condition of the patient. Beta-blockers, calcium channel blockers, digoxin, and class I and III antiarrhythmics all are useful in the treatment of this dysrhythmia; if hemodynamic instability is present, emergent electrical cardioversion is necessary.

Ventricular Tachycardia

Ventricular tachycardia (VT), defined as three or more ventricular beats in a row, is a highly lethal dysrhythmia. Perfusion, blood pressure, and pulse can be maintained, especially when only a few beats at a time occur, or cardiac output can be lost, in which case it presents as cardiac arrest due to "pulseless VT" (see Chapter 13, "Basic ACLS"). The electrical impulses arise from single or multiple foci in the ventricle. More than half the patients who present with VT have ischemic heart disease as the underlying problem; congestive or hypertrophic cardiomyopathy is the second most common cause. Sustained or nonsustained VT is a common dysrhythmia after an MI and should be suspected if syncope or hypotension suddenly occurs in this setting.

Diagnosis

The rate in ventricular tachycardia is between 70 and 250 beats per minute. The EKG pattern is often obvious but can be confusing; because of the lethality of VT, **any wide-complex tachycardia** (QRS duration of greater than 120 msec) **should be considered VT until proved**

Figure 14.3
Ventricular tachycardia.

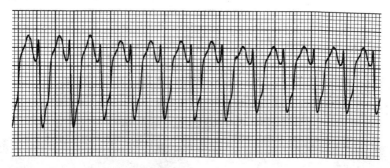

otherwise. The characteristic EKG pattern is that of a widened, ill-defined QRS complex, fusion beats reflecting activation of the ventricle from 2 foci, capture beats (conducted supraventricular foci), and AV dissociation. Regularity is common, but multifocal foci and variable QRS complexes can be seen.

Treatment

Management of sustained VT, whether perfusing or not, is emergent. A precordial thump, cardioversion, and antiarrhythmic drugs all may be used. Non-sustained or paroxysmal VT is treated by chemical or mechanical means. Amiodarone is a useful antiarrhythmic; correction of coronary artery disease or implantation of an automatic cardioverter/defibrillator, as indicated, are options (see Chapter 36, "Cardiac Surgery"), as is electrophysiologic ablation of pathologic extra-anatomic electrical pathways.

Ventricular Fibrillation

Ventricular fibrillation (VF) never produces a measurable cardiac output and leads to death within a few minutes if not corrected; the best prognosis occurs if defibrillation is accomplished within the first minute. This dysrhythmia is most commonly associated with coronary artery disease and is a leading cause of sudden death. The "rate" in ventricular fibrillation is between 150-300 beats per minute, but this is of academic interest only.

Figure 14.4
Ventricular fibrillation transforming to ventricular tachycardia (contrast Figure 14-3).

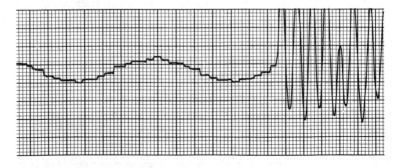

(continued)

The rhythm on the monitor is almost flat-line, consisting of irregular, low amplitude undulations of varying shape, which at times is easily confused with asystole. Prognosis is worse if the waves are less than 0.2 millivolts in amplitude. Management of VF is emergent, and similar to that of VT (see Chapter 13, "Basic ACLS").

Atrioventricular Block (Heart Block)

Prolonged or transient disturbance of impulse conduction through the AV node is referred to as **heart block**.

1° Block

First degree block is defined as conduction **delay** (PR interval greater than 200ms) through the AV node. All impulses are conducted, and every P wave has a related QRS. No treatment is needed in an asymptomatic patient, but if hemodynamic instability is present, pacing is required.

Figure 14.5
First-degree AV block. Apart from the prolonged P-R interval (greater than 200 ms), the rhythm is normal.

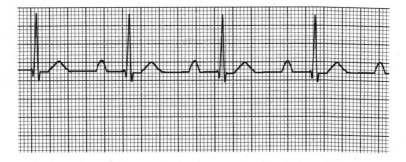

2° Block

Second degree block is divided into two types. **Mobitz type I** or **Wenkebach** is characterized by progressive prolongation of the PR interval with each beat until one P-wave is not conducted; the sequence then begins again at that point. This is also a benign dysrhythmia; no treatment is needed in a stable patient. **Mobitz type II** is characterized by the occasional, random loss of the QRS complex (nonconducted P-wave) without discernible lengthening of the PR interval. Progression to complete block is likely; thus, pacing is often required.

Figure 14.6
Mobitz type I (Wenkebach) second-degree AV block. Note the progressively lengthening P-R interval, until a dropped beat occurs.

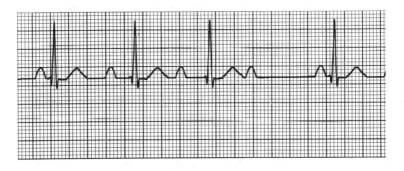

3° Block

Third degree or **complete block** is also known as **AV dissociation**; the relationship between the P wave and QRS complex is lost. By definition, a latent AV nodal pacemaker (junctional rhythm) or an idioventricular pacemaker must take over in order for cardiac output to be maintained. The rate, if junctional, is generally 40-60 beats per minute, the QRS is narrow, and there is complete AV dissociation. In a ventricular escape rhythm, in contrast, the rate is characteristically less than 40 beats per minute, QRS complexes are wide, and hemodynamic compromise is common. Treatment is by means of a temporary external (Zoll) or permanent implantable pacemaker. ■

Figure 14.7
Third-degree AV block. There is no consistent relationship between the P wave and QRS complex (which is wide, reflecting its ventricular origin).

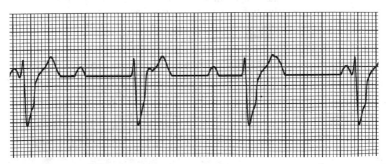

15 Ischemic Heart Disease and Chest Pain

Chest pain is one of the most common presenting complaints in any emergency department, and can be completely benign or be a true emergency. Many conditions making up the differential diagnosis, such as pulmonary embolus, trauma, or pneumonia, are covered elsewhere. This chapter focuses on the rapid identification and management of **myocardial ischemia**, and the recognition and long-term management of **coronary artery disease**.

Some Definitions

Angina pectoris is chest pain, pressure, or discomfort due to myocardial ischemia. Ischemia is caused by **oxygen demand that exceeds oxygen supply**. Increased demand commonly results from exercise, tachyarrhythmias, or hypertension (causing an increased cardiac workload), while deficient supply most commonly is the result of coronary artery stenosis. Most often, components of both coexist when acute symptoms occur.

Unstable angina

Stable angina refers to the classic symptoms of angina predictably brought on with exertion and relieved promptly with rest. To be classified as "stable," the frequency of attacks, the level of exertion required to cause discomfort, and the character and duration of pain must all be relatively constant.

Unstable angina describes a **change** in the patient's typical anginal pattern. New-onset angina, angina at rest, angina that occurs with significantly less exertion than in the past, or anginal attacks of significantly lengthening duration may all be classified as unstable. **Unstable angina carries a higher risk of death or ischemic complications than does stable angina**.

An anginal equivalent refers to other symptoms, commonly dyspnea or nausea, that may occur with myocardial ischemia in patients without classic angina.

MI

A **myocardial infarction (MI)** is actual irreversible ischemic necrosis and cellular death of myocardial tissue, most often caused by sudden occlusion of a coronary artery, and is commonly full-thickness or transmural. A **non Q-wave myocardial infarction** is death of subendo-cardial tissue only.

Acute Myocardial Infarction

While the differential diagnosis of acute chest pain is broad, the most important initial decision point is **whether or not an MI is occurring**. The reason for this urgency is that as time progresses heart muscle is being progressively lost. In other words, damage does not occur immediately or in an "all-or-none" fashion, but is dependent on the duration of ischemia. **The sooner the patient is diagnosed and receives appropriate therapy, the more functioning heart muscle is saved**.

Initial diagnosis

The diagnosis of myocardial infarction should ideally be made within the first 5-15 minutes of first seeing the patient. "Classic" symptoms of an MI are substernal, "crushing" chest pain or pressure radiating to the neck or left arm, diaphoresis, nausea, palpitations, lightheadedness, and dyspnea. The most important initial data are whether or not there is a **history of any symptoms of coronary artery disease** and the result of the **electrocardiogram (EKG)**. Ask the patient if the pain is similar to typical anginal pain or a previous MI; many patients can make this distinction quite accurately. The other information urgently required (while simultaneously recording an EKG) is the duration of the pain and the presence of associated lightheadedness or shortness of breath. Duration is important; most studies show a clear benefit of thrombolytic therapy if begun within 6 hours after **onset of symptoms** (**not** hospital arrival).
Lightheadedness and dyspnea can be signs of an arrhythmia or decreased cardiac output, both of which significantly alter prognosis and therapy. Assessing the patient's response to sublingual nitroglycerine takes only a minute or two and can also help to establish the cardiac nature of the pain.

EKG

By the time these few questions are asked, the EKG should be complete. First look for changes consistent with ischemia. **ST segment elevations** are characteristic of transmural infarction and are the EKG criteria used to determine candidacy for thrombolytic therapy, while **ST segment depressions** are more typical of myocardial ischemia or subendocardial infarction. Other, less specific indications of ischemia are **peaked T waves** seen in early myocardial infarction, and **inverted** or **"flipped" T waves** sometimes present in ischemia or infarction. Especially if these less specific changes are present, it is helpful to compare the current EKG with a previous tracing to see if new changes have occurred. **Q waves** suggest a prior MI, but are less helpful in the setting of acute chest pain. Rate and rhythm are important because tachyarrhythmias can cause or worsen ischemia by increasing oxygen demand. **Bradycardia** or a **heart block** are often caused by inferior wall infarction leading to increased vagal output or ischemia of the conduction system.

If acute transmural infarction is diagnosed by EKG, treatment (see below) should be instituted **immediately**, **before** completion of the full history and physical. If the EKG is nondiagnostic, further history and physical examination, with selected radiologic testing and laboratory evaluation as appropriate, assist in determining if the chest pain is cardiac in origin.

Differential diagnosis

If it does not appear that the patient is having an acute MI, workup can be more complete. Noncardiac causes for chest pain should be considered. Obviously, recent trauma is significant; pneumothorax can be delayed in occurrence and/or presentation. A "tearing" sensation in the chest or mid-scapular region of the back in a hypertensive patient is the classic presentation of a thoracic aortic dissection (which is not the same as an abdominal aneurysm; see Chapter 37, "Vascular Surgery"). Dissection itself can cause ischemia if it causes occlusion of the coronary arteries. Pleuritic chest pain (that which changes with respiration) in association with a cough or fever point toward a pulmonary process such as pneumonia or pulmonary embolus. Association of pain with eating, complaints of substernal burning, a sour taste in the mouth, or relief of pain with antacids all suggest a gastrointestinal source. Esophageal spasm can present with symptoms very similar to angina; cardiac risk factors can help determine the probability that a particular patient has coronary artery disease.

Exam

Initial **physical exam** should include vital signs. Tachycardia or hypertension will increase cardiac workload. A difference in blood pressure between the arms can be seen with aortic dissection, although subclavian atherosclerosis is not uncommon in these patients. Signs of cardiac compromise such as an elevated jugular venous pressure, rales heard on auscultation of the lung, an S3 gallop or new murmur suggestive of papillary muscle dysfunction, or peripheral edema should be specifically sought for. Chest pain that is reproducible with palpation of the chest wall is suggestive of a musculoskeletal cause, but does not rule out ischemia.

Enzyme changes

While initial presentation and EKG are most important in the setting of acute chest pain, silent or painless ischemia is common, and angina and non-Q wave MIs can occur without any EKG changes. Certain enzymes are released preferentially by damaged myocardial cells, and their levels show characteristic changes in the hours following an MI. **Creatinine phosphokinase (CK)** levels are the most useful. Isozyme determination is vital; the **MB** fraction is most specific for myocardial necrosis. CK-MB levels begin to rise approximately 6 hours after infarction and peak at 18-24 hours. An elevated total CK and CK-MB is very specific for heart muscle damage. Aspartate aminotransferase (AST) and lactic acid dehydrogenase (LDH) also have characteristic patterns of elevation after an MI, but are much less specific. AST will be elevated 12-48 hours after infarction, while LDH levels increase within a day of infarction and persist for up to a week. The finding of elevated LDH isoenzymes -1 and -2 can be helpful in determining whether an MI has occurred more than 24 hours after the acute event.

A **chest x-ray** should be obtained in every patient with chest pain. Although of very little use in the diagnosis of an MI, it is essential to rule out such conditions such as pneumothorax, pneumonia, congestive heart failure, or aortic dissection or aneurysm. Oxygen saturation should always be checked, even if the patient is not overtly short of breath.

Echocardiography

An **echocardiogram** is occasionally useful in the setting of acute chest pain to look for wall hypokinesis suggestive of ischemia or infarction. It is also indicated if acute valvular dysfunction is suspected. One limitation of the echocardiogram is that without a previous study there is no way of determining the age of any abnormality discovered. **Transesophageal echocardiography** (**TEE**) is crucial if a thoracic aortic dissection or aneurysm is suspected.

Management of Acute Myocardial Infarction

Thrombolytic therapy

If an acute MI is suspected on the basis of the history and EKG findings, treatment must begin immediately to save as much threatened heart muscle as possible. Myocardial infarction is almost always due to an acute occlusion of a coronary artery, usually from **sudden thrombosis of a chronically diseased vessel**; thus urgent restoration of patency is the prime objective. Heparin only prevents new clot from forming; in the setting of an acute MI, **thrombolytics** are needed. The most commonly used agent in the United States is **tissue plasminogen activator**, which, when given systemically, usually lyses the thrombus and restores flow in 30-60 minutes. **Streptokinase** (**SK**) is also widely used. **Urokinase** (**UK**), the other commonly available agent, is most effective if given directly into the clot. Criteria for the use of thrombolytics are clear transmural myocardial infarction as demonstrated by ST segment elevation, and onset of symptoms within 6 hours. Thrombolytics are not specific for pathologic clot, but will lyse any recent clot in the body. Therefore, contraindications to thrombolysis are any condition that places the patient at high risk of **uncontrollable** bleeding (such as trauma, recent stroke, intracranial neoplasm, or active GI bleeding); relative contraindications include recent surgery (two weeks is probably sufficient), malignant hypertension, and diabetic retinopathy; age over 75 is no longer believed a contraindication. The early use of systemic thrombolytics in the setting of a suspected acute MI has clearly been shown to reduce morbidity and mortality and is the current standard of care.

PTCA

If available, primary **percutaneous transluminal coronary angioplasty** (**PTCA**) is at least as effective as thrombolytic therapy in the treatment of acute MI. PTCA involves passing a catheter into a coronary artery via a percutaneous vessel in order to dilate a stenotic or occluded lesion with an inflatable balloon. If PTCA can be performed within a reasonable amount of time it is preferable to thrombolytic therapy, especially in patients with cardiogenic shock or who are at particularly high risk for bleeding.

Other therapy

Reperfusion is the cornerstone of therapy for acute myocardial infarction, but other medical therapy is beneficial. **Aspirin** should be given early in an acute MI for its antiplatelet effect to reduce further thrombosis. **Heparin**, however, has not proved as beneficial, and is used only as part of a thrombolytic protocol or after PTCA. **Beta-blockers** reduce heart rate and blood pressure, and **nitrates** decrease preload and afterload and promote coronary vasodilatation. Both of these reduce workload and oxygen demand, and thus can minimize ischemia and reduce infarct size.

In addition to reperfusion, much of the initial management of acute myocardial infarction involves managing potential complications. **Arrhythmias**, particularly ventricular tachycardia, are common in the first 24-48 hours. Continuous cardiac monitoring is essential (see Chapters 13 and 14, "Basic ACLS" and "Cardiac Dysrhythmias"). The other common complication is **congestive heart failure** from either valvular dysfunction or "pump failure" (cardiogenic shock).

Management of Unstable Angina

Patients with unstable angina generally do not have complete occlusion of a vessel, but rather an unstable atheromatous plaque. Therapy is generally similar to that of an MI, with the exception that because no occlusive clot is present, thrombolytics are not needed.

Treatment

Aspirin is clearly beneficial in reducing the risk of thrombus formation, as is **heparin**, which should be administered at diagnosis and continued as a constant infusion. Both of these will reduce the chances of acute thrombosis of the unstable plaque, which will convert unstable angina into an acute MI. Because imbalance between oxygen supply and demand is a prominent feature of unstable angina, medications that reduce cardiac workload play an extremely important role. Sublingual **nitroglycerine** should be used initially, with early conversion to constant infusion via the IV route planned if pain control is not quickly achieved. Enough IV nitroglycerine should be given to completely relieve symptoms if the blood pressure allows. **Beta-blockers** should also be instituted early. IV administration is recommended, with a target heart rate around 60 beats/minute as the goal. **Morphine** has anxiolytic, cardiosuppressive, analgesic, and mild vasodilatatory effects, and **calcium channel blockers** can reduce heart rate and blood pressure if adequate control is not achieved by beta-blockade. Oxygen administration to maintain high arterial saturations is also beneficial.

IABP

If symptoms persist or the patient is in cardiogenic shock, an **intra-aortic balloon pump** (**IABP**) can be inserted. The "ultimate inotrope," it not only decreases afterload, thus decreasing cardiac workload, but also augments coronary perfusion during diastole, thus increasing myocardial blood supply.

Early cardiac catheterization with PTCA is not as clearly beneficial as in myocardial infarction. If symptoms cannot be controlled or recur with aggressive medical therapy, however, urgent cardiac catheterization is indicated to treat the stenotic lesion with angioplasty or stenting, or to suggest the need for operative bypass.

Chronic Angina

Chronic **angina pectoris** is caused by a relative imbalance between oxygen supply and demand, but, by definition, supply is adequate at rest. The atheromatous coronary artery lesion, however, does not dilate when demand is increased by exercise, and thus ischemia and pain result. With rest demand drops to baseline, and oxygen supply again becomes adequate. By definition, the anatomy and symptoms are stable.

Diagnosis

Patients with chronic, stable angina often present with fairly typical complaints: substernal chest pressure with radiation to the jaw or left arm, shortness of breath, diaphoresis, and/or nausea; classically precipitated by typical activities such as exercise, large meals, emotional distress, or cold weather, and relieved promptly by rest or sublingual nitroglycerine. Known **cardiac risk factors** are male sex, age greater than 55, a family history of coronary artery disease before age 65, tobacco abuse, hypertension, hyperlipidemia, peripheral vascular disease, and diabetes mellitus. Interestingly, a carotid bruit is more predictive of significant coronary artery disease than it is of significant carotid artery stenosis.

Exam

Physical examination will often be normal in patients with stable angina, or will be significant only for signs of atherosclerosis in more accessible locations. Signs of hypertension, congestive heart failure, or valvular dysfunction should be sought. Laboratory screening for risk factors such as hyperlipidemia and precipitants such as anemia should be performed. A resting EKG may reveal a previous MI and will serve as a baseline for future evaluation. It is unlikely to reveal acute ischemic changes such as ST depression, elevation, or T wave inversion, though, in a patient who is pain-free.

Stress testing

Functional tests are often valuable in a patient with stable angina. In an **exercise stress test** a patient walks on a treadmill while the heart rate, blood pressure, and EKG are monitored; administering an inotrope such as dobutamine can accomplish the same effect (cardiac stress) without exercise. A stress test is valuable because it reproduces the symptoms of chest pain and objectively documents myocardial ischemia by EKG changes at a fairly reproducible level of stress in a controlled setting. Moreover, if pain or EKG changes do not occur with adequate cardiac work, a search for noncardiac causes can be carried out.

Catheterization

The major anatomic test is **cardiac catheterization**, which is valuable in the patient with known angina because of its ability to direct therapy. It is critically important to remember, however, that the mere presence of a stenosis does not mean that it needs to be corrected (by surgery or PTCA); the anatomic findings must be correlated with symptoms and the overall clinical scenario. A normal coronary angiogram, on the other hand, is fairly reassuring.

Stress echo-cardiography

Combination tests such as a **stress thallium** test or **stress echocardiogram** give both functional and anatomic information. Thallium is a radioisotope that is taken up by the myocardium in proportion to perfusion; areas supplied by narrowed coronary arteries (which are ischemic) will take up less thallium. Scarring (indicative of an old MI) will show up as "cold" areas; if delayed images are compared to images taken immediately after exercise, an initial "cold" appearing area will become normal after the radioisotope **redistributes** to healthy, but underperfused, myocardium. These areas of reperfusion indicate ischemic tissue at high risk for outright infarction, and redistribution seems to predict risk more than does a fixed defect. Stress echocardiography allows examination of the the heart's wall motion and overall function in the stressed state, which is more predictive of future risk than is resting function.

Management

Principles of management are similar to those of unstable angina, although with lesser urgency. Acute anginal episodes are treated primarily with sublingual nitroglycerine and rest. Long-term therapy is aimed toward prevention of symptoms. **Long-acting nitrates**, administered as pills or a transdermal patch, are the mainstay of treatment, acting to reduce cardiac work during the active hours. Because tolerance develops quickly, a nitrate-free period of 10-12 hours (usually overnight) is provided. Oral **beta-blockers** and **calcium channel blockers** also reduce cardiac work and reduce the frequency and severity of symptoms. Emphasis is placed on risk factor modification, including cessation of smoking, lowering of cholesterol and lipids, weight loss, and control of hypertension and diabetes. Daily **aspirin** has been shown to greatly reduce the risk of MI in patients with coronary artery disease and is strongly recommended, although the optimal dose (325mg versus 85mg) is unclear. While anti-anginal therapy minimizes symptoms, actually reducing the progression of atherosclerotic disease may provide the greatest benefit in terms of longevity.

Definitive treatment

When symptoms occurring with a reasonably normal lifestyle are no longer controlled with medical therapy, a more aggressive approach is warranted. Treatment of coronary artery stenosis clearly can reduce symptoms. Until recently, treatment of single vessel disease was primarily achieved with PTCA. Recent innovations such as **coronary artery stenting** and **rotational atherectomy**, however, are now being used with success. Stenting appears to lower the fairly high rate of restenosis seen after PTCA (30% at 6 months), although evidence is incomplete. Multi-vessel angioplasty is also being used as an alternative to surgery in selected cases.

CABG   **Coronary artery bypass grafting (CABG)** is the last resort for patients whose symptoms are uncontrolled or whose coronary disease is not amenable to angioplasty (see Chapter 36, "Cardiac Surgery"). Fairly firm indications in the appropriate clinical setting include isolated left main and three-vessel coronary artery disease, because patients in these categories have better overall prognosis with CABG. Surgery can provide longterm symptom relief in one- or two-vessel disease, but it may not reduce mortality. For any intervention to be appropriate, whether medication, PTCA, or surgery, **the benefits must outweigh the risks.** ■

16 Dyspnea

Dyspnea is the **subjective sense** of shortness of breath. It is a symptom, not a diagnosis. The presence of dyspnea does not imply any particular physiologic abnormality, and no single clinical finding is universally present in the dyspneic patient. Dyspnea may be chronic or acute, or it can be the acute manifestation of a worsening chronic condition such as anemia. What a patient might initially describe as weakness or fatigue can, often after close questioning, be best categorized as dyspnea on exertion. Dyspnea can even be caused by psychological factors—dyspnea that improves with exercise is more likely to be psychologically based.

It is the severity of the dyspnea rather than the cause that is most important on initial presentation. In any patient with dyspnea, there are four potentially life-threatening conditions to consider: acute bronchospasm (asthma or chronic obstructive pulmonary disease, COPD), pulmonary edema as a consequence of congestive heart failure, pulmonary embolus (PE), and pneumonia. All patients with dyspnea should have a thorough **history** and **physical exam**. Many others, depending on the clinical situation, should also have a **chest x-ray, EKG, arterial blood gas**, and/or **pulmonary function testing**. Rather than by diagnosis per se, dyspnea may best be approached by considering the components of the workup individually and how they provide clues to the underlying diagnosis.

History

Dyspnea that is long-standing (often since childhood) or associated with cold, exercise, or environmental allergens suggests **asthma**. There is an association between asthma and aspirin sensitivity, nasal polyps, and atopic dermatitis, and asthma tends to run in families.

Emphysema and **chronic bronchitis** (defined clinically by chronic expectoration for at least 3 months per year for 2 straight years) are strongly associated with a long history of tobacco abuse. Onset of emphysema at a young age, especially if a family history is present, raises the prospect of the inherited disease alpha-1-antitrypsin deficiency.

The presence of **congestive heart failure (CHF)** is suggested by a history of peripheral edema, orthopnea (increased dyspnea when prone), or dyspnea that occurs paroxysmally at night. The major cause of CHF is **coronary artery disease**, so it is vital to ask about cardiac risk factors and typical symptoms such as chest pain or palpitations (CHF can be caused by an arrhythmia). A recent change in diet (typically an ill-advised "splurge" with a high-sodium item such as pizza or potato chips) can provoke an acute episode of failure.

Ninety percent of patients with an acute **pulmonary embolus (PE)** have an obvious historical risk factor. A swollen leg suggests the presence of a deep venous thrombosis (DVT) of the lower extremity, especially if acute dyspnea (suggesting PE) is present. Interestingly, the predictive value of leg swelling (or lack thereof) for a DVT alone is only about 50%. Inquire about risk factors for Virchow's triad: poor blood flow (sedentary lifestyle, a recent long trip), blood vessel wall damage (prior DVT, smoking), or hypercoagulable states (pregnancy, birth control pills, or malignancy). Deficiencies of protein C, protein S, and anti-thrombin III are strong risk factors for PE, and resistance to activated protein C, possibly an even more common condition, is being actively studied as a risk factor for hypercoagulable states in general.

Pulmonary infarction following a PE can lead to hemoptysis or pleuritic chest pain. Patients with **pneumonia** also can have pleuritic chest pain, especially if an **empyema** has developed. Patients with pneumonia describe a cough productive of green, yellow, or brown sputum, although atypical pneumonia, especially due to mycoplasma, may not be associated with sputum production. Fever and rigors (teeth-chattering chills) are classically seen with pneumococcal pneumonia. Bloody sputum suggests **tuberculosis**, and severe dyspnea is the classic presenting symptom of **pneumocystis carinii pneumonia (PCP)** seen in patients with AIDS. Any dyspnea occurring after an injury to the chest, no matter how minor, should be considered a **pneumothorax** until proved otherwise (see Chapter 28, "Trauma").
(continued)

Medicine
Dyspnea *continued*

Physical Exam

The presence of **chronic obstructive pulmonary disease (COPD)** is suggested by decreased breath sounds, prolonged expiration, barrel chest, nail clubbing, nicotine stains or tobacco odor, and wheezing, if an acute flare-up is present. New wheezing and decreased breath sounds, however, especially in a patient with nasal polyps or a rash, suggest **asthma**.

Hypertension (along with coronary artery disease) is still one of the most common causes of **CHF**. Distended neck veins, rales, peripheral edema, or decreased basilar breath sounds (indicating a possible effusion) are commonly seen with CHF, and an S_3 heart sound or displaced point of maximal impulse signify a dilated heart.

The patient with a **PE** will often be tachypneic, tachycardic, and anxious, but may have few physical findings other than a swollen leg, if that. Fever, especially if associated with rhonchi and localized dullness to percussion on lung exam, suggest a lobar **pneumonia**.

Chest X-ray

Hyperinflation (low diaphragms, long or large thorax) is the characteristic finding in chronic **asthma** or **COPD**. Bullae and decreased pulmonary markings as the result of emphysematous destruction of lung parenchyma are also seen in COPD. **CHF** leads to increased interstitial marking, cephalization, pulmonary effusions, peribronchial cuffing, and fluid in the fissures.

The chest x-ray is usually normal after a **PE**, but can demonstrate atelectasis. A wedge-shaped peripherally-based infiltrate can be seen after a true infarction has occurred, but this is pretty rare. Infiltrates and consolidation are seen in lobar pneumonia, while the lung can have a ground-glass appearance in **PCP**.

Bilateral hilar adenopathy, especially in a dyspneic patient, is commonly caused by **sarcoidosis**. This is a relatively common disease, especially in young African-American women, and is associated with nonspecific lab abnormalities such as elevated serum calcium and angiotensin converting enzyme.

EKG

An EKG is essential if **myocardial ischemia** or an **arrhythmia** is suspected. Nonspecific sinus tachycardia can be a clue that a **PE** has occurred, but dyspnea in general causes an elevated heart rate. New atrial fibrillation can tip a borderline patient with heart disease into CHF because the atrial "kick" is lost and the left ventricle does not fill properly.

Arterial Blood Gas

An arterial blood gas (ABG) can be very helpful early in the evaluation of any patient with dyspnea (see Chapter 2, "Acid-Base Disorders"). It does not necessarily suggest a diagnosis, but is invaluable in determining to what degree a primary respiratory problem exists. The three critical values, usually reported in order, are the pH, the pCO_2, and the pO_2. There are thus three things to consider with every blood gas: acid-base status, ventilation, and oxygenation. A critical point to remember is that oxygenation and ventilation are separate and vary independently of each other.

The pH describes the overall acid-base status of the body. This number, however, is affected by both metabolic and respiratory factors, and represents the balance between them. CO_2 can be viewed as an acid. If the pH changes appropriately with changes in pCO_2 (e.g., decreased pH with high pCO_2 and vice versa) then the primary disorder is respiratory. If pH and pCO_2 both fall, however, a primary metabolic acidosis with respiratory compensation must exist. More complex acid-base disturbances such as elevated pCO_2 and pH usually represent not compensation but rather superimposed, often unrelated problems.

Ventilation describes the ability of the lungs to exchange air (excrete CO_2), and thus is measured by the pCO_2. Interpretation is straightforward; if the $pCO2$ is too high, there is a problem with ventilation. Acute hypercarbia causes respiratory acidosis and is always pathologic, because a compensatory metabolic alkalosis has not had time to occur. Chronic hypercarbia with normal pH, however, is commonly seen in patients with longstanding COPD whose kidneys save bicarbonate to compensate. *(continued)*

Medicine
Dyspnea *continued*

There are two important questions to ask when considering a patient's oxygenation status. First, is hypoxemia present? At a paO_2 of 60mmHg about 90% of the hemoglobin is saturated; below this the curve drops off and the chance for tissue hypoxia increases precipitously. Second, is there an abnormal alveolar-arterial oxygen difference (A-a gradient)? The A-a gradient is equal to the partial pressure of oxygen in the alveolus (A) minus the partial pressure of oxygen in the artery (a). The alveolar partial pressure is calculated from the simplified alveolar gas equation as:

$$A = \textbf{(atmospheric pressure-partial pressure of water)} \times FIO_2 - 1.25 \times pCO_2$$

So, on room air, at sea level, the alveolar pO_2 is:

$$A = (760-47) \times 0.21 - 1.25 \times 40 = 99\text{mmHg}$$

and thus, with an arterial pO_2 (a) of 95, the A-a gradient will be about 4mmHg (which is normal).

The utility of the A-a gradient is twofold. First, simple hypoventilation can be differentiated from ventilation-perfusion mismatches and shunts, and second, ventilation-perfusion mismatches and shunts can be separated from each other based on the way that the A-a gradient responds to increasing concentrations of inspired oxygen.

Differentiating hypoventilation from shunts and mismatches is simple: in hypoventilation there is **not** an increased A-a gradient, while with a shunt or ventilation-perfusion mismatch there **is** (for example, hypoventilation to pH = 7.10, pCO_2 = 88, pO_2 = 40 on room air produces a gradient of only 5). Both shunts (for example, a right-to-left intracardiac shunt) and ventilation-perfusion mismatches (as occur in pneumonia, for example) produce elevated A-a gradients, but if supplemental oxygen is given the gradient **will** improve if a mismatch is present, but **will not** if the problem is a shunt (because the shunted blood never "sees" the increased oxygen delivered to the lung).

Pulmonary Function Tests

Pulmonary function testis (PFTs) are useful for diagnosis in the patient with chronic dyspnea, and for prediction of risk with a planned intervention (such as surgery). Although multiple tests are reported, the most important are the forced vital capacity (FVC) which is the amount of air that can be expelled after a full inspiration, and the timed forced expiratory volume (FEV_1) which is the air that can be forcibly expelled in the first second. PFTs will usually determine whether the lung disease is restrictive or obstructive.

In restrictive lung disease, inhalation is difficult, due to decreased compliance, while exhalation is typically not a problem. Neuromuscular or chest wall disease, as well as interstitial fibrosis, can lead to a restrictive picture. Most or all absolute values are less than predicted, while the ratio of FEV_1 to FVC is typically normal. In obstructive lung disease such as **COPD**, the lungs have lost their elastic recoil. Inhalation is not a problem, but expiration is slowed due to airway collapse resulting from the loss of ability to hold the airways open. Thus, FEV_1 is decreased. By repeating the PFTs before and after treatment, one can determine whether bronchodilators will help.

The Acutely Dyspneic Patient

As with any symptom or sign, new or acutely worsened dyspnea is potentially much more serious than is chronic. The absence of wheezing in a patient with asthma or COPD can be an ominous sign. The lungs may not be "clear," rather, the patient may simply not be moving enough air to wheeze! A jugular venous pulsation clearly visible above the clavicle with the patient's head at 45° suggests an elevated right atrial pressure. A new murmur associated with acute dyspnea is a very serious finding, because an acute myocardial infarction with papillary muscle dysfunction and mitral regurgitation or ventricular septal defect can be the cause.

The key to the diagnosis of pulmonary embolism is to think of it! In a ventilation/perfusion lung scan, the pulmonary distributions of inhaled and injected radionuclides are compared for mismatches, suggesting areas of the lung that are ventilated but not perfused (because of the obstructing embolus). Multiple, large segmental defects indicate a high probability for PE, while a normal scan effectively rules out a clinically significant embolism. If the scan is indeterminate (non-diagnostic), consideration should be given to a pulmonary angiogram if it will change management.

Therapy

In **acute asthma** the patient should be easy to oxygenate; if not, a separate process such as a pneumonia may be present. Use nebulized beta-agonists (to relieve bronchospasm) until the patient gains relief or until severe tachycardia or tremulousness is seen. Nebulized anticholinergics (antibronchospasmic) and IV steroids (anti-inflammatory) are helpful. Don't use epinephrine in the setting of chest pain: if cardiac in origin, the resultant tachycardia and increased contractile state will worsen myocardial ischemia.

Chronic asthmatics benefit from periodic home measurements of peak expiratory flow; low flows merit a check with their physician. Inhaled steroids are effective in preventing attacks, and inhaled cromalyn sodium will stabilize mast cell membranes in patients with an allergic component. Theophylline has a narrow therapeutic window and interacts with many drugs, and is used less and often. Chronic beta-agonist use seems to be associated with decreased mortality, although the mechanisms behind this relationship are not clear. Respiratory infections should be treated early and aggressively.

Therapy for **acute COPD** is similar to for asthma, but especially in these older patients, an underlying lower respiratory infection (such as pneumonia) should be ruled out. In **chronic COPD**, inhaled anti-cholinergics are most useful. Low flow home oxygen has survival benefit for patients with a room air pO_2 of 55 or less.

Therapy for **acute CHF** revolves around decreasing venous return. In the past, revolving tourniquets and phlebotomy were the mainstays of treatment, but better choices these days are nitrates, morphine, and diuretics. Through a venodilatory effect, furosemide provides relief even before diuresis occurs. Gentle afterload reduction can be used if blood pressure is elevated, and, if suspicion is present, a myocardial infarction should be ruled out. Significant failure can require inotropic support to increase cardiac output.

Therapy for **chronic CHF** includes a low-salt diet, reducing the risk factors for myocardial ischemia, controlling blood pressure, and diuretic administration. Angiotensin-converting enzyme inhibitors have been shown to be useful, especially in patients with low left ventricular ejection fractions, and digitalis has long been used for its modest inotropic effect. Stress the need for compliance with medicines and diet; noncompliance often tips the patient over into a decompensated state.

The acute therapy for a **PE** is IV heparin. Although it does not lyse the clot, it prevents extension of thrombosis and allows intrinsic thrombolysis to occur. In the (very small) subset of patients who are still alive but critically ill because of pulmonary arterial obstruction, thrombolytics or operative embolectomy is an option. An intensive work-up for an occult malignancy in patient with a DVT or PE is seldom fruitful if the history, physical exam, and detailed review of systems are not suggestive of a source. ■

17   Hematology

Hematology is the study of malignant and non-malignant diseases of the blood, including neoplastic diseases such as leukemia, lymphoma, and multiple myeloma, myeloproliferative disorders such as polycythemia vera and essential thrombocytosis, anemia, bleeding and clotting disorders, hemoglobinopathies, and immune-mediated disorders of the blood such as immune thrombocytopenic purpura. Although many of these disorders render the patient acutely ill, many patients are also relatively asymptomatic and are detected only by laboratory evaluation performed for other reasons.

This chapter focuses on **leukemia** and the common **hereditary bleeding disorders**. See Chapter 54, "Pediatric Hematology and Oncology" for discussion of anemia, thalassemia, and sickle cell disease, and Chapter 8, "Hemostasis, Thrombosis, and Transfusion," for a discussion of the coagulation system in general.

Leukemia

The **leukemias** make up a diverse group of diseases that arise from malignant transformation of hematopoietic stem cells marked by abnormal proliferation and accumulation of lymphoid and non-lymphoid malignant white blood cells (WBCs) within the bone marrow and bloodstream. Many of the leukemias are associated with well-defined chromosomal abnormalities, affecting genes that encode for proteins regulating cell growth and differentiation. The cause of leukemia in most patients is not known.

The most straightforward way to approach the leukemias is to divide them into **acute** and **chronic** forms and by cell of origin (**lymphoid** or **non-lymphoid**).

Acute Leukemia

Acute lymphoblastic leukemia (ALL) is more common in children, and **acute myelogenous leukemia (AML)** is more common in adults, but either can occur at any age. Although the specific chemotherapeutic agents are different, the presentation and initial approach to management of both types of acute leukemia are similar.

Presentation

Patients with **acute leukemia** almost always come to medical attention because they are acutely ill. Symptoms usually arise because of **pancytopenia**, a reduction in the number of circulating cells of all three types – red blood cells (RBCs), WBCs, and platelets. Severe anemia causes fatigue, pallor, and dyspnea, thrombocytopenia causes bleeding and petechiae, and leukopenia or malfunctioning WBCs often lead to fever. Symptoms due to tissue infiltration by leukemic cells occur but are less common; patients with monocytic or myelomonocytic leukemia, for example, can have gingival infiltration causing painful hypertrophy of the gums or headache and cranial nerve abnormalities due to meningeal infiltration. **Leukostasis** (occlusion of small blood vessels by WBCs) can occur when there is a massive number of circulating myeloid leukemic cells, causing priapism, central nervous system (CNS) symptoms, and injury to the heart, kidneys, and lungs.

CBC and bone marrow

While the complete blood count (CBC) usually demonstrates anemia and thrombocytopenia, **the WBC can be low, normal, or elevated.** The peripheral smear in most patients with acute leukemia demonstrates **abnormal myeloblasts** or **lymphoblasts**, depending on whether the patient has AML or ALL, respectively, with few normal mature white cells. Leukemic blasts in the blood are absent in approximately 10% percent of patients; these patients are said to have **aleukemic leukemia**. A **bone marrow aspirate** and **biopsy** are usually required and are sufficient for diagnosis. The morphologic appearance of the abnormal cell is usually adequate to determine its origin, but cell marker studies can help if in question. The diagnosis of acute leukemia is usually not subtle, but delay can occur due to interpreter inexperience or absence of leukemic blasts. Immature cells can be seen on the peripheral smear in a variety of other conditions, including sepsis, infection, or any condition causing a "fight-or-flight" response, bone marrow infection with fungus or mycobacteria, or a non-hematologic malignancy that has metastasized to the marrow.

Immediate problems

Control of infection, bleeding, and leukostasis are the most important concerns in the initial evaluation of the patient with acute leukemia. If the patient is febrile and neutropenic or if the patient appears septic, IV broad spectrum antibiotics (including coverage against

Medicine
Hematology *continued*

Pseudomonas) should be started immediately. Platelet transfusions should be given if there is active bleeding or if the platelet count is less than 10-20,000/mcL. If a patient with AML has a peripheral blast count greater than 100,000/mcL or symptoms of leukostasis are present, leukapheresis should be performed. In many cases, chemotherapy needs to be started within a day or two after presentation.

Neutropenia

The best marker of the risk for infection is the **absolute neutrophil count (ANC)**, which is the percent neutrophils **and** bands multiplied by the total WBC; for example, a patient with a WBC of 2,300/mcL with 45% neutrophils, 6% bands, 34% lymphocytes, and 15% monocytes therefore has an ANC of 2,300 x (.45 + .06), or 1173/mcL. "**Neutropenia**" is usually defined as an ANC of less than 500 and usually means that certain infection control and antibiotic protocols must be followed. This number, however, is not absolute. A patient with an ANC of less than 1000 whose count is falling rapidly, for example, may best be treated by adherence to neutropenic protocols, while a patient who is recovering from chemotherapy and has a rising ANC, even if under 500, may not require further antibiotic therapy.

Chemotherapy

After control of any acute problems present at presentation, most patients with acute leukemia are treated with **myeloablative chemotherapy**. In most cases, patients require a prolonged hospital stay for the chemotherapy itself and for treatment of ongoing infectious and bleeding complications while their bone marrow recovers. Patients who go into remission, as demonstrated by serial bone marrow biopsies, are treated with additional courses of chemotherapy. Bone marrow transplantation is an option in both AML and ALL.

Most patients with acute leukemia do not survive; even those who go into complete remission usually relapse. **Bone marrow transplantation** can be curative, but is associated with a high incidence of graft-versus-host disease, which can be lethal.

Chronic Leukemia

Unlike the acute leukemias, the two types of **chronic leukemias, chronic myelogenous leukemia (CML)** and chronic lymphocytic leukemia (CLL), differ tremendously in presentation, prognosis, and treatment. All patients with CML will eventually transform into an **accelerated** or **blast** phase, a condition that behaves like acute leukemia. If untreated, all such patients will die of progressive leukemia. CLL, on the other hand, is a more indolent disease that usually occurs in older patients, and mortality is as likely to be due to other problems as it is to be due to the leukemia itself.

CML

CML is a myeloproliferative disorder of the pluripotential stem cell. Most patients with CML have the **Philadelphia chromosome**, an abnormal chromosome 22 arising from reciprocal translocation of material from chromosome 9. CML invariably progresses to acute leukemia, and is divided into three phases: **chronic**, **accelerated**, and **blast**. Many patients with CML are asymptomatic at the time of diagnosis; the diagnosis is made only when an abnormally high white blood cell count is noted on routine bloodwork. If symptoms are present, they are often nonspecific (fatigue, modest weight loss, fevers, and night sweats). Moderate splenomegaly is present about half the time at diagnosis, and is usually the only abnormal physical finding. Anemia, if present, is mild and rarely symptomatic; an occasional patient will have polycythemia.

Diagnosis

The WBC count in patients with CML can be as high as 1,000,000/mcL. There is often thrombocytosis, but anemia, if present, is mild. **In contrast to the patient with acute leukemia, the patient with CML (in the chronic phase) will have the full spectrum of myeloid maturation.** In other words, the patient will have an increased number of immature forms **without** a significant decrease in the numbers of mature neutrophils and bands. An increase in eosinophils and basophils is also characteristic of CML (basophilia is associated with a poorer prognosis). Because of the cell burden, the urate and lactate dehydrogenase may be elevated in the patient with CML. Again, bone marrow biopsy and aspirate are required for morphologic diagnosis and chromosomal analysis. Polymerase chain reaction can be used to detect the fusion gene (bcr/abl) in most of those patients in whom the characteristic Philadelphia chromosome is not identified (only about 10%). The **leukocyte alkaline phosphatase (LAP)** score can be used for prompt diagnosis. After staining, 100 cells are assigned a value from 1-4 based on the number and intensity of granules positive for leukocyte alkaline phosphatase, an enzyme found in neutrophilic leukocytes. CML produces a low LAP score; if high, a leukemoid reaction due to severe stress or another myeloproliferative disorder is probably present. As patients progress to the accelerated and blast phases, they can develop progressive anemia, fatigue, fever, and weight loss, marked splenomegaly, and adenopathy and bony pain. Patients with full-blown **blast crisis** have the same complications of pancytopenia as do those with acute leukemia. While the majority of cases of CML transform into AML, one-third will transform into acute **lymphoblastic** leukemia.

Treatment

Patients with CML in chronic phase can be followed without specific therapy, but nearly all require treatment to control the WBC count. Hydroxyurea effectively controls both WBC and platelet proliferation, and is well-tolerated by most patients. Alpha-interferon can also be used in the chronic phase and appears to reduce the number of cells with the Philadelphia chromosome. **Thus far, however, the only treatment that has significantly altered the natural course of CML is allogeneic bone marrow transplant**; approximately 60% of patients undergoing transplant achieve apparent cure. Patients who are otherwise in good health and who have a matched sibling donor should be considered for transplantation.

The accelerated and blastic phases are difficult to treat. Progressive difficulty controlling the WBC count is, in fact, one of the hallmarks of progression to the accelerated phase. Intensive chemotherapy usually fails to induce a true remission. Bone marrow transplantation is also much less effective once the patient has progressive disease.

CLL

Although it is unusual to hospitalize patients for **chronic lymphocytic leukemia** (**CLL**), it is actually the most common leukemia in adults, comprising about a third of cases. **CLL is a clonal disorder of B-lymphocytes that results in the accumulation of mature-appearing but functionally abnormal lymphocytes.** These lymphocytes are found throughout the hematopoietic system, including the peripheral blood, bone marrow, lymph nodes, and, often, spleen. CLL usually occurs in older patients (median age 60), and trisomy 12 is the most common chromosomal abnormality seen. Abnormalities of the patient's blood counts and immune system, including hypogammaglobulinemia, impaired cellular immunity, autoimmune hemolytic anemia, and thrombocytopenia, are common and account for many of the clinical problems.

Diagnosis

As is the case with CML, the diagnosis of CLL is often made in an asymptomatic patient who is found to have an elevated white blood cell count during evaluation for an unrelated problem; when symptoms are present, they are nonspecific or result from splenomegaly (left upper quadrant fullness or early satiety). Patients with CLL have reduced immunoglobulin levels and impaired cellular immunity. **Because fever and night sweats are uncommon in CLL, such complaints should prompt evaluation for possible infection**. Physical examination can be entirely normal, but careful examination of the lymph nodes and spleen must be done to assist in staging.

The diagnosis of CLL requires a lymphocyte count over 5,000/mcL. Anemia and/or thrombocytopenia can be present, but significant metabolic abnormalities such as hyperuricemia are not usually seen. Because cell marker studies can be performed on peripheral blood samples, a bone marrow biopsy is not required, (although it can help evaluate the patient's reserve of normal marrow elements). Patients should have a quantitative immunoglobulin analysis to rule out significant hypogammaglobulinemia and a direct Coombs test to rule out the presence of anti-red cell antibodies. Certain viral infections such as mononucleosis and Cytomegalovirus and infection with Toxoplasmosis gondii can sometimes be confused with CLL. These, however, give rise to a **polyclonal** population of lymphocytes, easily documented by cell marker studies.

The **Rai** and **Binet** staging systems are both used to stage CLL. Both define early stage disease (Stages 0 and A, respectively) as isolated blood and bone marrow lymphocytosis. Median survival is greater than 7 years from the time of diagnosis. The presence of lymphadenopathy, splenomegaly, and non-immune anemia or thrombocytopenia indicate advancing disease (Stages IV and C, respectively); median survival in this situation is less than 2 years. Richter's transformation (rare) denotes transformation to a high-grade lymphoma.

Treatment

Early, asymptomatic CLL does not require specific treatment. Autoimmune hemolytic anemia and thrombocytopenia are treated with steroids. Intravenous immunoglobulins (IVIg) may decrease the incidence of recurrent infections in the patient with known hypogammaglobulinemia. Regular immunoglobulin therapy does not appear to prolong survival, but may decrease the need for hospitalization in patients with a history of recurrent serious infections. Advanced stage disease is usually treated on an outpatient basis. Steroids and chlorambucil are the most commonly used drugs; combination chemotherapy is also successful. Younger patients with CLL have undergone bone marrow transplantation in experimental protocols in an attempt to improve long-term survival.

Hemophilia

The **hemophilias** are inherited defects that result in decreased levels of factors VIII (**hemophilia A**) or IX (**hemophilia B** or **Christmas disease**); the two are clinically indistinguishable. Both cause spontaneous hemorrhage into joints (hemarthrosis) and soft tissues, and can produce ongoing hemorrhage after even minor trauma (see also Chapter 8, "Hemostasis, Thrombosis, and Transfusion"). Depending on the amount of coagulant activity, hemophilia is classified as **severe** (less than 1%), **moderate** (1%-5%), or **mild** (greater than 5% coagulant activity). As many as 20% of patients with hemophilia A have antibodies against factor VIII.

Diagnosis

The diagnosis of hemophilia is usually made because of a positive family history. Because the condition is transmitted in a sex-linked, recessive manner, only male patients are typically affected (females are carriers), although an occasional female carrier can have unusually low factor levels, and, very rarely, a homozygous, affected female can be born to a hemophiliac father and a carrier mother. **In patients with mild hemophilia, the family history can be negative.** Severe hemophilia usually leads to spontaneous hemorrhagic manifestations early in life (shortly after infancy), while milder disease may not be apparent until after trauma or an operative procedure.

Complications

Hemarthrosis is the most common spontaneous bleeding complication. Recurrent bleeding into the joints leads to pain and deformity, and often eventually necessitates fusion or replacement. Bleeding within a limb can produce a compartment syndrome, and ecchymoses, retroperitoneal hematomas, troublesome oral or nasal bleeding, and gastrointestinal hemorrhage are all common. Intracranial hemorrhage, which can occur spontaneously or after trauma, is the most common cause of death from bleeding. Because of the need for blood products, as many as three-quarters of patients with hemophilia have evidence of infection with hepatitis B or C, and cirrhosis and the complications of portal hypertension contribute significantly to morbidity and mortality. Patients who received blood products and factor concentrates in the late 1970s and early- to mid-1980s have a high rate of infection with the human immunodeficiency virus, much rarer today; many such patients have died from complications of AIDS.

Most patients with hemophilia have an **elevated partial thromboplastin time (PTT)**, although the prothrombin time (PT) and bleeding times are normal. Patients with mild hemophilia can have a normal PTT. Direct assays of both factors VIII and IX levels can be done to measure the coagulant activity in the patient's blood.

Treatment

"Never make a hemophiliac wait"; a symptomatic patient should be evaluated immediately to prevent loss of life or limb. **Physical examination often underestimates the severity of bleeding.** Factor VIII and IX concentrates are used for treatment with dosage based on weight. Factor concentrates are usually given every 8-12 hours with the goal of reaching 50%-100% of normal coagulant activity. Management of hemarthrosis requires orthopaedic surgery consultation, and any suspicion of a compartment syndrome requires prompt surgical evaluation. If a known hemophiliac is to undergo operation, coagulant levels should be brought to 50%-100% of normal preoperatively, and treatment continued for up to 7 days after operation. Patients with inhibitors (antibodies to factors VIII or IX) may require immunosuppression. *(continued)*

Home factor replacement, given as soon as symptoms appear, has been used with great success. Because of prompt therapy, most young patients with hemophilia do not have the joint deformities seen in the past.

von Willebrand's Disease

von Willebrand's disease refers to a group of heterogeneous hereditary coagulation disorders that arise because of abnormal synthesis or release of von Willebrand factor (vWF) from endothelial cells, a molecule required for platelet adhesion to subendothelial surfaces and stabilization of factor VIII. The most common form of the disease, Type I or "classic" von Willebrand's disease, is inherited as an autosomal dominant trait and thus occurs in both men and women.

von Willebrand's disease characteristically causes mucocutaneous bleeding (epistaxis, gingival bleeding, and menorrhagia) and easy bruisability. **Variability of bleeding, both in the same patient and in the patient's family, is characteristic of the disease.** Therefore, while bleeding after surgery, childbirth, or dental extractions is common, the patient may not have a consistent bleeding history. Laboratory findings are also variable; thus, if the clinical situation is suggestive despite a negative workup, laboratory testing should be repeated at a later time.

The bleeding time, **a measure of platelet function**, is often prolonged in von Willebrand's disease. The coagulant property of factor VIII (termed factor VIIIC), stabilized by vWF, may be reduced, and the PTT is often (but not always) elevated. Ristocetin, a clinically obsolete antibiotic that causes platelet aggregation in the presence of von Willebrand's factor, can be used for diagnosis.

von Willebrand's disease can be treated with cryoprecipitate (which contains vWF) or factor VIII products "contaminated" with vWF. Patients with Type I von Willebrand's disease, in which secretion of normal vWF is impaired, may respond to DDAVP (an analog of vasopressin) which stimulates release of vWF from endothelial cells, although in a less common form of von Willebrand's disease, type IIB, it can cause abnormal platelet aggregation and is therefore contraindicated. ■

18 **Infectious Diseases**

Fever and infection are common problems in almost every field of medicine, and several relevant issues, including the inappropriate overuse of antibiotics, have emerged among the most pressing problems in medicine today. This chapter focuses on the basic concepts behind the treatment of infections, the use of antibiotics, fever, and several specific infections that are not covered elsewhere. HIV infection and AIDS are covered in the following chapter.

Basic Concepts

Infection and colonization are two very different things. **Colonization** is the mere presence of bacteria, and is thus ubiquitous. A wound can be colonized and heal normally. **Infection**, on the other hand, is defined as the presence of bacteria that are causing a clinically relevant problem. The point at which colonization becomes infection is not sharply delineated, and depends on the virulence of the bacteria themselves, their number, the blood supply to the tissues, the presence of devitalized tissue or a foreign body, the immunologic status of the host, and other factors. For example, a healthy patient with vancomycin-resistant enterococcus (VRE) is simply colonized and not presently at risk. If a true infection develops with this organism, it will be harder to treat, although the **risk** of such an infection developing (all things being equal) is no different than in a person colonized (everybody else) with vancomycin-sensitive enterococcus.

There are several general principles in the treatment of infections. **Antibiotics are dependent on adequate blood flow for delivery to the site of action**. Thus, any dead and devitalized tissue must be removed, and abscesses must be drained (see Chapter 29, "Wounds") before antibiotics can be expected to work. Because the presence of antibiotics in a sample can sterilize it, **cultures should be drawn before antibiotics are started**. In an emergency, however, **antibiotic administration takes priority over obtaining cultures**. Since cultures take time (generally at least 24-48 hours), the offending organism is usually unknown at the time treatment is begun. Start with an educated guess as to the most likely organisms based on the site of infection, epidemiologic data, and so on, and choose antibiotics appropriately. Antibiotics at this point are often "broad-spectrum," that is, designed to kill a variety of bacteria so that there is a high likelihood the bacteria responsible for the current infection will be covered. Later, when identification and specific antibiotic sensitivities are known, coverage can be "narrowed" to target the specific bacterium present. Finally, **antibiotics, like any intervention, have risks**. In addition to cost and the risks of allergic reactions, by altering the normal balance of flora antibiotic use can lead to overgrowth of normally suppressed or resistant strains, producing specific (pseudomembranous colitis; see Chapter 22, "Gastroenterology") or resistant infections (vancomycin-resistant enterococcus).

Fever

The hallmark of an infection is **fever**, generally defined in an adult as a temperature greater than or equal to 38.0° Celsius. **Fever does not always imply infection is present, and infection is not always heralded by fever**. Fever is caused by **pyrogens**, either **exogenous** (produced by the pathogen) or **endogenous** (produced by the host). The best-known exogenous pyrogen is **endotoxin** or **lipopolysaccharide** (**LPS**), a soluble product of many Gram negative bacteria. There are many endogenous pyrogens, mostly **cytokines**, substances released by immunocompetent cells (often macrophages; see Chapters 4, "Response to Injury," and 10, "Immunology"). The most important are interleukins-1 (IL-1) and -6 (IL-6) and tumor necrosis factor (TNF); TNF and IL-1 seem to be the mediators of endotoxin-induced septic shock. Cytokines are released in generalized inflammatory states and in response to neoplasms also. The mechanism of fever production by cytokines is not known, but they most likely cause release of prostaglandins in the anterior hypothalamus, increasing the body's thermoregulatory setpoint.

Fever probably evolved because parts of the immune system act more efficiently at higher temperatures. The costs to the patient, however, such as increased myocardial work due to tachycardia and increased oxygen and energy consumption, are high. **The best treatment for fever is** to treat the source, but numerous methods exist to acutely lower the temperature. Aspirin and nonsteroidal anti-inflammatory drugs (NSAIDs) block prostaglandin E_2 (PGE_2), which seems to be the molecular messenger for fever at the level of the hypothalamus; acetaminophen (Tylenol) and steroids can also reduce fever.

Sepsis & SIRS

Sepsis is the clinical syndrome of overwhelming bacteremia; if a clear infectious focus is not found, the patient is said to have **systemic inflammatory response syndrome (SIRS**; see Chapter 4, "Response to Injury"). Clinical manifestations of both are caused by cytokines released as part of the host's response to an insult, whether bacterial endotoxin (sepsis), or trauma, tissue ischemia, or other, non-infectious insult (SIRS). The syndromes are characterized, in part, by inappropriate systemic vasodilation and increased capillary permeability, resulting in edema, relative hypovolemia, tissue hypoperfusion, and hypoxia. **Infected patients, especially if elderly, can present with altered mental status and hypothermia**, and septic patients characteristically develop metabolic acidosis caused by lactic acid.

Specific, localizing symptoms suggest specific infections. **Common causes of fever in outpatients** include viral illnesses, urinary tract infections (UTIs), pulmonary infections such as pneumonia or infected pleural effusions (bronchitis rarely causes fever), skin infections such as cellulitis, wound infections, or decubitus ulcers, and bacteremia from any source. Meningitis and encephalitis, although less common, are life-threatening illness and should be suspected in any febrile patient with headache, stiff neck, cranial nerve abnormalities, or mental status changes. **Empiric antibiotics** (that is, antibiotics given when the source of infection is not definitively known) **can be started in this situation** based on an educated guess as to the likely source combined with knowledge of the patterns of organisms and their sensitivities within the community. Patients with relapsed or recurrent infections should be cultured before antibiotics are started.

General treatment

Some patients require hospital admission, either for administration of IV antibiotics or because they are "too sick" to go home (which usually implies the need for IV antibiotics). The decision to admit a previously healthy febrile patient to the hospital is based on the degree and duration of the fever, the site of the infection, the ability of the patient to take adequate fluids by mouth, the need for operative intervention (such as drainage of an abscess or removal of an organ), the presence of hemodynamic instability or severe pain, and confidence in the clinical diagnosis. **The empiric use of antibiotics in those admitted to the hospital should be avoided in most stable patients**. In this situation, empiric antibiotics decrease the "true-positive" rate of cultures, change the body's flora, risk selecting resistant organisms, and confound the diagnosis: did the patient get better because of or despite the antibiotics? **Ideally, a stable, admitted patient should be fully cultured and worked up before antibiotics are started**.

Several groups of patients **should** receive antibiotics right away. First, obviously, are those in whom the diagnosis of a problem requiring antibiotics is clear. Also, patients with suspected meningitis and those who are septic, "toxic," hemodynamically unstable, or who are immuno-suppressed (including those who are receiving immuno-suppressive medication) require antibiotics as soon as possible. Unusual pathogens, such as mycobacteria, fungi, and viruses (particularly cytomegalovirus), should be considered in immunosuppressed patients.

Although infection is by far the most common cause of fever, many other conditions can be associated with temperature elevation, including collagen vascular diseases, solid and hematologic tumors, drug reactions, and granulomatous diseases such as sarcoidosis or Crohn's disease.

Fevers in inpatients

Patients **hospitalized for other problems** who develop fevers pose additional problems. A careful review of the hospital course, including procedures and medications received, will often suggest the culprit. Fever the first 48-72 hours after a surgical procedure is common and almost always due to pulmonary atelectasis; such a fever requires no specific treatment other than efforts to expand the lungs and bring up secretions ("pulmonary toilet"). Any indwelling device significantly increases the risk of infection in the body cavity (i.e., bladder) or device itself (central venous catheter). Febrile episodes are commonly the result of drug reactions and can be the only manifestation of a transfusion reaction. Fever and diarrhea in a patient who has received antibiotics raises the possibility of pseudomembranous colitis, and fever in a patient with any fluid collection suggests infection of the collection. Most infections in hospitalized patients arise from their own flora, often altered as the result of treatment and a variety of other factors. Hospitals, unfortunately, teem with bacteria, and essentially every patient, if hospitalized long enough, will develop a nosocomial infection.

FUO

The diagnosis and treatment of **persistent fever** or **fever of unknown origin** (**FUO**) in a patient who has been cultured and maintained on a reasonable antibiotic regimen includes incorrect identification of the source, inadequate antibiotic coverage, a closed-space infection or infected foreign body, endocarditis, a non-infectious source for the fever, or a drug fever from the antibiotics. This situation can obviously be difficult to sort out. Repeat cultures, including **cultures of any abnormal fluid collections** should be obtained, all catheters and other devices that enter the body should be changed and cultured, the patient's record and hospital course carefully reviewed, and formal infectious disease service consultation considered. In this situation it is often useful to stop all antibiotics, not only to prove or disprove the presence of drug fever, but also to increase the culture yield and allow the problem to "declare itself."

Antibiotics

Antibiotics can be used in a prophylactic or therapeutic sense. **Prophylactic** antibiotics, by definition, are used to prevent an infection that has not yet occurred; the classic example is an antibiotic given before an operation. To be used correctly, the antibiotic has to be effective against the expected organism(s), and **adequate tissue levels must be present at the time infection is likely to occur**. In practical terms the antibiotic must be given **before** the operation begins. **Therapeutic** antibiotics, on the other hand, are those given when an infection already exists (or is thought to exist). Antibiotics are generally classified as **bactericidal** if they kill living bacteria, and **bacteriostatic** if they merely prevent further growth and/or replication. Four basic classes of antibiotics exist.

Mechanisms of action

First, there are antibiotics that **attack the cell wall**. These are bactericidal and generally effective against Gram positive bacteria. Many have a beta-lactam ring, including

Medicine
Infectious Diseases *continued*

penicillin, ampicillin, methicillin, the cephalosporins, Imipenem, and aztreonam. Many bacteria, especially Staphylococcus, produce enzymes that attack the ring (beta-lactamases); oxacillin and methicillin, resistant to this enzyme, are useful against such bacteria, as is vancomycin, a non-beta-lactam antibiotic in this class. Second, many antibiotics **inhibit the ribosomal phase of protein synthesis**. This group is less homogeneous, and includes the aminoglycosides, erythromycin, clindamycin, and tetracycline. Third, the sulfa drugs, including trimethoprim-sulfamethoxazole (TMP-SMX; Bactrim) act as **inhibitors of folic acid**, and, fourth, several drugs such as metronidazole and ciprofloxacin act by **inhibiting DNA synthesis**.

Bacteria, being prokaryocytes, are relatively easy to selectively kill. For example, not only do they have cell walls (which human cells do not), but their ribosomes and DNA structure are different from ours. Unfortunately, fungi are much more similar to human cells and are more difficult to selectively harm. Amphotericin is the "gold-standard" antifungal agent, but is quite toxic. There is accumulating evidence that fluconazole, a well-tolerated drug, may be equally effective. Antiviral chemotherapy is fairly limited, although acyclovir and gancyclovir are effective against herpes simplex and varicella zoster viruses and cytomegalovirus, respectively.

Antibiotic usage varies widely depending on institutional preferences and organism susceptibility, but a simplified, general scheme for remembering antibiotic choices is helpful:

Organism/ Situation	"Classic" Antibiotics	Alternatives for Resistant Organisms
Gram positives	Penicillin, 1st generation cephalosporins	
Staph aureus	Methicillin oxacillin	Vancomycin (ORSA)
Staph epidermidis	Vancomycin	
Enterococcus	Ampicillin, vancomycin	NONE (VRE)
Gram negatives	Aminoglycosides, aztreonam, 3rd generation. cephalosporins, ciprofloxacin	
Pseudomonas	Antipseudomonal PCN and aminoglycoside	
Anaerobes	Metronidazole, clindamycin, ampicillin-sulbactam	
"Triple coverage"	Ampicillin, gentamicin, and metronidazole	
"Broad spectrum"	Imipenem, timentin	
Fungi	Fluconazole, amphotericin	
Surgical prophylaxis "Skin" Bowel/biliary	1st generation cephalosporin 2nd generation cephalosporin (see Chapter 32, "Colon and rectum")	

Sanford's *Guide to Antimicrobial Therapy*, updated and published every year and distributed free of charge by a variety of pharmaceutical companies, has become the pocket "bible" of infectious diseases for the non-specialist. It is incredibly detailed, covers every conceivable situation, and is one of the very few books (other than this one) that every physician caring for acutely ill patients should have in their pockets at all times.

Some Specific Infections

UTI

A **urinary tract infection (UTI)** is defined as the presence of bacteria in the urine. UTIs are divided clinically into lower and upper tract infections. Lower tract infections include **urethritis**, **cystitis**, **prostatitis**, and **epididymitis**, while upper tract infection is synonymous with **pyelonephritis**, an inflammatory process of the renal parenchyma itself. The classic "rule of thumb" (in adults) is that a UTI associated with fever indicates pyelonephritis, while one without fever indicates the presence of a lower tract infection. Signs and symptoms of cystitis include dysuria, frequency, urgency, suprapubic pain, and, at times, hematuria. Men with epididymitis classically present with testicular pain, and those with prostatitis often complain of perineal pain and discomfort. Pyelonephritis, on the other hand, classically causes fever, shaking chills, and costovertebral angle pain and tenderness.

Obviously, the urinalysis, Gram stain, and culture are the basis for diagnosis. Sterile pyuria (leukocytes without bacteria) suggests urethritis, but can also be seen with a foreign body or tumor of the urinary tract. Cystitis and pyelonephritis usually cause pyuria and bacteriuria. The responsible organisms most commonly arise from perineal and fecal flora, typically Gram negative bacteria; E. coli accounts for about 80% of all UTIs. Any of the antibiotics active against Gram negative bacteria can be used, although pyelonephritis may require IV administration (see also Chapter 64, "ED Gynecology" for a discussion of the the treatment of sexually-transmitted diseases, and Chapter 56, "Pediatric Nephrology" for additional information on UTIs in children).

Pneumonia

Although usually easy to recognize and treat, **pneumonia** still is associated with significant morbidity and mortality, because it often strikes patients who are already critically ill or otherwise immunosuppressed. Pneumonia is an infection of the lung parenchyma caused by microorganisms that have been inhaled, aspirated, or acquired via

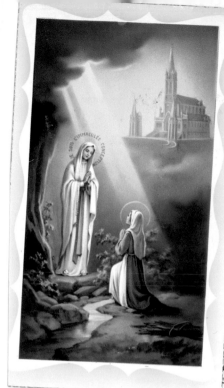

The hallmark for diagnosis is an
am-stained sputum specimen and
d sputum sample can be distin-
vhich is of no use for diagnosis) by
in the former and epithelial cells

d bacterial pneumonia is usually
pneumoniae (pneumococcus),
zae, or mixed normal flora.
aphylococcus aureus or Klebsiella
ess often. Pneumococcal pneumonia
winter and early spring, in otherwise
present with a single, "teeth-chatter-
luctive cough, and pleuritic chest
s most frequent in the winter and
ds to a slowly progressive and milder
cal pneumonia commonly occurs
n; affected patients usually present
pain and multiple chills, and the
c. Finally, Klebsiella pneumonia usu-
ts debilitated by alcohol, diabetes, or
e; the right upper lobe is the most
common ection because it is the most dependent
portion if aspiration occurs while supine, an event common to many of these patients.

"**Atypical pneumonia**" refers to pneumonia in the
absence of leukocytosis. The term is usually used to
denote pneumonia caused by Mycoplasma ("walking
pneumonia"), but technically also refers also to that
caused by Legionella ("Legionnaires' Disease") and
Chlamydia. All are gradual in onset; patients present with
low-grade fevers, nonproductive cough, headache, and
myalgias. The respiratory exam is typically unrevealing.
Legionnaires' disease commonly occurs in the summer;
air conditioners are a primary source of infection. Patients
classically present with a one day prodrome of myalgia
and headache; severe illness and even death can occur.
Chlamydia occurs most commonly in college students,
adolescents, military recruits, and the elderly.

Hospital-acquired pneumonias are typically caused by
resistant or unusual organisms in patients who are
immunosuppressed, critically ill, malnourished, or require

mechanical ventilation. The widespread use of antacids and H$_2$-receptor blockers (see Chapter 34, "Peptic Ulcer Disease") have unquestionably lowered the incidence of stress ulceration and hemorrhage, but, by increasing gastric pH, allow bacterial overgrowth in the normally sterile stomach. Because repeated, low-level aspiration of gastric contents occurs in any patient with an endotracheal tube, some believe that this has led to higher rates of iatrogenic pneumonia. Broad-spectrum antibiotics, including those active against Pseudomonas, may be required for a patient with hospital-acquired pneumonia.

Some **viruses** cause pneumonia, including influenza A, parainfluenza, and respiratory syncitial virus. Viral pneumonia itself tends to be relatively innocuous, but since the very young and the elderly are at highest risk, outcome can be poor. Problems may be due to superimposed bacterial pneumonia rather than to the virus, per se.

Soft tissue infections

The major **soft tissue infection** of clinical relevance is **cellulitis**, an infection of the connective tissue. By definition, no hypoperfused "pocket" of necrosis (**abscess**) exists. Blood supply, in fact, is excellent, and response to antibiotics is usually prompt. Cellulitis presents as an area of **erythema**, **warmth**, and **pain**. If bacteria extend proximally up the lymphatics, red streaks are seen (**lymphangitis**). There may be a history of a previous wound (traumatic or surgical), but this can be absent. **Erysipelas** is a superficial cellulitis with prominent lymphatic involvement; Staph and Strep are the most common causative organisms. Cellulitis, lymphangitis, and erysipelas usually respond to penicillins or early-generation cephalosporins within a day or so. An important exception is cellulitis (or any other infection or wound) in a poorly-perfused lower extremity, which will not heal until the blood supply is improved (see Chapter 37, "Vascular Surgery").

Necrotizing cellulitis is a virulent infection superficial to the fascia, usually caused by group A Streptococci, recently sensationalized in the lay press as "flesh-eating bacteria." **Necrotizing fasciitis** is infection involving the fascia, and is often caused by group A Streptococci or mixed flora, including anaerobes. **Clostridial myonecrosis**, or "gas gangrene," is a true anaerobic necrosis of the muscle and is very rare today. All three of these are extremely rapidly-moving infections that require surgical debridement of **all** infected tissue, up to and including amputation. Most such infections are sensitive to the penicillins (and anti-anaerobic drugs, if applicable) **provided that adequate operative debridement has taken place.**

Meningitis

Meningitis is inflammation of the meninges; fever, headache, a change in mental status, and nuchal rigidity or resistance to passive movement are the hallmarks of this disease. Bacterial meningitis is a severe and often fatal disease; if suspected, a lumbar puncture for examination of cerebrospinal fluid (CSF) is required. Typical CSF findings include a high white blood cell count with a high number of segmented cells, and high protein and low glucose levels. The most common causative organisms include Streptococcus pneumoniae, Neisseria meningitidis, Listeria, and Hemophilus influenzae; ampicillin and a 3rd generation cephalosporin are typically used for treatment. ■

19 **HIV Infection and Acquired Immunodeficiency Syndrome**

N.B.: The practice of medicine is constantly changing; no field is currently as fluid as that of the study and treatment of HIV disease. This chapter reflects knowledge and opinions as of early 1996, and the reader is cautioned always to pursue information from the most contemporary sources. As one reviewer put it, "some things here change by the minute."

Millions of people throughout the world are infected with the **human immunodeficiency virus (HIV)**, the virus that causes **acquired immunodeficiency syndrome (AIDS)**. The disease was first recognized as a specific syndrome in 1983 in homosexual men. Since then, other high-risk groups that have been identified include intravenous drug users who share needles, people who received contaminated blood products, and children born to mothers with HIV infection. The risk of acquiring HIV infection in health care workers is low and has generally occurred after deep intramuscular injection with contaminated hollow needles; there have also been rare cases of patients acquiring infection from their health care providers. **Heterosexual transmission is rapidly increasing in frequency**; in Africa, the country with the highest incidence of HIV infection, heterosexual transmission is the most common route of infection. Transmission via contaminated blood products is extremely rare in the US today, recently estimated at 1 per 500,000-1,000,000 units transfused.

HIV is transmitted by contact with blood and, less often, other body fluids. A variety of other factors, not all of which are understood, play a role in acquisition of the virus and development of the disease.

Pathogenesis of HIV Infection

HIV is a **retrovirus** that codes for an RNA-dependent DNA polymerase, thereby causing incorporation of the viral RNA into the host's DNA. The virus enters and injures cells of the hematopoietic system (primarily CD4 T lymphocytes and macrophages; see Chapter 10, "Immunology"), brain, and skin; colon and kidney cells have also been found to have virus particles within them. By entering and depleting the host lymphocytes, the virus causes impaired **cellular** immunity which is the primary reason for the high prevalence of (eventually fatal) infectious and neoplastic complications that characterize HIV infection and AIDS.

Diagnosis of HIV Infection

HIV testing, risk assessment, and risk reduction are all areas that should routinely be addressed as part of health maintenance in healthy patients. People with known risk factors or who suspect their partner(s) might have participated in high-risk behavior should be encouraged to be tested for HIV infection. Pre-test counseling is important, and ideally should take the form of a dialogue between patient and provider. After explaining the risks and benefits of testing, the provider should allow the patient to ask questions and express concerns and fears. It is important for the provider to ask "what will you do if the test is positive?" and "with whom will you share the news?" After blood is obtained, a followup appointment is scheduled to discuss the test results. Sharing the news by phone, whether positive or negative, is inappropriate. If the test is positive, it is essential to allow the patient time to react and ask questions. If negative but risk is believed to be high, the patient should be counseled again and retested 3 and 6 months later.

Diagnosis

The diagnosis of HIV infection is made by detecting antibodies to the virus, first with an **enzyme-linked immunoabsorbent assay (ELISA)** and then with a confirmatory **Western blot** (98% sensitive and 99.8% specific in combination). Measurement of viral nucleic acids by means of polymerase chain reaction (PCR) and measurement of the surface **antigen p24** are useful if results are needed immediately after presumed infection (100% sensitive within 18 days of infection). At the time of diagnosis, lymphocyte subset counts should be drawn to assess levels and establish a baseline, if normal.

HIV versus AIDS

A patient who is found to have antibodies to the virus, PCR positivity, or p24 antigenemia is **infected with HIV, but does not (necessarily) have AIDS. AIDS is a syndrome defined by the presence of specific features occurring in an HIV-positive person; the patient does**

not have AIDS until there is a history of characteristic infections or other diseases, termed "AIDS-defining illnesses." Examples are Pneumocystis carinii pneumonia, candidiasis of the esophagus, trachea, or bronchi, tuberculosis, cytomegalovirus (CMV) retinitis, recurrent bacterial pneumonia, progressive multifocal leukoencephalopathy, lymphoma, Kaposi's sarcoma, and wasting syndrome. As of early 1996 it is believed that essentially every person with HIV infection will eventually develop AIDS, although there is a small group of people who have been HIV-positive since 1980 and still have CD4 counts of more than 500.

Clinical Manifestations of HIV Infection and AIDS

Once an acute and rapidly fatal disease that was often diagnosed shortly before death, AIDS now behaves in a much more chronic fashion. Antiretroviral therapy, prophylaxis against common infections, clinical expertise, and other advances have improved the quality and length of life in patients with AIDS.

Clinical manifestations of HIV disease depend on the stage of infection. Many patients (50%-93%) will have an acute illness at the time of seroconversion; this is called **primary HIV infection** and typically occurs 2-4 weeks after infection takes place. The most common symptoms (fever, lethargy, malaise, myalgias, photophobia, lymphadenopathy, and rash) are nonspecific and reflect the tendency of the virus to infect the lymphocytic and neurologic cells of the host. The illness may be confused with mononucleosis, viral hepatitis, and other acute infectious processes. Since the antibody test is usually negative at that time, the great majority of patients are not diagnosed at the time of primary HIV infection. When patients do eventually seek medical care, symptoms usually depend on the degree of immunodeficiency present. It is not unusual for patients to present with CD4 counts of less than 50, indicating advanced disease.

Because of impairment in both cellular and humoral immunity, common complications of HIV disease and AIDS are **opportunistic infections** with fungi, protozoa, and viruses. Herpes zoster is often the first manifestation. Any organ system can be involved, and more than one process can occur in the same patient. The general rule in medicine of trying to find a single, unifying diagnosis to explain all symptoms (Occam's Razor) does not apply in patients with HIV infection. While opportunistic pathogens are very significant, it is important to remember that **common bacterial pathogens are also important causes of morbidity and mortality** in patients with AIDS; with the advent of better prophylactic measure against opportunistic infections, in fact, bacterial pathogens account for a higher proportion of problems. Such infections are associated with higher rates of bacteremia and relapse after appropriate antibiotic treatment than they are in the general population.

Pulmonary Manifestations

In the early years of AIDS, pneumonia caused by the fungus **Pneumocystis carinii** was a common and often rapidly fatal infection; early recognition of P. carinii pneumonia (**PCP**) and long-term prophylaxis, however, have made PCP a much less significant infection. Patients with CD4 cell counts less than 200/mcL require prophylaxis, preferably with trimethoprim-sulfamethoxazole (Bactrim) or dapsone. Patients with PCP typically describe a several-day history of cough, fever, and dyspnea; the organism is identified on silver stain of sputum or bronchoalveolar lavage fluid (pentamidine prophylaxis increases the rate of intrapulmonary infection, thus, transbronchial biopsy can be required). PCP is treated with oral or IV trimethoprim-sulfamethoxazole or intravenous pentamidine; severe hypoxia warrants the addition of steroids.

In addition to PCP, other pulmonary diseases that need to be considered in HIV-positive patients include **bacterial pneumonia, tuberculosis, lymphoma, histoplasmosis, coccidiomycosis, blastomycosis, aspergellosis,** and, rarely, **Kaposi's sarcoma**. Such patients can also develop severe chronic obstructive pulmonary disease.

Gastrointestinal Manifestations

Nausea and anorexia are common complaints in patients with HIV and AIDS. Other common symptoms and signs include oral **candidiasis (thrush), esophagitis, diarrhea, right-upper-quadrant abdominal pain,** and **oral or esophageal lesions** caused by cytomegalovirus (CMV) and herpes simplex virus (HSV). Severe esophagitis occa-

Medicine
HIV Infection and Acquired Immunodeficiency Syndrome *continued*

sionally causes formation of a **tracheoesophageal fistula**, causing recurrent pneumonia. Lymphoma and Kaposi's sarcoma are occasionally found on endoscopy in patients with esophageal disease, and **idiopathic esophageal ulceration** where no pathogen is identified is common.

Pathogens that commonly cause **diarrhea** include cryptosporidium, microsporidia, Mycobacterium avium-intracellulare (MAI), and CMV. Every effort should be made to reach a diagnosis to allow specific therapy. **Malabsorptive** diarrhea can be caused by small bowel lymphoma or Kaposi's sarcoma. AIDS-associated **cholangiopathy**, which leads to jaundice, is usually caused by similar micro-organisms, but the pathogen often goes unidentified.

Neurologic Manifestations

HIV infection can affect the both the central (CNS) and peripheral nervous systems. **Meningitis**, **parenchymal brain lesions**, the **AIDS dementia** complex, **neuropathy**, **myopathy**, and **myelopathy** (e.g. transverse myelitis) can all occur. The virus itself can cause neuropathy and meningitis in the early and late stages of infection, respectively. CMV retinitis causes **blindness** if patients are not treated promptly. Meningitis can also be caused by Cryptococcus neoformans, other fungi, M. tuberculosis, and syphilis. Because of the high risk of mass lesions within the brain in these patients, a stable patient with neurologic symptoms should undergo head CT before a lumbar puncture is performed.

Cerebral mass lesions common in patients with HIV and AIDS include **cerebral toxoplasmosis, central nervous system lymphoma, crytococcomas,** and **abscesses**. Radiographic appearance and cerebral spinal fluid analysis, unfortunately, are not always helpful in making the diagnosis, although a new radionuclide scan is promising. In a patient with antibodies to toxoplasmosis and a ring-enhancing lesion on CT, anti-toxoplasmosis therapy (primarily with pyrimethamine and sulfadiazine) can be started and the patient followed with serial CT scans over 1-2 weeks; corticosteroids should not be given because they might produce a response if the cause is lymphoma, thus confusing the picture. **Encephalitis** from herpes viruses and varicella-zoster virus are unusual but can also occur. **Progressive multifocal leukoencephalopathy**, most likely caused by a papovavirus (JC virus), is a rare, and, as yet untreatable complication of AIDS.

The **AIDS dementia complex** usually occurs in patients who have had opportunistic infections but can occur before the appearance of other systemic manifestations of AIDS (i.e., as an "AIDS-defining illness" in a person who, thus far, has only been considered "HIV-positive"). Such patients develop cognitive, motor, and behavioral dysfunction. Symptoms include forgetfulness and difficulty concentrating, clumsiness, ataxia, motor slowing, altered personality, and, in later stages, global dementia, paraplegia, and mutism, and is often preceded by seizures of unexplained etiology (presumably due to HIV itself). Treatment with high doses of antiretroviral agents such as zidovudine (AZT) can improve symptoms.

Neuropathy in patients with AIDS can be due to the effects of the virus itself, to those of other viruses such as HSV and CMV, or, commonly, as a side effect of treatment. Patients usually experience painful burning in their feet (causalgia) occasionally associated with sensory loss. **CMV retinitis** occurs in up to a quarter of patients with advanced AIDS. Regular ophthalmoscopy is helpful, and any patient with AIDS who has visual complaints, particularly those with low CD4 counts (less than 50 cells/mcL), should undergo immediate ophthalmoscopic examination. Treatment with ganciclovir or foscarnet is effective. Retinal abnormalities recur if treatment is discontinued, so lifelong therapy is mandatory.

Hematologic Manifestations

HIV has **direct myelosuppressive effects** on the bone marrow, thereby causing depression of white cell, red cell, and platelet counts. **Infiltration of the bone marrow from infectious or neoplastic processes** will further decrease cell counts. Bone marrow culture and microscopic examination can be helpful in making the diagnosis of Mycobacterium avium-complex (MAC), Pneumocystis carinii, and parvovirus B19, but are usually not helpful if a lymphoma or other malignancy is present. MAC and parvovirus B19 are often associated with isolated anemia.
(continued)

Medicine
HIV Infection and Acquired
Immunodeficiency Syndrome *continued*

HIV-associated thrombocytopenia was one of the earliest recognized complications of HIV infection. This is an immune-mediated peripheral destructive process caused by platelet-associated antibodies; the marrow responds appropriately by producing more megakaryocytes. Therapeutic options in the treatment of HIV-associated thrombocytopenia include steroids (which must be used with caution because of the further risk of immunosuppression), intravenous immunoglobulin therapy, splenectomy or splenic radiation, and the antiretroviral drug zidovudine.

Many of the medications used in the treatment of patients with AIDS cause **iatrogenic myelosuppression**. The antiretroviral agents can all cause myelosuppression, as can ganciclovir, an agent used in the treatment of CMV retinitis, and trimethoprim-sulfamethoxazole, pentamidine, and antineoplastic agents. The development of colony-stimulating factors (e.g., erythropoetin and granulocyte-colony stimulating factor; G-CSF) has allowed the ongoing use of such myelosuppressive medications in patients with cytopenias related to HIV or to the drugs themselves.

Cutaneous Manifestations

Patients with HIV infection and AIDS have striking problems with pruritis, dry skin, and a variety of cutaneous complications. They often develop recurrent skin infections of the hair follicles (**folliculitis**) with Staphylococcus aureus; the face, trunk, and groin are common sites. Other common dermatologic manifestations of AIDS include **herpes zoster** (**shingles**) and **molluscum contagiosum**. Less common are **bacillary angiomatosis** and **Kaposi's sarcoma** (**KS**). KS, now believed to be caused by a newly described herpes virus (KHSV or HHV8), is far less common now than in the early 1980s.

HIV-Associated Malignancies

Malignancy arising in the setting of HIV infection can be viewed as "**opportunistic**," arising and proliferating because of **defective host immunity**. While there is a slight increase in many types of malignancy in patients infected with HIV, the most commonly seen malignancies are **Kaposi's sarcoma, lymphoma,** and **anogenital malignancies** such as invasive cervical carcinoma.

Kaposi's sarcoma in AIDS is much more common in homosexual men than in IV drug users, probably because KHSV is a sexually transmitted virus. KS can be confined to the skin or involve visceral organs such as the lung or GI tract. Cutaneous KS presents as raised, purple-colored lesions ranging in size from millimeters to a centimeter or so. Oral lesions are common. Lymphatic obstruction is also common, and can cause painful edema of the lower extremities and, occasionally, the arms and face. Therapeutic options include radiation, laser ablation, systemic chemotherapy, cryotherapy, and intralesional injection of vinblastine, a vinca alkaloid chemo-therapeutic agent.

Up to 95% of **non-Hodgkin's lymphomas** in HIV-positive patients arise in extranodal sites. Patients with relatively high CD4 counts can be affected. Response rates to chemotherapy are much lower than in non-HIV-infected patients, remission duration is generally shorter, and concurrent cytopenia often makes the use of standard-dose chemotherapy difficult. CNS lymphoma is usually best treated with cranial radiation, although many such patients are so debilitated that specific treatment is not rational. **Cervical neoplasia** is much more common in HIV-infected women; those with concurrent human papilloma virus (HPV) infection are at especially high risk. Most patients with AIDS and cervical neoplasia do not develop true invasive cervical carcinoma, most likely because of the long period of time (years; see Chapter 66, "Gynecologic Malignancies") required for its development.
(continued)

Health Maintenance of the HIV-Infected Patient

When the diagnosis of HIV infection is made, the patient should be seen by a health care provider familiar with the care of HIV-infected patients. Emotional needs and coping mechanisms should be addressed.

CD4 count

In the absence of symptoms, therapy is guided by the CD4 count. Patients with CD4 counts **greater than 500cells/mcL** should be seen approximately every 6 months; CD4 counts are checked at each visit. As the count falls closer to 500, repeat counts should be done every 2-3 months. Once the CD4 count falls **below 500**, antiretroviral therapy with zidovudine (AZT) should be started at a dose of 500-600 mg each day in divided doses (e.g,. 200 mg three times a day). The patient should be seen after 2-3 weeks to assess side effects (headache, nausea, and insomnia, among others), for which symptomatic treatment is usually adequate, and return for followup visits every 2-3 months. Liver function and blood counts should be checked at each visit; anemia, granulocytopenia, or myopathy (manifest as proximal muscle weakness and wasting) require dose reduction or a change in therapy. The CD4 count is checked every 6 months; more frequently as it approaches 200cells/mcL. When the CD4 count falls **below 200**, PCP prophylaxis is started. If thrush or systemic complaints occur before the CD4 count drops to 200, PCP prophylaxis should be considered.

Immunizations

Immunizations for adult HIV-positive patients can help reduce the likelihood of acquiring common viral and bacterial illnesses. Patients should receive Pneumovax (active against Streptococcal pneumoniae), influenza, hepatitis B, and possibly the measles, mumps, and rubella (MMR) vaccination (although this is a live virus). **Yearly PPD** skin testing should be done until the patient becomes anergic (an area of induration measuring 5mm or more is considered positive in an HIV-positive patient). **Yearly or twice-yearly Papanicolaou (Pap) smear testing** (see Chapter 66, Gynecologic Malignancies) for cervical dysplasia should be done in women with HIV infection, and sexually active patients are tested for sexually transmitted diseases including syphilis, gonorrhea, and chlamydia (see Chapter 64, ED Gynecology).

The topic of **antiretroviral therapy**, although important, is so labile and, at times, controversial that it will not be discussed further in this text. The reader is urged to pursue currently evolving information on this topic.

Pediatric HIV Infection and AIDS

"Pediatric" HIV infection and AIDS are defined as those involving children under 13; current estimates are that between 15-20,000 children are infected in this country. Most acquire the disease by vertical transmission during labor and delivery, less often by intrauterine infection, and nearly all the rest, via contaminated blood products. **Early detection of HIV infection greatly improves longevity and quality of life.**

Maternal HIV antibodies are passively transferred to the neonate, making **ELISA and Western blot testing falsely-positive;** viral culture or PCR are preferred in children under 18 months of age. Transmission is affected by poorly characterized factors; only 23% -35% of infants born to HIV-positive women develop the infection.

The diagnosis of HIV infection in infants and children born to mothers without known infection requires a high index of suspicion. **HIV infection should be suspected in any child with symptoms or signs suggestive of immunodeficiency**. Identification of risk factors (in both parents and children) is crucial. **Persistent mucocutaneous candidiasis with failure to thrive is a common early presentation**; generalized lymphadenopathy and hepatomegaly are also common. Recurrent bacterial or opportunistic infection, lymphoid interstitial pneumonia, and developmental delay with or without milestone regression can also be seen. Children infected at birth have a shorter incubation period and more rapid disease progression than do individuals infected later in life. In contrast, children infected by transfusion of contaminated blood products or shared bodily fluids have an inverse relationship between age at seroconversion and time to onset of symptoms—children infected at a younger age have a longer incubation period. The absolute CD4 count is less useful in infants, and infections can occur when the CD4 count is high.
(continued)

Medicine
HIV Infection and Acquired Immunodeficiency Syndrome *continued*

Infectious problems in children are similar to those in adults. PCP is a common pulmonary pathogen, although viruses and bacteria are also common. **Diarrhea** can be caused by Salmonella, Shigella, Campylobacter, MAI, Clostridium difficile, CMV, rotaviruses, adenoviruses, cryptosporidium, Isospora belli, Giardia, and microspordia, although the pathogen causing the diarrhea may never be identified.

Neurologic manifestations, ranging from mild developmental delay to HIV encephalopathy, are nearly universal in children, although secondary infections and CNS tumors are less common than in adults. Encephalopathy can be stable or chronically progressive, and can be associated with weakness, microcephaly, seizures, and ataxia. **AIDS-associated cardiomyopathy** is the most prominent cardiac manifestation of AIDS in children. The dilated cardiomyopathy can lead to heart failure, arrhythmias, and sudden death. **AIDS-associated malignancies** are rare; as survival in HIV-infected children improves, an increase in the incidence of opportunistic malignancies might occur.

Issues surrounding the use of **antiretroviral agents** are similar to those in adults. **Vaccination recommendations** are complicated by the observation that vaccine-related measles pneumonia and non-paralytic poliomyelitis have developed in children with immune system suppression given live vaccines. The inactivated polio virus vaccine (IPV) should be administered to HIV-positive children instead of the commonly used live vaccine (OPV), although there is no adequate substitute for the MMR. Pneumococcal and influenza vaccination are recommended only for children with symptomatic HIV infection.

Prophylaxis for PCP (trimethoprim-sulfamethoxazole) should begin at age 4-6 weeks in all children born to HIV-positive women (before that time, risk is low), and continue through age 12 months in HIV-infected children. After 12 months, the decision to continue prophylaxis is based on CD4 counts and previous history of PCP. Inhaled pentamidine can be used in children older than 5 if trimethoprim-sulfamethoxazole is not tolerated. ■

20   Neurology

Neurology is the study of diseases of the central and peripheral nervous systems. The most commonly encountered problems include stroke, seizures, dementia and delirium, peripheral neuropathy, headache, and vertigo.

Stroke

A **stroke** (or **cerebrovascular accident, CVA**) refers to a disorder of the cerebral circulation that results in damage to the brain. Stroke is categorized as **ischemic** (resulting from decreased blood flow) or **hemorrhagic** (actual bleeding into the brain). Ischemic strokes are subdivided by etiology into embolic, thrombotic, and hypoperfusion types, while hemorrhagic strokes are subdivided on the basis of location into subarachnoid and intracerebral hemorrhage.

Embolism

An **embolic stroke** can present in one of several ways. A transient ischemic attack (TIA) is a set of focal or global neurologic deficits that resolve within 24 hours. A true stroke can resolve fully, but usually results in a permanent deficit. Onset of symptoms is usually sudden, and deficits are usually focal. The CT scan can be initially normal, but hypodense lesions are usually seen if the scan is performed later than 24 hours or so. Sources of emboli include carotid artery atherosclerosis or cardiac mural thrombus from atrial fibrillation or ventricular aneurysm. TIAs are commonly precursors to true stroke, and their presence should lead to aggressive investigation of possible sources, starting with the carotid arteries. Patients with 60% or greater narrowing of the carotid artery, whether symptomatic or not, have been shown to have a higher risk of stroke if the atherosclerotic plaque is not removed surgically (see Chapter 37, "Vascular Surgery").

Thrombosis

Large artery **thrombosis** usually injures the cortex and is manifest by "stuttering," stepwise, focal symptomatology. Small vessel thrombosis (more common if hypertension or diabetes are present) can also produce fluctuating symptoms, but often involve deeper brain structures such as the basal ganglia, cerebral white matter, thalamus, pons, or cerebellum. Lacunar infarcts can produce pure motor hemiplegia (pons, internal capsule), pure sensory deficits (thalamus), clumsy hand-dysarthria (pons, internal capsule), or ataxic hemiparesis (pons, internal capsule), depending on the area injured.

Hypoperfusion

Hypoperfusion strokes occur in patients with compromised delivery of oxygenated blood to the brain, most often after cardiac arrest or hypotensive episodes. The "watershed areas," or regions between the major arteries with most tenuous blood supply, are most often involved.

Hemorrhagic

A hemorrhagic stroke results from intracranial bleeding. A **subarachnoid hemorrhage** occurs in patients with hypertension, coagulopathies, drug use, or an intracerebral aneurysm. Onset of symptoms is usually sudden and can occur at times of exertion or during sleep. Symptoms include severe headache (the hallmark of the diagnosis), vomiting, confusion and/or loss of consciousness; there may be no focal deficit. CT scan will usually demonstrate subarachnoid blood, but a lumbar puncture should be done if the scan is negative and suspicion is high.

As with subarachnoid hemorrhage, an **intracerebral hemorrhage** can occur in patients with hypertension, a coagulopathy, or amyloid angiopathy. Symptoms develop gradually and may include headache, nausea, vomiting, altered mental status and/or seizures. Hemorrhage may involve the ventricles. CT reveals hyperdense lesions corresponding to intraparenchymal blood.

Diagnosis

Diagnosis of a stroke begins with an appropriate level of suspicion based on presenting complaints. A thorough history and general physical exam is essential, with particular attention to the cardiac and vascular systems. A complete neurologic exam entails evaluation of mental status, speech and language, memory, cranial, motor, and sensory nerve function, coordination, and reflexes, with the objective of pinpointing the site of damage. Strokes affecting the anterior circulation (anterior and middle cerebral arteries) commonly produce deficits such as hemiparesis, hemiplegia, hemisensory loss, homonymous hemianopsia, aphasia syndromes (left hemisphere) and neglect syndromes (right hemisphere). Strokes affecting the posterior circulation (posterior cerebral, cerebellar, and vertebrobasilar arteries) may cause altered level of consciousness, dizziness, vertigo, ataxia, dysarthria, dysphagia, or visual field cuts, as well as any of several specific brain stem syndromes. CT or MRI imaging remain the standard studies to directly visualize the brain. If embolization is suspected, the carotid arteries should be imaged using ultrasound. If a cardiac mural thrombus is suspected, transthoracic or transesophageal echocardiography can directly visualize a clot, while EKG and 24-hour Holter monitoring can identify the arrhythmias that commonly coexist.

Treatment

Treatment depends on the cause. Two general principles to keep in mind include the need for gentle fluid hydration and tolerance of some hypertension (mean arterial pressure of up to 130-140mmHg) in thrombotic or embolic strokes to maintain high cerebral perfusion pressures. Labetalol is a good agent for blood pressure control in this situation because it can be given intravenously as a bolus or titrated as a continuous drip, does not increase intracranial pressure, and can be administered orally. Anticoagulation with heparin is indicated in patients with a risk for further emboli, although hemorrhagic transformation is a potential complication.

Seizure

A seizure is the onset of abnormal electrical activity in the brain, causing changes in motor activity, sensory phenomena, behavior, or level of consciousness. A **partial seizure** produces focal symptoms, and may be either **simple** (no impairment of consciousness) or **complex** (altered consciousness). Although partial seizures can secondarily generalize, the observation that a seizure was initially focal is important for accurate diagnosis and treatment. **Generalized seizures** produce global, symmetrical symptoms, usually with an impaired level of consciousness. Included in this category are **absence seizures** (impairment of consciousness only), **myoclonic seizures** (single muscle contraction or repetitive contractions), and **tonic-clonic seizures** (sustained muscle contraction followed by repetitive muscle contractions of all extremities). **Status epilepticus** refers to the presence of successive seizures without regaining consciousness.

Seizures result from functional or structural disease of the brain. Idiopathic epilepsy is thought to result from a combination of genetic predisposition and neurotransmitter imbalance. Seizures associated with fever, stress, menses, drugs, alcohol-withdrawal, sleep deprivation, syncope from any cause, or metabolic derangements can also occur in the absence of structural brain pathology. In contrast, seizures can also be associated with structural lesions (such as a tumor).

Workup

A thorough history, including birth and development, recent trauma, drug use, current medications, sleep pattern, co-morbid illnesses, and physical and emotional stressors is critical. Detailed description of the seizure is very important, including the setting in which the event occurred, early observations (i.e., partial or generalized), behavior changes, duration of symptoms, incontinence, loss of consciousness, and postictal behavior. Physical examination should focus on the cardiovascular, pulmonary, and neurologic systems, although clues to the etiology of a seizure can be found in other parts of the exam as well. Laboratory evaluation should focus on the identification of a metabolic or other non-cerebral cause, especially reversible conditions such as hypoxia, hypoglycemia, or intoxication. Imaging usually begins with a CT scan, which will detect most major anatomic abnormalities. MRI is indicated if CT is negative or inadequate, or when subtle anatomic abnormalities are suspected. EEG may provide useful data about seizure activity, focus, and/or susceptibility, but a normal study does not rule out seizure activity unless it is performed during the event. Simultaneous video and EEG monitoring is useful for difficult cases.

Treatment

Treatment strategies are aimed first at immediate therapy for the seizing patient, and second at long term management of the patient with seizures. Status epilepticus is a medical emergency. Immediate concerns include airway protection, prevention of trauma, and IV access. Hypoglycemia must immediately be excluded; if a glucometer is unavailable, dextrose should be given empirically because hypoglycemia severe enough to cause a seizure will cause permanent damage if not immediately corrected. Intravenous benzodiazepines are very effective agents for the initial management of status epilepticus. Long-term treatment of a seizure disorder depends on the cause. Many types of idiopathic epilepsy respond to anticonvulsant therapy with agents such as carbamazepine, phenytoin, phenobarbital, valproic acid and others. Combinations of agents may be superior to single agents, but adequate monotherapy with available agents should be attempted first. Surgery can benefit some seizure patients with refractory disease and surgically amenable seizure foci.

Febrile seizures

Febrile seizures occur, by definition, in children between 6 months and 6 years of age who do not have a known underlying neurologic problem or previous non-febrile seizure. Febrile seizures are not indicative of underlying brain pathology, but seem to occur because the febrile young brain is abnormally sensitive to electrical impulses. In order to be classified as a febrile seizure, the temperature must be over 38°C and CNS infections and acute metabolic abnormalities must be absent.

Febrile seizures are classified as one of two types based on clinical presentation: **simple** febrile seizures last less than 15 minutes, manifest no focal signs, and usually occur only once in the course of a single febrile illness, while **complex** febrile seizures last more than 15 minutes, display focal features or postictal paresis, and can occur several times during the febrile episode. Most febrile seizures are of the simple type, usually occur on the first day of the illness, and depend more on the rate of rise rather than maximal temperature.

The main conditions to exclude after a febrile seizure are **meningitis** or **encephalitis** (see Chapter 49, "Pediatric Infectious Diseases"). Infants display few, if any, reliable symptoms or signs to help in clinical assessment; a high index of suspicion must therefore always be entertained in this age group. The only way to diagnose meningitis is by examination of cerebrospinal fluid. Routine examination of CSF after a febrile seizure is not generally performed because the incidence of meningitis in patients with febrile seizures is low. Examination of CSF is indicated, however, if the child is less than 6 months of age, has an abnormal neurological exam or concerning physical finding (for example, petechiae or bulging fontanelle), or if an adequate neurological exam cannot be performed. A lumbar puncture should not be done on a patient who has evidence of increased intracranial pressure (for example, headache with vomiting, papilledema, prominent downward gaze) because of the risk of herniation. Head CT should be performed in this situation to rule out a mass lesion; antibiotics should be given prior to CT if suspicion for meningitis is high.

Delirium and Dementia

Delirium and dementia are two very different entities. **Delirium** refers to the presence of a fluctuating level of consciousness, while **dementia** refers to the presence of altered cognitive function with preserved consciousness.

Delirium

Delirium is very common in hospitalized patients, especially the elderly, and is manifest by behavior anywhere along the scale from lethargy to agitation. Patients exhibit a decreased attention span and disorganized thinking, decreased level of consciousness, perceptual disturbances, sleep-wake disturbances, increased or decreased psychomotor activity, disorientation, and/or memory impairment. The causes of delirium are multiple, and include toxic or metabolic disturbances, infection, stroke, cerebral mass lesions, malignancy, and the postoperative state. Drug effects and early sepsis are perhaps the most common causes in hospitalized patients, and initial workup must be designed to rule these out. Review the medication list; anticholinergics, benzodiazepines, antiepileptics, analgesics, and steroids are common culprits. Particularly important is the observation that an infection often first presents with altered mental status, particularly in the very young and the elderly. Postoperative delirium is very common, particularly in elderly patients who require ICU care. Therapy is directed at the specific underlying cause and toward minimizing polypharmacy.

Dementia

Dementia is a condition or process of global, progressive decline in cognitive function with a preserved level of consciousness. Memory loss, personality changes, and the development of language deficits are all seen. Functional impairment socially or occupationally is a hallmark of this disease. The dementias have been categorized in various ways, but an approach that focuses on the reversibility the underlying process is probably the most helpful. Potentially reversible causes of dementia include toxic or metabolic derangements, endocrinopathies, nutritional deficiencies, mass lesions, infections, hydrocephalus, and psychiatric disturbances. Irreversible causes of dementia include Alzheimer's disease, Pick's disease, and processes associated with fixed structural defects such as multi-infarct dementia, posttraumatic dementia, and mass lesions. Multiple causes of dementia can co-exist in one patient.

It is essential to make the distinction between delirium and dementia, and to identify any potentially reversible process. In all cases, appropriate education, counseling, alteration in living environment, and trials of pharmacologic therapy need to be considered. Discussion of future options, goals, health care proxy, and code status with the patient and/or caretakers is very important early in the disease.

Other Neurologic Problems

Peripheral neuropathy

A **peripheral neuropathy** is a problem with the peripheral nervous system (arbitrarily encompassing the cranial nerves, after they exit the brainstem, and nerves exiting the spine). Peripheral neuropathies can be caused by numerous systemic or local processes, such as diabetes, alcohol abuse, nutritional deficiencies, ingestion of toxic metals or drugs, hematologic or hepatic disorders, endocrine abnormalities, renal failure, nerve compression syndromes, or tumor (paraneoplastic neuropathy). A focused history along with a thorough physical exam (with particular attention to the sensory, motor, and reflex components of the neurologic exam) should make it possible to classify the neuropathy into one of 2 anatomic types: symmetric generalized polyneuropathy or focal mononeuropathy. **Symmetric polyneuropathies** can be sensory, motor, or both, and typically affect the distal extremities first. **Mononeuropathies** are asymmetric, sometimes painful, and more commonly (than polyneuropathies) affect the cranial nerves. Nerve conduction velocity studies help identify demyelination and conduction blocks, while electromyography (EMG) helps identify acute and chronic denervation. Nerve biopsy can be done if needed. Treatment varies depending on the underlying cause. Medical therapy, physical therapy, and surgery can all be appropriate.

Headache

Headache is an extremely common problem. Fortunately, most headaches are not life-threatening. The severity and character of the headache are helpful in the evaluation of a headache, especially if it is described as "the worst headache of my life," in which case a subarachnoid hemorrhage must be ruled out. Prodromal events and symptoms are important to note, as are the relation of the headache to medication, alcohol, food, or exertion, aggravating or relieving factors, and any family history.

New headaches, in general, are potentially more serious than are chronic. A subarachnoid hemorrhage is typically very severe and sudden in onset, often associated with loss of consciousness, emesis, and meningismus, although some patients remain completely awake and alert without focal neurologic deficits. The initial test of choice is a CT scan, but, if negative, a lumbar puncture (to look for blood) is diagnostic. A post-concussive (traumatic) headache is usually throbbing in nature, and is associated with nausea, vomiting, lightheadedness, vertigo, poor concentration, memory deficit, fatigue, and irritability. Usually self-limited, it can persist for months to a year. Patients with a history of minor head trauma can eventually develop chronic recurrent headaches similar to migraines. Patients with meningitis will usually be febrile, and will often describe severe headache, neck stiffness, photophobia, nausea, and vomiting. If meningitis is suspected, a lumbar puncture should be performed provided a mass lesion has been ruled out.

When patients with AIDS present with headache and fever, it is important to rule out acute sinusitis, meningitis, encephalitis, and CNS lymphoma, as well as toxoplasmosis, cryptococcal meningitis, and herpes simplex encephalitis. A sinus headache is often localized to the areas of the frontal, ethmoidal, and maxillary sinuses, with coexistent fever, congestion, postnasal drip, cough, and tenderness over the affected sinuses. Headaches secondary to mass lesions can be mild or severe, and also are associated with nausea, vomiting, and anorexia. A key feature of this type of headache is that often it is present every morning at awakening or it awakens the patient from sleep. Focal neurologic signs, signs of increased intracranial pressure, or mental status changes on exam are highly suggestive. A post-lumbar puncture headache, secondary to a persistent leakage of CSF, can be treated with an epidural blood "patch."

Many drugs can produce a headache, including vasodilators, oral contraceptives, indomethacin, theophylline, cimetidine, and oral hypoglycemics. Caffeine, alcohol, tobacco, monosodium glutamate, ice cream, chocolate, cheese, and tyramine containing foods also can cause headache, by use or withdrawal. Finally, temporal arteritis, an inflammatory blood vessel disease in older patients, can lead to headache over the temporal arteries, jaw claudication, fever, fatigue, weight loss, and weakness.

Chronic or recurrent headaches are usually less worrisome. Tension headaches may be caused by muscle contraction, are intermittent or continuous (often refractory to analgesics), and are usually bilateral. A migraine headache is common (5% of the population), hereditary, and is felt to be secondary to changes in cerebral blood flow. During the prodromal phase of a migraine, there is vasoconstriction; the actual headache phase occurs during vasodilation of the vessels. A cluster headache consists of unilateral stabbing pain in the eye, orbit or cheek, often with associated autonomic symptoms, and often occurring a few hours after the patient has gone to bed.

Vertigo

Vertigo is the subjective sensation of motion. Peripheral vertigo occurs when there is an abnormality in function of the vestibular system peripheral to and including the VIII nerve (external, middle, inner ear), and is often associated with tinnitus, deafness, nausea, vomiting, pallor, and diaphoresis. The most common causes of peripheral vertigo include benign positional vertigo, ear infections, labyrinthitis, vestibular neuritis, cerebellopontine angle tumors (acoustic neuromas), and Meniere's disease. Central vertigo occurs when there is an abnormality in the vestibular system proximal to the VIII nerve (brainstem and cerebellum). It is less common than peripheral vertigo, and can be caused by drugs (alcohol, tranquilizers, barbiturates, anticonvulsants), vertebrobasilar ischemia, or cerebellar hemorrhage. Acute vertigo always is associated with nystagmus. ■

21   Nephrology

Nephrology is the study of normal and abnormal kidney function. Patients with reduced glomerular filtration have elevated serum creatinine (Cr) and blood urea nitrogen (BUN) levels, a condition termed **azotemia**; symptomatic azotemia is called **uremia**. Kidney failure can occur over days (**acute renal failure**), weeks (**rapidly progressive renal failure**), or months to years (**chronic renal failure**).

Patients with acute renal failure can be anuric or can have reduced, normal, or supranormal urine output. Acute renal failure is often reversible, and function in many instances can normalize. Chronic renal failure results from progressive and irreversible loss of glomerular function. Death usually is not due to uremia per se, but rather is the result of electrolyte derangements (especially potassium), infection, or multisystem organ failure caused by whatever insult precipitated the renal failure itself.

This chapter covers acute and chronic renal failure and dialysis. See Chapter 56, "Pediatric Nephrology," for a discussion of hematuria, proteinuria, and the various intrinsic renal diseases.

Acute Renal Failure

Acute renal failure (ARF) is defined as an abrupt decline in renal function. It can be associated with no urine output (**anuric**), low urine output (**oliguric**; urine output less than 400 mL/day) or normal or high urine output (**nonoliguric**). The decline in renal function is manifest as increased BUN and Cr levels as the result of the fall in glomerular filtration rate (GFR) – **adequate urine output does not mean kidney function is normal, and life-threatening effects of renal failure can occur in the face of a normal urine output**. If acute renal failure occurs in the setting of otherwise normal metabolism, BUN and Cr rise about 7-9 and 0.5-1.75mg/dL per day, respectively. If the increment is greater, overproduction (due to rhabdomyolysis or an increased protein load from GI bleeding, for example) is probably occurring. In general, GFR is adequate even with only one normal kidney. Any insult, therefore, usually must be bilateral before clinically apparent renal failure occurs. Because creatinine is completely filtered, not reabsorbed, and secreted, its clearance (CrCl) is a close approximation of GFR. The CrCl can be calculated using data derived from a timed urine specimen (typically over 24 hours):

$$\text{GFR} = \text{CrCl (mL/min)} = \frac{\text{(urine Cr x urine volume)}}{\text{(serum Cr x time)}}$$

Alternatively, CrCl can be estimated by the empiric formula:

$$\text{CrCl (mL/min)} = \frac{\text{[(140-age) x weight]}}{\text{(72 x serum Cr) (x .85 for women)}}$$

Prerenal azotemia

The best way to classify ARF is according to the location of the insult. **Prerenal** azotemia is caused by diminished renal blood flow, most often caused by reduced cardiac output; hypovolemia is the most common underlying problem. Prerenal azotemia is suggested by a BUN/Cr ratio of 20 or greater, and a fractional excretion of sodium (see below) of less than 1.0.

Renal azotemia

Renal azotemia is caused by problems intrinsic to the kidney. **Glomerular** diseases are the result of damage to the glomeruli themselves (glomerulonephritis), **tubulointerstitial** problems are those due to damage to the renal tubules (acute tubular necrosis; ATN) or interstitium (acute interstitial nephritis), and **microvascular** problems are due to inflammation of the microvasculature supplying the renal parenchyma and glomeruli (vasculitis, thrombosis, and many drug effects). Direct renal injury is suggested by a fractional excretion of sodium of greater than 1.0. ATN can be caused by a hypovolemic or hypotensive (prerenal) insult.

Postrenal azotemia

Postrenal azotemia is usually the result of bilateral obstruction, most commonly by a bladder carcinoma or prostatic hypertrophy. Physiologic problems such as neuromuscular disorders or neuropathies producing inadequate bladder emptying can also cause postrenal azotemia. Postrenal azotemia is almost always associated with dilated ureters and renal pelvices (depending on the level of obstruction). Obstruction must be bilateral to pro-

Medicine
Nephrology *continued*

duce a noticeable fall in GFR, unless the other kidney is abnormal or hypofunctional.

Workup

When faced with a patient in acute renal failure (rising BUN and Cr, whatever the renal output) the history should be explored for recent sources of volume loss, cardiac failure, mechanical trauma, or hypotension, and for symptoms of diseases such as prostatic hypertrophy. Recent drug ingestion, whether prescribed, over-the-counter, or illicit, is particularly important; nonsteroidal anti-inflammatory drugs, antibiotics, diuretics, and angiotensin-converting enzyme inhibitors are common culprits. The most important functions of the physical exam in this situation are to assess volume status and tissue perfusion, and to rule out obstruction (a Foley catheter must be placed, if not already present). Examination of the extremities can reveal muscular pain suggesting rhabdomyolysis or skin lesions commonly seen with certain intrinsic renal diseases. Patients with ARF are often in an intensive care unit setting; accurate assessment of intravascular volume status can be accomplished fairly easily in this situation (see Chapter 6, "Basic Hemodynamics and Invasive Monitoring").

Serum BUN and Cr are obviously important, but must be evaluated in light of the overall clinical situation. The possibility of abnormal production must be kept in mind: elderly or thin patients with little muscle mass can have low Cr levels despite an impaired GFR, and patients experiencing upper gastrointestinal bleeding can have a high BUN due to absorption of cellular protein from digested blood. Patients with ureteral leaks (after traumatic or iatrogenic injury) can have azotemia due to peritoneal reabsorption in the face of a normal GFR. The urinalysis (UA), urine electrolytes, and urine osmolality are the mainstays of laboratory workup. One of the functions of the kidney is to concentrate the urine by reabsorbing sodium. Patients with **prerenal azotemia** have an intact renal concentrating mechanism, and will therefore have a low urine sodium and high urine osmolality. The UA is usually unremarkable, although hyaline casts can be present. Concentrating ability of the kidney in **renal azotemia** is impaired; patients usually have a high urine sodium and **isotonic** urine. ATN characteristically causes granular casts (which indicate tubular damage), and interstitial kidney disease produces red and white cells and possibly eosinophils. The UA in **postrenal azotemia** is usually unremarkable, although cytology can reveal malignant cells, if present. CT and/or renal ultrasound must be performed in nearly all cases and can help localize and characterize the problem. Fresh urine should always be examined, because casts break up within minutes. When the UA suggests an intrinsic renal problem a biopsy should always be considered because it is the only way to diagnose a potentially treatable acute glomerulonephritis.

In any patient with unexplained azotemia, simultaneous urine and blood samples should be obtained before giving the patient a diuretic. Using the sodium and creatinine levels, the fractional excretion of sodium (FENa) can be calculated:

$$FE_{Na} = [(urine_{Na}/urine_{Cr}) \times (serum_{Cr}/serum_{Na})] \times 100$$

Prerenal azotemia is characterized by a high Uosm and low UNa (less than 20 meq/L) and FE_{Na} (less than 1), **ATN** by a high U_{osm}/U_{Na} (greater than 40 meq/L), and FE_{Na} (greater than 1), and **acute glomerulonephritis** by a high U_{osm}/ low U_{Na} (less than 20meq/L) and low FE_{Na} (less than 1).

Treatment

Treatment of ARF depends on the cause; obviously, correctable things (such as hypovolemia or obstruction) need to be corrected. For many conditions (glomerulonephritis, ATN) no specific therapy exists other than optimization of tissue perfusion by ensuring adequate volume status, cardiac output, and renal blood flow. Laboratory data need to be monitored frequently; electrolytes (especially potassium), BUN and Cr, calcium, phosphate, albumin, and hematocrit all are significantly affected by renal failure. Elimination of any potentially nephrotoxic drug and adjustment of the doses of any required medications according to the GFR is crucial. Intake of potassium, phosphate, magnesium, and protein should be restricted, and fluid balance closely monitored. Dialysis (see below) is instituted to treat volume overload, significant electrolyte abnormalities or acidosis, or significant uremia. *(continued)*

Normal renal function, rather than urine output, is the goal—if function is normalized, output will follow. Patients with **non-oliguric renal failure**, however, tend to be easier to manage and to have a better prognosis, in part because volume overload is not a problem. Therefore, as long as volume status and renal perfusion have been optimized and efforts are underway to correct whatever underlying problem is present, diuretics can be administered in an attempt to maintain urine output and normal volume status.

Chronic Renal Failure

Chronic renal failure (CRF) is a **progressive** and **irreversible** decline in the number of functioning nephrons and, therefore, GFR. The most significant (and common) causes are **diabetes mellitus** and **hypertension** (see Chapter 39, "Transplantation"). The most important part of treating CRF is, thus, prevention of the underlying problem and/or delay of renal damage. Microalbuminuria in diabetics (and perhaps hypertensives) is the earliest clinical sign of renal damage. It has been recently shown that treatment with an angiotensin converting enzyme (ACE) inhibitor at this early stage will significantly delay onset and progression of renal insufficiency.

Initiation of dialysis

A fundamental question in CRF is when dialysis should be started. There is no one algorithm that applies to every patient, but, in general, uremic symptoms such as pruritus, somnolence, nausea, vomiting, pericardial effusion, asterixis, or mental status changes mean that dialysis is required. Less common indications for beginning dialysis in CRF are uncontrollable electrolyte, acid-base, or volume abnormalities. The decision whether and when to initiate dialysis can often be made in a controlled, "elective" manner. Eligibility and desire for renal transplant should be addressed at an early stage (see Chapter 39, "Transplantation").

Management of ESRD

Management of the patient with CRF and **end stage renal disease** (**ESRD**) can be quite complicated. There are some basic guidelines fundamental to the care of any patient on dialysis:

Diet: 2-4gm Na, 3gm K, without strict protein restriction.

Vitamins: Berocca or Nephrovite (containing vitamins B and C and folate).

Erythropoietin (Epogen) and iron: Epogen is usually given IV (because it produces less discomfort than when given subcutaneously) during hemodialysis. Most patients require supplemental iron, usually 325mg of $FeSO_4$ given twice a day. Iron must be given between meals, because absorption is inhibited by PO_4 binders. Adequate iron stores are necessary for Epogen to be effective.

Transfusions are given only while the patient is undergoing dialysis because of the risks of volume overload and hyperkalemia. If the patient requires blood in an emergency, or the patient is not on dialysis, blood should be given slowly (this does **not** apply to trauma or acute hypovolemia due to bleeding). Many patients are transplant candidates; therefore, try to minimize transfusions and give leukocyte-depleted ("filtered") RBCs in order to minimize the development of immunoreactivity against common blood antigens.

Bleeding: uremia causes platelet dysfunction, possibly because of low levels or abnormal function of von Willebrand's factor, the molecule mediating platelet-subendothelial attraction, or because of uremic by-products. DDAVP, a synthetic analogue of antidiuretic hormone that increases levels of von Willebrand's factor, will often correct bleeding in uremic patients.

Calcium and phosphate: patients with ESRD have low calcium and, often, high parathyroid hormone (PTH) levels (secondary hyperparathyroidism; see Chapter 9, "Endocrinology") along with high PO_4, which can be toxic. Calcium- ($CaCO_3$) and aluminum hydroxide ($Al(OH)_2$) lower serum PO_4 levels by binding to PO_4 in the GI tract, decreasing absorption; increasing serum calcium levels will decrease PTH secretion. The product of the two (Ca x PO_4) can be used to guide dosage. If the

Medicine
Nephrology *continued*

Ca x PO_4 product is between 40-70, 650mg-1300mg $CaCO_3$ should be given three times a day (with meals); if greater than 70, the risk of Ca and PO_4 precipitation is high and binding agents such as aluminum hydroxide ($Al(OH)_2$; Alternagel or Amphogel) should be used. The hazard of chronic aluminum use is osteomalacia and central nervous system toxicity, thus, it should not be administered unless the Ca x PO_4 product is high. Vitamin D is given orally (Calcitrol) or parenterally (Calcijex).

Antibiotics: some antibiotics, including most cephalosporins and penicillins, are removed during hemodialysis, and must therefore be given after each dialysis, if required. Gentamicin is dialyzed, and can therefore be given as a single dose after each dialysis treatment (predialysis blood levels should be followed). Vancomycin is not removed during dialysis; random levels should be followed with re-dosing when levels fall to the normal "trough" range of 5-10mg/dL (about every 5-7 days in the typical patient). Dosages of all antibiotics need to be adjusted according to the GFR.

Dialysis

Dialysis is the means whereby the blood is artificially filtered. It is used primarily to treat volume overload, hyperkalemia, refractory acidosis, or symptoms of uremia. It can be used in the chronic setting in patients with ESRD, or in ARF while renal function is recovering.

Hemodialysis

Hemodialysis consists of physically removing the blood from the body, filtering it in a machine, and returning it. A route for intravenous access must be established that allows the high flows (typically 300cc/minute) required. **Dialysis access catheters** are double-lumen tubes inserted into a central vein; different models with different insertion requirements (bedside or operating room) are used depending on the anticipated duration of use. Although the terms "arterial" and "venous" ports are commonly used, the catheters lie within the vein only, and the ports are schematically interchangeable. "Permanent" access is accomplished by means of an **arteriovenous** (**AV**) fistula, most commonly created by connecting the cephalic vein and radial artery in the wrist or by using a tube of artificial material (beneath the skin) to connect an artery with a vein elsewhere in the arm. The connection between artery and vein simply establishes the presence of a chronic, high-flow situation allowing easy cannulation, durability, and high flow rates during dialysis.

Hemodialysis is efficient. Sessions typically last about 4 hours, and patients are dialyzed 3 times a week. Near-normal volume and electrolyte status can be achieved, although hypotension sometimes occurs during treatment. Hypoperfusion-related bowel ischemia can occasionally occur; this should be kept in mind when evaluating a patient on hemodialysis who develops abdominal pain.

Peritoneal dialysis

Peritoneal dialysis is performed by the instillation of dialysate into the peritoneal cavity through a surgically-placed catheter, allowing the peritoneal surface to act as the dialysis membrane. It is also effective, but is not as efficient as is hemodialysis, and patients typically require daily sessions. Its advantages are that it is self-administered at home and patients can travel. A recognized complication is the development of **spontaneous bacterial peritonitis (SBP)**, often caused by Staphylococci or Streptococci that typically respond to antibiotics alone. Removal of the catheter is occasionally required, but laparotomy is not, unless another problem exists.

Hemofiltration

Continuous hemofiltration (arteriovenous or venovenous; **CAVH** and **CVVH**) is a method of continually removing volume and uremic toxins in critically ill patients with ARF. It does not generally cause severe hypotension, and is thus better tolerated by these very sick patients. ∎

22 Gastroenterology

Gastroenterology is the study of diseases or abnormal conditions of the gastrointestinal (GI) tract, such as inflammatory bowel disease, gastroesophageal reflux, and disorders of elimination (diarrhea and constipation). Diverticular disease (Chapter 32, "Colon and Rectum"), jaundice (Chapter 24, "Jaundice"), and gastrointestinal bleeding (Chapter 40, "GI Bleeding"), also issues gastroenterologists frequently face, are covered elsewhere.

Inflammatory Bowel Disease

Inflammatory bowel disease (IBD), a chronic inflammatory disorder of unknown origin involving the GI tract, is divided into two major categories: ulcerative colitis and Crohn's disease. IBD is a disease of young adults, most commonly affecting those ages 15-35. Although many theories have been put forth, its cause remains a mystery.

Ulcerative colitis (UC) is a diffuse inflammatory process involving colonic and rectal mucosa. It almost always begins in the rectum and extends to a varying distance proximally in a continuous fashion. Although the disease process is occasionally limited to an ulcerative proctitis, the most common form of presentation is involvement of the entire colon. The ileum is believed not to be directly involved with the underlying disease process, although nonspecific inflammation ("backwash ileitis") can occur. Colon cancer is common in longstanding, untreated UC. **Crohn's disease (CD)**, in contrast, can affect any portion of the GI tract; notably the small bowel and anorectal areas. Moreover, "skip lesions" are common, with intervening regions of normal bowel. Although the symptoms can "burn out" with advancing age, CD is essentially incurable.

Therapy (especially surgical) differs fundamentally between the two conditions. Although sometimes difficult, it is important to be able to distinguish the two:

	Ulcerative Colitis	Crohn's Disease
Histology	Mucosa and submucosa	Transmural
	Crypt abscesses	Granulomas
Distribution	Rectum and colon (variable)	Entire bowel, "skip" areas
Fistulization	Rare	Common, especially anal
Clinical presentation	Bloody diarrhea	Diarrhea, chronic illness, malabsorption
Acute complications	Toxic megacolon	Bowel obstruction, abscess
Risk of carcinoma	High (if pancolitis present)	Low (but not zero)

Disease involving the small bowel is almost surely CD, but disease isolated to the colon could be either. Endoscopy seems quite reliable, but histologic examination of either a biopsy specimen obtained at endoscopy or a resected surgical specimen is best. Unfortunately, no method is absolutely perfect (although the larger the specimen, the more reliable the interpretation), and ultimate differentiation really rests on longterm behavior of the disease.

Medical management

Initial treatment of IBD is **medical**, although most patients with severe disease eventually require surgery. Initial goals are to control inflammation and replace nutritional losses. For more than 30 years, sulfasalazine and steroids have been the mainstays of therapy for UC and CD. Sulfasalazine is effective for acute and maintenance therapy of UC; it is less effective in the treatment of CD. About 25% of the sulfasalazine is absorbed; the remainder metabolized in the colon into 5-aminosalicylic acid (5-ASA) and sulfapyridine, the latter responsible for its side effects (anorexia, dyspepsia, headache, and vomit *(continued)* ing). Maintenance therapy prevents symptom recurrence in 85% of patients with UC. Both enteral (including per rectum) and topical steroids are also commonly used to treat IBD. The roles of antibiotics (metronidazole) and immunomodulators (such as azathioprine, 6-mercaptopurine, methotrexate, and cyclosporine) are currently being investigated.

Surgical management

Surgical therapy is commonly required for both UC and CD, although indications and treatment fundamentally differ, making differentiation vital. 20%-25% of patients with UC will require a colectomy during the course of their disease, whether for failure of medical management to alleviate symptoms, because of a complication such as toxic megacolon, or because of the risk of cancer. Severe dysplasia (or frank carcinoma) seen during colonoscopic surveillance biopsy suggests that colectomy is required, and many patients will opt for prophylactic colectomy. Total colectomy (including removal of all rectal mucosa) is curative for UC. A variety of reconstructive techniques are possible, including direct ileoanal anastomosis, because the sphincter mechanism can be preserved in UC (because it is not a transmural process). CD, in contrast, cannot be cured. Well over half those with CD will require surgery at some point in their lives: a general rule of thumb is that surgery should be reserved for the treatment of complications such as a fistula, bowel obstruction, abscess, or failure of medical management to provide an acceptable quality of life. CD has a high recurrence rate, and each operation creates more adhesions, becomes more difficult, and requires removal of more and more bowel; thus, the cardinal objective is to avoid surgery whenever possible. Continent reconstruction is not advisable after colectomy because perianal recurrence is very common (due to the transmural nature of the disease); a permanent ileostomy is usually the best option.

Gastroesophageal Reflux

Gastroesophageal reflux (GER) is the reflux of gastric (or duodenal) contents into the esophagus. Intermittently present in almost everyone, **GER disease (GERD)** is said to be present if any symptoms or esophageal mucosal damage occur. Nearly half the US adult population has "heartburn" at least once monthly. Apart from the production of symptoms, the major longterm problem created by untreated GERD is the risk of developing cancer of the esophagus.

LES

An abnormal lower esophageal sphincter (LES) is the principal causative factor for GERD. The LES is complex: not an anatomic structure per se, it is an area of distal esophagus that maintains a high basal resting muscle tone, partially due to its intra-abdominal position. Increased gastric volume, increased intra-abdominal pressure, delayed gastric emptying, and impaired esophageal clearance during swallowing also contribute to GE reflux. Most patients with moderate to severe esophagitis have a **sliding hiatus hernia**, but the issue of causality (i.e., which came first) is murky. Interestingly, it is becoming apparent that bile reflux into the esophagus (all the way from the duodenum) may play a role in the disease.

Manifestations

Symptoms of GERD include classic "heartburn" that is most commonly described as an intermittent retrosternal chest pain, often worse with recumbency or after certain specific meals. Patients complain of regurgitation, dysphagia or a "lump in the throat," or "water brash" (hypersalivation induced by acid reflux). A classic history alone is sufficient to allow a trial of therapy, but if the history is atypical, symptoms are refractory to treatment, or complications of esophagitis are believed present, specific diagnostic testing is warranted.

Workup

An **upper GI series**, or radiologic examination of the esophagus and stomach with contrast material, is of low sensitivity for detecting GERD. It might reveal thickened esophageal folds, irregularity or thickening of the esophageal wall, or luminal narrowing. It is a good test for the evaluation of esophageal compliance, suspected stricture, or mechanical problems such as rings or webs. It is also useful to evaluate swallowing in real-time. If GERD is suspected, perhaps the most important test, however, is upper GI endoscopy (**esophagogastroduodenoscopy, EGD**). EGD provides a direct view of mucosa and allows for biopsy if needed. Esophagitis is suggested by the presence of erythema, erosions, or epithelial hyperplasia. **Barrett's esophagus** is present when epithelium of the distal esophagus undergoes columnar transformation in response to acid (and probably bile). 12% of patients with persistent symptoms of GERD will have a Barrett's esophagus, the presence of which can confer a 30- to 40- fold risk for the development of esophageal adenocarcinoma (depending on the degree of atypia).

Ambulatory pH monitoring is useful to quantify the degree of reflux by measuring pH changes in the esophagus as patients go about their daily routines. Closely related is the **Bernstein test**, a provocative test to see whether acid infusion reproduces the patient's symptoms, if the diagnosis is unclear. **Esophageal manometry** is used to assess the function of the LES in difficult cases or in cases where surgery is contemplated.

Medical management

Initial treatment is medical. First, **lifestyle modifications** are made. The patient should change physical factors that promote reflux (by elevation of the head of the bed, weight reduction, avoidance of straining, stooping, tight clothes, and large, late meals) and avoid foods, medications (such as caffeine, chocolate, theophylline, alcohol, calcium-channel blockers, or anticholinergics), and behaviors (such as smoking and late exercise) that promote reflux. By increasing the pH of the refluxed gastric contents, **antacids** inactivate pepsin and probably reduce the direct damage done by acid. Next, histamine (H_2) receptor antagonists and/or prokinetic agents are tried. The **H_2 receptor antagonists** (cimetidine, ranitidine, famotidine, nizatidine) inhibit gastric acid secretion by competitively blocking H_2 receptors on the parietal cells. Esophageal mucosal healing rates are inversely proportional to the severity of esophagitis. While 50%-70% of symptomatic patients have partial or complete resolution of reflux symptoms, such resolution does not correlate with esophageal mucosal healing. **Prokinetic agents** (Bathanechol, metoclopramide, and cisapride) seem to be of benefit primarily by increasing resting LES pressure and esophageal clearance rather than by affecting gastric emptying or small bowel motility. If GERD persists, the next line of therapy is the $Na^+/K^+ATPase$ inhibitor **omeprazole**, which produces a prolonged and highly effective inhibition of both basal and stimulated gastric acid secretion. In studies comparing the two, omeprazole yields healing rates almost twice those of the H_2 blockers. Omeprazole is not the first line of treatment, however, due to its expense and the theoretic concerns of the production of gastric bacterial overgrowth and elevated gastrin.

Surgical management

If medical treatment fails, **surgical therapy** is the next option. Surgery is indicated for "failure of medical management" (not rigorously defined), those with significant respiratory tract complications, or those in whom severe Barrett's esophagitis is present (surgery will not eliminate the Barrett's, but will reduce further damage). Principles of surgical repair include tightening the diaphragmatic hiatus, return of the LES into the abdomen, and some sort of gastric wrap to add "tone" to the LES. Several procedures can be done through either the abdomen (Nissen fundoplication) or the left chest (Belsey Mark IV). Early experience with laparoscopic repair has been quite favorable.

Complications

Complications of longstanding GERD include **esophageal stricture**, which causes dysphagia. If severe, it may require balloon dilatation or, occasionally, resection and replacement. Barrett's esophagitis is a major risk factor for **esophageal cancer**, which must be ruled out when dysphagia is present. If severely dysplastic esophageal mucosa is found the risk of cancer is so great that prophylactic esophageal resection is warranted even if actual cancer is not (yet) present.

Diarrhea

Diarrhea is said to be present when there is an **abnormal increase** in daily stool **weight**, **liquidity**, or **frequency**. The definition of diarrhea ultimately depends on each patient; what is troublesome in some may be tolerated and even perceived as normal by others. Nine liters of fluid a day pass into the duodenum. The small bowel resorbs 90% of this fluid; the colon, 90% of what remains. Only about 100cc of fluid per day is normally excreted in the stool—it seems remarkable that diarrhea isn't more common than it is! Diarrhea is usually classified into one (or more) of several possible mechanisms.

Osmotic diarrhea is due to the accumulation of a nonabsorbable solute in the colonic lumen, such as lactose in patients with lactase deficiency. The solute causes impaired water resorption with resultant increased liquidity. The hallmark of osmotic diarrhea is that it **stops** or **decreases** with **fasting** (because the solute is no longer present). **Secretory** diarrhea, in contrast, is caused by active secretion or malabsorption of substances such as bile, fatty acids, hormones such as VIP or gastrin, or water and mucus in conditions such as inflammatory bowel disease, sprue, or intestinal lymphoma. The critical observation that suggests that secretory diarrhea might be present is that the diarrhea **does not stop** with **fasting**. The **fecal solute gap** (conceptually similar to the anion gap) is also useful; a high solute gap is suggestive of osmotic diarrhea; a low gap suggests secretory diarrhea:

Fecal solute gap = fecal osmolality-[2 x (Na + K)]

Infectious diarrhea is diarrhea due to toxins produced by certain pathogens, such as seen in cholera or pseudomembranous colitis. Pseudomembranous colitis is caused by overgrowth of **Clostridium difficile** bacteria in the colon, usually due to iatrogenic destruction of the normal colonic flora that keep it in check. Although clindamycin is the "classic" culprit, it can be caused by virtually any antibiotic. This is an extremely common cause of diarrhea in hospitalized patients, can be fatal, and should be suspected in any patient who has received any antibiotic within the past few weeks or so. Diarrhea also can be due to **deranged intestinal motility**. Decreased peristalsis (or the presence of functionally blind loops after surgery or with disease) can promote bacterial overgrowth, and increased motility (caused by drugs such as caffeine, for example), causes diarrhea by decreasing stool transit time. Finally, diarrhea can be caused by accumulation of **blood** or **protein** in the lumen. Blood in particular is a very strong cathartic; this effect is useful in gastrointestinal bleeding because any significant amount of intraluminal blood usually produces a bloody bowel movement soon afterward.

These divisions are fairly arbitrary. A patient with diabetes (reduced motility), for example, may have bacterial overgrowth (infectious), osmotically-active products stimulate abnormal water secretion (secretory); attempted treatment of the infectious source might produce pseudomembranous colitis. The best strategy in a patient with diarrhea is to look at the big picture to identify potentially treatable causes. Generally, in situations that are not clear, a brief fast, measurement of the fecal solute gap, appropriate stool cultures (for pathogenic bacteria not normally present), assay for Clostridium difficile toxin, and examination of the stool for fecal leukocytes (suggesting inflammation) are cost-efficient first steps.

Toxic Megacolon

Toxic megacolon is a condition where the colon acutely dilates in conjunction with severe systemic illness ("toxicity"). It can occur in a variety of conditions, including IBD and infectious colitis (commonly pseudomembranous colitis). Much of the systemic toxicity probably results from translocation of bacteria and endotoxin across the bowel wall into the body itself. The cecal diameter is the critical variable: according to LaPlace's law, the cecum (largest diameter) dilates the most in response to a given intracolonic pressure. A cecal diameter greater than 9-12cm (if acute) indicates accumulating risk of full-thickness necrosis and impending perforation (chronic dilation is less dangerous).

A distinction must be made between colon dilation due to obstruction or ileus and colon dilatation due to true toxic megacolon. If the intestinal wall is viable, nonoperative decompression (via colonoscopy) can be successful. In toxic megacolon, however, the intestinal wall is usually necrotic to a variable degree, and the situation is usually irreversible. Resection (colectomy with ileostomy) is usually required, though if full thickness necrosis is not present, a short trial of nonoperative therapy is acceptable.

Ogilvie's Syndrome

Ogilvie's Syndrome is a unique entity. It is essentially a localized ileus of the left and sigmoid colon, with impressive proximal dilation, believed due to impaired parasympathetic sacral outflow. It is classically seen in elderly patients at prolonged bedrest or in those with psychiatric problems, and presents as an impressive clinical and radiologic large bowel obstruction. Notably, however, these patients are very comfortable (and often hungry). Bowel rest, correction of malnutrition, dehydration, and electrolyte disturbances, and reduction of medications that impair motility (such as narcotics) will usually allow the situation to resolve.
(continued)

Medicine
Gastroenterology *continued*

Endoscopy

Endoscopy refers to the techniques used to examine the interior of the GI tract. **Esophagogastroduodenoscopy (EGD)** uses a forward-viewing endoscope to examine the esophagus, stomach, and duodenum, and is useful both for diagnostic and therapeutic interventions. In the latter role, EGD allows one to cauterize a bleeding ulcer and inject sclerosant into esophageal varices. **Endoscopic retrograde cholangiopancreatography (ERCP)** is the technique of cannulating the common bile duct from within the duodenum using a side-viewing endoscope (note that this requires a different instrument from conventional EGD). Contrast material can be injected, the sphincter of Oddi can be widened, stones can be removed, and stents can be placed.

Anoscopy requires an anoscope or one of several retractor-type instruments to examine the anus, while **rigid sigmoidoscopy** uses a scope 25cm long to examine the rectum (it is difficult to see much of the sigmoid, despite its name). Both can be performed at the bedside. **Flexible sigmoidoscopy** and **colonoscopy** require sedation and special equipment, and are thus almost always done in a specialized endoscopy suite. Flexible sigmoidoscopy is used to examine the left colon (up to 50-60cm or so); an experienced colonoscopist can usually reach the cecum. Flexible sigmoidoscopy is valuable because the majority of colon tumors occur within its reach. ∎

23 Geriatrics

Geriatrics is the part of internal medicine concerned with the care of elderly patients. The term was originally used by Ignaz Nasch in 1903; geriatrics was first recognized by a separate credentialing exam in 1988. The definition of the geriatric patient is varied and somewhat arbitrary. The most common defining age in the United States is 65, since this qualifies a citizen for Medicare. This age is an historical carryover from Kaiser Wilhelm's Germany, however, and is not based on any medical, epidemiologic, or actuarial data. Senescence (aging) is a process, not an event, and a patient's chronologic and physiologic ages can be quite disparate.

Demographics

Currently more than 30 million Americans, representing almost 13% of the population, are 65 or older. This group is responsible for greater than 30% of the health care expenditures in this country, and approximately a third of all patients seen by primary care physicians are 65 or older. This "graying of America" is not an isolated blip in the population distribution, but an ongoing shift in the population curve. During the next 35 years (your professional career) this group is expected to grow to a quarter of the population. The fastest growing subset is made up of those over 80, who already number over 3 million and are expected to grow to 4.6 million by the end of the decade.

Approach to the Geriatric Patient

The history and physical, while often more difficult and time consuming, are of even greater importance in the geriatric patient than in younger patients. The focus in a geriatric patient is **function**, that is, how successful the patient is at interacting with the world. The goal is more often to maximize patient function and quality of life than to cure.

History

The **history** starts with the **history of the present illness**. Older patients tend to underreport symptom; geriatric patients will often report symptoms only when directly questioned. Patient complaints are often multiple, vague, and nonspecific. The most difficult task might be deciphering and defining the significance of the various complaints; keeping a list is helpful. Patterns may emerge that guide workup or treatment, and a change in the list might be the first sign of a new problem. Starting with the **past medical history** can often focus the interview. The **surgical history** is variable and should be specifically sought; operations in the remote past are often omitted by patients. Obtain records whenever possible, record dates, and look for patterns. Look for precipitating factors that might have led to significant changes in the patient's health or life, such as a specific injury, death of a spouse, or change in medication.

Medications are best managed by the ALL principle: ALL patients should be instructed to bring ALL medications from ALL doctors to ALL their appointments—this is your best chance to find out what your patients are actually taking. Quiz the patient (or person giving the drugs to the patient) about dose, frequency, and even route of administration of their medications. If an **allergy** is reported, find out both the exact culprit and the reaction it caused; don't eliminate the use of a medication simply because the patient experienced a common side effect. The **family history** can be very important in younger geriatric patients, but as patients age, family history is often more interesting than helpful. The **social history** is critical. Is the patient married? If divorced or widowed, how long ago, and how is the patient adjusting to the change? Does the patient have children or grandchildren? Is the patient employed; if not, how are the days spent? These factors all influence patients' ability to travel and live in the community, get to appointments, and occupy their time.

Things to look for in the **review of systems** are recent changes and current functional status. Sexual function needs to be included; don't assume that older patients are sexually inactive (or even monogamous). If you have not already done so, this is the time to document the patient's abilities to carry out **activities of daily living**, such as bathing, toileting, eating, ambulating, transferring, and dressing, and **instrumental activities of daily living**, such as cooking, driving, cleaning, public transportation use, shopping, management of finances, and telephone use.

Exam

By the time the history is complete you should have a clear picture of the patient. Start the **physical exam** by documenting the patient's general appearance (e.g., frail, obese, cachectic, or disheveled), hygiene, ambulation status, and so on. A careful examination of the **skin**, especially sun-exposed areas, for malignant and premalignant lesions should be performed; don't overlook the feet and intertriginous areas. While assessing **head and neck** function, note assistive devices, such as glasses, hearing aids, and dentures. Arcus senilis is common and rarely significant, but cataracts, while also common, are very important. Assess dental health carefully, because most of the current geriatric population did not go through life with the benefits of fluoride and regular dental care. The status of the mucosal membranes will help determine hydration status. **Cardiovascular** assessment includes documentation of jugular venous distention and pulses. Remember that coronary and peripheral vascular disease are both very prevalent in these patients. Document the presence or absence of cardiac murmurs and carotid bruits.

Similarly, breast cancer is very prevalent in this age group. Geriatric patients should all have annual **breast** exams (including men) and mammograms. The **abdomen** should be examined carefully for the presence of masses (including aneurysms) and scars. A bruit may be the only sign of renal or mesenteric occlusive disease. Signs of an acute abdominal problem can be much more subtle in the older patient. The **genitourinary** system should be carefully examined for the presence of hernias, testicular masses, and prostatic enlargement in males, and for vulvar lesions and dry atrophic vaginal mucosa (a cause of dyspareunia) in females. Women of this age require annual pelvic exams and Pap smears (see Chapter 66, "Gynecologic Malignancies"); if they do not see a gynecologist, you are their source. Do not assume that any part of the **neurologic exam** is normal. Test all aspects completely, especially gait and mental status. All new patients should have a formal mental status screening. Dementia is not a natural consequence of aging, but is a sign of a pathologic state.

In every encounter with an elderly patient, such a detailed approach will not be feasible. "A Simple Procedure for General Screening for Functional Disability in Elderly Patients" has been developed by Lachs and colleagues, which focuses on assessment of function. It is only a screening instrument; any deficiencies detected mandate complete evaluation.

While organ systems vary in their response to senescence, the general pattern is that of **increasingly tenuous homeostasis**. Physiology in the elderly is more easily disturbed, is able to compensate to a lesser degree, and recovers more slowly. **The geriatric patient often presents in an atypical fashion**, and many common problems present in similar ways.

Altered Mental Status

A change in cognitive function is a common complaint with which geriatric patients come to medical attention, whether in the emergency department, office, or inpatient setting. Several questions are helpful to guide your workup. What is the patient's baseline? Is this an acute change? Is it dementia or delirium?

An **acute change** means an **acute process**; find it. Look at the vital signs carefully. Hypotension can be caused by blood loss, cardiac disease, or dehydration; hypertension can cause encephalopathy. Tachycardia is nonspecific but abnormal, and may be the only sign of infection, while bradycardia, if not pharmacologically induced, is almost always due to a primary cardiac process. Tachypnea often indicates hypoxia, but may also be caused by anxiety or infection. Temperature is an unreliable sign in the elderly since the febrile response is generally dampened; a temperature of 38.0° in an elderly patient should be considered a fever. A complete physical exam is obviously very important. Two very common causes of altered mental status in the elderly are **infection** and the effects of **medication**: don't forget to check the urine and the patient's medication list.

Dementia

The process should be categorized as dementia or delirium, because causes and treatment vary (see Chapter 20, "Neurology"). **Dementia** is characterized by progressive memory loss with retention of a fairly normal ability to interact with the world; it usually is of insidious onset and is progressive, worsening gradually over months to years. The incidence of dementia, like heart disease, increases with age. **Alzheimer's disease** represents the most common form of dementia, but can only be definitively diagnosed by autopsy. Onset is insidious and compensatory social graces remain intact, allowing the patient to mask the problem in the early stages. Progressive impairment of memory, speech, and judgment interfere with daily activities until the patient is unable to function alone. Affected patients often become active or agitated at night and are prone to wander.

Pseudo-dementia is the term used to describe a reversible form of dementia secondary to depression. Neurovegetative signs of depression (see Chapter 76, "Mood Disorders") are present. Mental status testing will suggest dementia, but missed questions are usually answered with "I don't know," rather than incorrect responses.

Delirium

Delirium is a change in the level of consciousness and is characterized by a decreased ability to maintain attention to external stimuli, and disorganized thinking. Onset is characteristically fairly rapid (hours to days), and the degree of impairment generally fluctuates. The patient's **medication** list will often reveal an **iatrogenic** cause; metabolic problems (electrolyte disturbances, renal or liver failure, or hypoglycemia) or infection are other common causes. Delirium and dementia can overlap in the elderly, which is why baseline status is so important. Both are increasingly common with age, but neither is normal.
(continued)

Incontinence

Incontinence is quite common in the elderly. Patients who report leaking urine during cough or exertion are said to have **stress incontinence**, usually caused by an abnormally low outlet resistance. This can be due to pelvic floor relaxation in females after childbirth, and may be exacerbated by obesity. Kegel exercises and estrogen creams may help, but surgical repair may be necessary.

Patients who report a sudden overwhelming urge to void but are unable to get to the bathroom in time have **urge incontinence**. These patients generally report large volume urine loss and often withdraw socially for fear of having a public "accident." Urge incontinence is related to detrusor dysfunction, which can be secondary to obstruction, neurologic problems, diabetic neuropathy, or peripheral nerve damage from a herniated disc or pelvic surgery. Treatment varies according to the cause, but generally is nonoperative unless obstruction from a mechanical source is the problem. Incontinence can be caused by several more easily reversible causes. Many are described by the mnemonic **DIAPPERS**: **delirium** or **dementia**, **infections** of the urinary tract, **atrophic vaginitis** or urethritis, **pharmaceuticals** such as sedatives, diuretics, or anticholinergics, **psychologic problems** such as depression or behavioral disturbances, **excess urine output**, **restricted mobility**, and **stool impaction**.

Falls

35%-40% of people over 65 suffer at least one fall per year. Falls in the elderly are serious events; they cause significant morbidity, worsen function, and, in some studies, lead to increased mortality. **A fall is a symptom, not a diagnosis**. Falls should be distinguished from syncope. A fall is a change in position, usually from vertical to some variant of horizontal, while syncope is a transient loss of consciousness with spontaneous recovery. Syncope in an upright person usually leads to a fall, but not all falls are due to syncope.

The mnemonic **DDROPP** can be helpful in guiding workup of patients who have fallen. **Diseases** such as macular degeneration, cataracts, peripheral neuropathy, vestibular dysfunction, arthritis, hypotension (orthostatic or postprandial), cardiac arrhythmias, transient ischemic attack or stroke, Parkinson's disease, normal pressure hydrocephalus, orthopedic injury or deformity, and dementia are a few of the obviously protean clinical entities that can lead to falls, as can **drugs** such as psychotropics, anti-arrhythmics, antihypertensives, anticonvulsants, and alcohol. A very important issue to investigate is that of the patient's **recovery**. Was it spontaneous, or was intervention required? How long was the patient "down?" Was there post-fall confusion (suggesting either seizure as a cause or neurologic injury as a result) or weakness? And, very importantly, was there any secondary injury produced by the fall? Other issues to explore are the **onset** of the symptoms—gradual versus sudden—the presence of any **prodromal** symptoms such as dizziness, chest pain, palpitations, or "aura," and the presence of **precipitants** such as a loose rug or other environmental hazard or abrupt change in posture. Obviously, a fall with a clear precipitant ("I tripped") is much less worrisome than is a spontaneous syncopal event.

The history and physical is directed at separating a fall from an actual loss of consciousness and at discovering the cause of the problem, while treatment is directed at both the cause and the consequences of the fall.

Elder Abuse

Many elderly people find themselves dependent on others for basic needs; this dependency makes them very vulnerable to abuse. Such abuse can take many forms: physical, verbal, psychologic, or financial. It may be abuse through neglect.

Signs of elder abuse are not greatly different from child abuse (see Chapter 58, "Child Abuse"). The victim may appear frightened or intimidated and is reluctant to report the abuser. Frequent injuries of varying ages or injuries inconsistent with the reported mechanism may be present, and illnesses may fail to respond to appropriate therapy because prescribed treatment was never given. The situation commonly is one in which a caregiver with poor social skills or support is faced with severe psychosocial stressors; the caregiver may have been a victim of abuse as a child. Drug or alcohol abuse creates a high-risk

Medicine
Geriatrics *continued*

environment. Unfortunately, elder abuse can also occur in long-term care institutions. Like most diagnoses, the key to diagnosing elder abuse is to think of it. Most localities have adult protective services to aid in confirming or clearing your suspicions.

Medicare and Medicaid

Even as a student or resident, you can't escape being affected by the two federal insurance programs. The intricacies of federal and state health insurance fill volumes and are likely to change, and as a trainee you do not need to know every detail. But, there are a few basic points that are extremely helpful to understand.

Medicare is a federal program that provides health insurance to all citizens 65 or older. There are no income or need requirements. Some younger people with long-term disabilities are also covered by Medicare, but prescription drugs and long-term care are **not** covered.

Medicaid is a federal program of health insurance for the poor. It is run by the states, with state and federal funding. Eligibility requirements and benefits vary from state to state; medicaid usually pays for medications and long-term care, and usually pays for over-the-counter medication if a prescription is written. ■

24   Jaundice

Jaundice and **icterus** are synonyms that refer to the presence of an elevated bilirubin level. Hyperbilirubinemia is significant because it is often (but not always) due to a progressive, correctable problem.

Metabolism

Bilirubin is normally present in the blood at levels ranging from 0.5-1.0mg/dL. Serum bilirubin is in equilibrium with tissue bilirubin due to simple diffusion across capillary membranes. Serum and tissue levels correlate, although if an acute change occurs equilibration is delayed 24 hours or so. When tissue levels increase to greater than about 3mg/dL, skin, eye, and tissue discoloration become clinically apparent (depending on the experience of the examiner).

Bilirubin formation

Most bilirubin is derived from breakdown of the heme ring of senescent red blood cells, which occurs in the reticuloendothelial system (RES) of the spleen, liver, and bone marrow. Red blood cells (RBCs) are taken up by the RES, where **hemoglobin** is liberated and subsequently broken down into a **heme** group, globin, and iron. Heme is then cleaved to form **biliverdin**, which in turn is oxidized to form **bilirubin**. Bilirubin is a non-polar molecule, and is therefore insoluble. It is released into the plasma where it binds to albumin ("unconjugated").

Excretion

Bilirubin cannot be excreted until it is conjugated in the liver. Hepatic bilirubin metabolism is divided into three phases: uptake, conjugation, and excretion. The bilirubin-albumin complex circulates through the hepatic sinusoids where the bilirubin is taken up by hepatocytes. Within the hepatocyte, bilirubin can be complexed with storage proteins or can be immediately **conjugated** with glucoronic acid by glucuronyl transferase. This conjugation polarizes bilirubin, making it water-soluble. The conjugated bilirubin is secreted into the bile cannaliculi leading to the hepatic and bile ducts by an active, energy-requiring process. Conjugated bilirubin mixes with lecithin and cholesterol to form **bile**. Bile is stored in the gallbladder between meals, and expressed into the duodenum after stimulation of the gallbladder by cholecystokinin in response to food where it is required for fat digestion. Conjugated bilirubin is finally converted into **urobilinogens** by gut bacteria. Although most is excreted, up to 20% of the urobilinogens are reabsorbed and undergo enterohepatic circulation, in effect recycling the bilirubin to be used again. The urobilinogens impart the dark color to stool; complete absence of bile will produce pale, **acholic** stools.

Figure 24.1
Bilirubin metabolism.

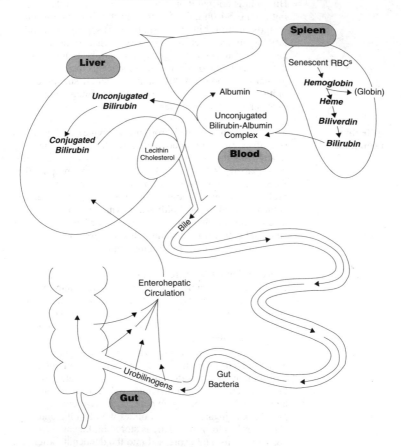

Causes of Jaundice

There are two ways of thinking about the causes of jaundice. In a biochemical sense, it is important to determine whether the hyperbilirubinemia is **conjugated** or **unconjugated**. In a clinical sense, the goal is to determine whether the hyperbilirubinemia is "**medical**" or "**surgical**." Although these overlap, they are not strictly comparable—it is best to think about each division in turn.

First is the question of whether conjugated or unconjugated hyperbilirubinemia is present. Conjugated bilirubin is water soluble, while unconjugated bilirubin is not. The amount of free-floating, conjugated bilirubin in serum can be measured directly, as can the total bilirubin. Unconjugated bilirubin can thus be determined by subtracting the amount of conjugated from the total. Consequently, the amount of **conjugated** bilirubin is called **direct** because it is directly measured, while that of **unconjugated** bilirubin is called **indirect** because it is a calculated value.

Unconjugated hyper-bilirubinemia	**Unconjugated** hyperbilirubinemia means one of several things: either hepatic uptake or conjugation is abnormal, or overproduction of bilirubin is overwhelming the excretion mechanism. Impaired hepatic uptake, a passive (but saturable) process, is usually seen in combination with other causes of jaundice. Impaired conjugation of bilirubin results from genetic or acquired defects, such as Crigler-Najjar and Gilbert's syndromes. Hepatitis and liver failure cause jaundice, although the bilirubin may be conjugated, as well, if impaired secretion coexists. Hepatocellular damage from any cause typically leads to the release of various enzymes such as serum aspartate aminotransferase (AST) and serum alanine aminotransferase (ALT). AST is less specific because it is also released by muscle tissue, while ALT is much more specific for liver damage (an AST:ALT ratio of 2:1 or more is suggestive of alcoholic liver disease).

Overproduction is usually the result of hemolysis, either intravascular (hemolytic anemia) or extravascular (reabsorption of a hematoma). This type of jaundice is typically mild, with bilirubin levels in the range of 5mg/dL. Sepsis in general, or liver failure due to multiple systemic

Medicine
Jaundice *continued*

organ failure/systemic inflammatory response syndrome (SIRS) can also cause unconjugated hyperbilirubinemia.

Conjugated hyper-bilirubinemia

Conjugated hyperbilirubinemia is more difficult to evaluate at times. In this situation the hepatocyte's ability to conjugate bilirubin is normal; the defect lies "distal" to this step. There is either a defect in hepatocyte secretion (Dubin-Johnson and Rotor syndromes, viral or drug-induced hepatitis, for example), cholestasis (seen sometimes with parenteral feeding or in the postoperative state, for example), or a mechanical obstruction in the biliary tree.

"Surgical" and "Medical" jaundice

Because of both laboratory and clinical variability and the overlap with impaired secretory function, conjugated and unconjugated hyperbilirubinemia do not always correspond directly with surgical and medical jaundice, respectively. Nonetheless, **surgical** or **obstructive** hyperbilirubinemia is most often reflected by a high conjugated fraction. The cells are working properly, but there is a mechanical obstruction to the flow of bile after it leaves the liver: conjugated bilirubin is excreted, but has nowhere to go, and is reabsorbed into the tissues. The two classic causes are gallstones obstructing the common bile duct (but **not** the cystic duct—see Chapter 33, "Biliary Tract") and a tumor of the pancreas or biliary tree. Surgical jaundice implies that correction may be possible. **Medical** jaundice, in contrast, is what's left over. Usually reflected by an excess of unconjugated bilirubin, this implies that physical correction is not possible, except perhaps by liver transplant.

The Jaundiced Patient

The first step is the recognition that jaundice is present. While obvious if the bilirubin level is very high, lower levels of hyperbilirubinemia can be subtle. Examination under normal sunlight, if possible, is best. Yellowed sclera or discoloration beneath the tongue are sometimes more obvious. In general, jaundice that is mechanically correctable will be severe and fairly easy to recognize.

H&P

Careful attention to drinking history and possible hepatitis exposure are important. A history of biliary colic or pancreatitis in a nonalcoholic patient suggests the presence of gallstone disease. All such patients should be asked about the color of their urine and stool. Conjugated bilirubin, because it is water soluble, can be excreted in the urine, imparting a dark color to it. Bile duct obstruction leads to a lack of bilirubin and urobilinogens in the stool, imparting a light, acholic color; thus dark urine and light stools suggest obstructive jaundice. Close evaluation of the abdomen for liver size and the presence of a palpable gallbladder are important. Tenderness is nonspecific and often indicative of acute infection, such as cholangitis (a surgical emergency) or hepatitis; cholecystitis usually does not produce jaundice, because the cystic duct, not the common bile duct, is obstructed. A palpable, **nontender** gallbladder or right upper quadrant mass **in the presence of jaundice (Courvoisier's sign)** is suggestive of a malignancy obstructing the biliary tree.

Laboratory workup

Obviously, the direct, indirect, and total bilirubin levels are obtained. Again, although helpful, the specific cause of jaundice cannot reliably be determined by the relative levels of conjugated and unconjugated bilirubin. Evaluation of liver synthetic function and biliary tree and hepatocyte damage are helpful. Common bile duct obstruction is typically associated with elevations of alkaline phosphatase, while elevations in AST, ALT, and lactate dehydrogenase (LDH) suggest hepatocyte damage. Decreased albumin and elevated prothrombin time (PT) imply an impairment in liver synthetic function. Viral studies to rule out hepatitis ("hepatitis screen") should be obtained, if appropriate. Screening tests for rarer diseases (such as serum iron, transferrin, and ferritin for hemochromatosis, ceruloplasmin for Wilson's disease, antimitochondrial antibodies for primary biliary cirrhosis, or alpha-1 antitrypsin for alpha-1 antitrypsin deficiency) are obtained as indicated.

Radiologic workup

If a "surgical" problem is suspected, **ultrasonography** is useful. It is fast, usually available, inexpensive, and noninvasive. Common bile duct (CBD) obstruction (of more than a few hours duration) is usually associated with ductal dilation. A normal CBD diameter is between 7-10mm; anything larger than a centimeter is usually abnormal. A **radionuclide liver scan** (DISIDA or HIDA scan) assesses overall excretory function from uptake to delivery into the duodenum and is an excellent means of diagnosing cystic duct obstruction (i.e., cholecystitis; see Chapter 33, "Biliary Tract"), but is not terribly useful if the CBD is obstructed. A **CT scan** is very useful to assess the head of the pancreas if malignancy is suspected. **Endoscopic retrograde cholangiopancreaticography** (**ERCP**), cannulation of the common bile duct from within the duodenum, and **percutaneous transhepatic cholangiography** (**PTC**), the passage of a needle through the skin and hepatic parenchyma in order to cannulate an intrahepatic duct, are both useful techniques to access the ductal system. ERCP and PTC are **complementary** studies, the choice of which depends on the level of obstruction (or lack thereof), the degree of dilation of the intrahepatic ducts, and the skill and experience of the physicians involved. Both can be used to obtain a cholangiogram, insert a stent, and to remove gallstones:

Figure 24.2
Evaluation and treatment of suspected "surgical" jaundice.

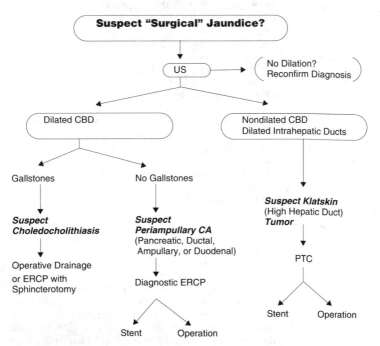

Percutaneous **liver biopsy** is sometimes useful if the cause remains obscure.

Treatment

"Surgical" jaundice is caused by obstruction of the hepatic or common bile ducts, thus accurate localization and delineation of the ductal anatomy is important. Treatment consists of the provision of mechanical relief via ERCP, PTC, or surgery. A stone in the CBD can be removed, or the duct can be bypassed by anastomosis to the duodenum or jejunum. Cholangitis can be a true emergency and usually indicates the need for urgent drainage. Tumors are problematic. Many tumors of the distal CBD or duodenum can be resected, along with the duodenum, distal CBD, and head of the pancreas (Whipple operation). Cancer of the head of the pancreas, however, is almost uniformly metastatic at the time of diagnosis, and thus simple palliation (bypass of the blocked bile duct and sometimes GI tract) is advocated by many surgeons because of its lower morbidity. Malignant obstruction of the CBD can also be palliated by placement of a stent through the lesion by ERCP or PTC.

Cirrhosis cannot be reversed, but the process can be arrested by abstinence from alcohol. If the patient is truly abstinent (and several other criteria are met), liver transplantation is an option. For most cases of "medical" jaundice, however, no cure is possible. Goals are palliation of pruritis, elimination or retardation of ongoing liver damage, and the reduction of toxins in the blood (for example, phlebotomy for hemochromatosis or copper chelation for Wilson's disease). ■

25   Abdominal Pain

Abdominal pain is usually caused by a problem with an abdominal organ, but can be the result of cardiac, pleural, metabolic, hematologic, or psychiatric pathology. Workup of patients with abdominal pain must be thorough and directed if the correct diagnosis is to be made. Silen's *Cope's Early Diagnosis of the Acute Abdomen*, in its 19th edition (1996), is the historic and current "bible" of abdominal pain.

General Concepts

Pain that is sharp, "cutaneous," and well-localized ("**somatic**" pain) is usually caused by localized irritation of the highly sensitive parietal peritoneum, while pain that is poorly localized, deep, dull, and diffuse ("**visceral**" or "**splanchnic**" pain) is usually caused by distension of a hollow viscus. The viscera do not respond to cutting, touch, or any of the stimuli that cutaneously innervated tissue does, but are exquisitely sensitive to **stretching**; the most common cause of visceral pain is obstruction of a viscus leading to **distension**. Because its recognition within the brain is poorly mapped, visceral pain is perceived by the sufferer to originate in the midline. Its cranio-caudal perception parallels embryonic neural development. Disorders affecting the ileum in the region of the embryonic midgut loop are referred to the periumbilical region. Problems with organs proximal to this (stomach, duodenum, and proximal small bowel) produce epigastric discomfort, and problems in organs distally (colon and appendix) produce peri- or infraumbilical pain. By definition, however, perception of this type of pain is ill-defined and widely variable.

Generalized inflammation of the peritoneum gives rise to **peritonitis** (discussed below). Pain can be **referred** based on central convergence of sensory nerves; irritation of the diaphragm by pus or gastric juice, for example, is perceived as shoulder pain. Pancreatitis, an expanding aortic aneurysm, or kidney stone can cause pain in the flank or mid-back because of the retroperitoneal location of their respective organs.

Location of pain

The abdomen is traditionally divided into four parts, the right and left upper and lower quadrants (**RUQ**, **LUQ**, **LLQ**, and **RLQ**). These are, of course, not anatomically separate; the terms are used for convenience of communication. When supine, the pelvis and subdiaphragmatic spaces are most dependent; thus, fluid tends to accumulate in these areas. Further, the diagonal course of the mesenteric root (from LUQ to RLQ) tends to channel fluid from the upper abdomen to the RLQ, especially if the patient is upright, explaining why a perforated ulcer can present as RLQ pain.

While there is a myriad of problems that can occur, evaluation of a person with abdominal pain is easiest if you keep in mind what is **most common**:

Location of Pain	Responsible Organ(s)	Most common causes	Where Discussed
RUQ	Gallbladder	Cholecystitis and biliary colic	Chapter 33
	Liver	Hepatitis	-
LUQ	Spleen	Rare-infarction, trauma	-
LLQ	Sigmoid colon	Diverticulosis	Chapter 32
	Left ureter	Kidney stone	Discussed Below
	Left adnexa	Pelvic inflammatory disease	Chapter 64
RLQ	Appendix	Appendicitis	Discussed Below
	Cecum	Obstructing colon cancer	Chapter 32
	Right ureter	Kidney stone	Discussed Below
	Right adnexa	Pelvic inflammatory disease	Chapter 64
Midline or Variable		Gastritis	Chapter 25
		Gastroenteritis	Discussed Below
		Peptic ulcer disease	Chapter 34
		Pancreatitis	Discussed Below
		Bowel obstruction or ischemia	Chapter 41
		Early appendicitis	Discussed Below
		Symptomatic aneurysm	Chapter 37
		Inflammatory bowel disease	Chapter 22
Diffuse peritonitis		Any longstanding process involving spillage of intestinal fluid or tissue necrosis	Discussed Below

Medicine
Abdominal Pain *continued*

History

Although assigned a lesser degree of importance in some areas of medicine, the history and physical examination remain critically important components of the evaluation of a patient with abdominal pain. First, ask the patient about the pain itself. Pain should be **characterized**:

- **Sharp pain** suggests localized peritoneal irritation or a cutaneous problem;
- **Dull** suggests visceral, stretching pain;
- **Constant** suggests an advanced process, possibly with tissue necrosis;
- **Intermittent** suggests hollow viscus (bowel, gallbladder, ureter) obstruction;
- **Improvement when lying still** suggests peritoneal irritation, while
- **"Can't get comfortable"** (**colic**) suggests biliary or ureteral obstruction.

The patient should be asked to **point to the area of pain**. A useful trick is to have patients point with one finger only – if they can, local peritoneal irritation is probable; if they vaguely wave their hand over a broad area, visceral pain or diffuse peritonitis is probably present. **Time of onset, worsening or improvement over time**, and **duration** of pain should also be determined. **Acuity of onset** is important: severe pain that begins suddenly or awakens the patient from sleep often indicates a more serious process or sudden change in the structure of an organ, while pain that gradually increases suggests a more slowly developing problem. It is important to know whether the patient has had similar pain before, and its cause, if known. The **association** of the pain with other events is often very helpful. For example, exacerbation by eating can be seen with gastritis, peptic ulcer disease, or chronic intestinal ischemia, while pain during the car ride to the hospital (going over bumps) is common in patients with peritoneal irritation.

The presence of **associated signs and symptoms** such as fever, anorexia, nausea, vomiting, diarrhea, jaundice, pruritus, or distention is important. Vomiting that precedes pain often signals a "medical" problem, while vomiting that follows pain often is seen with "surgical" conditions. The patient should be asked about recent illnesses in family members and exposure to viral or bacterial illnesses. Progressive constipation or change in stool caliber in the recent past is a clue that a growing colon cancer, now presenting as obstruction, could be present.

The **past medical history** alone can suggest the diagnoses. History of any suspected or uncorrected intra-abdominal problem obviously increases the chance that a recurrence of this problem is present; obviously, another, unconnected problem can occur. **Atrial fibrillation** and, independently, **digitalis** use are risk factors for mesenteric artery embolism and intestinal infarction, and patients with systemic atherosclerosis, who are critically ill from another problem, who may be hypercoagulatable (including those with malignancy), and on hemodialysis are at risk for embolic, occlusive, or low-flow intestinal ischemia. Knowledge of the patient's **medication** list is mandatory. For example, non-steroidal anti-inflammatory drugs (NSAIDs) can cause peptic ulcer disease or gastritis, and steroids can blunt the pain and other symptoms of acute abdominal pathology. Critically important to elicit, if present, is a **history of a previous abdominal operation**. Any operation increases the risk of adhesions and bowel obstruction (see Chapter 41, "Bowel Obstruction"), and, of course, if an organ such as the appendix was removed, the relevant diagnosis is effectively eliminated.

Physical Exam

The first move is to observe the patient's general appearance. Patients with peritoneal irritation **tend to lie very still**, because any movement jars the peritoneum and causes significant pain, while patients with renal or biliary colic usually **move about** in an attempt to find a comfortable position. Peritoneal irritation is often partially relieved by **bending the knees** to decrease peritoneal stretch. Pallor and wasting can be seen in patients with chronic anemia or cancer cachexia, while visible jaundice suggests cholangitis or hepatitis.

Tachycardia and hypotension are signs of hypovolemia caused by third-spacing (see Chapter 7, "Basic Fluids and Electrolytes" and 27, "Postoperative Care") or sepsis. **Fever** is common and nonspecific; its absence, though, does not rule out a problem. Pulmonary exam may reveal a pleural effusion or atelectasis caused by a subdiaphagmatic process, while atrial fibrillation raises the possibility of embolization.

The abdomen should first be **inspected**. The presence of distension, scars and their location, visible peristalsis, and obvious abdominal wall hernias are particularly important. **Auscultation** is only sometimes helpful. True absence of bowel sounds is characteristic of peritonitis, although a "false-positive" exam is common if you don't listen long enough, and high-pitched, "tinkling" bowel sounds or "rushes" corresponding to waves of pain are characteristic of mechanical bowel obstruction. Other than in the settings of diffuse peritonitis and bowel obstruction, however, the information gained by listening to bowel sounds or by noting their "location" is fairly minimal; bowel sounds are transmitted throughout the entire abdomen, and "where" they are heard really depends on where you're listening when they occur.

Maneuvers to elicit pain should begin by asking the patient to cough; jarring the bed or asking a standing patient drop from the toes down to the heels will accomplish the same thing. These maneuvers, as well as light **percussion**, will jar the peritoneum and cause pain if inflammation is present. **Rebound tenderness** is a technique designed to separate pain of visceral and peritoneal origin. Press down slowly; discomfort will occur whatever the source. Let things settle down, then suddenly release the pressure. If there is a sudden, sharp, often fairly severe stab of pain, **worse on the way out**, peritoneal irritation or inflammation is probably preset. Such patients will exhibit **guarding**, voluntary or involuntary abdominal muscle contraction to minimize pressure transmitted to the painful structure beneath.

Patients with peritoneal inflammation are usually in significant pain. Therefore, start with the gentlest maneuvers, work your way "upward," and **stop when you have a diagnosis**. It is cruel to persist and try to elicit rebound tenderness, for example, if it is already clear that the patient needs an operation. In the experience of many examiners, cough or percussion tenderness is most helpful, and checking for rebound tenderness is rarely necessary. **Palpation** should first be light and proceed to deep as the patient tolerates. Begin palpation away from the pain and work toward it; deep palpation should be used to assess subtle tenderness and feel for masses.

Peritonitis A word about "**peritonitis**" is appropriate. The term technically indicates inflammation of the peritoneum. It is commonly used, however, to denote the condition of widespread, diffuse peritoneal irritation due to pus, gastric juice, or other irritative or infected fluid, while the term "**localized peritonitis**" is best used to denote localized inflammation. "**Peritoneal irritation**" is the term denoting pain of peritoneal origin, in general (including "peritonitis"), that can be caused by non-surgical bowel obstruction, a kidney stone, gastroenteritis, and so on. Why are these terms significant? Because "peritonitis," whether localized or diffuse, generally means that a "surgical" condition is present, while "peritoneal irritation" is less discriminatory. The maneuvers used to assess irritation of the peritoneum—cough and percussion tenderness, rebound tenderness, and so on—are not specific for "peritonitis" or need for operation, but indicate that pain of peritoneal origin is present.

Continuing the exam, inspect the inguinal and femoral areas for hernias. The rectal exam is useful to identify tenderness, masses, or occult blood in the stool. Women with abdominal pain require a bimanual pelvic exam to identify cervical motion tenderness, adnexal pain, and masses; if suspicion for pelvic inflammatory disease is present a formal speculum exam with cultures must be performed.

Several maneuvers are helpful in specific situations. Pain on passive hip extension or active flexion suggests the presence of an inflammatory process irritating the psoas muscle ("**psoas sign**"). Inspiratory arrest with deep right upper quadrant palpation (or ultrasonic compression) suggests inflammation of the gallbladder ("**Murphy's sign**"), and "referred" RLQ pain during deep palpation of the LLQ suggests appendicitis ("**Rovsing's sign**").

Keep in mind that **elderly patients** and those receiving **steroids** can have significantly less pain than they "should" based on their true problem.
(continued)

Medicine
Abdominal Pain *continued*

Laboratory and Radiologic Workup

The white blood cell count (WBC) is often elevated during any acute inflammatory process, with a preponderance of neutrophils and bands; this is a **nonspecific** reaction to stress caused by vascular demargination. Therefore, while often useful, a high WBC does not automatically denote infection, and a normal or low WBC can be present even during significant illness in patients who are too ill or immunosuppressed to mount a proper response. Electrolyte abnormalities are common and reflect fluid shifts or actual losses from vomiting; abnormal renal chemistries in an otherwise healthy patient usually denotes severe hypovolemia. Elevated amylase and lipase are suggestive of (but not diagnostic for) acute pancreatitis, and elevated bilirubin reflects either obstruction of the biliary tree or a hepatocellular problem (see Chapter 24, "Jaundice," and 33, "Biliary Tract").

Radiographs of the abdomen show dilated bowel loops with air-fluid levels (see Chapter 41, "Bowel Obstruction") if intestinal obstruction is present. Free air anywhere in the abdomen, typically under the diaphragms on upright chest x-ray, indicates perforation of a hollow viscus and is essentially an absolute indication for operation. Ultrasound, contrast studies, endoscopy, and CT scanning all can be helpful depending on the specific problem.

Specific Problems

Kidney stones

Kidney stones are fairly common and, if on the right, can mimic appendicitis. The usual patient is young and describes significant pain starting in the flank and radiating to the appropriate lower quadrant and, if male, testicle. Pain results from ureteral obstruction and spasm; the patient will roll around in bed in an attempt to get comfortable, and typically has a significant vagal response leading to nausea and emesis. Pain is typically extreme, and peritoneal irritation is often seen. Significant hematuria (greater than 40 red blood cells (RBCs) per high power field) will usually be seen, but kidney stones can occur without hematuria, and RBCs can be seen in the urine of patients with appendicitis (see below). Kidney stones tend to recur, and many patients can thus tell you exactly what's going on.

A patient with a suspected kidney stone should have a plain abdominal x-ray; approximately 85% of kidney stones are radio-opaque. If a stone is seen or if the diagnosis is clear, an initial trial of pain control and vigorous hydration frequently leads to spontaneous passage. If the diagnosis is not clear or if pain persists, an intravenous pyelogram (IVP) is needed. If significant obstruction is present or if conservative treatment is unsuccessful, referral to a urologist for definitive treatment is appropriate.

Appendicitis

One of the most common conditions requiring urgent abdominal surgery is **appendicitis**. Pathophysiology is fairly straightforward: the small lumen of the appendix becomes obstructed by a fecalith, inflamed lymphoid tissue, or other process, causing, in sequence, distension, inflammation, and eventually infection. Perforation results if the appendix is not removed or if the obstruction fails to spontaneously resolve. While presentation can be variable, especially in patients at the extremes of age, the "classic" patient initially describes **poorly localized periumbilical visceral pain** caused by distension of the appendix. As the outer surface of the appendix becomes inflamed and irritates the parietal peritoneum, **the pain shifts in both quality and location, becoming sharp, cutaneous, and worse in the RLQ, and becomes associated with signs of peritoneal irritation ("localized peritonitis")**. Only if true rupture occurs will true diffuse peritonitis be present. The patient will classically sit with the knees bent to minimize peritoneal stretch, and will complain that bumps on the car ride to the hospital caused significant pain.

Anorexia with nausea and an episode or two of vomiting are usually present. If the patient is truly hungry or emesis is protracted, another diagnosis should be considered. Moderate **fever** (usually below 39°) and **leukocytosis** (usually less than 18,000 wbc/mL^3 or so) are later findings. Diarrhea is uncommon and, if present, suggests gastroenteritis. Auscultation of the abdomen often reveals normal bowel sounds. A useful trick is the administration pressure with your stethoscope to covertly assess the degree of pain in a patient whose nervousness interferes with an adequate exam. Radiographs are usually not helpful in the diagnosis of appendicitis per se, but can exclude other conditions.
(continued)

Medicine
Abdominal Pain *continued*

PID

Conditions that commonly mimic appendicitis are pelvic inflammatory disease (PID) and other gynecologic problems (see Chapter 64, "ED Gynecology"), gastroenteritis, and kidney stones. Right-sided PID is especially difficult to exclude because the pathophysiology and resultant physical and laboratory findings are essentially identical to those of appendicitis; in difficult cases, laparoscopy can be very useful both for diagnosis and therapy. Female patients should be thoroughly queried about their menstrual and sexual histories; pain with ovulation ("mittelschmerz") or due to a ruptured cyst often occurs at midcycle. If visible pus is seen at the cervical os or clear cervical motion tenderness is present, PID is fairly likely. It is very important to remember that appendicitis can produce microscopic hematuria and pyuria because of ureteral irritation.

Appendicitis usually evolves over 18-36 hours, with the risk of perforation increasing as time progresses. Perforation is rare if symptoms have been present for less than 12 hours, but risk is higher in the pediatric and geriatric populations.

History, physical exam, and laboratory analysis are usually sufficient to make the diagnosis. Appendectomy can be performed through a conventional RLQ incision or using laparoscopic techniques. A false negative appendectomy rate of 10%-15% is desirable: if any lower, there is a good chance that you are inappropriately reluctant to operate and missing some patients with appendicitis.

Gastroenteritis

Gastroenteritis is a fairly nonspecific term used to denote pain resulting from a mild gastrointestinal infection, irritation, or other upset. It is usually a diagnosis of exclusion, and specific testing is rarely required. Essentially by definition, gastroenteritis resolves without specific treatment. Patients with gastroenteritis typically complain of mild to moderate, diffuse abdominal pain, nausea, diarrhea, vomiting, and hyperactive bowel sounds, and have minimal, nonprogressive peritoneal irritation. Most such patients are never admitted to the hospital. Patients with gastroenteritis can have an elevated temperature and WBC, and, when they do, are typically evaluated for appendicitis. This diagnosis is applied, among other situations, when a patient operated on for appendicitis has no demonstrable tissue pathology.

Pancreatitis

Acute pancreatitis is usually the result either of alcohol abuse or of passage of a gallstone through the ampulla of Vater. Although the pathophysiology is not completely clear, in both situations there seems to be inappropriate liberation and intraglandular activation of pancreatic digestive enzymes. Pancreatitis usually produces severe, upper abdominal, midline pain, radiating to the back. Signs vary from tachycardia and tenderness to overt shock. Mild fever and leukocytosis are often present, vomiting is common and often protracted, and some degree of abdominal distension due to ileus usually occurs. Amylase and lipase levels are usually elevated. Unless clearly due to alcohol, workup should include an ultrasound to rule out gallstone disease.

Treatment is usually supportive, including bowel rest and IV fluids; nasogastric drainage is used if vomiting persists. Although patients with pancreatitis generally do not require operation, two exceptions exist. First, if the pancreas is infected (as determined by needle biopsy), serial operative debridement offers the only chance of survival. Second, if passage of a gallstone was the inciting factor the gallbladder should be removed during the primary admission. Cholecystectomy is not done to treat the **current attack** in any way, but is done to **prevent future episodes**. Thus, although early cholecystectomy can be safe in mild pancreatitis, it is usually deferred until the acute attack is over.

Acute abdomen

The term **"acute abdomen"** is used in a clinical sense to describe the situation where a sudden, potentially life-threatening situation requiring immediate operation exists. Synonyms include "abdominal catastrophe" and "diffuse peritonitis," and the urgency of the situation often mandates surgical intervention before a definite diagnosis is made. The most common conditions creating diffuse peritonitis include perforation of a viscus (usually a duodenal ulcer or colonic diverticular lesion), perforated appendicitis, longstanding bowel ischemia with infarction, or gangrenous cholecystitis. Reflex paralytic ileus is almost universal. Severe peritoneal irritation produces **involuntary** rectus muscle spasm; the classic "board-like" abdomen usually means perforation of a viscus has occurred.
(continued)

Initial **resuscitation** of a patient with an acute abdomen includes volume restoration with fluids, correction of electrolyte abnormalities, bladder catheterization to accurately assess hydration status (see Chapter 5, "Shock"), and nasogastric tube decompression. Definitive treatment usually requires operation, but, unless uncontrolled intra-abdominal bleeding exists, **a patient cannot be subjected to general anesthesia unless intravascular volume is normal.** ■

Surgery

Karl A Illig
Section Editor

26 Preoperative Care

The first step in any patient encounter, including the pre-operative evaluation, is the history. In general, apart from the specific problem the patient is being treated for, your **history** should identify issues that specifically increase the risk of anesthesia or surgery. Ask about:

– Personal or family history of bleeding problems,
– Personal or family history of problems with anesthesia,
– Recent changes in stable symptoms (such as angina, etc),
– Smoking and alcohol history,
– Aspirin or other anticoagulant use,
– Steroid use,
– Other medications.

Similarly, during the **physical exam**, look especially for things that would affect your planned surgical procedure or increase morbidity or mortality—such as evidence of cirrhosis, bleeding problems, heart or lung disease, obesity, previous scars, and so on. Do not assume the attending surgeon or anesthesiologists know every detail!

Preoperative Laboratory Evaluation

In the past, essentially everybody got the full "battery" of tests. It is becoming more and more apparent, however, that not only are most such labs unnecessary, but they also are costly and, if falsely positive, can lead to unnecessary delay and workup. The bottom line is that requirements vary from hospital to hospital, surgeon to surgeon, and anesthesiologist to anesthesiologist (and day to day!). Unfortunately, medicine remains an anecdotally-driven profession, and individual preferences will vary. In general, the following guidelines for preoperative testing are useful in **healthy, asymptomatic** patients undergoing **elective** surgery:

Age	Men	Women
Children	None	None
< 40	None	Hct
40-50	EKG	Hct
50-60	EKG	Hct, EKG
> 60	EKG, CBC, electrolytes	
> 75	EKG, CBC, electrolytes, and CXR	

A CXR is probably not routinely necessary in patients younger than 75.

Although routine "shotgun" laboratory evaluation is discouraged, patients with specific disease states have special needs. Numerous studies have demonstrated the lack of predictive value and the cost-ineffectiveness of checking coagulation parameters (platelet count, prothrombin and partial thromboplastin times) in healthy patients. If a history of bleeding is present, if the procedure carries high risk or incidence of bleeding (cardiac or vascular surgery), or if even minor bleeding would be catastrophic (neurosurgery), checking these factors as well as the bleeding time is important. Uremic patients have a high incidence of platelet dysfunction (although platelet number may be adequate), thus a bleeding time is useful. Coagulation studies (PT and PTT) should be done if liver dysfunction is suspected. Glucose should be checked in diabetics. Consider a sickle cell screen in black patients who have not already been checked, as surgery can cause significant sickling and resultant morbidity. A preoperative room air arterial blood gas provides a useful baseline value in a patient in whom you feel might have respiratory difficulties postoperatively.

Preoperative risk evaluation

Cardiac risk

In general, the first step beyond the routine history and physical to evaluate **cardiac** risk is an EKG. Unfortunately, most of the "traditional" risk factors such as angina, hypertension, hypercholesterolemia, smoking, and so on do not predict risk very well. The best clinical predictors, interestingly, are a recent myocardial infarction or current congestive heart failure episode, a previous coronary artery bypass graft, or planned peripheral vascular procedure. It's best to be too safe rather than too

Surgery
Preoperative Care *continued*

cavalier, thus, age over 40 or so, any evidence of atherosclerosis, or any stable cardiac symptoms should prompt
an EKG. New or unstable symptoms, EKG changes, high
clinical suspicion, congestive heart failure, valvular disease, or need to operate within six months after a heart
attack should prompt a cardiology consult. As with any
consult, ask a specific question: In this case, "is the
risk great enough to warrant delay in surgery," or "how
do we decrease the risk of an adverse cardiac event,
assuming that surgery cannot be delayed?" Even if
operation is required and maximal monitoring and ICU
postoperative care is already planned, merely having a
cardiologist follow the patient can improve and simplify
postoperative care.

Recent MI

Operation soon (6 months) after a myocardial infarction
is a special problem. Operation is certainly not "prohib-
ited"; the decision to operate or not is a judgment call,
based on risk-benefit analysis, and should be jointly made
by the patient, surgeon, and consultants (probably in that
order). The "classic" data show that operation 0-3 months
after a heart attack carries a 30% mortality, while operation 3-6 months after carries a 15% mortality. After 6
months, the risk is essentially baseline. Things have
improved, however, such as better monitoring and perioperative awareness and care. Current numbers are closer to
6% mortality at 0-3 months, and 3% at 3-6 months.
Truly elective cases should be deferred until 6 months
after a heart attack, but emergency surgery can be
performed earlier, depending on whether the risk from a
new infarction or from the untreated problem is believed
to be greater.

Pulmonary risk

Smoking, advanced age, or entering a major bodily cavity
(abdomen or chest) increase the risk of postop
pulmonary problems. Preoperative incentive spirometry
teaching and cessation of smoking are the minimum
requirements if risk is present. Baseline room air arterial
blood gas analysis is quite useful, both to predict risk and
also to compare in the postoperative period. Pulmonary
function tests help to determine whether the patient will
tolerate the surgery or respond to bronchodilators if doubt
is present.

Neurologic problems

Neurologic problems are also possible. Signs and symptoms of cerebral ischemia (see Chapter 37, "Vascular Surgery") mandate noninvasive carotid testing. High-grade carotid stenosis may increase the risk of a perioperative stroke, but the issue of whether to correct lesser degrees of carotid stenosis preoperatively is unresolved. A bruit (audible turbulence) does not necessarily predict a significant carotid stenosis, and usually need not alter surgical plans in the absence of symptoms, but if found should lead to noninvasive testing postoperatively (interestingly, the presence of a carotid bruit is a better predictor of postoperative **cardiac** rather than cerebral morbidity). Pay attention to drug and alcohol use, because these increase the chance of postoperative neurological problems. Postoperative unexplained tachycardia may be the first symptom of delirium tremens (alcohol withdrawal).

Metabolic disorders

Severe **metabolic** disorders need to be corrected as much as possible before surgery is safe, again using a risk/benefit analysis. Hepatic disease, especially cirrhosis, predicts a surprisingly high morbidity and mortality and must be diligently searched for. Preoperative renal insufficiency is also an important predictor of adverse outcome, particularly for elective and emergent abdominal aneurysm repair.

ASA classification

It is quite useful to have a general sense of the American Society of Anesthesiologists' (ASA) risk assessment grading system:

Grade	Description	Overall Mortality
I	No significant disease	Essentially none
II	Mild-moderate disease	< 1%
III	Severe disease	2%
IV	Incapacitating or life-threatening disease	8%
V	Moribund (not expected to survive 24 hours)	10%

An "E" is added for emergency operations (with correspondingly increased mortality rates).
(continued)

Surgery
Preoperative Care *continued*

Preoperative Check

Every patient should have a "preoperative check" in the chart on the night before surgery. The note helps organize your thinking, ensures that you haven't missed anything, and communicates important data to the anesthesia and nursing staff.

☐ **Consent:** Document that you discussed the problem, proposed procedure, risks, benefits, and alternatives with the patient (and family, if present), and that the patient understands and **consents**.

☐ **NPO after midnight** (to empty stomach).

☐ **Antibiotics** for potentially contaminated cases, or for clean cases where infection would be catastrophic (implantation of prosthetic materials, for example).

☐ **IV fluids** are not always necessary, especially for an early case. You may want to run IV fluids at low rate starting in the morning if the case will be later in the day, or you may want to hydrate the patient overnight if significant blood loss is possible, if preoperative dehydration exists, or if you have dehydrated the patient with a bowel prep, for example.

☐ Check **labs, EKG,** and **chest x-ray** if you ordered them!

☐ **Bowel preparation:** For esophageal, gastric, and especially colon surgery (see Chapter 32, "Colon and Rectum").

☐ **DVT prophylaxis:** Subcutaneous heparin should be started before surgery in patients at risk (those who are obese, have a malignancy, have had a previous DVT, or are to undergo an orthopaedic operation, for example). Subcutaneous heparin and pneumatic boots have been shown to reduce the incidence of DVT, but passive support hose probably are not of benefit.

☐ **Diabetics:** A common recommendation is to give half the usual dose of insulin in the morning and to perform the case early, but it is usually more convenient to write a sliding scale and check a fingerstick glucose level just before the operation. Serum glucose needs to be less than 200-250mg/dL for safe anesthesia and surgery.

☐ **Sterolds:** Anybody who received steroids for at least **2 weeks** in the past **2 years** needs stress-dose steroids, usually hydrocortisone in doses ranging from 25-150mg per day, depending on the magnitude of the procedure. Current data suggests that we don't need to be giving as much as we used to.

☐ **Medications:** Give beta-blockers and most cardiac drugs with a sip of water, but generally all other medications can be omitted. The anesthesiologist generally manages preoperative sedation.

Some Miscellaneous Caveats

A remote infection (suggested by a fever the morning of surgery) increases the risk of infection (i.e., always see your patients the morning of the procedure). With the exception of uncontrolled hemorrhage, no patient should be put under general anesthesia until they are making adequate urine (or more precisely, are euvolemic). Active hepatitis is an absolute contraindication to general anesthesia. And finally, don't assume that the patient has already been fully worked up—you may be the first to see abnormal labs or pick up significant findings. ■

27   Postoperative Care

Surgery is often an acute, predictable insult superimposed on fairly normal physiology, enabling the trained surgeon to make generalizations, to predict specific anticipated problems, and to plan their avoidance.

Fluids and Electrolytes

This topic is fully covered in Chapter 7, "Basic Fluids and Electrolytes." Consider the electrolyte composition of the most common intravenous fluids:

	Na^+	K^+	Cl^-	HCO_3^-	Osm	
Serum	140	4	100	26	300	
Lactated Ringer's	130	4	109	(28)	275	(Ca=3)
Normal Saline	154	0	154	0	308	

These figures demonstrate that LR (Lactated Ringer's solution) is nearly identical to serum. In the perioperative period, fluids are lost in a generally **isotonic** fashion, due to bleeding and, most importantly, via **"third spacing."**

Third Spacing

Intracellular ("first space") and extracellular ("second space") fluids are freely exchangeable. The "third space," by definition, is always pathologic, resulting from surgical stress, sepsis, or other problems, and can be thought of as fluid functionally separate and nonexchangeable with the normal intra- and extracellular fluid spaces. "Third-spaced" fluid exists within the body, but the body cannot recognize it nor can it use such fluid to perform useful "work" (such as restore intravascular volume and deliver oxygen to the tissues). In other words, a **normal** reaction to surgery is **total body fluid excess with normal or reduced intravascular volume**—the difference representing the **obligatory** "third space" losses into bowel lumen and wall, retroperitoneum, tissue (edema), etc. Unlike bleeding (a permanent loss), this fluid is still within the body and is lost only temporarily, and will eventually return to the intravascular space.

This "third spacing" occurs **isotonically**. Moreover, the associated hormonal and membrane changes occurring into the postoperative period result in continued, "third-spaced" fluid loss for several days following the procedure.

Peri- and postoperative fluid management can be divided into three phases:

Intraoperative period

Phase 1: Intraoperative losses (isotonic replacement). Fluids are given to replace estimated pre-existing volume deficits, intraoperative blood losses, evaporative losses, and losses due to third-spaced fluids—the last often being most significant. LR, being equivalent to serum, is used to replace volume, while blood itself (usually packed red cells) is used only to replace significant deficits in oxygen-carrying capacity. Although the anesthesiologist usually manages this phase, the surgeon should be aware of these issues to better judge the postop volume status of his or her patient.

Early postoperative period

Phase 2: Early postoperative period (isotonic replacement). For the first 24-72 hours after uncomplicated surgery, obligatory isotonic third-spacing occurs due to continued hormonal and cellular membrane alterations. This is often manifest clinically as "capillary leak." During this period LR continues to be the ideal replacement fluid as losses continue to be isotonic. This "third-spacing" produces mild, obligatory edema in all patients. Despite everyone's best theories concerning albumin, osmotic pressure, and so on, there's nothing you can do to alter this, and fluid replacement must be guided by clinical indicators of **intravascular volume** (see below), **not total body water!** This phase can be prolonged if the patient is sick, and this scenario is common in the ICU. Blood (again, packed cells) is given as needed to restore oxygen carrying capacity, recognizing that transfusions can transmit disease and can impair the immune system.

Late postoperative period

Phase 3: Late postoperative period (hypotonic fluids). About 24-72 hours after uncomplicated surgery the patient will begin to "mobilize fluids": as metabolism returns to normal the third-spaced fluids will begin to be "mobilized" back into the circulation as the cell membranes regain their normal function. This results in increased renal perfusion and resultant **diuresis.** This

Surgery
Postoperative Care *continued*

diuresis, therefore, signals that isotonic losses and thus the need for isotonic replacement has ended, and that the patient can be switched to **maintenance fluids** (if IV fluids are still needed).

Maintenance fluids

Maintenance fluids are easily calculatable from looking at **losses**:

Urine: Approx 1000cc/day, roughly isotonic or hypotonic
Insensible: 1000cc/day, usually very hypotonic
K^+: 40meq/day obligate urine loss

=2000cc half-isotonic fluid with $40/K^+$ each day...

Add sugar: **$D_5$1/2NS with 20 mEq/K^+/liter at 80cc/hr!**

Sometimes this normal fluid mobilization back into the intravascular space will lead to transient functional hypervolemia, especially in the elderly, even to the point of congestive heart failure. Close observation and timely diuretic administration will usually suffice.

Intravascular hypovolemia

As discussed above, because of perioperative third-spacing, intravascular hypovolemia can often exist despite total body fluid overload. In other words, the presence or absence of edema is irrelevant compared to intravascular volume status. With intravascular hypovolemia, a characteristic sequence of clinical signs develops. First, **urine output drops** as the kidneys compensate by reabsorbing sodium and water (normal urine output is 1/2cc/kg per hour, or 240cc per 8 hours in a normal adult). Next, **tachycardia** occurs as the heart compensates for the decreased stroke volume in an attempt to increase cardiac output. Finally, if the intravascular hypovolemia worsens, **hypotension** occurs, indicating that compensation has failed.

Thus, decreased urine output in the postoperative period is usually due to intravascular hypovolemia (even if edema is present), assuming that urinary retention, catheter malfunction, and ureteral or renal pathology have been ruled out. Therefore, the first step in this situation (probably the most common postoperative problem of all) is to replete the intravascular volume with fluids. Do not (initially) treat an edematous postoperative patient with oliguria with diuretics! **Urine output is a sign, not the**

goal—the artificial production of urine with diuretics in the early postoperative period only worsens the hypovolemia while doing nothing to treat the edema and third-spacing at all. Diuretics are rarely indicated in the first 48 hours postoperatively.

If there is no response to fluids or the situation is unclear, you may need more invasive monitoring (See Chapter 6, "Basic Hemodynamics and Invasive Monitoring").

"Is and Os"
Urine output and overall fluid intake and output should be monitored in essentially every postop patient. Intake does not need to equal output. In fact, as you know from the preceding discussion, after uncomplicated surgery intake should exceed output for the first few days because of ongoing, unavoidable third-space losses, while output will exceed intake during the later diuretic phase as fluids are mobilized. Remember that overall output will be underestimated because insensible losses, by definition, are not measured. Daily weights are the best indicator of acute fluid balance, and although probably not needed in uncomplicated cases, are invaluable after major surgery or when major fluid issues exist. Weight change in the short term (days) reflects fluid balance, not nutrition.

Ileus

Postop ileus is a functional paralysis of the intestinal tract, part of the "fight-or-flight" sympathetic response to stress. It is normal and expected after any surgery of significant magnitude to induce stress.

The bowel recovers at different rates. The small intestine recovers first, often within hours after surgery. Burned patients, for example, can be fed via the small intestine on the day of their injury. The stomach recovers next, often in 24-72 hours; the oropharynx and stomach secrete about 1-2 liters per day of fluid that need to go somewhere, even if the patient is NPO. The colon recovers last—heralded by the passage of flatus (stool is not a reliable sign—it can be evacuated early as a reflex, and can occur many days after the colon is ready to accept small intestinal contents). Recovery often occurs 3-5 days after bowel surgery.
(continued)

Decreased NG output and flatus are much more reliable indicators of resolving ileus than are bowel sounds or stool passage. Be very cautious with antiemetics after abdominal/bowel surgery, especially if an NG tube is not in, so as not to mask signs of obstruction or ileus (see also Chapter 3, "Nutrition").

Drains and Tubes

Many drains and related tubes can be conceptually lumped together; there are several general principles to remember.

Specific sites should be drained (stomach, bladder, or abscess cavity) rather than a diffuse area such as the peritoneal cavity. Drains provide an exit path for fluids, bacteria and debris, but can also provide an entrance for infection. Drains are not a substitute for hemostasis. They are useful for monitoring the integrity of an anastomosis, but they can mechanically damage anything they are in contact with. Finally, a drain should be removed as soon as its job is done.

NG tubes

Simple, single lumen tubes ("red rubber catheters") are rarely used for **nasogastric (NG) drainage** today, and require intermittent suction to prevent stomach mucosa from blocking the suction. Much more common are sump tubes which have a separate, sump lumen to allow air to enter and thus can be used with continuous suction. An NG tube can be set to suction to provide obligate removal of contents, but one should remember that drainage can be high even when the ileus has resolved. An NG tube that is simply placed to gravity drainage acts as an "overflow" drain, letting fluids pass distally if the bowel is ready to accept them; some surgeons use gravity drainage routinely with excellent results. This method may be less likely to cause erosive gastritis, and drainage that turns heme positive can often be treated solely by placing the tube to gravity.

An NG tube is used to prevent the obligate 1-2 liters per day of normal oropharyngeal and gastric secretions from passing into the small bowel during disease states such as small or large bowel obstruction, pancreatitis, or ileus from any source. The NG tube does not remove small bowel contents, but merely stops more fluid from arriving. Many surgeons believe that an NG tube is not needed after uncomplicated colon resection in most patients, and that it can be reserved for the minority of patients who develop postoperative nausea or vomiting. An NG tube is the solution to an acute gastric dilatation, often reactive to another process, which can be severe enough to mimic an acute abdomen. It is used to drain stomach contents before emergency surgery, to sample the stomach contents for blood, bile, or toxins, and to decompress the stomach for laparoscopy. An NG tube produces minimal morbidity and is invaluable in any situation where an obstruction or ileus might be present, but is uncomfortable, interferes with pulmonary toilet and ambulation, and can cause sinusitis or even esophageal perforation. Like any tube, it should be removed promptly when its job is done.

Foley catheter

A **bladder (Foley) catheter** is absolutely critical to monitor urine output when there is any question of volume status. Remember, "no urine output" in a patient without a Foley could range from total anuria to a brisk diuresis with a full (but obstructed) bladder—so the first move, in this situation, is to put one in. It is used to monitor urine output in real time, to act as a stent after prostatectomy or bladder surgery, and to prevent or relieve obstruction after hemorrhoid surgery, low sigmoid or rectal surgery, during epidural anesthesia in males, and in patients with prostatic hypertrophy. A Foley is, however, uncomfortable and interferes with ambulation. It also contributes to or causes urinary tract infections in virtually all cases if left in for a long enough period. In general, a urinary tract infection cannot be eradicated, only suppressed, until the Foley is removed. Incontinence is not a good reason for a Foley—use a condom catheter. The longer the Foley is in, the greater the risk of infection, and the greater the incidence of retention and recatheterization. Once again, remove the catheter as soon as its job is done.

"Surgical" drains

"Surgical" drains can be open to the atmosphere, such as Penrose, gauze, or sump drains, or closed, such as Jackson-Pratt ("JP"), or Hemovac drains. Drains are used to reduce the risk of seroma formation after surgery involving lymph node basins, to drain accumulating fluids under flaps to improve adherence, and to allow egress of pus and debris from a frank abscess or contaminated space. In an infected situation a drain is often left in

Surgery
Postoperative Care *continued*

longer, and is withdrawn slowly to allow closure from below. Although discouraged, drains are sometimes indicated in special circumstances in the general peritoneal cavity, such as after an emergency splenectomy (if one is worried about pancreatic injury), a cholecystectomy for severe cholecystitis, or a low colon anastomosis. In this situation it is important to remember that the drainage may stay high; normal peritoneal fluid accumulates continuously, and thus the drain can be removed even if drainage continues. Finally, drains are used in situations where even a slight amount of drainage could be dangerous, such as within the enclosed spaces of the neck.

Chest tubes

Chest tubes (see Chapter 35, "Thoracic Surgery") are used in two ways. In the short term, chest tubes are used to drain air (pneumothorax) or blood (hemothorax) from the chest after trauma or surgery, or after spontaneous or neoplastic problems have arisen. They must remain tightly sealed, are removed when the accumulation has stopped, and are pulled quickly to avoid an iatrogenic pneumothorax. Pus in the chest (empyema), however, is often treated with chronic chest tubes ("empyema tubes"). These can be left open to air as the lung is adherent to the chest wall, and are withdrawn slowly, over days or weeks, to allow a tract to form and closure to take place from within.

Miscellaneous Postoperative Issues

Lab workup

Laboratory values should be checked for specific reasons only—healthy patients after uncomplicated surgery do not need routine labs.

Assess the hematocrit after re-equilibration if significant losses were encountered, or serially if continued loss is possible. The white blood cell count is often elevated with infection, but can also be increased after stress due to vascular demargination. The platelet count and tests of coagulation are rarely abnormal unless the patient is very sick (liver failure, disseminated intravascular coagulopathy) or has received a massive transfusion. Platelets should, however, be monitored routinely while a patient is on heparin to identify heparin-induced thrombocytopenia/thrombosis. Electrolytes should be followed in the setting of massive fluid shifts, fistulas, prolonged IV hyperalimentation, renal or acid-base abnormalities, and so on.

Prealbumin and albumin are useful in the assessment of long-term nutritional status. Glucose levels should be followed closely in diabetics. A sudden rise in glucose levels or insulin requirements could signify insulin resistance due to occult sepsis. In diabetics in the postoperative period it's most convenient to check finger-stick glucose levels every 6 hours and cover with an insulin sliding scale. Their normal regimen can be resumed when the patient is tolerating regular food.

Antibiotics

Antibiotics should also be used only for specific reasons. **Prophylactic antibiotics** are used when infection, although not present, is a risk (bowel or groin surgery) or when infection, although unlikely, would be catastrophic (insertion of a heart valve or vascular graft, for example). The principle is to obtain an adequate tissue level **at the time of surgery** with a drug effective against most common pathogen(s), and stop administration quickly after. Many choices exist. For enteric pathogens commonly found during bowel or biliary procedures, a 2nd generation cephalosporin such as cefoxitin or cefotetan is often used. A 1st generation cephalosporin such as cefazolin is often used when skin flora are expected to be the primary pathogens, and vancomycin and gentamycin are often recommended in the setting of prophylactic heart valves.

Therapeutic antibiotics, on the other hand, by definition are used when an infection already exists. In general, one starts with broad coverage after an "educated guess" as to the likely pathogen(s), with coverage subsequently narrowed when further data accumulates.

Postoperative fevers

Virtually all **postoperative fevers** within the first 2-3 days after surgery are due to atelectasis, and therefore these patients rarely need to be cultured or worked up. Especially in the obese, elderly, and those with thoracic or high abdominal incisions, periodic coughing, deep breathing, and early and frequent ambulation are vital to prevent significant atelectasis and subsequent pneumonia. Fever occurring beyond the first few days should be worked up, and not attributed to atelectasis unless other sources have been ruled out. Common sources include wound infections, urinary tract infections, drug reactions, pneumonia, anastomotic leaks, abscesses, and so on. A common source and one that is often overlooked is indwelling intravenous and intraarterial catheters, which need to be changed or removed if the source of the fever is obscure. It is very rare for a wound infection to occur in the first few days unless infected before the operation. Important exceptions are the anaerobic, gas-forming organisms such as anaerobic strep and clostridia.

Deep venous thromboses

Deep venous thromboses are very difficult to diagnose. Homan's sign (pain in the calves with dorsiflexion) is highly variable and of little value whether present or not. Perioperative prophylaxis is problematic. Sequential compression stockings work well, probably by activation of fibrinolysis as well as by augmenting venous flow. Likewise, low-dose subcutaneous heparin works well, and does not seem to cause increased bleeding. Passive support hose and, in fact, early ambulation have not been shown to reduce risk. A ventilation-perfusion (VQ) scan can suggest a pulmonary embolus, but the gold standard is pulmonary arteriography. A high level of suspicion is required to make the diagnosis. Unfortunately, about half the patients who die of a pulmonary embolus have no antecedent symptoms or signs of deep venous thrombosis.

"Stress" bleeding

Significant bleeding from **stress ulcers** and **gastritis**, both significant problems in the past, have been virtually eliminated by the liberal use of histamine receptor blockers and antacids. One or the other should probably always be used after operations of any magnitude, and in any patient who requires ICU care. A recent study showed negligible major bleeding rates in patients not on a ventilator for more than two days or without a coagulopathy, and suggests the elimination of routine prophylaxis for all but these groups, but this opinion is not yet universally accepted. ■

28   Trauma

Trauma is the leading cause of death in the first four decades of life. The care of the acutely injured patient proceeds in a rigorous, methodical fashion as dictated by the **Advanced Trauma Life Support (ATLS) protocol** developed and taught by the American College of Surgeons.

Mortality from trauma follows a trimodal distribution.

Figure 28.1
Trimodal distribution of trauma deaths. The focus of ATLS is the period of time shortly (minutes to hours) after injury and arrival in the emergency department.

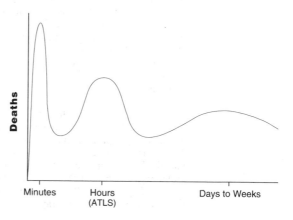

Immediate deaths (minutes) are unpreventable by the surgeon, and are best addressed by political, public health, or safety professionals. Likewise, late deaths (days to weeks), often occurring in the ICU, are not the focus of ATLS or this chapter. ATLS was designed to standardize and improve care in the so-called "golden hour" of initial resuscitation in the trauma room, and to act as a guideline to prioritize the steps to be taken. The key to management of trauma patients is an approach predicated on prioritizing injuries by their life-threatening potential. Injuries that can kill in minutes are addressed first (the "primary survey"), while more minor injuries are left until later ("secondary survey" and "definitive care"). With well-trained teams, many steps, including resuscitation, can be done simultaneously.
(continued)

The mnemonic "ABCDE" is the guide to caring for injured patients.

Airway

Securing the **airway** is the first and most important step in caring for any trauma patient—blood is no good if it isn't carrying oxygen, and oxygen can't get into the blood unless it first gets into the lungs (see Chapter 1, "Airway and Ventilator Management"). Cervical spine injury is assumed present until proved otherwise, and can be worsened by neck extension. A person needs a definitive (mechanical) airway if unconscious, needs positive pressure ventilation, can't breathe effectively, or has structural damage to their oropharynx. Oro- or nasotracheal intubation is the first choice. Occasionally the upper airway will be impossible to manage and these patients will require a surgical airway (cricothyroidotomy).

Breathing

After the airway is controlled, adequate **ventilation** must be assured. The most common causes of inadequate ventilation are an improperly placed (i.e., esophageal) endotracheal tube or a pneumo- or hemothorax. If significant pneumothorax, massive hemothorax, or tension pneumothorax is suspected clinically, immediate chest decompression is performed (by needle thoracentesis or chest tube) without waiting for x-ray.

Circulation

Control of obvious external **hemorrhage**, obtaining **intravenous access**, and **fluid resuscitation** are the next priority. A minimum of 2 large bore (16 or 14 gauge) IVs should be placed peripherally, always proximal to any extremity injury. In situations where peripheral access is not possible, large bore venous access (8.5 Fr. introducer sheath) may be placed in the femoral, subclavian, or internal jugular veins, or the saphenous, femoral, or brachial veins can be accessed by surgical cutdown. In children, intraosseous infusion (tibia, femur) is a good alternative if IV access is not possible.

Fluid resuscitation is begun with 2 liters of isotonic lactated Ringer's solution in adults, 20 cc per kilogram in children. Further fluid and/or blood requirements are determined by the subsequent course. Obviously, if no pulse is detectable, external cardiac compressions are performed. Cardiac arrest in trauma, especially if blunt, carries a dismal prognosis.

Disability (Neurologic Assessment)

Having secured airway, breathing, and circulation, a **brief** exam is performed to determine the extent of **neurologic injury**. This includes determining mental status (level of consciousness) and pupillary reaction. The "AVPU" scale is a crude but convenient method of defining mental status: the patient is described as being alert (A), responsive to verbal stimulus (V), responsive to painful stimulus only (P), and unresponsive (U). The Glasgow Coma Score (GCS) is most useful for comparing serial neurologic exams, and is predictive of recovery. It is a scale ranging from 3-15 that includes scoring of best eye opening, verbal, and motor responses.

Exposure

Expeditious but complete re-examination of the patient from head to toe is next to discover any other injuries. **Removing all clothing** (with efforts to avoid hypothermia) is important. **Look at the back** to avoid missed injuries.

At this time other catheters (nasogastric tube, Foley catheter, other venous access) and monitoring devices such as EKG leads and the oxygen saturation monitor are placed. Appropriate blood, urine, and radiographic studies are obtained. Initial portable radiographs include chest and pelvis, and often C-spine (but a normal single lateral does **not** rule out significant injury). Definitive radiographs are deferred until the patient is stable.

Specific Injuries

Chest trauma accounts for approximately 25% of all civilian trauma deaths. Airway control and tube thoracostomy effectively treat the majority of these patients, while thoracotomy is required in only 10%-15% of cases.
(continued)

Surgery
Trauma *continued*

Rib fractures

Rib fractures are the most common thoracic injury and are usually adequately treated with analgesics and muscle relaxants. The associated pain can impair pulmonary toilet and lead to retained secretions, atelectasis, and pneumonia. Fractures of any of the first 3 ribs, clavicle, or scapula suggests that significant force has been applied to the chest; this raises the suspicion that occult vascular trauma is present. When 2 or more ribs are fractured in 2 or more places, a free-floating segment of chest wall exists. This is called a **flail chest** and produces paradoxical chest wall motion. Ventilation and oxygenation may be so compromised that intubation and mechanical ventilation is required. Injury to the underlying lung tissue is termed **pulmonary contusion**. Typically, there is alveolar edema and hemorrhage, leading to shunting and decreased compliance (increased stiffness) of the lung.

Pneumothorax

Pneumothorax is the accumulation of air in the potential space between the visceral and parietal pleura. This results when there is disruption of the chest wall, pleura, or tracheobronchial tree. If the chest wall defect is sufficiently large, air can move in and out through the chest wall defect, a so-called open pneumothorax or "sucking chest wound." If the accumulated air in the pleural space is under positive pressure, then a **tension pneumothorax** exists. This may lead to rapid hemodynamic and respiratory failure as lung is collapsed and mediastinal structures are forced toward the contralateral hemithorax, "pinching off" the cava at the diaphragm. This is a clinical (not radiologic) diagnosis that requires immediate needle decompression followed by tube thoracostomy. **Hemothorax** is the accumulation of blood in the potential space between the parietal and visceral pleura. Tube thoracostomy with large (36 French) chest tubes is sufficient treatment in the majority of patients with hemothorax. An initial blood loss of 1-2000cc or ongoing blood loss of 1-200cc per hour is generally an indication for exploratory thoracotomy.

Myocardial injury

Direct trauma to the heart and subsequent cardiac injury is called **myocardial contusion**. This is usually an electrical rather than a mechanical problem; the extent of cardiac dysfunction is variable and the most common presenting sign is dysrhythmia. The EKG is almost always abnormal, while cardiac enzymes (CPK-MB) are of no value in diagnosis. If a new-onset dysrhythmia is present then continuous telemetry (but not necessarily ICU care) is required. Treatment is generally supportive, and outcome good. **Cardiac tamponade** is the accumulation of blood (or other fluid) within the pericardial sac that impairs filling of the heart. Pericardiocentesis is both diagnostic and temporarily therapeutic, but formal thoracotomy is required.

Aortic tear

An **aortic tear** results from a shearing force at the ligamentum arteriosum where the aorta is tethered to the pulmonary artery and typically occurs after a deceleration injury (car crash or fall). Most patients exsanguinate and die immediatcly, but perhaps 20% have a contained hematoma and survive to hospital arrival. A suggestive mechanism of injury and mediastinal widening by chest x-ray should raise suspicion and should prompt angiography (CT has not been as accurate). The **diaphragm** is several times more likely to sustain injury from penetrating rather than blunt trauma. Regardless of mechanism, diaphragmatic herniation may later occur, so this injury always requires repair. Diaphragmatic hernias are not always identifiable on radiographs, can go undiagnosed for months or years, and may then be discovered serendipitously at laparotomy for other intra-abdominal conditions.

Abdominal trauma

The history and physical examination are sufficient to evaluate the **abdomen** of an awake, alert, responsive, unintoxicated, and unmedicated patient with isolated abdominal trauma. In any other situation, such as the presence of an equivocal abdominal examination or a patient in whom the exam is unreliable (intoxication, significant other injuries, spinal cord injury, need for general anesthesia), workup in the form of a diagnostic peritoneal lavage (DPL) and/or CT are indicated. DPL is the study of choice in the hemodynamically unstable multiply-injured trauma patient (quick, cheap, and highly accurate). Unfortunately, DPL does not yield any information about the retroperitoneum, and is overly sensitive (mandating a significant number of "positive but unnecessary" laparotomies). CT (slow, expensive, but very accurate and specific) is only indicated in the hemodynamically stable patient. The management of **stab wounds** is individualized. Observation with serial exams is acceptable if the patient is stable and has no evidence of peritoneal irritation or hypotension. **A gunshot wound to the abdomen**

Surgery
Trauma *continued*

mandates exploration due to the large amount of kinetic energy transferred to the intra-abdominal contents.

Spleen

The **spleen** is one of the most commonly injured intra-abdominal organs. The choice of splenic salvage versus splenectomy is made weighing the risks of increased blood loss with observation or repair versus late post-splenectomy sepsis after splenectomy, respectively. Kerr's sign, referred pain to the left shoulder from diaphragmatic irritation secondary to splenic injury, should not be missed. A classic radiographic finding suggestive of subcapsular splenic hematoma is medial displacement of the gastric bubble.

Liver

The **liver** is the other most commonly injured organ following blunt trauma. Fifty percent of liver injuries are nonbleeding at time of exploration. Significant bleeding can be controlled by inflow occlusion (Pringle maneuver), compressing the hepatic artery and portal vein. If inflow occlusion is unsuccessful, one must assume retrohepatic caval injury, hepatic vein injury, or juxtacaval intraparenchymal hepatic vein injury. In this dire circumstance, emergent atrial-caval shunting is often required and mortality exceeds 50%.

Small bowel

The **small bowel** is the most commonly injured organ in penetrating abdominal trauma. During laparotomy the entire small bowel should be meticulously examined. Simple lacerations are debrided and repaired. With more extensive or multiple localized injuries, bowel resection is considered; reanastomosis is generally safe.

Colon

Treatment of **colon** injuries is individualized. Primary repair is generally acceptable only in the stable patient with minimal contamination, intact vascularity, minimal tissue loss, and few other injuries. There is a general trend to primarily repair right colon injuries, stab wounds, and low-velocity gunshot wounds. More significant injuries or those with significant fecal spillage are typically treated with resection and proximal colostomy, but primary anastomosis with a diverting colostomy to protect the anastomosis may be considered. **Rectal injuries** proximal to the dentate line require diverting colostomy and drainage.

Duodenum

Penetrating **duodenal injuries** are typically diagnosed at exploratory laparotomy. Blunt duodenal injuries are generally occult and the associated delay in diagnosis may be lethal. There is an approximately four-fold increase in mortality if diagnosis is delayed more than 24 hours. Serum amylase is useful as an initial screen but is unreliable. If suspicion exists, Gastrografin swallow or CT with intraluminal contrast are helpful. Most duodenal injuries may be repaired primarily, but many require "exclusion" (stapling of the pylorus with proximal diversion through a gastrojejunostomy). Intramural **duodenal hematomas** do not usually require operative intervention, but respond to nasogastric suction and hyperalimentation. If the resulting obstruction persists, operative evacuation of the hematoma is indicated.

Vascular abdominal trauma

The mortality from **vascular abdominal trauma** is variable—greatest for aortic injuries, less so for superior mesenteric and iliac vessels, and least for caval injuries. Approximately one third of patients with vascular abdominal trauma present in shock; management priorities are concomitant resuscitation and emergent control of hemorrhage. This is nearly always best accomplished in the operating room. **Midline** hemorrhage is most complex as the source could involve aorta, celiac axis, mesenteric vessels, portal vein, or the inferior vena cava with possible associated gastric, duodenal, or pancreatic injuries. Proximal aortic control may be achieved by direct compression of the supraceliac aorta or through a left anterolateral thoracotomy. Retrohepatic caval injuries are highly lethal. **Lateral** hematomas are most often due to renal parenchymal or renovascular injuries. The approach to **pelvic** hematomas depends on the mechanism of injury, with those due to blunt pelvic fractures controlled nonsurgically (external stabilization or embolization), but those following penetrating trauma requiring exploration. In general, midline hematomas require exploration, while lateral hematomas in the setting of a normal "one-shot" portable intravenous pyelogram (documenting bilateral renal perfusion) and pelvic hematomas in the setting of pelvic fractures do not.

GU trauma

Hematuria does not correlate well with severity of injury to the **genitourinary system**. As a result, one must rely on mechanism of injury and other physical exam findings. If urethral injury is suspected (blood at the meatus, massive pelvic fracture, "high riding" prostate, urinary retention, bladder distention), a retrograde urethrogram is indicated prior to foley placement. In the hemodynamically unstable trauma patient, the upper urinary system can be assessed with a "one-shot" IVP. If stable, then the CT scan is very accurate.

Pelvic fracture

Anterior **pelvic fractures** are relatively benign, while posterior fractures are highly morbid. Massive blood loss can occur into the retroperitoneum from pelvic fractures. Approximately 25% of trauma patients with pelvic fractures have intra-abdominal injury. In this setting, the DPL should be performed via the supraumbilical approach to avoid a false-positive result from properitoneal blood. If stable, a pelvic CT is useful. Treatment is external fixation; operation is avoided.

Neurologic injury

The severity of **neurologic injury** is easily assessed by determination of level of consciousness, pupillary exam, and lateralized sensory-motor changes. In general, any evidence of head injury mandates a CT. Global injury ("concussion," contusion) is treated supportively, while space-occupying hematomas and depressed skull fractures generally require surgery. Secondary injury prevention consists of the prevention of cerebral hypoxia by optimizing cerebral perfusion pressure (arterial pressure minus intracranial pressure, ICP) and arterial oxygen content. Generally, ICP is controlled with hyperventilation, fluid restriction and osmotic diuresis (if the patient's overall condition allows), and the reverse Trendelenberg position.

All patients sustaining blunt trauma are presumed to have **spinal injury** until proved otherwise. Spinal immobilization is instituted early and is maintained until specific injuries are excluded. Incomplete spinal cord injury typically presents with mixed sensory and motor deficits which tend to improve over time. Complete spinal cord injuries are characterized by complete sensory and motor loss below the level of injury, and these patients will likely not improve function beyond one cord level above the initial injury. Intravenous steroid therapy for the first 24 hours, although still controversial, is currently the standard of care in acute spinal cord injury due to blunt trauma.

Neck trauma

Trauma to the anterior triangle of the **neck** that penetrates the platysma is associated with a high probability of tracheal, esophageal, or vascular injury. Conversely, penetrating injuries to the posterior triangle are much less likely to involve important structures. The anterior neck is divided into three regions. Zone I is the infraclavicular neck (essentially thorax) and injuries at this level carry the greatest mortality due to the proximity of major vascular and thoracic structures. Zone II is the area of the neck located between the clavicles and the angle of the mandible and is the most common location for penetrating neck injury. Trauma to the mid neck carries the least mortality as injuries are easily identified and exposure is readily accomplished. Zone III is the region of the neck cephalad to the angle of the mandible where the distal carotid artery and the pharynx are at risk. Operative exposure is particularly difficult in this region of the neck. Zone II injuries that penetrate the platysma mandate either exploration or full radiographic and endoscopic examination of the arteries, esophagus, and trachea.

Extremity trauma

Extremity trauma involves soft tissue, bone, nerves, and vessels. Penetrating trauma tends to directly disrupt blood vessels, whereas blunt trauma can cause intimal injury with later thrombosis; a normal vascular exam does not rule out a vascular injury. The most conservative view is that any injury in the proximity of major blood vessels (especially penetrating trauma) deserves operative or angiographic evaluation regardless of the physical examination. Many vascular and trauma surgeons, however, feel that in the setting of a normal vascular exam without hard signs of unstable vascular injury (expanding hematoma, continued hemorrhage, pulsatile hematoma, bruit, etc.) observation alone is sufficient. Duplex ultrasonography has emerged as a valuable tool in this setting.

Long bone fractures

Long bone fractures are associated with fat embolization syndrome and resulting pulmonary damage. The mechanism is poorly understood, but there is strong evidence that early (within hours) operative stabilization of major fractures improves morbidity and mortality. Soft tissue injury is treated by debridement of devitalized tissue and copious irrigation. Often the involved soft tissue will be ischemic or inadequate to cover vital structures (nerves, tendons, and vessels). This situation requires revascularization of the ischemic tissue and/or grafting tissue to cover the traumatic defect. The most important prognostic factor in these injuries is the limb's neurologic status. Nerves will rarely regenerate. If irreversibly denervated, consideration is given to primary amputation. ■

29 Wounds

Wounds differ by cause, chronicity, degree of contamination, and so on, and their management can seem complex and difficult to conceptualize. Experience resolves much of the difficulty, but as a starting point one can lump all wounds (traumatic defects) together in a biologic and even therapeutic sense.

Pathophysiology

Basically, all acute wounds have in common disruption of the endothelium. A characteristic sequence of events occur.

Wound healing

First is **hemostasis** (see Chapter 8, "Hemostasis, Thrombosis, and Transfusion"). Vasoconstriction occurs initially, followed by platelet aggregation, thrombosis and fibrinolysis. Subsequent vasodilatation, increased capillary permeability, and chemotactic mediators (most importantly products produced in the compliment cascade) lead to the **cellular phase** of healing, when inflammatory cells such as neutrophils and macrophages enter the wound, followed by fibroblasts and myofibroblasts. The fibrin created during coagulation acts as a scaffolding to support the influx of cellular components (but also entraps bacteria, protecting them from antibiotics). This lasts several days, and is known as the "lag phase" because strength of the wound is minimally affected. From about 5 days to 3 weeks or so, **collagen deposition** (synthesized and secreted by the fibroblasts) occurs, and gain in strength is high ("log phase"). Finally, from 3-4 weeks to 6-12 months after injury, the **collagen remodeling** phase occurs. During this phase the amount of collagen does not change, but the strength of the wound continues to increase as a result of remodeling due to collagen cross-linking. These events account for the clinical observations that the strength of most wounds does not start to significantly increase until several days after injury but is high after several weeks, that gain in strength continues for 6-12 months, and that a healing wound that is disrupted after a few days and reclosed will regain strength much faster because the "lag phase" (cellular infiltration) has already occurred.

Treatment

Again, in the most fundamental sense, there are three types of wounds. Simple wounds with little or no tissue loss that are **clean**; the same wounds but **dirty**; and complex wounds that involve actual **tissue loss**. Clean and dirty are relative terms, defined only by specific situations and experience of the clinician.

Clean wounds

There are two major issues in an uncomplicated, relatively small **clean** surgical or traumatic wound—strength, and barrier function, i.e., resistance to bacterial invasion. The strength of a wound is obviously nil to start—this is why we suture and staple. Strength starts to increase significantly after a few days, once collagen deposition begins, but this varies with age of the patient, the clinical milieu, and the anatomic location. Cosmetic concerns affect decision making. The trade-off is between native strength and scarring produced by the artificial materials used to hold the wound together. A wound's barrier function is also zero to start, but very quickly (by 24-36 hours after injury) an epithelial monolayer grows over the wound, rendering its resistance to infection quite strong. This is why the initial sterile dressing applied in the operating room or emergency department is usually left undisturbed for the first day or so. The dressing can be removed, for example, leaving the wound open, on morning rounds the second postoperative day. The patient can even shower at this point (but bathing or soaking may not be a good idea until the staples or sutures have been removed).

Dirty wounds

The above applies to wounds closed primarily ("healing by primary intention"). If an operation is **"dirty"** or the risk of infection is otherwise high, the wound can be left open to heal by "secondary intention." Leaving a wound open is a little bit of a misnomer. The fascia (or strength layer) of the abdomen is quite resistant to infection and is almost always sutured closed. It is the overlying, relatively avascular fat that is prone to infection and is left open. This open wound is treated with dressings designed to provide gentle mechanical debridement and to protect the wound. The wound is not sterile, but dressings should be to keep it as clean as possible.
(continued)

Surgery
Wounds *continued*

The fate of a wound left open can follow several courses. If it is clean on the fourth or fifth postop day, it can be loosely closed with sutures or steristrips ("delayed primary intention"). Unclosed, it will contract and heal, leaving a scar (which can be surprisingly small in some cases). Finally, if anticipated closure is too slow, a split-thickness skin graft can be placed if the underlying tissue is clean and healthy.

A surgical wound closed primarily that becomes infected (redness, warmth, pain, etc.) should usually be reopened (at the bedside), both to allow drainage of any pus, if present, and to prevent the almost inevitable later abscess if not. Antibiotics are used to treat the associated cellulitis, but simple opening and drainage alone is probably adequate for any abscess.

Tissue loss

Wounds that involve **loss** of enough **tissue** to make primary or secondary closure impossible, such as burns or lower extremity ulcers, are the final major group. In these wounds, especially burns, one must also consider the issue of loss of thermoregulatory and barrier function and treat the patient accordingly, often with high volumes of fluid, external warming devices, and so on. Again, these wounds are not sterile, but should be covered with sterile dressings changed at frequent intervals to keep the wound as clean as possible. These wounds, by definition, require some form of surgical closure (discussed below).

General principles

The treatment of **any** wound can be conceptually simplified to encompass a few consistent principles.

First, **identify the cause**, and **correct or plan to correct it**, if possible. This step is vitally important, for example, when dealing with decubitus ulcers, where removal of pressure is the essential first step, or arterial ulcers, where surgical revascularization is necessary for healing.

Second, **drain all infected spaces (abscesses)**. This can be done at the bedside, in the emergency room, or in the operating room as dictated by the size and sensation of the wound. A route must be kept open for continued removal of debris, by means of a large opening or a drain. If the skin is allowed to close too soon, the abscess will reform. Again, the wound is not sterile—it can usually be washed with soapy water between dressing changes—but should be kept clean with a sterile dressing.

Third, **debride all dead tissue**. This can be done both grossly and microscopically. Gross debridement can be done at the bedside with a scalpel, suture removal kit, or any other tool, or can be performed in the operating room as a formal procedure, again depending upon the size and sensation of the wound. Microscopic debridement is best accomplished by a simple "wet-to-dry dressing." This is ideal for most cases, the principle is that as the inner layer dries, dead tissue will adhere and be debrided when the dressing is changed. The dressing should be "moist"; a "soupy" wound should be avoided. Such wet, oozing wounds are best treated with dry dressings alone, using the same principle. In general, most solutions other than saline do more harm to tissues than to bacteria (Dakin's, Betadine, etc). The simpler the better—there is probably little advantage to complicated sprays and so on.

Fourth, **fight infection**. Antibiotics, usually targeted against gram positive skin flora, are routinely used for cellulitis (diffusely infected soft tissue). Any abscess **must be opened and drained**. Although antibiotics are often given as a "knee-jerk" reaction, if adequate drainage has been established and there is minimal cellulitis, antibiotic coverage is not required for most abscesses. A wound that is open and receiving good care in a healthy patient is resistant to infection.
(continued)

Finally, **close the defect**. Wounds that involve little or no loss of tissue can be closed by primary intention if clean, or by delayed primary or secondary intention if dirty, given time, good local care, correction of the underlying cause, and good local blood supply and nutrition. Wounds with significant loss of tissue require more complex definitive treatment. If clean, such a wound with **granulation tissue** (red, meaty appearance due to ingrowing capillary buds) can be closed with a split-thickness graft—split-thickness signifying that epidermis and some dermis (with enough endothelial precursors left in both the donor and recipient sites to allow endothelial regeneration) is autotransplanted. This is generally left absolutely undisturbed for about 4 days to allow capillary ingrowth. If structures that won't support a skin graft (by "supplying" capillaries) such as bone or tendon are exposed, a "macrovascularized" composite graft must be used for coverage. The flap's native blood supply may be carefully saved by rotating it on a pedicle, or the flap may be cut entirely free and transferred to the recipient site, with microvascular anastomoses (arterial and venous) done to convenient nearby vessels.

Special Cases

Lower extremity ulcers

Most **lower extremity ulcers** are one of three types. **Venous stasis ulcers** are caused by chronically elevated venous pressure resulting from venous valvular damage secondary to a previous deep venous thrombosis. These ulcers are often pretibial or malleolar, clean, and shallow. A venous ulcer is associated with stigmata of chronic venous stasis ("brawny," pitting edema due to chronic hemosiderin and other protein extravasation). In a sense, these wounds are due to hypoxia due to the increased distance required for oxygen to diffuse from the capillaries, and the most vital treatment therefore is elevation and compression wraps to reduce the edema. Wet-to-dry dressings or medicated wraps (Unna Boots) are used for local debridement and cleaning. Lower extremity ulcers can also result from **arterial insufficiency** (see Chapter 37, "Vascular Surgery"). These are usually deep, dirty, and infected, and occur distally, often on the toes. Their presence indicates a high risk of a major amputation if not corrected, and surgical arterial revascularization is usually necessary to save the limb. Finally, lower extremity ulcers can exist in **diabetic patients** with normal arterial supply (although many diabetics have impaired arterial inflow, as well). These ulcers are often located on the balls of the feet ("malperforans ulcers") and are multifactoral, due to chronic trauma in the setting of diabetic neuropathy and to poor intrinsic wound healing due to impaired immune and inflammatory function.

Burns

Burns are due to heat (damage from frostbite is conceptually similar). **First degree burns** involve damage to epidermis only, and healing is spontaneous. **Second degree burns ("partial thickness")** involve damage to varying levels of dermis, but again, spontaneous healing is expected from epithelial regeneration from the hair follicles. Deep second degree and **third degree ("full thickness")** burns, by definition, involve loss of enough dermis to make epithelial regeneration impossible. These must, again by definition, be closed with a skin graft. A surgical split-thickness skin graft is a second degree wound. Only second and third degree burns are physiologically significant, and only these are counted when describing the total body surface area burned.

Burns can be devastating. Early excision of eschar and early grafting of deep wounds improves overall outcome. Intact blisters due to second degree burns are sterile and provide an ideal milieu for healing, probably containing high local concentrations of growth factors, and thus should usually be left alone (but dead tissue should be debrided once the blister has opened). A second degree burn can be converted to a full-thickness wound requiring grafting if infection is allowed unchecked, thus topical antibiotics are universally used. Silver sulfadiazine (Silvadene), a topical antibiotic, is the traditional and ideal treatment for burns or any extensive open wound. Interestingly, systemic antibiotics given early have been shown to worsen outcome and should not be used in a prophylactic sense; these should be reserved for specific infectious complications. ■

30   Hernia

Abdominal wall hernias are the most common medical condition requiring major surgery. "Hernia" means "rupture" (Latin) or "bud" (Greek). It is defined as a protrusion of anything (here, omentum, bowel, or fat) through an opening in the wall of the cavity in which it is normally contained. Groin hernias are much more common in men due to the larger opening required for passage of the spermatic cord.

Background

The hernia **orifice** and **sac** are two different entities, and are a hernia's most important features. The orifice corresponds to the fascial defect itself, while the sac is an actual outpouching of peritoneum. The neck of the hernia sac protrudes through the defect. The term **hernia** is used clinically to describe the defect itself whether or not anything actually protrudes at the time of examination. Having the potential for a hernia (fascial weakness) does not mean that a hernia sac will necessarily develop. Other factors must be present to cause failure of the abdominal wall to retain its contents, such as humans' erect stance and the effects of gravity, muscular weakness, chronic connective tissue stress from coughing due to smoking or chronic lung disease or persistent straining at urination due to prostatic hypertrophy, aging, intrinsic connective tissue disease, or chronic abdominal distention due to ascites or peritoneal dialysis. Abdominal wall hernias usually occur in areas where aponeurotic tissue is devoid of the protective support of skeletal muscle. Such sites exist both normally and pathologically at areas of muscular atrophy or surgical incisions. Common hernia sites include the groin, the umbilicus, and the linea alba.

Terminology

Hernias are described in several ways. A hernia is **reducible** when the protruding contents can be returned to the abdomen by external manipulation, and irreducible or **incarcerated** when they cannot. A **strangulated** hernia is one in which the vascularity of the protruding contents (omentum or bowel) is compromised, typically by constriction at the neck, most commonly with hernias that have small orifices and voluminous sacs. Incarceration is

253

usually necessary for strangulation (most incarcerated hernias eventually strangulate), but not all incarcerated hernias are strangulated when first seen. A **Richter's** hernia is any hernia in which only a part of a viscus (usually the antimesenteric wall) is trapped and strangulated, without obstruction. A **sliding** hernia is one in which a normally retroperitoneal viscus (e.g., the cecum) "slides" out with the peritoneal sac; a wall of the sac is thus bowel, and it cannot simply be ligated and amputated.

Finally, if the properitoneal fat accompanies the herniating peritoneum in an indirect hernia, a **cord lipoma** is said to exist.

Symptoms

While most hernias are asymptomatic, they can produce a wide variety of nonspecific discomforts related to pressure in the sac and on adjacent structures. Typically, a hernia sac enlarges and transmits a palpable impulse with palpation of the inguinal canal when the patient coughs or strains. In contrast, actual strangulation produces intense local pain and tenderness, intestinal obstruction, and, if uncorrected, perforation. Often the strangulated hernia produces local erythema. Small bowel resection is typically required once a hernia strangulates.

In general, since hernias do not spontaneously improve, and frequently progress to strangulation, all asymptomatic hernias should be electively repaired if the general medical condition permits. All incarcerated hernias should be urgently repaired (but not necessarily in the middle of the night) to avoid strangulation. It is generally safe to attempt to reduce all but obviously strangulated hernias; if an incarcerated hernia is truly strangulated it will not be reducible because of edema (in other words, the risk of reducing dead intestine intraperitoneally is fairly remote). *(continued)*

Surgery
Hernia *continued*

Inguinal Hernia

The groin is one of the natural weak areas in the abdominal wall and is the most common site for abdominal herniation. The anatomy of this area is surprisingly complex.

Figure 30.1
Simplified view of the right inguinal region seen from the front, showing the spermatic cord running from the abdomen out to the testicle. On the left, note the indirect hernia protruding through the internal ring lateral to the inferior epigastric vessels. On the right, there is a direct hernia protruding through the weakened transversalis fascia medial to the vessels (Hasselbach's triangle). From Wantz, GE. Atlas of Hernia Surgery. New York: Raven Press, 1991. Reprinted with permission.

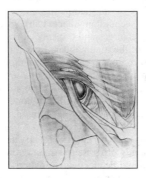 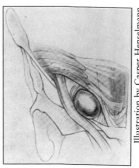

Illustration by Casper Henselmann

The path of the inguinal canal through the abdominal wall is oblique. The anterior wall of the inguinal canal is formed by the aponeurosis of the external oblique, and the (superficial) external ring is the medial divergence of its fibers just before they reach the pubic tubercle. The posterior wall ("floor") is the aponeurosis and fascia of the transversus abdominis muscle, while the (deep) internal ring is a direct opening in this fascia laterally. The inferior epigastric vessels define the medial wall of the internal ring. The middle layer, the internal oblique muscle, arches over (cephalad to) the internal ring and forms the so-called "shutter" mechanism, because it normally contracts and closes over the internal ring with straining. The spermatic cord begins at the internal ring and contains the vas deferens, testicular artery and vein, lymphatics, and nerves, and is surrounded by fibers of the internal oblique, called here the **cremaster** muscle. Several nerves pass through this area, in variable locations. The iliohypogastric and ilioinguinal nerves are sensory to the skin of the groin, medial upper thigh and the base of the penis, while the genital branch of the genitofemoral nerve innervates the cremaster muscle and the skin on the lateral aspects of the scrotum or labia.

A useful concept is that of the **musculopectineal orifice**. When viewed as a whole, the weak area in the groin is bounded by the internal oblique muscle and **conjoint tendon** superiorly and **Cooper's Ligament** (the periosteum covering the pectin pubis) inferiorly, bisected by the **inguinal ligament.**

Figure 30.2
**Anterior, somewhat schematic view of the musculopectineal orifice. The inguinal ligament bisects the opening bounded by the abdominal wall muscles and conjoint tendon, iliopsoas muscle, and periosteum of the pubic bone (Cooper's ligament). Inguinal hernias pass through this orifice above the inguinal ligament, and femoral hernias, below. From Wantz, GE. Atlas of Hernia Surgery. New York: Raven Press, 1991.
Reprinted with permission.**

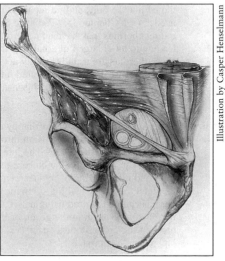

Illustration by Casper Henselmann

(continued)

Surgery
Hernia *continued*

Hernias arising above the inguinal ligament (passing into the inguinal canal) are **inguinal** and those arising below (passing into the femoral triangle of the thigh) are **femoral.** Inguinal hernias may be direct or indirect. **Indirect** inguinal hernias arise lateral to the epigastric vessels and pass through the internal ring, thus usually lying within the spermatic cord. **Direct** hernias arise medial to the epigastric vessels, within **Hesselbach's triangle**, directly through the weakened floor, and usually lie outside the cord. Hesselbach's triangle is bounded by the rectus abdominis medially, the inguinal ligament inferiorly, and the epigastric vessels laterally. Physical examination is poor at distinguishing between direct and indirect inguinal hernias. When both a direct and indirect hernia occur ipsilaterally and simultaneously, a **pantaloon** hernia is said to exist, with the inferior epigastric vessels forming the "crotch" of the trousers.

Inguinal hernias can be congenital or acquired. Indirect hernias are usually primarily congenital, resulting from a patent processus vaginalis left over from testicular descent. Essentially all pediatric hernias are indirect, with no true fascial defect at all: treatment involves ligation of the hernia sac only, and no repair of the ring or floor is needed (see Chapter 38, "Pediatric Surgery"). In adults, indirect hernias may have an acquired component as well, leading to an enlarged internal ring that must be fixed. Direct hernias are usually wholly acquired, due to a combination of weakness and elevated intraperitoneal pressure. Both indirect and direct hernias in adults are usually repaired similarly.

Goals of repair

The goals of inguinal herniorrhaphy are to reduce the sac and to prevent further protrusion through the abdominal wall by repairing the defect. The integrity of the abdominal wall can be restored by closure of the aponeurotic floor and internal ring or replacement or reinforcement of the defective tissues with a synthetic prosthesis. In adults, hernias can be repaired using native tissue only, by placing prosthetic mesh in the groin, or by placing prosthetic mesh in the properitoneal space (via a properitoneal or laparoscopic approach).

Classic repair

Classic herniorrhaphies utilize only native tissues to effect repair of the hernia, and can easily be performed with local anesthesia only. Classic repairs encompass several steps: dissection of the inguinal canal and cord, identification and reduction of the sac(s), repair of the internal ring, and reconstruction of the inguinal floor (the round ligament can be sacrificed and the internal ring obliterated in women). The Marcy repair ("ringoplasty") consists of tightening the internal inguinal ring only, and is indicated in patients who have small indirect defects with strong fascia and minimal disruption of the deep ring. The Bassini and Shouldice repairs consist of ligation of the hernia sac and approximation of the conjoined tendon to the shelving edge of the inguinal ligament. These produce good results and are applicable to both direct and indirect defects, although do not address femoral herniation and, at times, can produce excessive tension. The McVay (or Cooper's ligament) repair, in contrast, closes the femoral defect, and thus is indicated for repair of inguinal or femoral herniation. Here, the conjoint tendon is sutured to Cooper's ligament medially, and not to the inguinal ligament (except laterally, to avoid the femoral vessels). The point at which the suture line passes from Cooper's to inguinal ligament is called the "transition stitch."

Prosthetic mesh

All classic repairs have the potential for excessive tension. **Prosthetic mesh** patches have been used for years to reinforce classical repairs without significantly improving results. When the prosthesis is implanted without reapproximation of the weakened tissues, however, eliminating tension, results improve dramatically (Lichtenstein repair). For successful tension-free patch hernioplasty, the prosthesis must be reasonably large, sutured to the inguinal ligament and rectus sheath, extend medially beyond the pubic tubercle and laterally beyond the internal ring, and snugly encompass the spermatic cord at the internal ring. The prosthetic mesh acts as a "scaffolding" for ingrowth of native tissues. The tension-free patch hernioplasty is easy to perform with local anesthesia, recovery is rapid, and results are excellent. Good results have been reported after the elimination of all suture material entirely, with only a simple plug of mesh stuffed into the defect.

(continued)

Surgery
Hernia *continued*

Properitoneal repair

Mesh can also be placed "behind" the defect in the properitoneal space. The **Stoppa** procedure ("Giant Prosthetic Reinforcement of the Visceral Sac," or GPRVS) consists of placement of a prosthetic patch properitoneally such that it adheres to the herniating visceral sac and renders the peritoneum inextensible. As a result, the peritoneum cannot protrude through the area of weakness. This procedure is usually performed through a transverse abdominal incision, avoiding inguinal dissection, and thus may be useful in the repair of recurrent inguinal herniation.

Laparoscopic repair

Finally, **laparoscopic** herniorrhaphy is similar to the Stoppa procedure (in that the mesh is placed properitoneally), except that access is gained via the peritoneal cavity using the laparoscope. The most common technique involves creation of an inferiorly-based flap of peritoneum, reducing the sac, and covering the defect from within with mesh. The increased morbidity of the repair itself (general anesthesia is needed) is thought to be balanced by a shorter recovery period. Definitive data, including recurrence rates, are not yet available.

Complications

Ischemic orchitis, neuralgia, and recurrence are the most common complications of inguinal herniorrhaphy. The etiology of ischemic orchitis is usually thrombosis of the spermatic cord with subsequent venous congestion; excessive dissection is most often the culprit. The testicle may survive without complication or may atrophy; gangrene requiring orchiectomy is rarely necessary. Chronic neuralgia may result from surgical dissection (i.e. neuroma, transection) or from entrapment by scar tissue during the healing phase. Recurrences are typically caused by excessive tension on the repair, deficient tissues, or inadequate hernioplasty, and tend to occur at the pubic tubercle or internal ring. Recurrence rates are notoriously difficult to accurately assess. Most published series are by experts or teams with unusually low rates, and a substantial number of hernia patients in any practice are lost to followup. Probably 5%-10% of all hernias recur, although some very low rates have been reported by routine users of mesh.

Femoral Hernia

Femoral hernias also result from a weakness in the floor of the canal (analogous to a direct inguinal hernia), but the sac passes **beneath** the inguinal ligament into the thigh medial to the femoral sheath. They typically present as a mass in the thigh, inferior to the inguinal crease and medial to the femoral vein. These hernias are uncommon, occurring most often in elderly women. A strangulated Richter's femoral hernia is associated with significant morbidity and mortality because the diagnosis is often difficult and delayed, producing minimal local signs, no "classic" inguinal bulge, and no evidence of intestinal obstruction (despite the presence of ischemic bowel wall). Femoral hernias are generally repaired by obliterating the medial aspect of the femoral canal with either a Cooper's ligament repair or a prosthetic mesh plug.

Ventral Hernia

The **umbilicus** is a common site of herniation and is more frequent in women in general, multiparous women, obese patients, and patients with ascites. Strangulation of the colon and omentum is not uncommon. The classic repair is the Mayo herniorrhaphy consisting of a "vest over pants" imbrication of the superior and inferior aponeurotic flaps, but repair is usually individualized based on size and anatomy. **Epigastric** hernias are protrusions of properitoneal fat and peritoneum through the decussation of the rectus sheath in the midline (linea alba) between the xyphoid and umbilicus.

Incisional hernia

Post-incisional hernias can lead to surprisingly high morbidity. They tend to enlarge inordinately, can be difficult to repair, and are often accompanied by unrelated systemic disease. Obesity, local wound infection, and systemic illnesses are predisposing conditions for the original fascial disruptions. "Loss of domain" is an important concept to understand. In large abdominal hernias, there is a tendency to preferentially push the abdominal contents out into the hernia sac. Over time, as the hernia sac enlarges, the true peritoneal space diminishes. Eventually, the abdominal contents remain in the hernia sac preferentially. When herniorrhaphy is attempted, there is an inade-

Surgery
Hernia *continued*

quate intraperitoneal volume to accommodate the abdominal contents after the hernia sac has been reduced.

Forced closure of the abdomen may lead to respiratory compromise or impingement on the inferior vena cava. Planned progressive pneumoperitoneum has been used to prepare patients for incisional herniorrhaphy after loss of domain: it stretches the abdominal wall, creating a larger intraperitoneal volume, and thus facilitates the return of viscera to the abdomen. Mesh repair, however, can accomplish closure without undue tension, and is much easier. Prosthetic mesh repair is almost essential for large incisional hernias.

Parastomal Hernia

Parastomal hernias are herniation of bowel, omentum, or properitoneal fat beside a stoma. Paracolostomal hernias are more common than paraileostomal hernias. Both are more likely to occur when the stoma emerges through the semilunar line rather than the rectus sheath, and thus parastomal hernias are more likely to present on the lateral aspect of the stoma. Replantation of the stoma with complete closure of the entire original defect is more effective than local repair.

Uncommon Hernias

Spigelian hernias are ventral hernias occurring through the semilunar line and the lateral border of the rectus sheath. The sac protrudes between the muscle layers of the abdominal wall. They are rare and, unless large, are difficult to diagnose because they are intraparietal and contained by the aponeurosis of the external oblique muscle. **Lumbar** hernias are extremely rare congenital, spontaneous, or traumatic herniations through the posterior lumbar triangles. Hernias also occur in the obturator fossa, the greater and lesser sciatic foramen, and in the perineum. These are all very rare and typically occur in elderly, cachectic women. The **obturator** hernia is the most common of the pelvic hernias. Pressure on the obturator nerve causes pain in the region of the hip, knee, and inner aspect of the thigh (Howship-Romberg sign). ■

31   Breast Cancer

One of the most common problems in general surgery is the evaluation of a breast mass, and one of the most common specific disease entities surgeons deal with is breast cancer. One in nine women will develop breast cancer during her lifetime–only lung cancer will cause more cancer deaths. Because it is so common, involves an organ so visible and cosmetically important in Western society, and has been so extensively discussed in the past few decades, breast cancer is perhaps the most emotionally-charged pathophysiologic entity a physician will face. Although many physicians (commonly primary care physicians, surgeons, radiologists, oncologists, and plastic surgeons) are involved in the treatment of breast cancer, it is the surgeon who most often bears primary responsibility for providing definitive diagnosis and treatment, and it is the surgeon who causes the greatest scarring (both physically and mentally). It is incumbent upon the physician to approach patients who may have breast cancer with a great deal of sensitivity and kindness, as well as with a thorough and up-to-date knowledge base so that all possible treatment options and prognostic information can accurately be transmitted to the patient.

Patients with a suspicion of breast cancer will present in one of three ways: with a **palpable mass**, a **positive mammogram**, or **nipple discharge**. Each is initially approached in the same fashion.

Diagnosis

As in all of medicine, a good **history** is the first step. Risk factors for breast cancer should be well known: increasing age, previous breast carcinoma, early menarche, nulliparity, obesity, late first pregnancy, and late menopause. Many of these, at least teleologically, have in common prolonged exposure to unopposed estrogen. A family history of breast cancer, particularly in a first-degree relative (mother or sister) is also significant, particularly if these relatives had premenopausal cancer or bilateral disease. Birth control pills have not been shown to be associated with breast cancer, but a high intake of fat has. The location, duration, and characteristics of the lump, and quality of any nipple

Surgery
Breast Cancer *continued*

discharge, if present, should be ascertained. Critical to note are the presence of axillary masses, or signs or symptoms of potential metastatic disease.

The **physical exam** should be performed with the patient in both the supine and sitting positions. Visual inspection is followed by careful, systematic, and complete exam of the breast and axilla. Palpation of the axilla and the tail of the breast can be aided by placing the patient's ipsilateral hand behind the head. The presence or absence of the following should be noted:

– Skin Changes
  including dimpling, thickening, erythema, or ulceration
– Nipple Changes
  including retraction, discharge, desquamation, or inversion.
– Masses
  if present, mobile or fixed, size, and position.
– Axillary adenopathy
  if present, mobile, matted, or fixed.
– Arm edema
  present or absent.

All patients, if not done already, should undergo **bilateral mammograms**. These will help in the diagnosis of a palpable lesion and rule out (or identify) synchronous lesions in the same or opposite breast. Lesions that might represent carcinoma include those containing clustered microcalcifications, localized soft tissue masses, and those causing architectural distortion (commonly stellate lesions). Ultrasonography can identify cysts (which are rarely malignant).

If suspicion is very low, a brief period of observation (2-3 months) is safe for young women. All persistent masses, however, require that a definitive **tissue diagnosis** be made, with the twin goals of differentiating benign from malignant lesions, and, if malignant, of identifying the specific lesion so that the best treatment can be planned. Tissue can be obtained from palpable lesions in one of two ways: by means of fine-needle aspiration (FNA) or surgical biopsy.

Tissue diagnosis

Fine needle aspiration (FNA) refers to the process of obtaining a tissue sample by means of a small needle (typically 22 gauge) under local anesthetic in the clinic or office. A "chunk" of tissue is not obtained as it is with a core biopsy needle, rather, unconnected cells are the result; the pathologic technique to examine these is termed cytology. Results are quite good, but interpretation must be approached with a clear knowledge of the limitations of the test. Generally, the pathologist will err on the side of conservatism. Thus, a report of "definite cancer" or "definitely not cancer" is usually accurate. If the report is at all equivocal, however, or the sample is not adequate, a formal biopsy must be done. A **surgical biopsy** is simply the removal of a discrete piece of tissue containing the lump. This can be done under local or general anesthetic, or in the clinic or the operating room, depending on resources, and can consist of removal of the entire lump ("excisional biopsy") or, rarely, just a piece ("incisional biopsy") if the mass is very large. This has the twofold advantage of providing a definitive tissue sample for the pathologist to make the most accurate diagnosis, and, in some cases, providing definitive local control of the disease (see below). The biopsy incision should be planned so that a subsequent mastectomy, if needed, will encompass the entire tract from skin down.

If the lesion is nonpalpable (i.e., detected by mammogram), essentially the same two options are available. A **stereotactic core needle biopsy** is performed by passing a larger needle (typically 14 gauge) through the area of suspicion under precise mammographic visualization. Finally, a **needle-localization surgical biopsy** is performed by placing a localizing needle in the lesion, again under mammographic control. The surgeon then excises the area at the tip of the needle with generous margins, and full excision of the lesion is confirmed by radiography of the excised specimen before the wound is closed (the previously seen mammographic lesion should be present in the specimen).

Putting it all together, patients with suspected breast cancer will present with either a palpable mass or a positive mammogram. **All persistent lesions should be sampled by needle aspiration or formal surgical biopsy**. Patients with a positive mammogram (but no palpable mass) should also have a tissue sample obtained, either by stereotactic or needle-localization surgical biopsy. There is an aphorism that says roughly, "any breast lump (or abnormal mammographic lesion) belongs in a jar in the pathologists' lab." This may be too strong as an absolute rule, but the message is that because breast cancer is so common, one must have an extremely low threshold for biopsy of any breast lesion. The ability to know when to **safely** watch such a lesion can only be gained with extensive experience.

Pathology

The goal of obtaining tissue for diagnosis is to differentiate benign from malignant lesions, and to identify the specific histologic subtype. Obviously, actual tissue is required for histologic identification. None of these can be reliably identified without a biopsy.

Benign lesions

The two most common benign lesions that produce breast masses are **fibrocystic change** and **fibroadenomas**. The term "fibrocystic change" (better than fibrocystic "disease") refers to a spectrum of benign proliferative lesions of the breast. If a lump is found in a young women, changes in size, is tender, or occurs in the setting of diffusely "lumpy" breasts, a fibrocystic lesion is most likely. These come in multiple histologic variants, almost all of which have no risk of leading to cancer. The one important exception is the lesion classified as containing "atypical hyperplasia" by the pathologist. These should usually be removed; "atypia" is a dirty word when dealing with potential cancer. A true cyst is present if, on FNA, clear or greenish fluid is obtained. If the cyst disappears and does not reaccumulate, no further treatment is needed. No matter how much diffuse fibrocystic change is present within the breast, however, if there is a dominant or persistent lump, it should be biopsied. A benign fibroadenoma also presents as a discrete lump. An experienced physician, especially with the help of FNA or stereotactic biopsy, can often identify a fibroadenoma, but because differentiation based on clinical characteristics is not perfect, however, surgical biopsy is often needed to exclude malignancy. No further treatment is necessary.

Malignant lesions

True breast cancer comes in many histologic variants, the most common being **infiltrating ductal carcinoma** (about 80% of all breast tumors). This is "classic" breast cancer, and, unless otherwise specified, treatment strategies (including those discussed below) are directed toward this subtype. The other common form of invasive breast cancer is **lobular carcinoma**. This has a higher chance of being multicentric within the breast at diagnosis, and true mastectomy rather than conservative excision (see below) may be more strongly considered. There are two common in situ tumors of importance. **Ductal carcinoma in situ (DCIS)** seems to be a true in situ lesion that can later progress to invasive carcinoma. Breast conservation therapy may be adequate, but the data are not as firm as for invasive ductal carcinoma. **Lobular carcinoma in situ (LCIS)**, however, does not seem to act as a true in situ precursor lesion. Rather, it seems to be a marker for increased risk of subsequent invasive carcinoma, in much the same way as does a positive family history. The fascinating points are, however, that the subsequent cancer is usually ductal, not lobular, in origin, and that the risk in both breasts is equal! In other words, local excision or even mastectomy is of no benefit. Both breasts must be treated in identical fashion. Usually, this means close observation, but bilateral simple mastectomy is sometimes appropriate if risk is high.

Breast cancer can present, in addition to a lump, in several unique ways. **Paget's disease** is an intraepithelial form of invasive ductal or lobular carcinoma that presents as an exzematoid nipple lesion. This has a relatively good prognosis (perhaps because of earlier diagnosis), but **inflammatory breast cancer** does not. This variant results when dermal lymphatics are blocked, producing erythema and the classic peau d'orange ("orange skin") skin changes. These two are essentially clinical syndromes, and do not imply any specific histologic subtype. There are multiple other histologic variants of adenocarcinoma, all with subtly different prognoses, and sarcomas and lymphomas also can originate in breast tissue.

Breast cancer also occurs in men, at a rate of approximately 1% that in women. After controlling for later diagnosis (probably due to a lower level of suspicion), breast cancer in men is treated and behaves in exactly the same way as it does in women.
(continued)

Surgery
Breast Cancer *continued*

Staging

Staging of breast cancer is used to determine treatment and to predict outcome. Staging can be confusing. It is done both clinically (based on the history and physical) and pathologically (based on actual tissue retrieved), and both are useful as long as you clearly specify which you are referring to. In practice, a clinical stage may be assigned based on initial evaluation, which then may be modified after tissue samples of the tumor and lymph nodes are obtained.

The TNM system is used to stage breast cancer. It is surprisingly simple to remember. **Stage I** tumors are less than 2cm in maximal diameter without involved axillary lymph nodes. **Stage II** tumors are 2-5cm or those with lymph nodes that are palpable (clinically) or histologically positive for cancer (pathologically) but not fixed to each other. **Stage III** tumors are greater than 5cm or those with fixed axillary nodes, and **Stage IV** refers to the presence of metastatic disease beyond the lymph nodes. The single factor that best correlates with outcome is the number of involved lymph nodes.

In general, patients with either Stage I or Stage II disease are candidates for breast-conservation procedures to treat their tumors. Patients with Stage III disease are fairly rare today, and in those with Stage IV disease (metastatic), the goal is, by definition, palliation.

Treatment

The history of therapy for breast cancer is fascinating both from a historical perspective and because it clearly illustrates the evolving understanding of the biologic behavior of the disease.

Radical mastectomy

The symbol for cancer, the crab, arose from descriptions of breast cancer. Originally considered incurable, little was done to treat breast cancer until the late 1800s. Halsted was one of the first physicians to approach treatment of the disease in a rational way. He formulated the hypothesis that breast cancer arose in a discrete area of the breast, spread to nearby lymph nodes next, and finally to the rest of the body, all in an orderly and temporally non-overlapping fashion. He believed that cure was possible if the breast, contiguous muscles, and nearby lymph nodes were removed en bloc before metastatic spread occurred, a procedure termed **radical mastectomy**. This procedure includes removal of the pectoralis major and minor muscles with the overlying breast tissue and axillary contents and is very rarely done today.

Modified radical mastectomy

In the 1960s and 70s it became apparent to many surgeons that most breast cancers were presenting at an earlier stage, with involvement of the pectoralis muscles much less common. The **modified radical mastectomy (MRM)** consists of removal of the breast, nipple and areola, and axillary contents only, leaving the muscles and most of the overlying skin alone. No difference in local or distant recurrence can be demonstrated between these procedures. There is no paradigm shift between the radical and modified radical mastectomy, however, merely a difference in scale, mostly related to the earlier stage at presentation in modern times. The modified radical mastectomy was still conceived with the assumption that the cancer progresses first to the axillary nodes, then to the rest of the body, and cure is possible if caught at the right time.

Breast-conserving therapy

In the 1980s, however, a shift in thinking occurred. Because of both empiric evidence and evolving knowledge of tumor behavior, many began to believe that breast cancer, while arising from a discrete area in the breast, "metastasizes" simultaneously to both regional lymph nodes and distant sites. Cancer in a lymph node is thus not invariably required before distant spread, and removal of the nodes will not necessarily forestall metastases. Positive lymph nodes are, however, excellent markers of the degree to which the cancer may have disseminated, and thus are excellent prognostic indicators. From this, and from the observation that more conservative local treatment of the primary tumor is safe, the concept of **breast-conserving therapy**, notably by Veronesi, in Italy, arose. This, in essence, consists of local treatment of the primary tumor by "lumpectomy" and postoperative irradiation to kill any microscopic foci that have been missed, and axillary dissection to obtain prognostic information (whether or not the nodes are involved, and how many). It is important to realize that axillary dissection is not done for treatment or cure, but for prognostic and therapeutic information (if nodes are clinically positive, local palliation is also a goal). In multiple prospective randomized clinical trials with huge patient populations, this mode of therapy has been shown to be as effective in producing long-term survival as MRM in the treatment of Stage I and II breast cancer. Local recurrence is slightly more common, but local failures can be easily be managed with re-excision or conversion to modified radical mastectomy, illustrating the fact that it is not the local effects but rather the distant disease that kills the patient. Current debate focuses on whether the initial excisional biopsy is adequate definitive lumpectomy, and whether axillary dissection need be done at all. As discussed above, breast conservation therapy is most appropriate for infiltrating ductal carcinoma and DCIS. Invasive lobular carcinoma is more apt to be multicentric, and relatively more weight should be given toward MRM. LCIS is a predictor of overall risk and therefore requires no specific treatment other than observation.

Adjuvant therapy

Surgery and radiation are local therapies, designed to treat local disease. As discussed above, current evidence suggests that the tumor has the potential for systemic spread right from the beginning. The question of which patients benefit from systemic adjuvant therapy (chemo- or hormonal therapy) to treat potential systemic micrometastases is confusing and, at present, controversial. For current purposes a useful generalization is that all patients with positive nodes benefit, because spread to a regional node is a marker of the potential for distant spread. Some patients with negative nodes also benefit, such as those with especially "malignant" tumors (in a biologic sense). Factors such as aneuploidy, rapid growth, poor nuclear grade, or aggressive histologic subtype may all suggest that adjuvant therapy may be helpful, but this topic is an area of active research and debate.

In general, premenopausal and estrogen receptor-negative postmenopausal patients should receive standard chemotherapeutic drugs, while postmenopausal patients with positive estrogen receptors should receive the anti-estrogen tamoxifen. ■

32   Colon and Rectum

Surgery of the colon and rectum can be surprisingly complex. Although an integral part of general surgery, many surgeons pursue advanced training in the field, and limit their practice to colorectal surgery alone. Surgeons with an interest in this area of the body also often pursue advanced training in endoscopy. Diagnosis and treatment of inflammatory bowel disease, diverticular disease, colon cancer, and anorectal disorders, and the performance of endoscopy make up the bulk of a colorectal surgical practice.

Surgical Anatomy

The large intestine, which makes up approximately 20% of the length of the gastrointestinal (GI) tract, begins at the ileocecal valve, and consists of the colon and rectum. The rectum is not an anatomically discrete organ, but is a continuation of the colon. The rectum is said to begin where the longitudinal teniae coli disappear (approximately at the level of the sacral promontory); using this definition, the rectum consists of the last 15 cm of the colon. The first third is intraperitoneal, the middle third free anteriorly, and the distal third entirely retroperitoneal.

The anal canal begins where the terminal part of the rectum passes through the levator ani muscles, ends at the anal verge, and measures about 4 cm. The dentate line marks the transition between the inside (visceral innervation, portal venous drainage) and outside (somatic, cutaneous innervation, systemic venous drainage) of the body; a point of importance when dealing with anorectal disorders. The superior mesenteric artery (SMA) supplies the colon to the splenic flexure, the inferior mesenteric artery (IMA) to mid-rectum, and branches of the internal iliac arteries supply the distal rectum and anus. Collateralization is extensive, accounting for the ability of the left colon to survive when the IMA is ligated during aortic surgery.
(continued)

Surgery
Colon and Rectum *continued*

Diverticular Disease

Diverticular disease is an extremely common condition in Western society. A **diverticulum** is an outpouching of the mucosa and muscularis through the serosa of the colonic wall ("false" diverticulum), typically at the site of a perforating blood vessel's entry at the edge of a tenia. Low dietary fiber is thought to lower stool bulk, which leads to increased intraluminal pressure causing herniation at sites of weakness. **Diverticulosis** is the presence of diverticula, while **diverticulitis** refers to the clinical syndrome that results when infection results. Diverticulosis is usually asymptomatic and presents as an incidental radiographic finding. Symptoms, if present, include recurrent left lower quadrant pain, constipation, or diarrhea. High fiber intake helps prevent the development of diverticula, and seems to reduce symptom recurrence and the development of complications. Diverticula are much more common in the left and sigmoid colon.

Lower GI bleeding

One of the most significant complications of diverticulosis is **lower GI bleeding**. For reasons that are not entirely clear, bleeding almost always arises from noninflamed diverticula—in other words, diverticulosis bleeds, diverticulitis does not. Also, right-sided diverticula, which are less common than those on the left, seem to have a relatively greater propensity to bleed relative to their distribution. Most episodes of diverticular bleeding stop spontaneously; workup and treatment of bleeding is covered in more detail in Chapter 40, "GI Bleeding."

Diverticulitis

Diverticulitis results when the neck of the diverticulum is obstructed, resulting in an inflammatory or frankly infectious process. Obstruction causes micro- or macroperforation that results in inflammation and edema. Most episodes of perforation lead to a contained abscess within the mesentery or pericolonic tissues; true intraperitoneal perforation is not as common. Clinical presentation varies widely depending on the degree of inflammation, the presence or absence of perforation or abscess, and, obviously, the general health of the patient. Classic symptoms of relatively uncomplicated diverticulitis or a small, contained abscess mimic appendicitis (fever, leukocytosis, anorexia, and localized abdominal pain), but occur in the left rather than right lower quadrant. Larger abscesses will tend to produce a greater degree of toxicity, while frank perforation will quickly produce true peritonitis. CT scan is very accurate in the diagnosis of diverticulitis. Complications of diverticulitis include late obstruction due to scarring and fistula formation. Pneumaturia (air bubbles in the urinary stream) is the classic, unmistakable sign of the presence of a colovesical fistula.

Uncomplicated diverticulosis requires no treatment other than observation and dietary education (encourage fiber, discourage items with small, undigestible seeds that are thought to easily block the diverticular neck). Diverticulitis in the absence of perforation or a large abscess usually responds to conservative treatment consisting of antibiotics and bowel rest; small abscesses often will resolve, but larger ones must be drained (surgically or percutaneously). Perforation, obstruction, or uncontrolled sepsis require laparotomy (discussed below). The decision is largely subjective whether and when to remove the involved bowel after attacks of diverticulitis (or bleeding) have been easily controlled. Resection of the involved segment usually is not performed until several episodes of inflammation or bleeding have occurred. Diverticulitis behaves in a much more "malignant" fashion in patients younger than 40, however, and elective resection is generally a good idea after the resolution of any complication of diverticular disease, no matter how minor, in a patient younger than this.

Inflammatory Bowel Disease

Inflammatory bowel disease (IBD) refers to either of two clinical entities (both of unknown etiology): **Crohn's disease (CD)** and **ulcerative colitis (UC)**. This topic is more fully covered in Chapter 22, "Gastroenterology," but a few points are of special importance to the surgeon. UC is essentially always limited to the colon and almost always leads to cancer, if present for long enough (decades). Colectomy, which is curative, is thus often eventually needed for severe UC. In contrast, CD is a chronic, incurable condition potentially affecting the entire GI tract (most commonly small bowel). Since cure is not possible, operative intervention is reserved for the treatment of complications only. A cardinal rule when dealing with CD is to avoid operation, if at all possible. *(continued)*

Surgery
Colon and Rectum *continued*

Differentiation between the two conditions, which can present in very similar fashion, is of utmost importance but is frequently difficult.

Colon Cancer

Colorectal cancer is the third leading cause of cancer death after lung, breast (women), and prostate (men) in the United States. Strongest risk factors are advancing age and diet, particularly those high in animal fat or low in fiber. Rectal cancers appear to be more prevalent in men, while colon cancers are more commonly seen in women. Genetic factors are also important: about 15% of affected patients have a family history of "sporadic" colorectal cancer, while the (rarer) familial polyposis and Gardner's syndromes clearly are premalignant conditions. Finally, UC and, to a lesser degree, CD, clearly increase the risk of eventual cancer.

Polyps

Colon cancers are thought to arise from certain types of **colonic polyps.** Polyps can be histologically described as pseudopolyps (inflammatory polyps without malignant potential), hamartomas such as those associated with juvenile polyposis and Peutz-Jeghers syndrome (also essentially without malignant potential), and true adenomas. Adenomas can be further classified into 3 subtypes: **tubular**, **tubulovillous**, and **villous**. Tubular and tubulovillous adenomas are usually pedunculated (rounded and attached to mucosa by a stalk) whereas villous polyps are usually sessile (flat and intimately attached to mucosa). In general, the more villous component, the greater the risk of eventual malignancy.

Screening

Screening for colon cancer is a problematic issue. Colonoscopy is highly accurate, but expensive, time-consuming, and invasive. In contrast, although screening for occult blood in the stool is cheap and easy, it is not terribly sensitive or specific. Current recommendations of American Cancer Society are that low-risk patients older than 40 have a yearly rectal examination and fecal occult blood testing, and subsequently undergo sigmoidoscopy every three to five years beginning at age 50. Those with major risk factors (family history, polyps, previous colon cancer) should have complete colonoscopy or barium enema (BE) with sigmoidoscopy beginning at age 40 and every three to five years thereafter.

Manifestations   The cecum and right colon are large and contain relatively liquid stool. Cancers that arise on the **right side** therefore usually grow to a large size without producing obstruction, and present with **occult bleeding** and iron-deficiency anemia. Stool in the left colon, in contrast, is more solid, and the colon's diameter is smaller. Cancers of the **left** and **sigmoid colons** thus tend to present with **obstruction**, often producing the classic "apple core" lesion seen on BE. Rectal cancers often present with small amounts of bright red blood per rectum.

Staging   Once a cancer is suspected, complete evaluation of the entire colon is required to make the diagnosis and to rule out synchronous lesions. This can be done with either BE or colonoscopy; a tissue diagnosis is not necessarily required if suspicion is high, especially if resection must occur anyway (for example, if obstruction is present). Tumor staging, almost always done after resection, is of strong prognostic significance. The system traditionally used is the modified Dukes staging, but formal TNM staging is rapidly gaining favor. Although the details are not included here, they are both generally similar. Stage I (Dukes A) refers to a tumor that has not penetrated the muscularis mucosa (essentially carcinoma in situ), stage II (Dukes B) refers to one that has penetrated into or through the wall but with normal nodes, stage III (Dukes C) refers to one that has "metastasized" to regional lymph nodes, and Stage IV (Dukes D), to a tumor with distant metastatic disease. Colon cancer is somewhat unique in that resection of the primary is essentially **always** indicated to avoid death by bowel obstruction, no matter how much spread has taken place, and thus routine abdominal CT scans are **not** needed prior to resection.

Resection   The astute observer will realize that much more normal colon is resected than would seem to be needed to remove microscopic intramural spread (only a few centimeters). This is a direct result of the need to remove the regional lymph node drainage along with the specimen. Since lymphatic drainage follows the regional arterial supply, the artery supplying the involved colon is ligated and removed as close to the source as is practical. Therefore, all resultant devascularized bowel must be removed! Tumors of the cecum and ascending colon require ligation of the right colic artery, requiring anatomic **right hemicolectomy** that includes part of the

Surgery
Colon and Rectum *continued*

distal ileum and hepatic flexure. Similarly, left colon lesions are treated by **left hemicolectomy** from the transverse colon just proximal to the splenic flexure to the sigmoid colon, because the left colic artery is ligated and removed.

Terminology of more distal resections is confusing. A **left colectomy, sigmoid colectomy**, and **low anterior resection** describe procedures that lie along a spectrum, removing more distally-located tissue as one progresses. All are, however, done through a midline abdominal incision. In contrast, however, an **abdominoperineal resection (APR)** refers to the situation required to remove an extremely distal tumor (within a few centimeters of the anal verge). This operation, done in the lithotomy position, involves both abdominal resection of as much rectum as possible, and transperineal excision of the anus. The two dissections meet in the pelvis at the level of the levators, and the entire rectum, from sigmoid colon to daylight, is removed. By definition, a permanent colostomy is created and the skin surrounding the now-excised anus is sewn shut.

Postop surveillance

Surveillance is important after resection of a colon cancer, because recurrent lesions are both common and curable. Carcinoembryonic antigen (CEA) is a factor often synthesized by colon carcinoma, but also is elevated in several unrelated conditions. It is thus not useful as a screening test for colon cancer, but in the special situation where it normalizes after initial resection, a later elevation is a strong predictive factor for the presence of recurrence. Even if no tumor is found in this situation by radiologic and endoscopic investigation, blind exploratory laparotomy is usually performed. Until recently there was no good adjuvant therapy for colon cancer—surgery was the only helpful treatment. Within the past decade or so, however, 5-FU and levamasole have been shown to benefit patients with node-positive (stage III) tumors.

Rectal tumors

Cancers arising in the **rectum** behave in a generally similar fashion to those arising in the more proximal colon. The one important difference is that preoperative radiation (4500cGy over 5-6 weeks) is probably of benefit in patients with bulky, fixed rectal tumors, because it potentially can "downstage" an otherwise inoperable tumor to an operable and possibly curable one.

Transrectal ultrasound is an important diagnostic modality in the evaluation of rectal tumors; it can accurately demonstrate intramural and pelvic spread and thus predict the need for extensive resection.

Anal tumors

Anal tumors are rare, and behave differently from colorectal cancers. Presentation is often surprisingly late; mean size at diagnosis is 3-4 cm. Tumors of the anal margin are usually well-differentiated, keratinized squamous cell carcinomas that are manageable with local therapy. Epidermoid carcinomas are treated with preoperative irradiation and chemotherapy followed by excision; if residual tumor is present, abdominoperineal resection should follow. Adenocarcinomas usually require APR, but the safety of sphincter-saving local resection, in combination with chemo- and radiotherapy for invasive lesions, is an area of active research. Other tumors that arise in the anal canal include basal cell carcinoma and melanoma.

Colon Surgery

Bowel prep

Operation on the colon is clearly safest if done electively. The reason for this is that a **bowel preparation** can be performed. Bowel preparation consists of two parts. **Mechanical preparation** involves basically washing the stool and bacteria out of the colon. This is accomplished typically by first administering clear liquids for the two days prior to operation, then providing catharsis the day before surgery. This, in turn, can either be a true cathartic (typically magnesium citrate) or a solution such as polyethylene glycol that works by producing a high-volume GI lavage. **Antibiotic preparation**, in turn, is accomplished by administering oral antibiotics the day prior to surgery; typically erythromycin and neomycin base in several doses. Almost universally, IV antibiotics are given prior to skin incision, although there is no good evidence that this adds any protective benefit if an oral prep is done.

Emergent operations

Emergent operations pose complex problems. An emergent operation is one that is done without a bowel prep, either because of urgency (perforation or uncontrolled sepsis) or because an obstruction prevents preparation. Several options are available. The traditional "three stage" operation consists first of creating a proximal diverting colostomy, second, of resection and renanastomosis of the involved section of bowel, and finally, of takedown of the colostomy, all separated by weeks or months. This technique has several drawbacks, including the accumulation of substantial morbidity at each step and the period (between the first and second steps) when the problem (perforated diverticulum, for example) remains present within the body. Modern conservative practice typically consists of resection of the involved colon at the initial operation, leaving the proximal cut end of normal colon as an end-colostomy, and leaving the distal end closed within the abdomen (or exteriorized as a mucus fistula). This is known as a Hartmann's procedure; later, the colostomy is taken down and colonic continuity reestablished. Some surgeons advocate primary resection and reanastomosis at one stage with an "on-table" bowel preparation, irrigating the colon through a tube placed in the cecum.

Anorectal Disorders

Hemorrhoids

Hemorrhoids are vascularized cushions of tissue in the anal canal, thought to function to make stool elimination easier. They become problems when they enlarge, bleed, or become painful. An important distinction should be made between internal and external hemorrhoids; the former arise above the dentate line and, because of their visceral innervation, are painless. The two most common problems seen in the ED are thrombosis and prolapse. Both are extremely painful. Thrombosed hemorrhoids are hard with a dark clot within, and should be opened for clot evacuation under minimal anesthesia with extremely good symptom control. In contrast, prolapsed hemorrhoids are softer and pinker. If incised, these will bleed copiously. Instead, they should be manually reduced with prolonged, gentle pressure, sedation, if necessary, and lots of lubrication. When either acute problem has been controlled, initial treatment is conservative, and consists of sitz baths (soaking in a few inches of warm water) and stool softeners. If problems, including bleeding, persist, open hemorrhoidectomy (external) or transanal rubber banding (internal) is the next step.

Anal fissure

An **anal fissure** is a mucosal split, usually caused by the passage of a hard stool. Defecation is very painful, and the resulting constipation causes a vicious cycle because the stool becomes hard. Treatment is usually by partial sphincterotomy to reduce the tension on the fissure and allow healing.

Perirectal abscess

Perirectal and **perianal** abscesses are the source of much unnecessary confusion and anxiety to the uninitiated. Management is extremely simple. Like any abscess, they must be drained. If adequate anesthesia cannot be provided in the ED, formal operative drainage in the OR should take place. Much anxiety revolves around the sphincter mechanism and of the possibility of a late anorectal fistula. The sphincter is really not in jeopardy as long as a simple incision is made over the point of maximal tenderness and redness. An anorectal fistula is a late complication of an abscess. It occurs after approximately 50% of abscesses, but the method of initial drainage, or who does it (surgeon vs. ED physician, for example) does not affect this rate. Therefore, simple ED drainage is appropriate in most cases. The one helpful rule is to make the skin incision as close to the anal margin as possible, so that if a fistula develops, it will be easier to treat.

Anorectal fistula

An **anorectal fistula** is an abnormal connection between the anus (typically at the level of the anal glands near the dentate line) and the perianal skin. Several options are available. If the fistula does not surround the sphincters, it can be excised or flayed open, to better heal. If it does surround the sphincters, a seton can be used. This is a string or catheter placed through the fistula and gradually tightened over time (weeks), cutting through the tissue allowing healing to take place behind it, much as a hot wire will cut through but not divide a block of ice.

Stoma

Stoma are really quite simple; but because terminology is inconsistent, confusion results. A **colostomy** or **ileostomy** is present when the respective portion of bowel is brought out and sutured to the skin. Stool or succus, respectively, are collected in a bag (appliance). Because ileostomy output is so liquid, dehydration and electrolyte disturbances are common. An **end-ostomy** is present when the bowel is divided and the functional (stool-draining) end is brought out; a **loop** or **double-barrelled ostomy** means that the bowel is not divided, but a loop, with a hole cut in the side, is brought to the skin. It seems to work as well (in terms of fecal diversion) as an end-ostomy; and

Surgery
Colon and Rectum *continued*

has the advantage of easy construction and reanastomosis. A **mucous fistula** is really just the distal, defunctionalized end of the cut bowel sutured to the skin. No stool, only mucous drains. Note that a double-barrelled or loop ostomy is anatomically and topologically identical to a conventional ostomy and mucus fistula with an intervening posterior bridge of bowel wall present. Finally, any ostomy may also be called "**diverting**" if its function is to divert the fecal stream from progressing normally (for example, if a tenuous anastomosis or healing rectal wound is present). ■

33   Biliary Tract

Most problems that occur in the biliary tract are due to **gallstones**. Gallstones are usually composed primarily of cholesterol, and are almost always formed in the gallbladder when the bile becomes supersaturated. Terms and pathology can seem confusing at first, but things can be simplified by realizing that everything depends on the location of the stone within the biliary tree, and that the most vital piece of information is whether the **cystic duct** or **common bile duct** is blocked.

Definitions

Cholelithiasis is simply the presence of stones within the gallbladder. **Acute cholecystitis** denotes an inflamed gallbladder, and implies that a stone is impacted in and blocks the **cystic duct**. Often this is a sterile inflammation only.

Choledocholithiasis refers to the presence of a stone in the **common bile duct**. **Cholangitis** means that the common bile duct is infected, almost always from a common bile duct stone impacted at the Ampulla of Vater. Surprisingly, cholangitis from a tumor blocking the duct is rare. Choledocholithiasis often leads to cholangitis if not corrected, and cholangitis almost always implies the presence of choledocholithiasis.

Biliary colic refers to pain caused by any of the above, and usually implies the absence of infection or inflammation. It doesn't tell you where the stone is, but implies that whatever the problem, it's transient (in other words, "the stone passed").

Gallstone Pancreatitis is simply pancreatitis caused by gallstones, the pathogenesis of which is not entirely clear. It is likely that the passage of a stone inflames the orifice of the pancreatic duct, temporarily blocking it and causing pancreatitis. Removal of the gallbladder does not in any way ameliorate the current attack (indeed, may worsen it), but is performed to prevent a future attack from occurring.
(continued)

Surgery
Biliary Tract *continued*

The critical determinant of outcome, treatment, and so on, therefore, is whether the cystic or common duct is obstructed. As a general rule, obstruction of the cystic duct will not produce jaundice, while obstruction of the common bile duct will. Therefore, pain alone (biliary colic) that subsides means that the patient is passing a stone, or has transient cystic duct obstruction. This is not an emergency. Fever and leukocytosis and right upper quadrant pain **without** jaundice implies cystic duct obstruction, i.e., cholecystitis. This is also not an emergency, but usually requires admission and antibiotics. Mild elevations in bilirubin (<3.0) can be present in the setting of cholecystitis alone with a patent common duct. Fever and leukocytosis, right upper quadrant pain, and **jaundice ("Charcot's triad")** suggests that the patient has cholangitis due to common bile duct obstruction. This can be a surgical emergency, and usually requires urgent or emergent (depending on severity) surgical or radiologic drainage. Biliary colic with elevated amylase and/or lipase suggest gallstone pancreatitis, which usually requires admission, bowel rest, and later cholecystectomy.

Diagnosis

Characteristically patients will complain of right upper quadrant abdominal pain, often radiating to the back, worse or brought about by a fatty meal, and may describe similar episodes in the past. The pain of pancreatitis is often more severe and epigastric, but considerable overlap exists. On exam, apart from pain as above, the patient may demonstrate **Murphy's sign**, which is inspiratory arrest due to pain with right upper quadrant palpation as the tender gallbladder is pushed down on the examiner's hand (or ultrasound probe). Peritonitis is unusual, but if present may indicate gangrenous or perforated cholecystitis.

When evaluating a patient with right upper quadrant pain, obviously crucial are the white blood cell count and temperature (to differentiate simple colic from something more severe), the bilirubin level (to differentiate cholecystitis from cholangitis), and the amylase and lipase (to identify pancreatitis). Radiologic workup is likewise critical. In general, the two most useful tests are **ultrasound** and the **DISIDA scan**.

Ultrasound (US) provides **anatomic** information. The presence of acoustically dense stones, gallbladder wall thickening, or pericholecystic fluid imply cholecystitis. US can measure the diameter of the common duct, with a dilated duct (greater than 10mm) implying common duct obstruction. It is usually easy to obtain at night and takes only minutes, but interpretation is operator-dependent.

DISIDA scans provide **functional** information, with the key question being whether the cystic duct is obstructed. If so, the gallbladder will be **nonvisualized**, which strongly suggests the presence of cholecystitis. It is a slower test, taking hours for full examination, and is not usually available in the middle of the night.

In general, in a patient with presumed biliary colic, the presence or absence of stones may be all the information needed to plan treatment; thus, an outpatient US might be best. In a patient in the emergency room with presumed cholecystitis, either a positive DISIDA or US suggests the need for operation. If the US is normal but clinical suspicion is high, it would be reasonable to obtain a DISIDA to assess whether the cystic duct is blocked. In a patient with probable gallstone pancreatitis, again, the presence of stones would be important in planning treatment, but you wouldn't expect the cystic duct to be blocked (gallstone pancreatitis and cholangitis don't usually simultaneously coexist), thus an US to identify a stone would be the best test. Finally, in a patient with probable cholangitis, an US or CT scan might be the best initial study to define the anatomy and presence of ductal dilatation prior to definitive treatment.

Treatment

Again, the timing of intervention can seem confusing. The basic general principles are:

– Most asymptomatic gallstones stay asymptomatic.
– Symptoms usually precede life-threatening complications.
– Symptoms usually imply, however, that complications will develop.
–The risk of cancer is extremely low.
(continued)

Therefore, asymptomatic patients should be observed, but the occurrence of any symptoms definitely due to gallstones should lead to treatment. The treatment of biliary tract disease is to remove the stone-forming organ, i.e., **cholecystectomy** (lithotripsy and dissolutants don't seem to be panning out, in part because they leave the gallbladder in place).

Laparoscopic cholecystectomy

Laparoscopic cholecystectomy has been around for only half a decade or so, but has been revolutionary. It allows a faster recovery and is much more comfortable for the patient. It is usually easier in elective situations when cholecystitis is not present (the typical elective "lap chole" in a patient with outpatient biliary colic) but can be performed successfully in the setting of acute inflammation. The 5%-15% rate of conversion to open laparotomy and the higher rate of bile duct injury are balanced by quicker discharge and shorter recovery. Both conversion rate and injury rate seem to be decreasing with experience.

Open cholecystectomy

Open cholecystectomy is the classic method of removing the gallbladder. It is easier than the laparoscopic approach in the setting of acute cholecystitis. It also allows the best exposure for more complicated procedures such as exploration of the common bile duct, and allows better exploration of the rest of the abdomen, if necessary.

Ductal status

An **intraoperative cholangiogram**, or dye study of the ductal system, is done on a routine basis by some, and only if there are signs or symptoms suggesting the presence of a common duct stone (such as history of jaundice, pancreatitis, elevated liver function tests, and so on) by others. It requires cannulation of the cystic duct, and hence requires a fair degree of dissection. It can be done laparoscopically or open. These criteria are becoming indications for preoperative **endoscopic retrograde pancreaticoduodenoscopy (ERCP)** and stone removal, with cholangiogram and possible common duct exploration reserved for the 10% or so of patients in whom the ERCP is unsuccessful.

CBD exploration

A **common bile duct exploration** refers to the situation where the common duct contains stones, and is thus dissected free, opened, and cleared of stones using a variety of techniques. It is almost always done using the open approach, and the common duct is usually closed over a "T-tube" which exits the skin and stays in about six weeks. There are essentially three indications to explore the common duct: a positive cholangiogram, a palpable common duct stone, or cholangitis.

Timing of Surgery

Asymptomatic stones should be watched because most will stay asymptomatic. Some argue that asymptomatic stones in diabetics should be prophylactically removed. Although complications, if they occur, are more severe in diabetics, the **risk** of symptoms or complications seems to be no higher than in non-diabetics, and most surgeons would treat them like any other patient. Biliary colic with documented stones is treated by elective cholecystectomy. Acute cholecystitis usually mandates admission with bowel rest and antibiotics, followed by cholecystectomy when convenient, generally within 24-48 hours. In the past it was believed that operating after 72 hours of inflammation was unsafe, leading to the suggestion that cholecystectomy take place either within 72 hours of onset or deferred until after the inflammation subsided. This is no longer accepted, and operation is indicated even for inflammation longer than 3 days. Now that laparoscopic cholecystectomies are routine, a new but reasonable option is to allow a "cooling-off" period with later laparoscopy to lessen the chance of having to convert to open. This, however, is to be weighed against the increased risk of serious complications as operation is delayed.

Cholangitis usually is treated by urgent or immediate drainage of the common bile duct (radiologically by ERCP or by transhepatic percutaneous methods, or by surgical common duct exploration) and removal of the obstructing stone. Timing depends on the severity and overall patient condition. Cholangitis can be minor or can be life-threatening.

Gallstone pancreatitis is treated by admission and bowel rest, followed by cholecystectomy after acute attack subsides, usually during the same admission (because the risk of recurrent pancreatitis is high). Some feel that early cholecystectomy is safe if the attack is mild, but it is important to remember that removing the gallbladder has no impact on the acute pancreatitis, but is done to prevent

Surgery
Biliary Tract *continued*

later attacks; therefore there is no need to rush. There is some evidence that early ERCP with removal of an obstructing stone improves outcome, but this is still being investigated. Operation in pregnant patients with biliary tree pathology usually can be deferred until after delivery.

In some patients, especially the elderly and those with multiple stones or a dilated common bile duct, the safest and most "durable" operation (in terms of alleviating symptoms and risk) is anastomosis of the common bile duct to the duodenum or jejunum to allow unobstructed drainage (choledochoduodenostomy or choledochojejunostomy).

Malignancy

Courvoisier's law states that a painlessly dilated gallbladder (or painless palpable right upper quadrant mass) indicates malignancy in the pancreas or biliary tree until proven otherwise. Cancers obstructing the biliary tree usually cause **painless obstructive jaundice**. These tumors are best imaged using CT and ERCP (or percutaneous transhepatic cholangiography if the intrahepatic ducts are dilated) and can occur anywhere.

Ampulla of Vater or duodenal tumors have reasonable prognoses, perhaps because they tend to produce symptoms early. They often can be resected via a pancreaticoduodenectomy (Whipple procedure). Treatment of common bile duct or hepatic hilum (Klatskin's tumors) is complex and must be individualized. Pancreatic carcinoma (adenocarcinoma) is often incurable at presentation, although tumors occurring at the head of the pancreas and thus causing early symptoms (jaundice) via common duct obstruction can have more favorable outcomes. It is unclear whether curative operations (Whipple) really help, or whether palliative bypass (choledochoenteric anastamoses) is just as beneficial.

Gallbladder cancer is rare. It may not cause jaundice and often presents late. It can present as an incidental finding after routine cholecystectomy and in this special case can be cured. A calcified ("porcelain") gallbladder, although rare, indicates a high risk of malignancy, and this finding on x-ray, even if the patient is asymptomatic, suggests the need for elective cholecystectomy. ∎

34   Peptic Ulcer Disease

Ulcers of the duodenum and stomach are estimated to affect 10-20 million Americans. Although the incidence of gastric ulcers has not changed, over the last decade or so that of duodenal ulcers has been declining. Coincident with this trend has been a decline in the number of operations required for treatment of ulcers; interestingly, however, this seems to be independent of the rise in modern anti-ulcer treatment.

Ulcers, in general, are due to an imbalance between **acid production** and **mucosal barrier function** (provided by mucus and bicarbonate secretion and healthy blood flow). Duodenal ulcers can be due to either factor, but gastric ulcers usually are associated with normal or low acid states, implying that defective barrier function is the major problem. A critical point to remember when dealing with an ulcer is that duodenal ulcers are essentially always benign, while gastric ulcers can be malignant (in other words, not a true ulcer, but an ulcerated tumor).

Duodenal Ulcer

Duodenal ulcers are more common in men, especially during young adulthood and middle age (ages 20-45). Blood type O, gastric colonization with Helicobacter pylori (a gram negative rod found in 95% of patients with duodenal ulcers), chronic lung or liver disease, chronic pancreatitis, and alcoholism all are correlated with duodenal ulcers, but ulcers have not clearly been shown to correlate with the so-called "type-A" personality. Duodenal ulcers require normal (the majority) or excessive (about a third) acid production by the stomach—"no acid, no ulcer"—but impaired duodenal defenses probably play a significant role in their formation.

Manifestations   They occur most commonly (95%) in the duodenal bulb, within a few centimeters of the pylorus. They often cause burning, gnawing, epigastric pain aggravated by fasting and often relieved temporarily by food or antacids. The pain can awaken the patient from sleep. Ulcers can be chronic and uncomplicated, being manifest only by pain, or can produce a number of more serious complications. Duodenal ulcers can erode posteriorly or anteriorly, with

Surgery
Peptic Ulcer Disease *continued*

very characteristic results according to the relevant anatomy. The pancreas and gastroduodenal artery lie behind the second portion of the duodenum; **posteriorly** penetrating ulcers can cause pancreatitis or massive upper gastrointestinal hemorrhage. Likewise, the duodenum is unprotected anteriorly; **anterior** ulcers will perforate into the free peritoneal cavity.

Patients with symptomatic duodenal ulcers will present in one of four ways: **pain, bleeding, perforation,** or **obstruction**. If the pain is chronic, the diagnosis is often made by eliminating other sources of epigastric and right upper quadrant pain, such as cholecystitis, pancreatitis, indigestion, or esophagitis, for example. A bleeding ulcer will be manifest as a typical upper GI bleed (see Chapter 40, "GI Bleeding") with either hematemesis or melena. Bright red blood from the rectum from any upper GI source indicates that the bleeding is extremely rapid. Patients who perforate are classically very ill, usually demonstrating the classic "board-like," rigid abdomen of true peritonitis. A free air series (which includes abdominal films in varying positions and and an upright chest x-ray) will usually demonstrate free air under the diaphragms. A significant number (up to 25%) of patients who have perforated, however, will not initially demonstrate free air, and thus, if clinical suspicion is high, treatment (operation) should be initiated with or without this finding. Patients with an obstructing ulcer usually complain of symptoms of long duration, with recent emesis and inability to keep food or water down. They are commonly very ill and severely dehydrated, and demonstrate the classic hypochloremic, hypokalemic metabolic alkalosis (with paradoxic aciduria) of gastric outlet obstruction. Except in the setting of acute perforation, esophagogastroduodenoscopy (EGD) is crucial to make the diagnosis, to characterize, and possibly to treat the complication, if present, and to identify the location of the problem.

Gastric Ulcer

Patients with gastric ulcers are usually between ages 40-60. Just like those in the duodenum, gastric ulcers can be due to an imbalance between acid production and host defenses, and many gastric ulcers are probably identical to duodenal ulcers, only arising just on the other side of the pylorus. Most such true gastric peptic ulcers are located in the prepyloric region or along the lesser curvature of the stomach within a few centimeters of the transi-tion zone between the antrum and the body of the stomach. These ulcers, like duodenal, are almost always benign.

Other gastric ulcers, however, particularly those located in the body or along the greater curvature, are commonly associated with low-acid states (achlorhydria), and may be primarily due to a defective mucous barrier or Helicobacter pylori infection. Bile reflux from the duodenum can be part of the problem, as can nonsteroidal anti-inflammatory medications (NSAIDs). Critically important to remember, however, is the fact that these gastric ulcers have a significant risk of being malignant. Again, the ulcer does not somehow transform into a tumor, but rather was probably an ulcerated tumor from the start. These two groups (duodenal and gastric ulcers associated with high or normal acid states and gastric ulcers in the setting of achlorhydria) are two different entities.

Gastric ulcers present with similar symptoms as those in the duodenum (but are less likely to obstruct)—usually the location cannot be pinpointed based on the history alone. Gastric ulcers typically produce longer-lasting symptomatology, but the relationship to food (aggravating or relieving) is not constant enough to make a difference. Again, the diagnosis is made by direct visualization (usually by endoscopy). If a gastric ulcer is seen, multiple biopsies are taken to rule out a malignancy.

Medical Therapy

The majority of patients suffering from peptic ulcer disease can be satisfactorily managed with medical therapy. The first step is to make the diagnosis, usually by EGD or upper GI contrast study for workup of chronic epigastric pain or heme-positive stools (asymptomatic patients can also be diagnosed during evaluation for unrelated problems). Biopsies should be taken of most gastric ulcers, especially those that are associated with achlorhydria or are located in the body or along the greater curvature.

An initial trial of medical care is warranted in all patients with benign ulcers. Patients should avoid ulcerogenic agents, such as nicotine, alcohol, caffeine, aspirin, and NSAIDs. A variety of drugs can be used specifically to

Surgery
Peptic Ulcer Disease *continued*

treat the ulcer. **Antacids** are salts of aluminum, magnesium, or calcium which bind hydrogen and raise the pH (and may also augment defenses directly in as yet poorly understood ways). Side effects include constipation (aluminum-based antacids), diarrhea (magnesium-based), and poor compliance due to the need for frequent dosing. **Sulcrafate** (Carafate) is the aluminum salt of sucrose octasulfate. It adheres to and protects tissues, directly stimulating mucous production to augment barrier function. **Histamine receptor (H$_2$) antagonists** block the histamine receptor on parietal cells, thus diminishing acid secretion by both gastrin and vagally-mediated pathways. Antacids and H$_2$ receptor blockade seem to be about the same in their clinical efficacy (good), but the latter are more convenient for the patient. **Omeprazole** (Prilosec) blocks the H$^+$/K$^+$-ATPase proton pump of the parietal cell directly, inhibiting acid secretion, and also raising gastric pH. It is very effective, though costly. There is current interest in eradicating Helicobacter pylori infection directly with antibiotics, but it remains to be seen whether this technique will be useful.

Repeat endoscopy to document healing is usually not necessary after good clinical response to treatment of a duodenal ulcer (relief of symptoms within 4-8 weeks). Gastric ulcers are more difficult to heal (often requiring eight weeks or so) and recur more often than do duodenal ulcers. Because of the risk of malignancy, repeat EGD is thus essentially mandatory; nonhealing mandates resection.

Surgical Therapy

Surgical treatment of ulcer disease can be quite confusing. There are four indications for surgery for peptic ulcer disease: **bleeding, perforation, obstruction,** and **intractability** (failure of medical management). A fifth, malignancy, usually falls under the setting of failure of medical management, or failure to heal. The general principle of surgical management of these lesions is that different operations are necessary to treat different complications. The operation depends on the specific problem, the acute health of the patient, and the risk of cancer. There is no one "ulcer operation."

Bleeding ulcer

A patient who is **bleeding** needs the bleeding stopped. Endoscopic cautery is usually attempted first, but if bleeding persists, surgery is required. A visible vessel (bleeding or not) at endoscopy is a strong predictor of the need for operation. As discussed above, the vast majority of bleeding ulcers are those in the second portion of the duodenum that have eroded posteriorly, into the gastroduodenal artery. In a bleeding patient the duodenum is opened, the bleeding point oversewn directly, and the gastroduodenal artery ligated (watch out for the common bile duct!).

Perforated ulcer

A patient whose ulcer has **perforated** needs the hole sealed. Ulcers that perforate are those that have eroded anteriorly. Usually the tissues are edematous and friable, and the hole cannot be directly closed. In this case, a piece of omentum is brought up to patch the hole (Graham patch).

Obstruction

Ulcers that cause gastric outlet **obstruction** usually require resection of the antrum, scarred pylorus, and first part of duodenum, with continuity reestablished by direct gastroduodenostomy (Billroth I) or gastrojejunostomy (Billroth II).

Figure 34.1
Billroth I (left, direct gastroduo-denostomy) and II (right, gastroje-junostomy) reconstructions after gastric resection.

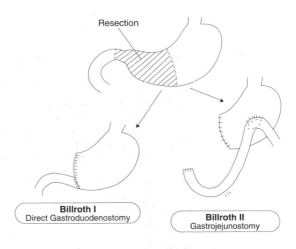

Resection

Billroth I
Direct Gastroduodenostomy

Billroth II
Gastrojejunostomy

Failed medical management

Ulcers that are chronic or have **failed medical manage-ment** are usually treated by means of an acid-reducing procedure alone (see below). Resection of the ulcer itself is not usually needed, but acid production must be reduced. *(continued)*

Acid reduction

In all of the above situations, the option of adding an **acid-reducing procedure** is considered, weighing, in each case, the ability of the patient to tolerate the additional operative time, the degree to which excessive acid production has contributed to the problem, and the other options available (such as medical management). In general, operations that reduce acid production show an inverse correlation between ulcer recurrence and morbidity. A simple operation will usually have a high recurrence rate, while a definitive operation can lead to substantial morbidity and mortality. The safest choice is a **truncal vagotomy** to eliminate vagally-mediated stimulation for acid secretion. Because the intact vagus causes relaxation of the pylorus, a **pyloroplasty** to avoid pyloric obstruction is also needed. More difficult but equally efficacious is a **highly selective** or **parietal cell vagotomy**, where only the nerves to the body of the stomach (containing the parietal cells) are sectioned. Although innervation to the antrum remains intact, recurrence (though greater than a vagotomy and antrectomy) is surprisingly low. Most morbid in the short-term, but associated with the lowest recurrence rates, are **vagotomy and antrectomy** (to eliminate all acid stimulation) and **subtotal gastrectomy** (eliminating all acid-producing tissue).

Gastric ulcers

Gastric **peptic** ulcers (prepyloric or lesser curve) can be treated according to the same principles as are duodenal ulcers. A major difference in the surgical therapy of **fundic** or **greater curve** gastric ulcers, however, is the advisability of resecting the entire ulcer to rule out malignancy (approximately 10% of gastric ulcers are malignant). If the entire ulcer cannot be resected, multiple biopsies should be obtained. Complicated ulcers (bleeding, perforation) located in the antrum or fundus are usually treated by wedge excision or hemigastrectomy if the patient can tolerate the procedure. Gastric ulcers that have not healed with good medical management (eight weeks) or that have been shown, by biopsy, to be cancer, are treated by aggressive gastric resection. A vagotomy is usually not needed in these cases because acid overproduction is not the problem.

Gastric ulcers located near the gastroesophageal junction present a particular problem. If the ulcer can be included in a hemigastrectomy, this is the procedure of choice. Other options include local excision, an acid-reducing procedure alone (if rigorous search has failed to document malignancy), or esophagogastrectomy if cancer is present.

Zollinger-Ellison Syndrome

Zollinger-Ellison Syndrome (ZES) is an uncommon cause of severe peptic ulcer disease. The pathophysiology is very simple: gastric acid hypersecretion is stimulated by excessive amounts of gastrin produced by an autonomous tumor (gastrinoma). These tumors are most often located in the pancreas or duodenum, and approximately 60% are malignant. This diagnosis should be considered in patients with severe duodenal ulcer disease refractory to optimal management, those with recurrent ulcers, or those with ulcers located in uncommon places (such as the jejunum or ileum). If ZES is suspected, a fasting serum gastrin level should be obtained. Secretin suppresses gastrin production by the normal stomach but causes a paradoxic elevation if a gastrinoma is present. Whenever possible the gastrin-producing tumor should be removed, although resection will be possible approximately a third of the time only. H_2 receptor antagonists, omeprazole, and octreotide (a somatostatin analogue) can be very helpful if resection is not feasible (or the tumor cannot be found), and even total gastrectomy to eliminate the target organ (parietal cells) can be palliative.

Post-gastrectomy Syndromes

Patients who have had gastric resection for any reason are prone to a number of specific problems. Most are late, remote enough from the operation that diagnosis is often difficult. The gastric resection, per se, is not the culprit—rather, it is usually the method of reestablishment of gastroenteral continuity (the anastomosis) that leads to these syndromes.

A patient who has had a blind end of duodenum stapled or oversewn (Billroth II gastrojejunostomy) is at risk in the early postoperative period for **duodenal stump blowout** due to increased intraluminal pressure from a proximal obstruction of the afferent limb. These patients are very sick, and develop acute, severe abdominal pain, fever, leukocytosis, and peritonitis 3-6 days after surgery. Reoperation is necessary to drain the leaking duodenal stump.

Surgery
Peptic Ulcer Disease *continued*

Several problems occur later (months to years after resection and gastroenterostomy of any configuration). **Early dumping syndrome** is a characteristic group of symptoms that occur **early** after the ingestion of a meal containing a high osmotic load (e.g., concentrated carbohydrates). Shortly after eating the meal patients experience anxiety, tachycardia, weakness, diaphoresis, borborygmi, and diarrhea, due to the rapid movement of intravascular fluid into the small intestine lumen (relative hypovolemia) and the release of several vasoactive substances (serotonin, histamine, glucagon, VIP, etc.). Treatment involves diet modification, to avoid large, highly osmotic meals and, in certain cases, conversion to a Roux-en-Y gastrojejunostomy. **Late dumping syndrome** (reactive hypoglycemia) is similar, but the patient experiences anxiety, tachycardia, weakness, and diaphoresis **later** (approximately 3-4 hours after eating). Patients usually do not experience GI symptoms or diarrhea because the etiology involves rapid changes in serum glucose and insulin levels. Treatment involves eating smaller more frequent meals. Bowel obstruction can occur just as after any abdominal surgery. If the **afferent limb** of a gastrojejunostomy is intermittently blocked, pancreatic and biliary secretions will build up and distend the loop, leading to severe abdominal pain that is relieved after decompression by vomiting (typically bilious). Obstruction distally is a typical small bowel obstruction, and is termed **efferent limb** obstruction. **Bile reflux gastritis** can develop when duodenal, pancreatic, and biliary secretion reflux into the stomach as the result of the (surgically) incompetent gastroenterostomy, leading to weakness, weight loss, nausea, abdominal pain, and perhaps recurrent ulceration. The margin of the anastomosis is particularly prone to develop recurrent ulceration **(marginal ulcer)**, especially if an acid-reducing procedure has not been performed. **Recurrent ulcer disease** can occur whenever acid producing cells are left intact. Often the cause is an inadequate first operation or vagotomy; Zollinger-Ellison syndrome should be ruled out.

Most of these problems, interestingly enough, can be cured by conversion of the existing gastroenterostomy to a Roux-en-Y configuration. ∎

35   Thoracic Surgery

Thoracic surgery is the care of patients with surgical problems of the thorax, **excluding** the heart and great vessels. During the two years following the general surgical residency, the cardiothoracic fellow treats both cardiac and thoracic problems; most such physicians, however, choose to do one or the other after they finish. The problems that thoracic surgeons face are surprisingly diverse. Although lung cancer is the most common pathologic entity, thoracic surgeons also treat infections of the lung and pleural space, tumors and other conditions of the esophagus and mediastinum, trauma, chest wall problems, and numerous other problems. This chapter focuses on understanding and interpreting **pulmonary function**, on **lung cancer** and pulmonary **infections**, on **esophageal cancer**, and on the mechanics and use of **chest tubes**.

Pulmonary Function Testing

In a patient who is being considered for major surgery, the ability of the lungs to successfully tolerate the planned insult is critical. This concept is applicable to any patient undergoing an **abdominal** as well as a **thoracic** incision, as well as to those undergoing prolonged general anesthesia or those with borderline pulmonary function to start with. Not every patient needs a full workup, but any patient with any question about pulmonary status should undergo evaluation. The goal of preoperative evaluation is to determine the operation of choice given the physiologic limitations of the patient. In some patients, this may mean no operation at all. Performing a pneumonectomy to remove a large lung tumor, for example, only to have the patient permanently dependent on a mechanical respirator is unacceptable. There is no formula or single test available for predicting postoperative success. Preoperative testing can stratify risk in a qualitative sense, but considerable clinical judgment is needed to choose the right treatment.

PFTs

Spirometry forms the basis of preoperative **pulmonary function tests** (**PFTs**) and should be performed on any patient with pulmonary risk factors such as heavy smoking, advanced age, malnutrition, or chronic obstructive

Surgery
Thoracic Surgery *continued*

pulmonary disease (COPD), scheduled to undergo major thoracic or abdominal surgery. Knowledge of lung volumes is essential to interpretation of PFTs:

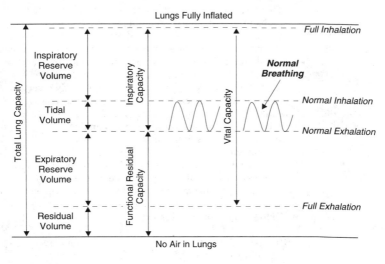

Lungs Fully Inflated

Figure 35.1
Review of lung volumes. Note that the vital capacity is the most air that can be moved in or out of the lung; residual volume and thus total lung capacity can only be measured using indirect means.

Three of the most useful indices are the vital capacity, forced expiratory volume accomplished in 1 second, and maximal ventilatory volume. **Vital capacity (VC)** is the total maximal volume of air that can be expelled from the lung. It is a static measure of volume and does not give much information regarding the strength of the respiratory muscles, lung and chest wall compliance, or underlying status of the airways. In contrast, **FEV_1**, the volume of air forcefully expelled from a deep inspiration in the first second of exhalation, is a dynamic measurement that takes these factors into account. In a healthy young adult, the FEV_1 is about 80% of the vital capacity. **VC is usually reduced in patients with restrictive lung disease** because their lungs and chest wall cannot fully expand, while **FEV_1 is reduced in patients with obstructive disease** because their resistance to dynamic flow is higher. FEV_1 is often improved after administration of bronchodilator therapy and, if so, bronchodilators can be used with success in the postoperative period. The other useful dynamic measure is **maximum ventilatory volume (MVV)**. The patient breathes as hard as possible for 10 seconds and the volume is multiplied by 6 to obtain a value in L/min; this helps predict the patient's ability to perform the sustained work of breathing. PFT results are expressed as a percentage of that expected for a healthy patient of the same size, sex and age. High-risk patients typically have a VC, FEV_1, and MVV less than 50% of that expected.

ABG

A preoperative arterial blood gas (ABG) analysis provides useful information as well (see Chapters 1, "Airway and Ventilator Management" and 2, "Acid-Base Disorders"). Perhaps most useful is its function as an indicator of the patient's baseline status. For example, patients with COPD may chronically retain CO_2; thus, a high pCO_2 in the postoperative state can be normal. pO_2 declines with age and smoking history.

Split function PFTs

Split function testing is sometimes useful if a pulmonary resection is planned. Radioisotopic techniques are used to lateralize gas exchange and perfusion to one lung or the other, the results of which can be used to predict residual function after resection. A patient with PFTs of only 50% of predicted, for example, would probably not be a candidate for pneumonectomy. If split function testing indicated that 90% of gas exchange was occurring in the "good" lung, however (i.e., the lung to be resected is essentially nonfunctional), the patient would be expected to tolerate the loss of the "bad" lung without much change in function. In general, the right lung accounts for about 55% of pulmonary "function" in a healthy adult.

Lung Cancer

Primary lung cancer is the leading cause of cancer death in both men and women in the US, killing 100,000 people a year. Cigarette smoking is the dominant causal factor in the great majority of cases; asbestos exposure and environmental pollutants also contribute. Cessation of smoking is clearly associated with a decreased risk of lung cancer (and cardiovascular disease). About 90% of patients with lung cancer are current or recently reformed smokers.

Histology

Lung cancer is usually classified by cell type. 95% of tumors are classified as **bronchogenic**, arising from epithelial cells lining the airways anywhere from the

major bronchi to the alveoli. Most bronchogenic carcinomas are one of four types: **squamous cell carcinoma**,
adenocarcinoma, **large cell carcinoma** (**LCLC**), and
small cell lung carcinoma (**SCLC**). The remaining 5%
include neuroendocrine tumors (**carcinoids**) and tumors
of mesenchymal cell origin (**sarcomas**).

Squamous cell carcinoma accounts for 30% of all lung
cancers. These are strongly associated with cigarette
smoking, are typically located near the hilum of the lung,
and are relatively slow to metastasize.

Adenocarcinoma also accounts for 30% of all lung cancers. These grow rapidly and arise from the subsegmental
bronchi, and are therefore located more peripherally than
are squamous cell tumors. **Bronchoalveolar carcinoma**,
a subset of adenocarcinoma, is notable for the fact that a
third of affected patients have no history of tobacco use.

Large cell carcinomas occur peripherally and are much
less common.

Small cell (**oat cell**) lung cancers make up 25% of lung
tumors. This is the most aggressive cell type, and is consequently associated with the poorest prognosis. Most
cases of SCLC have metastasized by the time of detection. Traditionally, lung cancers have been broadly classified as "small-" or "non-small cell," based on histologic
and biologic criteria. In general, patients with SCLC have
been believed to have no hope of cure or benefit from
surgery, but it is now recognized that some carefully
selected patients with SCLC will benefit from operation.

Many patients are asymptomatic. **Symptoms** caused by
lung cancer are an ominous sign, and can be due to local,
metastatic, or paraneoplastic factors. Median survival is
only 3 months once symptoms occur; incidental detection
on routine chest x-ray (CXR) examination carries a much
better prognosis.

Presentation   The most common symptoms are related to local invasion
of tumor into the airway and include cough, chest pain,
and **blood-streaked sputum**; massive hemoptysis is
extremely rare. Partial obstruction of an airway will cause
wheezing, while complete obstruction will lead to **atelectasis** (collapse of alveoli distal to the obstruction), bacter-

ial overgrowth, and infection. Invasion of the left recurrent laryngeal nerve as it loops underneath the aortic arch can result in hoarseness. Compression of the superior vena cava (**SVC syndrome**) causes marked facial, neck, and upper extremity edema, and almost always heralds malignancy. Tumors located in the superior sulcus can impinge on the brachial plexus and cervical sympathetic ganglion, causing shoulder and arm pain and Horner's syndrome (**Pancoast tumors**). Dyspnea can occur due to pleural effusion, phrenic nerve paralysis, or airway obstruction.

Lung tumors metastasize (in rough order) to regional lymph nodes, liver, adrenal glands, bone, brain, and kidney. Constitutional symptoms such as fatigue and weight loss usually signify metastatic disease.

Paraneoplastic syndromes are caused by secretion of hormone-like substances from the tumor. Although the effects are systemic, these syndromes do not necessarily indicate metastatic disease. The classic examples are production of Cushing's syndrome from ACTH-secreting oat cell tumors, and hypercalcemia caused by secretion of a PTH analog by squamous cell tumors.

Diagnosis

The primary diagnostic and therapeutic goals for the surgeon are to determine whether the lung tumor is amenable to resection and, if so, whether or not the patient will tolerate the planned procedure. After satisfactory PA and lateral CXRs have been reviewed, most patients require a CT scan of the chest. CT scanning of the upper abdomen and brain, bone scan, and alkaline phosphatase determination are often performed to detect metastases. Physical examination includes a search for lymph nodes suitable for biopsy. In most (but not all) cases, a tissue sample must be obtained to direct therapy.

Biopsy

Tumors near the hilus can be visualized and biopsied by means of flexible bronchoscopy. If located peripherally, beyond the reach of the bronchoscope, a percutaneous needle biopsy of the tumor can be performed. There is little or no risk of tumor cell implantation along the biopsy tract; the most common complication is simple, usually minor, pneumothorax. When needle biopsy is unsuccessful or deemed too risky because of proximity to vital structures, open biopsy may be required. Diagnostic thoracentesis ("pleural tap") should be performed if there is an effusion. Not all effusions in the presence of known lung cancer are malignant! Because the presence of malignant cells in pleural fluid usually excludes a patient from surgical treatment (see below), this is a crucial piece of information. Mediastinal lymph nodes on the right side can be biopsied via mediastinoscopy using a suprasternal incision; nodes on the left can be approached using a parasternal incision (anterior mediastinotomy).

The inability to obtain a tissue diagnosis by any or all of the above techniques should not prevent further evalua-tion or treatment. Thoracotomy for suspicious lesions without preoperative diagnosis is justified if reasonable efforts have been made to obtain tissue, the risk of cancer is believed to be high, and the benefits outweigh the risks.

Staging

Staging is necessary to determine treatment and progno-sis. The TNM classification is used. Briefly, **stage 0** indi-cates carcinoma in-situ. **Stage I** indicates the presence of a tumor of any size without lymph node involvement, metastases, or invasion of pleura or chest wall; if the ipsi-lateral hilar nodes are involved, the tumor is **stage II**. **Stage IIIa** indicates chest wall and/or ipsilateral medi-astinal nodal involvement, while stage **IIIb** indicates invasion of adjacent organs, pleural effusion, or involved contralateral nodes. Finally, **stage IV** indicates the pres-ence of distant metastases. Note that tumor size, per se, does not contribute to staging. Staging can be based on clinical (symptoms, x-rays, and biopsy) or pathologic (post-resection) data.

Treatment

Surgery represents the only potential curative treatment for lung cancer and is recommended for stage 0, I, II, and some IIIa NSCLC tumors; i.e., any non-small cell tumor limited to lung parenchyma or **ipsilateral** hilar nodes, and some tumors involving the chest wall. Pancoast tumors are included in this group. A few highly selected patients with peripheral small cell tumors can benefit from resec-tion, but **surgery is generally reserved for non-small cell tumors**.

Historically, surgery for lung cancer meant removal of the entire lung (**pneumonectomy**). The desire to preserve uninvolved lung tissue has led to the acceptance of **lobec-tomy** as standard treatment when tumor is isolated to a specific lobe. Limited **wedge resection** or anatomic **seg-**

mentectomy for focal tumors are options in patients with limited pulmonary reserve, although recent data suggests that these more limited resections may be associated with higher recurrence rates. Therefore, they should be reserved for patients who cannot tolerate a "major" operation. This topic is controversial at present, and it is hoped that ongoing studies will clarify this issue. **Video-assisted thoracoscopic surgery (VATS)** is a relatively new minimally-invasive procedure with great promise. Diagnostic and therapeutic maneuvers, including biopsy and limited lung resection, can be performed by placing a rigid camera and surgical instruments through one or more trocars into the thoracic cavity. Because of the rigidity of the chest wall, no insufflation is needed, but single-lung ventilation is usually performed.

Adjuvant chemo- and/or radiation therapy are recommended for most stage II and III lung cancers. Adjuvant therapy has not been shown to be of any benefit in metastatic disease, although research is ongoing.

Lung metastases

Many **lung metastases** (from non-pulmonary tumors) can be resected with overall survival benefit. For surgery to be of benefit, the primary tumor must be controlled, there should be no other known metastases, and the patient must be able to tolerate the thoracotomy. Multiple or bilateral lung lesions do not preclude resection.

The Solitary Pulmonary Nodule (Coin Lesion)

The presence of a solitary, peripheral, circumscribed lesion on routine CXR in an asymptomatic patient is relatively common and is understandably a cause for concern. The incidence of malignancy given a coin lesion is anywhere from 10%-50% depending on the population studied (cancer being most common in elderly smokers). Surgical resection for tumors at this stage have, by far, the best prognosis. Differential diagnosis includes granuloma, hamartoma, and pulmonary infarct. The first step in working up a coin lesion is to **obtain a previous CXR**, if one exists, for comparison. Factors increasing the risk of malignancy include new lesions (present for less than 2 years), calcifications in an eccentric, speckled pattern with irregular borders, age greater than 50, and a history of smoking. **Thoracotomy without further workup is recommended when any these criteria are present;**

negative results by needle biopsy and sputum cytology
are unreliable because sampling error cannot be excluded.
Vigilant observation alone is justified only when there is a
low risk of malignancy.

Pulmonary and Pleural Infections

Pulmonary infections, most notably tuberculosis, provided
the primary indication for thoracic surgery fifty years ago.
Today most of these conditions are managed medically.
Such problems include lung abscess (usually secondary to
aspiration pneumonia), bronchiectasis, tuberculosis, and
fungal infections. Surgery is principally reserved for
severe, refractory infection, and to rule out or treat malignancy. Pus in the pleural cavity (**empyema**) results from
direct extension of a parenchymal infection, trauma or foreign body, invasive procedures, or hematogenous seeding
of an effusion. A true empyema usually requires chest tube
drainage (see below). If tube thoracostomy is unsuccessful
or there are chronic, undrained collections, open thoracotomy with removal of the rind that forms on the lung
(**decortication**) and open drainage may be required.

Esophageal Cancer

Cancer of the esophagus usually carries a fairly poor prognosis. Most cancers are squamous in origin, but adenocarcinomas can arise near the gastroesophageal junction in
areas of columnar transformation (Barrett's esophagus)
resulting from prolonged gastroesophageal reflux (see
Chapter 22, "Gastroenterology"). "Severe dysplasia"
found on biopsy of a region of Barrett's esophagitis confers a high enough risk of cancer that prophylactic resection is indicated. Esophageal cancers often present with
dysphagia, and many are metastatic on presentation. Since
surgery confers significant palliation, resection is usually
indicated. Esophageal tumors can be resected using both
thoracotomy and laparotomy with reanastomosis in the
chest, or by blunt dissection via a transhiatal approach,
with reanastomosis in the neck. The stomach, based on
blood provided by the right gastroepiploic artery, is the
most commonly used esophageal substitute.
Esophagectomy carries with it substantial morbidity and
mortality. Preoperative chemo- and radiation therapy have
shown promise in improving resectability and local occurrence, but have not demonstrated improvement in survival.

Chest Tubes

Chest tubes are used to evacuate air, fluid, or infection from the pleural space. In health, the pleural "space" does not exist. The airtight nature of the intrapleural compartment maintains the visceral pleura of the lung in direct contact with the parietal pleura over its entire surface, separated and lubricated by a few mL of fluid. As the chest wall expands and the diaphragm is depressed, the lung expands concomitantly. Loss of this airtight seal due to injury or disease of the chest wall or lung will allow air and/or fluid to enter and create an actual space, interfering with respiratory mechanics. The most common cause of loss of chest wall integrity is penetrating trauma (see Chapter 28, "Trauma"); parenchymal air leaks are most commonly caused by lung lacerations from fractured ribs, needle sticks during central line placement, needle biopsy, or thoracentesis, and spontaneous rupture of emphysematous or congenital pulmonary blebs.

Terminology

If the pleural pressure, normally negative, becomes neutral with respect to the atmosphere, a **simple pneumothorax** results. Contralateral function is normal. If a situation creating a "one-way valve" effect occurs (fairly common, especially after trauma), the pleural pressure becomes increasingly positive with respect to the atmosphere with each breath. Known as a **tension pneumothorax**, this condition is much more serious because the pliable mediastinum can shift toward the opposite side, impairing contralateral function and systemic venous return. A tension pneumothorax can arise from a simple pneumothorax, especially if positive-pressure ventilation is used. A **hemothorax** exists if blood enters the pleural space.

Diagnosis

Pneumothorax is usually visualized on upright CXR as a clear space at the apex of the affected hemithorax. The diagnosis can often be made clinically by the presence of respiratory compromise, decreased breath sounds or crackles at the apex, and **subcutaneous emphysema** that gives the overlying skin a crunchy, "Rice Crispies" sensation (crepitus). Pneumothorax is traditionally "quantified" by the estimated percentage of lung volume loss. This is wildly subjective and inaccurate, and it is much helpful to simply state two factors: the distance between the thoracic apex and the apex of the deflated lung, and the distance the pneumothorax persists down the side of the chest wall. A small, asymptomatic, simple pneumothorax usually can be managed by observation and serial CXRs alone. A large or symptomatic pneumothorax, a pneumothorax that is expected to enlarge, or **any pneumothorax of any size when positive pressure ventilation is needed**, however, require chest tube placement.

The "Pleurevac"

Modern chest tubes are connected to a 3-chambered disposable container. Although individual brands vary in appearance, the essential components include a collection chamber for blood or fluid, an underwater seal that allows air to be evacuated with each expiration and not returned during inspiration, and a wall suction control chamber that regulates the amount of vacuum (commonly -20cm H_2O) applied to the lung:

Figure 35.2
Schematic view of a modern, "3-bottle" chest tube drainage apparatus. Any air that continues to come from the patient will move along "A" and bubble out through the air-leak chamber. The pressure within the suction control bottle, "B," "A," and the chest tube itself will be enough to pull the water to the bottom of the open straw only, whatever the degree of wall suction. Any more suction will merely bubble air through this chamber from the atmosphere. The suction control chamber should be bubbling, or else too little suction is being applied.

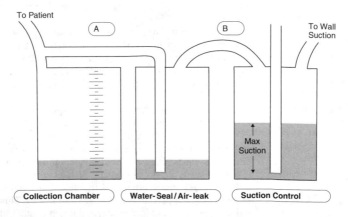

Chest tube management

It is not always necessary to connect chest tubes to wall suction, although it is common practice to do so initially. In the presence of a large, continuous air leak (ongoing entry of air into the pleural space), wall suction maintains a negative intrathoracic pressure to keep the lung expanded. Once the leak has abated, suction can be discontinued. Specifics of chest tube management are quite variable and depend on the surgeon's preferences. On rounds, the important information to convey includes whether the tube is connected to wall suction or simply to underwater seal, how much and what type of drainage has occurred over the previous time period of interest, and whether or not there is an air leak. The presence of an air leak can be determined by watching the water seal chamber, preferably while the patient coughs. Air bubbles passing through this chamber must have come from the pleural space (or through defects in the tubing). Note that on initial tube placement for pneumothorax there is always an air leak for a short period of time as the accumulated intrapleural air is evacuated. The suction control chamber always bubbles if the tube is connected to wall suction, but does not if the tube is to water seal only. Placing a tube to water seal means disconnecting its attachment with the wall. The connection between the patient and suction apparatus should never be disconnected because a pneumothorax will immediately result. When a chest tube is removed, it must be pulled out very quickly to avoid creation of a new pneumothorax via the side holes.

Thoracentesis

Thoracentesis is usually the initial procedure for treating and diagnosing symptomatic pleural effusions. Effusions that rapidly reaccumulate, particularly those caused by a tumor, can require chest tube drainage. Chemical sclerotherapy is performed for malignant effusions by instilling any one of numerous inflammatory agents through the chest tube to produce adhesions between the parietal and visceral pleura, thus preventing reaccumulation of fluid.

Empyema

An empyema is usually initially drained with a chest tube. If the lung re-expands to fill the pleural space, the tube can be removed. Many empyemas, however, especially if chronic, have a thick wall, preventing collapse of the cavity. In this case, the tube is simply cut at the level of the skin, left open to the atmosphere, and slowly removed over days to weeks as the abscess cavity closes behind it (see Chapter 27, "Postoperative Care"). Because of the walled-off nature of the cavity and widespread pleural adhesions, a significant pneumothorax will usually not occur when the tube is left open in this situation. ■

36 Cardiac Surgery

Cardiac surgery involves operating on or within the heart, usually for coronary artery disease, congenital or valvular heart disease, arrhythmias, tumors, or trauma. The field is relatively young, because the ability to safely and routinely operate on the heart did not occur until technology could provide oxygenated blood to the rest of the body and preserve myocardial tissue while the heart was stopped (late 1950s early 1960s). Cardiac surgeons also operate on the great vessels of the chest and on non-cardiac thoracic conditions (See Chapter 35, "Thoracic Surgery").

History

Although sporadic operations on the heart have been reported for centuries, the era of modern cardiac surgery began with the development of the heart-lung machine, an apparatus that temporarily takes over the pumping and ventilatory effects of the heart and lungs. First used in 1953, the early pioneers such as Gibbon, Lillihei, and Kirkland used the technology primarily to perform intracardiac procedures primarily for congenital heart defects.

The story of cardiac catheterization is interesting: in 1929 an intern self-cannulated his own brachial vein and passed a catheter into his right atrium, to prove it could be done—he then walked to the radiology suite to document his feat with an x-ray! With the ability to catheterize the coronary arteries, the importance of coronary atherosclerotic stenoses became apparent. In the 1930s and 40s efforts were made to improve blood supply to the myocardium by suturing muscle, omentum, and even the internal mammary artery to the heart tissue itself, but none of these proved effective. As refinements in the heart-lung machine and myocardial preservation techniques were made, interest in the definitive treatment of blocked coronary arteries grew. Such treatment initially consisted of coronary endarterectomy, but in 1967 the first coronary artery bypass graft (CABG) using a saphenous vein from the leg was performed by Favalaro. Reports soon arose from the US and Soviet Union point ing out the utility and durability of the internal mammary artery, now accepted as the conduit of choice for myocardial revascularization.

Coronary Artery Bypass Grafting (CABG)

The most frequently performed operation performed by the cardiac surgeon is coronary artery bypass grafting (CABG). Just like any part of the body, the myocardium is supplied by blood vessels that can become blocked by atherosclerosis. The heart, however, has an extremely high metabolic rate and oxygen requirement, and sudden depri-vation of blood produces immediate damage (within minutes).

Coronary anatomy

The major coronary arteries form two roughly perpendicular rings around the heart. The **right coronary** artery (RCA) and **left main coronary** artery arise from the sinuses of Valsalva in the root of the ascending aorta. The left main divides shortly after its origin into the **left anterior descending** (LAD) artery and the **circumflex** artery. A **posterior descending** artery arises from the RCA in 90% of patients ("right dominant"), and from the circumflex branch of the left main artery in the remaining 10% ("left dominant"); the RCA and circumflex form one ring, and the LAD and PDA form the second.

CAD

Coronary artery disease (**CAD**) is caused by atherosclerotic plaques within the coronary arteries. These lesions are typically focal (less than a centimeter in length) and involve the major epicardial vessels only, allowing surgical bypass to patent distal vessels. Disease in the left coronary circulation is usually limited to the more proximal branches (left main, proximal LAD, and circumflex, and their proximal branches, the diagonals and marginals), while right coronary artery disease can be more diffusely distributed. A stenosis that occludes greater than 70% of the vessel luminal area (50% reduction in apparent diameter on angiogram) reduces flow and causes a drop in distal pressure, and is thus considered "significant."

Myocardial ischemia and infarction

The coronary circulation responds to increased myocardial oxygen demand during stress and exercise by **vasodilation**. In CAD, the rigid, calcified plaque **cannot dilate**. Exercise-induced (stable) angina results when oxygen supply is thus inadequate to meet the increased demand that occurs with exercise. With time, the plaque can narrow the lumen enough so that flow is decreased even at rest, causing unstable angina. A calcified plaque can rupture, leading to thrombosis, acute occlusion of the artery, and infarction of the myocardium supplied by that vessel. **Myocardial infarction (MI**; see Chapter 15, "Ischemic Heart Disease and Chest Pain") can run the spectrum from small, inconsequential heart muscle damage to massive necrosis and ventricular failure. Congestive heart failure (CHF) can occur acutely during reversible episodes of ischemia, and chronically if enough ventricle is rendered nonfunctional. Infarcted tissue can provide a focus for arrhythmias, which are the leading cause of sudden cardiac death.

Symptoms

The natural progression and variable presentation of CAD runs the gamut from **pain** (stable and unstable angina) to **MI, CHF, arrhythmia**, and **sudden death**. Pain is by far the most common symptom; 75% of all patients with angina describe the classic symptom of substernal chest pressure, while others describe pain in the neck, jaw, teeth, or arms, without chest discomfort. An unknown number of patients have "silent" ischemia and initially present with one of the later symptoms of CAD or an abnormal EKG. The severity of cardiac symptoms, including angina, dyspnea, and fatigue, is classified by a system devised by the New York Heart Association:

Class I: symptom free
Class II: symptoms with moderate exercise or exertion
Class III: symptoms with minimal activity
Class IV: symptoms at rest; severe limitation of lifestyle

This classification system is extremely useful for patient selection and prediction of outcome after surgery. It can be applied to all patients with cardiac disease, including those with valvular pathology.

Ancillary testing

The diagnosis of CAD can often be made by history alone; physical examination will be unremarkable in the majority of patients who do not have CHF. The EKG will be normal unless there is ongoing ischemia, reflected by inverted T waves or ST segment abnormalities, or a past MI, reflected by Q waves (if transmural). Radionuclide studies provide anatomic and functional information. The exercise thallium "stress test" detects reversibly ischemic or infarcted myocardium in regions supplied by vessels unable to vasodilate (i.e., with atherosclerotic lesions) and is therefore useful in predicting which patients might benefit from bypass surgery. Gated blood pool scanning with technetium-99 and echocardiography are useful methods for assessing ventricular function at rest and during exercise.

Cardiac catheterization

Cardiac catheterization is the gold standard for diagnosis. Although invasive and expensive, it remains the most accurate and cost-effective study for CAD. Cardiac catheterization actually involves several separate studies performed simultaneously, including **coronary angiography** to visualize the location and severity of stenoses, **ventriculography**, in which dye is released into the ventricle to dynamically visualize wall motion abnormalities and valvular regurgitation; cardiac chamber **pressure measurements** with transvalvular gradients, and **calculations of cardiac output and valve area** by the Fick principle and Gorlin equations, respectively.

Who needs CABG

The decision to recommend surgical therapy (CABG) depends on three major variables: **symptomatology**, **CAD anatomy**, and **left ventricular (LV) function**. Symptoms refractory to medical treatment and/or significant disease in **three major vessels** or the **left main coronary artery** are better treated with surgery. There is data that supports CABG for one- and two-vessel disease, especially with **proximal LAD involvement**. Poor LV function in patients with CAD is an indication for CABG because of the dismal results with medical therapy. Patients with good preoperative LV function fare better than those with poor function after CABG, but the relative benefit of surgery compared with medical therapy is greater in the latter group. For this reason, **CABG should not be avoided in patients with left ventricular failure**. This includes patients with acute MI who are hemodynamically unstable.

Percutaneous transluminal coronary angioplasty

PTCA

PTCA is a relatively noninvasive technique for dilating coronary stenoses and improving distal flow. Although high re-stenosis rates (30% at 6 months) have limited its universal application, over 350,000 such procedures are performed annually (see Chapter 15, "Ischemic Heart Disease and Chest Pain"). Indications include patients with localized proximal single or double-vessel CAD, graft stenosis after CABG, and acute coronary artery occlusion. Emergent CABG is required in approximately 3%-5% of patients after failed PTCA, and carries an increased but acceptable mortality rate.

CABG

Every student should be exposed to coronary artery surgery during training. The operation clearly demonstrates a wide range of human physiology and is an excellent example of appropriately applied technology to clearly benefit sick patients. Moreover, the postoperative care is a further, real-life display of what you learned in the physiology classroom. In smooth cases, the excellent health of the patients within a few days is remarkable.

Access to the heart is obtained via a **median sternotomy**, a longitudinal division of the sternum with a saw. The incision is remarkably well tolerated and provides excellent exposure for most cardiac procedures. High doses of heparin are given to prevent clotting in the bypass tubing. Catheters for return of venous blood are placed, via the right atrium, into the inferior and sometimes superior vena cava. Venous blood is brought, via a collecting reservoir, to the **pump oxygenator**. After oxygenation, the warmed or cooled blood is returned, via relatively atraumatic roller pumps, to the ascending aorta through another catheter. With the "pump" on, oxygen is supplied directly to the blood, and the ventilator is turned off (one of the most unnerving parts of the operation to the neophyte). The heart is stopped using **hypothermia** and high-potassium blood **cardioplegia** with the aorta cross-clamped for the bypasses themselves. Bypasses from the ascending aorta and patent coronary vessel distal to the stenosis are performed using **reversed greater saphenous vein** harvested from the legs, and the **internal mammary artery** (left in situ proximally), which seems to be the most durable conduit; no artificial graft material has been produced with acceptable patency rates. The heart will resume beating with rewarming and release of the cross-clamp, although electrical pacing and/or inotropic agents are sometimes needed (including mechanical "inotropes" such as the intra-aortic balloon pump or artificial ventricular assist devices). The patient normally can be extubated the next day and is home in a week, if the case goes well.

The operative mortality for uncomplicated CABG is between 2%-3%. The benefits of operation are **relief of angina**, **improved LV function**, **decreased risk of MI**, and most importantly, **improved survival** compared with medical therapy if established indications are appropriately followed.

Valvular Disease

Most diseases of the heart valves are due to congenital lesions, rheumatic heart disease, or senile calcification. The major lesions are mitral and aortic valve stenosis and regurgitation, although other, less common problems are encountered.

Mitral stenosis

Rheumatic heart disease secondary to group A streptococcal pharyngitis is by far the most common cause of **mitral stenosis**. Symptoms of mitral stenosis are primarily those of increased left atrial and pulmonary pressure, such as **dyspnea**, **atrial fibrillation** due to atrial stretch, **decreased cardiac output** due to decreased ventricular filling across the stenotic valve, and **CHF**. The patient typically has a crescendo late diastolic murmur with an opening snap. Echocardiography demonstrates an enlarged left atrium, decreased leaflet mobility, decreased valvular area, and increased transvalvular pressure gradient. Surgery is indicated **as soon as symptoms appear**, because delay can lead to irreversible pulmonary hypertension. Although some patients can be treated initially with balloon valvuloplasty, the majority will require surgical treatment. There are two options, depending on the degree of stenosis and calcification: repair (commissurotomy) or replacement. More than half the patients who undergo mitral valve surgery can be treated successfully with commissurotomy, which is preferable because it better preserves native left ventricular function and avoids the need for systemic anticoagulation required with mechanical prostheses.

Mitral regurgitation

Mitral regurgitation can be caused by **rheumatic heart disease**, **ischemic papillary muscle damage**, **idiopathic calcification of the elderly**, **mitral valve prolapse**, or

Surgery
Cardiac Surgery *continued*

acute post-MI mitral regurgitation, the latter having an extremely high mortality rate. Again, the basic problem is that of volume overload and left atrial and pulmonary hypertension, and signs and symptoms, including **dyspnea**, **atrial fibrillation**, and **left ventricular dilatation** with eventual **failure**, are similar to those of mitral stenosis. The murmur is high-pitched, holosystolic, and loudest at the apex. Although echocardiography can demonstrate valve incompetence, regurgitation is best visualized by the dynamic ventriculogram during cardiac catheterization when dye can be seen refluxing into the left atrium during systole. The natural history of mitral regurgitation is more variable than mitral stenosis because of its numerous causes. Unlike mitral stenosis, **symptoms appear too late to be useful for timing of operation.** Catheterization and echocardiographic data, reflecting the degree of regurgitation and impairment of LV function, are imperative for planning surgery. Whether to repair or replace an incompetent valve depends on the etiology: rheumatic heart disease usually necessitates replacement because of fibrosis or calcification to the valve leaflets, while ischemic regurgitation can often be treated with coronary artery bypass grafting and reconstruction because the valve itself is not involved in the disease process.

Aortic stenosis

Aortic stenosis is caused by **idiopathic calcification** (common in the elderly), **rheumatic heart disease,** or **congenital malformations**. Aortic stenosis impedes cardiac output, decreases coronary perfusion pressure, and, as a result of ventricular hypertrophy, increases myocardial oxygen demand. Thus, pathophysiology and symptoms are similar to those of CAD: **dyspnea**, **LV failure**, **angina**, and **syncope**. A mid-systolic murmur at the left sternal border radiating to the carotid arteries is characteristic. Symptoms occur late in the disease process, and the stenotic valve should be corrected (usually by replacement) **as soon as possible after symptoms arise**, if possible. Echocardiography and/or cardiac catheterization to determine valve area and LV function should be performed; coronary angiography should be included to exclude CAD. A valve pressure gradient greater than 50 mmHg or a calculated valve area less than 1 cm2 (normally 3 cm2) are usually considered indications for surgery.

Aortic insufficiency

Endocarditis is now the most common cause of **aortic insufficiency** in the US, displacing **rheumatic heart disease** which has been steadily declining in frequency. **Collagen vascular diseases** (e.g., Marfan's syndrome), aortic dissection, and syphilis (quite rare) are other causes. The regurgitant diastolic blood subjects the LV to a large volume overload, causing dilatation, hypertrophy, and finally failure; symptoms are secondary to LV failure. Characteristically the pulse pressure will be widened due to regurgitation, and a high-pitched decrescendo diastolic murmur heard at the left sternal border. EKG will demonstrate LV hypertrophy, and echocardiography will accurately measure LV volume and document progressive dilation. The degree of regurgitation can be visualized by aortography or echocardiography. Aortic valve replacement is recommended before severe LV dilatation occurs to prevent long-term LV dysfunction; the development of symptoms is a strong indication for operation but usually reflects advanced disease.

Valve selection

The surgeon performing valve replacement must choose a mechanical or bioprosthetic valve; the latter being porcine or bovine valves fixed in gluteraldehyde, attached to a Dacron sewing ring. The critical issues in valve selection are durability and need for anticoagulation. The durability of mechanical valves is well-proven, usually greater than the life of the patient. All patients with mechanical valves, however, must be anticoagulated to protect against thromboembolism. Bioprosthetic valves, by comparison, have limited durability—generally 7-15 years, depending on position. Because of their inert biologic composition, however, they are less thrombogenic, and anticoagulation, in the absence of atrial fibrillation, is not essential. Patients with contraindications to anticoagulation, such as those over 70 (increased risk of cerebral hemorrhage) or women of childbearing age, would be considered for bioprosthesis insertion. Valve reconstruction is preferable to replacement whenever feasible to avoid the above complications.

Other Cardiac Surgical Issues

Many forms of **congenital heart disease** occur (see Chapter 52, "Pediatric Cardiology"), broadly divided into acyanotic (left-to-right shunts), obstructive, and complex or cyanotic (right-to-left shunts) lesions. Although tissue oxygenation is not a problem in left-to-right shunts, chronically elevated pulmonary flow eventually produces intractable pulmonary hypertension and reversal of flow due to elevated right-sided pressures (Eisenmenger's syndrome). Diagnosis, workup, and repair of these lesions are individualized and frequently complex.

Patients with recurrent, life-threatening ventricular arrhythmias can be treated with direct ablation of myocardial tissue shown to be the focus of such arrhythmias by electrophysiologic testing. Such patients also may be candidates for implantation (via thoracotomy) of an automatic cardioverter/defibrillator (**AICD**), which can be lifesaving. Patients with **penetrating cardiac injuries** can often be successfully salvaged, even if they arrive without vital signs. A patient who has some evidence of life (respiratory efforts or electrical cardiac activity) within a few minutes before arrival after penetrating chest trauma should be aggressively treated, usually by immediate lateral thoracotomy in the emergency department. Those with cardiac arrest after blunt injury elsewhere in the body have a uniformly fatal outcome. ■

37   Vascular Surgery

Vascular surgery is surgery of the non-cardiac and extracranial vascular system. Essentially all vascular problems (other than trauma and aneurysms) are caused by atherosclerosis. The best-accepted current theory of atherogenesis is that it is due to injury of the intima, the innermost layer of the blood vessels. This injury can be caused by abnormal blood flow patterns, a finding that helps to explain why atherosclerosis is often relatively limited to areas of branching (the carotid bifurcation) or repetitive stress (Hunter's Canal in the leg). A high-lipid diet and nicotine ingestion then provides the necessary milieu for progressive damage.

The cardinal concept is that atherosclerosis is a systemic disease – thus a typical patient being operated on for lower extremity ischemia is also likely to have coronary and renal artery disease as well. In vascular patients, most morbidity and mortality after operation is due to **cardiac disease**.

Evaluation and Workup

History, physical & ABI

Evaluation and workup vary considerably based on the problem at hand. Obviously, a complete history and physical directed toward the complaint and at other manifestations of atherosclerosis and ischemia is the first step. Often skin changes indicative of chronic extremity ischemia are evident, such as hairlessness, thin, brittle skin, thickened nails (due to slow growth), and, of course, ulcers and dry gangrene. A complete motor and sensory exam is important, and a complete assessment of all pulses by palpation and Doppler ultrasound is mandatory. These include the radial, carotid, femoral, popliteal, dorsalis pedis, and posterior tibial vessels. One should listen for bruits (suggesting turbulent blood flow), especially at the groins and within the abdomen. For any vascular patient, **an ankle-brachial index (ABI) is mandatory and is part of the physical exam, not the laboratory workup**. The ABI is simply the ankle blood pressure (with a cuff around the calf and Doppler interrogation of a pedal artery) divided by the brachial (arm) pressure. Normal values are 0.8-1.1. A value of less than 0.8 is usually associated with exercise-induced muscular pain (claudication), while a value of less than 0.5 is often seen in patients with **limb-threatening ischemia** (discussed below).

Noninvasive testing

The next step is to obtain information using any one of a number of techniques referred to collectively as the **noninvasive laboratory** examination. Most fundamental is Doppler ultrasound, which is the technique of measuring the movement of red blood cells by means of sound waves. Duplex and color duplex refer to technology that simultaneously images the two-dimentional tissue image (B-mode ultrasound) with cursor-directed Doppler ultrasound, allowing the user to see what is being imaged and to more precisely measure flow. It is important to remember that when you feel a pulse, you feel **pressure** – and actual **flow** need not exist. If you hear a Doppler signal, however, you know that actual flow of blood must be present.

Angiography

The noninvasive lab will usually provide extremely complete information regarding the problem, sometimes (as in carotid artery disease) allowing operation without further evaluation. In most cases, however, an **angiogram** is necessary before operation. Angiography gives precise anatomic information allowing the operative approach itself to be planned, or demonstrates that revascularization is hopeless and that operation should be aborted. **A general rule of thumb is that the decision to operate is based on the history, exam, and noninvasive laboratory results, and only after that decision has been made is the angiogram obtained as a "road map."**

A CT scan is vital in planning aneurysm surgery, while conventional ultrasound is excellent in the long-term surveillance of patients with aneurysms. Magnetic resonance angiography (MRI) and carbon-dioxide angiography are two newer imaging techniques designed to reduce the morbidity associated with angiography.

Chronic Ischemia of the Extremities

Chronic ischemia due to progressive atherosclerosis and narrowing of the supplying arteries is by far most common in the lower extremities, and is much rarer in the arms.

Claudication refers to the syndrome of reproducible aching pain in large muscle groups with exercise, eliminated by rest. Blood flow is adequate to supply tissues at rest, but inadequate to supply the increased demands imposed upon the muscles with exercise. Symptoms characteristically occur one level below the blockage, i.e., in the buttocks and thighs with aortoiliac disease, and in the calf with disease of the superficial femoral artery.

Rest pain exists when flow is inadequate to meet even resting needs. Pain occurs at rest and in the most distal part of the extremity, i.e., the foot. It is worsened by elevation and relieved by dependency, accounting for the remarkably constant observation that patients complain of pain most at night, and learn to dangle their foot off the bed to obtain relief.

Tissue loss, **ulceration**, and **gangrene** are similar to rest pain in that flow is inadequate to meet resting needs. In this case, an otherwise minor wound will not heal (and may worsen) because blood flow is inadequate to deliver inflammatory cells and other mediators to the wound.

Natural history

In three quarters of patients with **claudication**, symptoms will improve or stabilize with conservative care (including cessation of smoking and regular exercise). Since operation carries with it a risk of worsening the situation, it is reserved for those with **disabling claudication** – those whose symptoms are severe, have failed to resolve with conservative care, and that truly interfere with their lifestyle. Patients should be aware that the chance of actually worsening the situation by operating exists.

In contrast, patients who experience rest pain or tissue loss (any non-healing ulcer in the setting of insufficient blood flow) have a high chance of needing a major amputation if the problem is not corrected. For this reason, these problems are collectively referred to as **limb-threatening ischemia**, and such patients should be offered operation, if possible.

Collaterals

Patients often do well after gradual but complete occlusion of a main artery. This illustrates the key concept of **collaterals**—pre-existing vessels that dilate over time to supply enough flow around the blockage to preserve resting metabolism. As discussed above, however, when oxygen and blood requirements increase (e.g., when a wound requiring inflammatory mediators is present, or the patient is exercising) flow may not be adequate despite the collaterals, and symptoms occur.

Aortoiliac stenosis

Aortoiliac atherosclerotic disease and abdominal aortic aneurysms (AAA), discussed below, are separate problems; while the two can coexist, it is simpler to think of them separately. Aortoiliac atherosclerosis is suggested by thigh and hip claudication, diminished or absent femoral pulses, and impotence in males (Leriche Syndrome). The usual treatment is an aortobifemoral bypass graft, usually with synthetic material. This requires a major laparotomy, and in patients who might not tolerate the operation or clamping of their often brittle, friable aorta, an "extra-anatomic" bypass such as an axilliary-bifemoral (or femoral-femoral in the setting of unilateral iliac disease) is much less morbid, though at the expense of greater failure rates.

Infrainguinal stenoses

Infrainguinal disease refers to atherosclerosis of any vessel distal to the iliacs. It is suggested by calf claudication or limb-threatening ischemia in the setting of palpable femoral pulses. The usual treatment is bypass, often from the common femoral artery in the groin to a normal vessel distal to the problem. Saphenous vein is the preferred conduit, and can be used in a reversed or in situ fashion, the latter requiring lysis of the valves and ligation of large tributaries that otherwise would become AV fistulas and steal enough flow to cause failure of the graft. Synthetic grafts are used if vein is not available, especially if the bypass is limited to the above-knee position, but the results are clearly inferior to those seen with autologous vein. Very good results are achieved even with bypass to the dorsalis pedis artery in the foot.

Acute Ischemia of the Extremities

Acute ischemia caused by the sudden occlusion of a major artery is usually heralded by the **sudden** onset of symptoms, because collaterals have not had time to develop. Such occlusion can be caused by an embolus from the heart (often in patients in atrial fibrillation or who are taking digoxin), an embolus from a friable aortic plaque, or by acute thrombosis of a previously diseased vessel (in which case symptoms can be less severe, because some collaterals may exist). Acute limb ischemia is manifest by the classic "six P's":

- **Parasthesias** due to early neural ischemia,
- **Pain** caused by later neural and muscular ischemia,
- **Pulselessness** caused by the blockage itself,
- **Pallor** caused by reduced blood flow,
- **Paralysis** caused by late neural and muscle ischemia, and
- **Poikylothermia** (Greek for coldness) caused by reduced blood flow.

Parasthesias are caused by ischemia of the smaller, non-myelenated C-fibers, and often indicate reversibility. Paralysis, however, indicates damage to the larger motor fibers and muscles themselves, indicating that the situation may be irreversible. The rule of thumb is that you have about 6 hours to restore flow, although the sooner the better. Flow can be restored by embolectomy, bypass of the affected segment, or by fibrinolytic drugs.

Abdominal Aortic Aneurysm (AAA)

There is no end of confusion between **AAA** and **aortic dissection**. A dissection usually occurs in the thoracic aorta (but can extend to the belly), is manifest by crushing chest pain, is not usually associated with aneurysmal enlargement, and is associated with loss of flow to branch arteries (pulse deficits). The AAA, in contrast, is usually confined to the infrarenal abdominal aorta, is not usually associated with pulse deficits, and is asymptomatic unless growing rapidly or rupturing. Thoracic aneurysms and primary abdominal dissections occur, but in general, thoracic aortic dissection and AAA are two separate and unconnected entities.

Patho-physiology

Although AAA have been presumed to be caused by atherosclerosis, increasing data suggest that the underlying defect is one of connective tissue metabolism. This theory is supported by the observations that AAA are correlated with aneurysms elsewhere, with other diseases that may involve connective tissue defects such as COPD, and by the fascinating fact that patients with known, stable AAA are at increased risk of rupture following other unrelated major operations (when collagenolysis and elastase are more active during wound remodeling and healing).

Diagnosis

Aneurysms are often detected by the finding of a pulsatile mass on exam, or by calcification on a plain x-ray. A CT scan best characterizes the aneurysm and shows its relationship to the renal arteries (thus is usually needed before operation), while an ultrasound is the best screening test (because of its low cost) to determine whether an aneurysm is simply present, to measure its size, and to follow it over time. Interestingly, an angiogram is probably the least helpful exam. AAA usually have a thick layer of thrombus, thus the angiogram usually displays a somewhat normal-appearing aorta. An angiogram can give valuable information about the status of collateral and mesenteric vessels, however, and is necessary if there is associated aortoiliac or mesenteric occlusive disease.

Treatment

Because AAA are asymptomatic, they are repaired electively to reduce the risk of rupture. Aneurysm surgery itself carries with it a substantial morbidity and mortality. Therefore, the decision to operate is based on the ability to make the long-term benefit exceed the short-term risk. Formerly, the cut-off size when repair was felt to be justified was 6cm. With increasing awareness that rupture may occur at smaller sizes, and with increasingly sophisticated operative and postoperative care, almost all surgeons now consider 5cm an indication for repair, and many will operate on healthy patients with a 4cm aneurysm. Other indications for elective repair are any symptoms, rapid growth (more than half a centimeter in 6 months), associated aortoiliac ischemic disease, and a diameter greater than the patient's L3 vertebral body on CT scan (to index the aneurysm to the patient's size). Operative correction consists of opening the aneurysm and replacement of the aneurysmal segment with an artificial graft. Note that either an aneurysm or aortoiliac occlusive disease can be treated with an aortobi-iliac or aortobifemoral graft. Usually the inferior mesenteric artery is sacrificed, with the left colon then being supplied by collateral flow from the superior mesenteric artery.

Ruptured AAA

A ruptured aneurysm is a major surgical emergency. Any patient with a known (by history or exam) aneurysm or pulsatile abdominal mass with back pain or especially hemodynamic instability must be presumed to have a leaking or ruptured aneurysm until proven otherwise. In the most extreme cases a patient will be brought to the OR immediately (minutes) without further workup, accepting a certain risk of a negative laparotomy. If the situation is unclear, an ultrasound can often be obtained in minutes and will verify whether an aneurysm is **present** (but cannot tell if it's leaking; finding an aneurysm in such a situation mandates operation). If a leak or rupture is suspected, priorities should be obtaining **immediate** surgical consultation (a stat page is appropriate) and obtaining large-bore IV access. **These patients should not be sent to CT**. The mortality for patients who make it to the hospital alive is about 50%, while the mortality for elective repair is 2-4%.

Carotid Artery Disease

Atherosclerosis of the carotid artery is often sharply limited to the bifurcation of the common carotid into the internal and external carotid arteries. For this reason local endarterectomy, consisting of the removal of the atherosclerotic plaque (intima and part of the media) is most easily accomplished.

Symptoms

Symptoms are usually due to microemboli from the diseased area, and are classically manifest as **amaurosis fujax**, transient ipsilateral monocular blindness due to ophthalmic artery occlusion, **transient ischemic attack** (**TIA**), a neurologic event lasting less than 24 hours, or **cerebrovascular event** (**CVA** or **stroke**). These events all lie along a continuum, and CT changes can be seen even after some TIAs. In general, operation is not indicated and, in fact, is unsafe during an acute CVA, especially if neurologic status is deteriorating, but this is an area of debate and active investigation.

Treatment

Interestingly, however, although the pathophysiology of a stroke is the result of emboli, the variable that seems to best predict the need for an operation is the measured degree of stenosis. In the past decade there have been a number of well-designed, large, clinical prospective studies published. It is clear that patients with symptoms ipsilateral to a 70% or greater diameter stenosis (2-dimensional image seen on angiogram) do better with operation as compared to medical therapy alone, while those with minimal stenoses (less than 30%) should not be operated on (because of the small (2-4%) but significant stroke and death rate). Recent data, however, also strongly suggest that even asymptomatic patients with a 60% or greater diameter stenosis do better with operation as opposed to the "best" medical care, if the procedure can be performed with an acceptably low complication rate.

Operation is not without risk, as the carotid must be clamped. While clamped, blood flow to the brain can be maintained using a shunt (if you don't trust the Circle of Willis). One can shunt always, never, or selectively (based on one of several criteria), although results are essentially equivalent. Again, one must balance the short-term risk of operation against the long-term benefits of reducing the risk of stroke, hence the surgeon's and institution's skill is critically important in the decision making process.

Endovascular Techniques

In the past few years a great deal of interest has arisen in repairing vascular problems using various endovascular techniques. Unfortunately, many such procedures have been applied in poorly-controlled settings, and the situation is very murky. Percutaneous dilation of stenotic iliac arteries using balloons is clearly of benefit. There is insufficient data at present to fully assess the roles, long-term outcomes, and overall utility and future of most other such techniques, although this is an area of explosive research. ■

38   Pediatric Surgery

Surgical problems in children can be intimidating, because the anatomic and physiologic changes that occur during the course of development from fetus to adult require special consideration. Much of pediatric surgery involves familiar concepts and procedures, with adaptations made for the patient's age.

Common Outpatient Emergencies

Trauma is the leading cause of death in the pediatric population. Management of the pediatric trauma patient follows the same basic protocols of adult trauma care (see Chapter 28, "Trauma"). The high kinetic energy applied to the smaller mass of the child often leads to multisystem injury, and because of children's softer, more pliable skeletons, internal injuries can occur without overlying bony fractures. The larger surface-area-to-mass ratio also predisposes the victim to hypothermia. Further, the smaller size of the patient often creates problems regarding evaluation, intravenous access, and performance of other procedures.

Child abuse

Child abuse (see Chapter 58, "Child Abuse") is unfortunately a too-common problem. All caregivers must be able to recognize the syndrome. Common clues include a history that does not match the injury, a delay in bringing the child for treatment, or inconsistency in the parents' explanations. The finding of retinal hemorrhages, perioral, perianal or genital injuries, unusual types of injuries (bites or cigarette burns), or multiple injuries (or scars) of varying ages all are suspicious. The surgeon is legally and ethically obligated to report any suspected case to local authorities.

Foreign bodies

Infants and children have the propensity to place toys, coins, buttons, watch batteries, and so on into their mouths and thus often present with **foreign bodies** in their respiratory or GI tracts. Their presence is usually obvious by history and x-ray. Laryngeal foreign bodies can often be dislodged with backblow maneuvers if the airway is acutely compromised. If the airway is not obstructed, laryngoscopy is performed in a controlled setting. Blind finger sweeps should be avoided due to the

Surgery
Pediatric Surgery *continued*

risk of pushing the foreign body deeper. A deeper object (within the tracheobronchial tree), if not visible by x-ray, may be manifest by obstruction and air resorption leading to localized atelectasis or a high-riding diaphragm. Bronchoscopy is necessary to remove deeper foreign bodies. Esophageal foreign bodies can be seen on x-ray or visualized by contrast swallow. Removal is best carried out by rigid esophagoscopy, with perforation being the most feared complication. Objects that pass into the stomach will almost always pass through the entire GI tract in 24-48 hours without complication.

Esophageal injury

Esophageal injury secondary to the **ingestion** of a corrosive agent can lead to few signs or symptoms or can produce pain, drooling and oropharyngeal burns. If suspected, esophagoscopy is mandatory. In all but minor injuries, placement of a feeding gastrostomy tube is performed. Such injuries can lead to acute perforation or late stricture. In severe cases, the injured esophagus may need to be surgically excised and replaced with another conduit, such as colon or stomach.

Appendicitis

Appendicitis in children produces greater morbidity and mortality than in adults. Obstruction of the appendiceal lumen leads to distention, ischemia, bacterial overgrowth and ultimately, perforation. In children less than 2, the base of the appendix is wide and is less likely to obstruct. In older children the disease progresses more rapidly with perforation occurring earlier than in adults. The shorter, less developed omentum of the pediatric patient is less effective in walling-off the involved area, making peritonitis more common.

Children with appendicitis usually present with abdominal pain, but may not be able to describe the classic progression of diffuse pain localizing to the right lower quadrant. Anorexia, fever, leukocytosis, and vomiting are usually present and may be more severe than in the adult. Clues include ketones in the urine or an appendicolith seen on x-ray. A **Meckel's diverticulum** can become inflamed and mimic appendicitis, or can cause a massive lower GI bleed (the most common cause in children).

Intussusception

Intussusception describes the situation where a length of proximal bowel telescopes into a more distal segment, leading to pain and obstruction. It is more common in infants, and such patients often present with the sudden onset of colicky abdominal pain, frequently with drawn-up legs (presumably due to peritoneal irritation). Vomiting, fever, and the passage of bloody stool—classically described as "currant jelly"—often ensues, and the abdomen is distended with a sausage-shaped mass sometimes palpable in the right upper quadrant. Hydrostatic reduction can be attempted first by gentle barium enema under fluoroscopy. In the presence of pneumoperitoneum, peritonitis, or shock, or if hydrostatic reduction has been unsuccessful, exploration and surgical reduction is necessary.

Pyloric stenosis　　**Pyloric stenosis** is benign muscular hypertrophy of the pyloric channel. The classic presentation is one of nonbilious emesis progressing to projectile vomiting in a 6 week old male firstborn child. An "olive" (the hypertrophic pylorus) is usually palpable in the right epigastrium. Repeated vomiting usually leads to a hypochloremic alkalosis that requires correction before surgery. Repair is by pyloromyotomy, incising the hypertrophied muscle of the pylorus, leaving the mucosa untouched.

Malrotation　　During fetal development, the gut rotates such that the viscera comes to rest in the normal position. If this fails to occur, two problems can occur. Simple **malrotation**, although often asymptomatic, can lead to duodenal obstruction secondary to abnormal adhesions (Ladd's bands) in the right upper quadrant. Repair is simple lysis. More serious, however, is **midgut volvulous**. The malrotation (specifically lack of normal retroperitoneal attachments) increases the chance that the bowel can twist, leading to obstruction, vascular occlusion, and ischemia. In severe cases the entire midgut (from duodenum to cecum) is necrotic, requires resection, and leaves the child with short gut syndrome. Clinically important malrotation presents early: 33% within the first week of life, 85% by 1 year of age.

Common Neonatal Emergencies

NEC　　**Necrotizing Enterocolitis (NEC)** affects premature infants primarily. Impaired mesenteric blood flow due to stress (prematurity, shock, and so on) is believed to produce gut mucosal injury, leading to translocation of bacteria and endotoxin through the bowel wall, resulting in toxic colitis and further systemic compromise. Occult or gross blood in the stool, abdominal tenderness, and abdominal distention suggest the diagnosis, and x-rays often demonstrate obstruction, gas in the wall of the intestine (pneumatosis intestinalis), or gas in the portal vein. Most cases can be treated nonoperatively with broad spectrum antibiotics, close observation, and frequent exams and x-rays. Pneumoperitoneum (indicating perforation) or "failure of medical management" mandate exploration. The overall survival rate for NEC is between 60%-75%.

TE fistula

Tracheoesophageal (TE) fistulas are a group of congenital malformations of the trachea and esophagus, often associated with defects elsewhere. The most common type (90%) consists of a blind proximal esophagus and a distal TE fistula. Affected infants present at the time of birth with drooling, choking, and inability to feed. The diagnosis is suspected if an orogastric tube cannot be passed into the stomach. The immediate danger is respiratory infection arising from aspiration of gastric secretions through the fistula, thus, along with decompression of the proximal pouch, placement of a gastrostomy tube to empty the stomach is usually performed. Prompt definitive surgery is usually safe, and the defect is repaired directly (if short) or with interposed colon or stomach (if long).

Diaphragmatic hernia

Congenital diaphragmatic hernia results from a persistent pleuroperitoneal communication in the posterolateral aspect of the diaphragm (foramen of Bochdalek). The hernia itself is minor—it is the extent of pulmonary hypoplasia that has the greatest impact on the newborn's survival. It would seem that the presence of intestine in the chest during the lung's development produces the hypoplasia, but hypoplasia and herniation may be independent—both lungs are underdeveloped (more so on the affected side), suggesting the presence of a common primary genetic defect. These infants usually experience progressive acidosis and respiratory distress, often in the delivery room. Usually a markedly scaphoid abdomen is present, and auscultation reveals bowel sounds in the chest. These patients are sometimes ill, and need emergent repair, if severe. The diaphragm can easily be closed, but the problem remains one of pulmonary hypoplasia. In severe case extracorporeal membrane oxygenation (ECMO), essentially cardiopulmonary bypass, is used.

Intestinal atresia

There are numerous sites of **atresia** throughout the GI and biliary tracts. Duodenal atresia is suggested by bilious vomiting soon after birth, with a "double bubble" sign on x-ray (representing gas in the stomach and proximal duodenum). Jejunal atresia is thought to result from intrauterine mesenteric vascular ischemia leaving underdeveloped or absent sections of small bowel, also leading to progressive abdominal distension and vomiting. In general, the later the vomiting and greater the distention, the more distal the obstruction. **Imperforate anus** refers to a spectrum of problems, all having in common actual agenesis or malposition of the anus, usually with a fistula to the vagina or urethra. Treatment varies according to whether the proximal bowel ends above (colostomy with staged repair) or below (possible primary repair) the levators. Persistent neonatal jaundice suggests **biliary atresia**, or malformation and obstruction of the biliary tree. Correction by means of a portoenterostomy, or Kasai procedure, works only about half the time, and liver transplantation is the only option.

Hirschprung's disease

In **Hirschprung's disease**, a failure of normal neural crest cell migration leads to absence of ganglion cells in the distal gastrointestinal tract. The aganglionic segment, always extending proximally from the rectum, is aperistaltic and functionally obstructed (the proximal, dilated bowel is normal, a fact which has not always been appreciated). Presentation may be at birth, with failure to pass meconium, or may be more subtle, with constipation, malnutrition, and poor growth occurring later in childhood. Usually a proximal diverting colostomy is created to alleviate the obstruction, deferring definitive repair (resection of the aperistaltic segment with coloanal anastomosis) until the child is older.

Abdominal wall defects

Congenital abdominal wall defects can be dramatic. **Gastroschisis** is free evisceration of bowel in utero, usually to the right of the umbilical cord at the site of the resorbed right umbilical vein. **Omphalocele** is similar, but differs in that the herniated viscera is covered by peritoneum, protecting it from the amniotic fluid. Gastroschisis is not associated with other anomalies, but

Surgery
Pediatric Surgery *continued*

up to two thirds of neonates with omphalocele have associated defects (cardiovascular, urinary, gastrointestinal,
muscular) or chromosomal syndromes. Although details
differ, the goal is reconstruction of the abdominal wall. If
primary repair is not feasible (because the bowel, even
after being emptied of meconium, will not fit), a staged
closure using artificial material, slowly tightened, is used.

Nonemergent Problems

Inguinal hernias

Inguinal hernias in children are common. Unlike in
adults, where they are due to an acquired weakness (see
Chapter 30, "Hernia"), groin hernias in children are congenital, due to failure of the processus vaginalis to close.
The potential thus exists for abdominal viscera to herniate
through the internal ring (producing an indirect hernia).
Risks of incarceration or vascular ischemia and strangulation are present in children just as in adults. A **hydrocele**
is a collection of fluid in the distal (scrotal) processus
vaginalis. If a communication between the intraabdominal
cavity and the processus exists (communicating hydrocele), the scrotal fluid collection will change size over
time. Differentiation of a hydrocele from a hernia can
often be difficult. Inguinal hernias will not close on their
own, thus repair is indicated. Repair in children is simply
a ligation of the hernia sac (processus vaginalis); no procedure to reconstruct the internal ring is necessary.
Communicating hydroceles are topologically the same as
hernias, just with a narrower opening, and thus also
require intervention.

Umbilical hernias

Umbilical hernias consist of a peritoneal sac protruding
through a patent umbilical ring; the subcutaneous fat and
skin are intact (thus differentiating them from neonatal
abdominal wall defects). Incarceration and strangulation
are rare. Defects less than 2cm in diameter will usually
close in the first four years of life; persistence after four
means the hernia should be surgically repaired.

Branchial cleft cysts

Incomplete obliteration of the embryonic **branchial clefts**
may result in residual cysts, sinuses, fistulas, or cartilagi-
nous growths in the neck. The sinuses and fistulas may
produce a mucoid drainage. Eventual infection is the rule,
thus, surgical excision is recommended. Removal of the
entire sinus tract is necessary to avoid recurrence.
Branchial cleft masses present laterally, while **thyroglos-**

sal duct cysts, arising from incomplete obliteration of the thyroglossal duct, present as midline neck masses. Such cysts also may be infected, and are often associated with cutaneous sinuses. Again, the entire duct must be removed to the foramen cecum of the tongue, including the central portion of the hyoid bone through which it passes.

Cystic hygromas

Cystic hygromas arise from obstructed lymphatic channels. Most commonly arising in the neck, they can be detected by prenatal ultrasound, and usually enlarge after birth as lymph accumulates. Rapid enlargement can occur due to infection or intra-cystic bleeding, and airway obstruction can result. The best treatment is excision; sclerosing agents, steroids, and radiation are not effective.

GER

Gastroesophageal reflux (GER) is surprisingly common in infants, especially those who are neurologically impaired. In infants, episodes of choking, apnea, bradycardia, or recurrent pulmonary infections are common, while in children more than one the condition is usually first recognized as a failure to thrive. The initial treatment for GER is medical; surgery is indicated after failure of medical therapy or in the presence of life-threatening apnea, esophageal strictures, or severe hiatal hernia. Treatment is by conventional antireflux gastric wrap, but recurrence, especially in severely neurologically impaired children, is high. In these cases disconnection of the stomach from the esophagus with esophagojejunostomy has met with success.

Tumors

Wilms' tumor

Wilms' tumor, arising from the kidney, typically presents in children between the ages of 1-3. These children have a round, smooth abdominal mass, usually limited to one side of the midline, with associated hematuria and hypertension sometimes present. Other anomalies of the urogenital tract are often present as well. The tumor is unusual in that, in addition to metastasizing (to liver and lung), it locally invades the renal vein and vena cava. Surgery allows removal of the tumor and staging. Prognosis is good; patients with localized, unilateral tumors of favorable histology enjoy a 90% survival rate

when treated with adjuvant chemotherapy. In cases with
less favorable staging, both chemotherapy and radiation
therapy are used.

**Neuro-
blastomas**

Neuroblastomas, the other common childhood tumor, are
of neural crest origin and can be found arising in the
neck, posterior mediastinum, periaortic region, adrenal
medulla, pelvis, or from any other sympathetic ganglion
tissue. Half of these tumors present by 2 years of age.
These patients usually have an abdominal mass, which
(unlike Wilms' tumor) can cross the midline. Many of
these tumors will produce catecholamines that can cause
systemic symptoms. Unlike Wilms' tumor, neuroblastomas do not arise from but rather displace the kidney on
imaging studies. Treatment for neuroblastoma is surgical
removal; chemotherapy and radiation therapy are not dramatically effective. Cure can be achieved in most infants.
Survival rates are lower (less than 50%) in older children
and in cases of more advanced disease. ■

39 Transplantation

The field of transplantation has progressed remarkably since Dr. Joseph Murray successfully transplanted a kidney between identical twins in 1954. Advances in organ preservation, immunosuppression, prevention and treatment of infectious complications, tissue typing, and surgical techniques have led to the ability to routinely transplant solid organs from genetically disparate patients.

This chapter focuses on renal transplantation specifically, illustrating the basic immunologic concepts and techniques applicable to transplantation in general. As of December 1995 there were 31,045 patients on the waiting list for renal transplant in the U.S. This number continues to grow while the number of cadaveric organ donors remains relatively constant at approximately 4000. One of the greatest problems to solve in transplantation is the shortage of available organs.

Kidney Transplantation

Renal failure   What happens when a patient's kidneys fail and a transplant is needed?

The most common diseases leading to renal transplantation include insulin dependent diabetes mellitus (Caucasians), chronic glomerulonephritis (Asians and Hispanics), polycystic kidney disease, and hypertensive nephrosclerosis (African-Americans). There are few absolute contraindications for transplantation today other than incompatibility or a life expectancy short enough to erase any benefits of transplantation (such as active and uncontrolled malignancy or AIDS). Some of the more obvious relative contraindications are active infection or sepsis, prior malignancy, severe metabolic disturbances, ongoing noncompliance, or active psychosis.

Suitable patients diagnosed with chronic renal failure or end stage renal disease are referred to a transplant center. It is usually the patient's nephrologist, but may be their primary care physician, who makes this referral. The patient is initially evaluated by a transplant coordinator, nephrologist, and transplant surgeon. If the patient is found to be a suitable candidate, he or she is typed for

Surgery
Transplantation *continued*

HLA (see Chapter 10, "Immunology") and blood antigens (ABO). All the relevant information is then entered into local, regional, and national databases, so that the most closely matched donor organ can be located in the shortest amount of time.

Organ harvest

Transplant organs can be harvested from brain dead patients (cadaveric) or living related donors. Cadaveric donors can be hemodynamically stable brain dead patients (heart beating cadaveric donor), or patients who have recently lost all vital bodily functions (non-heart-beating cadaveric donor). To be eligible as a cadaveric donor, the patient must have sustained an injury or have a disease process that has or will lead to brain death but allows support of their other organs. Patients are often head trauma victims or have experienced anoxic brain injury (MI, drowning, stroke). Once a patient appears to be a possible organ donor, any member of the healthcare team (physician, resident, nurse) can initiate the donation process by notifying the organ procurement program. The transplant team will then contact the attending physician, review the chart, establish that a diagnosis of brain death is established, and coordinate notification and consent of the patient's family. The transplant team assists the medical staff in maintaining optimal organ support. The situation is more complicated with non-heartbeating donors because the patient's organs cannot be indefinitely supported, and organ retrieval must be accomplished in a much shorter time period—this area is still experimental.

HLA matching

In order to minimize the anti-allograft response and improve the outcome of cadaveric transplants, donors and recipients undergo preoperative HLA typing and cross matching. HLA matching consists of identification of the HLA A, B, and DR alleles of the donor and recipient. A direct relationship has been noted with increasing allograft survival rates with increasing degrees of HLA A, B, DR antigen matching. Cross-match testing detects the presence of donor specific anti-HLA antibodies and a positive cross-match (clumping due to antibody-antigen interaction) is an absolute contraindication (along with ABO incompatibility) to transplantation.

The potential recipient is contacted when a suitable donor is identified. The recipient must be available for operation within the time frame of tolerable ischemia for the organ in question and must be free of significant acute infection. A history and physical is performed, giving careful attention to possible occult infections. Seropositivity status to common viral agents (CMV, HIV, hepatitis) is ascertained. Electrolyte and/or acid-base abnormalities are frequently present, and dialysis is often required preoperatively.

Teams from other institutions may arrive to harvest organs depending on the institution's resources and the targeted recipient(s); this often determines the order of harvest and conduct of the operation. Once removed, the kidneys must be preserved during the extracorporeal phase. There are four major principles of organ preservation. **Hypothermia** is most important. Decreasing organ temperature slows the rate of degradation due to enzymatic catabolic reactions. Keeping the "warm ischemia time" as short as possible is critically important. Maintaining the cells' **physical environment** as normal as possible by reducing cell swelling and other structural changes caused by ischemia can be accomplished by using storage solutions with high osmotic pressures. Similarly, the **biochemical environment** is maintained using storage solutions with metabolites necessary to load cells with the substrates needed for normal intracellular function during storage and reperfusion. Finally, storage solutions include substances designed to reduce **reperfusion injury** secondary to oxygen free radicals and hydrolytic enzymes.

Transplantation

The recipient is brought to the operating room. After induction and patient preparation, the patient's bladder is irrigated and distended with antibiotic solution to facilitate identification of the bladder during the operation. An oblique right or left lower quadrant incision is made and a retroperitoneal dissection is carried down to the iliac vessels. Transplanted kidneys are most often placed in the right iliac fossa because the right external iliac vein follows a more superficial and direct course and the sigmoid colon does not interfere with exposure of the bladder, but this can be modified based on the presence of significant peripheral vascular disease or previous operation. The allograft renal artery is anastomosed to the recipient iliac artery, and the renal vein to the recipient iliac vein. The ureter is then anastomosed to the recipient bladder. It is important that the allograft kidney be kept cold with iced saline throughout the operation and that hemostasis be complete, to avoid a hematoma. Drains are not used, except for an indwelling Foley catheter.

Postoperative Concerns

The transplant patient can experience any postoperative complication experienced by the surgical patient in general, but there are problems of particular importance. A normally routine postoperative infectious complication can be catastrophic in the immunosuppressed patient because an infection can lead to eventual loss of the allograft, and even to death of the patient.

**Immuno-
suppression**

Currently the most common **immunosuppression** regimen is a combination of steroids, Cyclosporine A, and azothioprine. **Corticosteroids** (Prednisone, Solumedrol) suppress macrophage function, inhibiting the expression of cytokines, and thus, T-cell proliferation and T-cell dependent immunity. **Cyclosporine A** (CsA) is a fungus-derived peptide that blocks T-cell activation by inhibiting the production of IL-2 and IL-2 receptor expression by helper T-cells, and is the centerpiece of maintenance immunosuppression for renal, liver, heart, and heart/lung transplants. Unfortunately, nephrotoxicity is the most common and problematic side effect. CsA nephrotoxicity is suggested by increased serum levels of CsA, a paucity of other indicators of acute rejection, and renal biopsy. **Azathioprine** (Imuran) is a purine analogue, an antimetabolite that acts by interfering with nucleic acid synthesis, specifically inhibiting lymphocyte proliferation. Its major side effect is leukopenia, and the white blood count should be monitored daily on patients receiving this drug.

Other immunosuppressive agents include **Tacrolimus** (FK-506, Prograf), an antibiotic that blocks T-cell activation (similar to cyclosporine). It is approximately 500 times more potent than cyclosporine and is starting to be more widely used in liver, kidney, and small bowel transplants. **Antilymphocyte globulin** (ALG) is a preparation of polyclonal antibodies directed against T-lymphocytes. Patients develop antibodies to ALG rendering it less effective with subsequent use. It is usually reserved for episodes of rejection. **OKT3** is a monoclonal antibody directed against the CD3 cell surface antigen present on all mature T-cells, and also incites antibodies that limit its repeated use. Patients can experience severe allergic reactions with both ALG and OKT3, and premedication with steroids, antipyretics, and antihistamines can alleviate many of these problems.

Most modern immunosuppressive regimens consist of triple drug therapy with cyclosporine, azathioprine, and corticosteroids, using lower doses of each drug to minimize side effects (the immunosuppressive effects are additive, but the side effects are not). ALG and OKT3 can be used to induce immunosuppression immediately following transplantation to reduce the nephrotoxic effects of cyclosporine on the newly transplanted kidney, but more commonly are reserved (along with high dose corticosteroids) for episodes of acute rejection.

The successful transplant will often start to function immediately, and a brisk diuresis is expected. If a transplanted kidney begins to malfunction at any time (evidenced by decreased urine output, increased BUN and creatinine, hypertension, or hyperkalemia), a rapid approach to diagnosis and treatment of the disorder is essential. It is useful to divide the many possible etiologies of renal transplant dysfunction into prerenal, renal, and postrenal causes.

Transplant dysfunction

Prerenal causes include hypovolemia, common after any surgical procedure. Fluid challenges must be considered carefully because fluid overload is easily achieved in patients with renal failure. Technical problems such as anastomotic stenosis or thrombosis (either arterial or venous) are suggested by failure of optimization of fluid status to correct the dysfunction. A perfusion scan, Doppler ultrasound, or angiography can be used to evaluate renal perfusion. **Renal** causes of allograft dysfunction include acute tubular necrosis (ATN) due to ischemia, rejection, CsA nephrotoxicity, infection, or recurrence of the original disease (more common later). Urinalysis, urine culture, and nuclear scans are often helpful in making the diagnosis, but a renal biopsy may be necessary. Obstruction of the urinary collecting system leads to **postrenal** dysfunction. Obviously, a Foley catheter must be in place and patent, to rule out the possibility of obstruction due to blood clots (common postoperatively) or prostatic disease. Other sources of postrenal obstruction are technical problems at the neoureterocystostomy or ureteral obstruction due to hematomas or fluid collection. Treatment of obstruction includes urological evalua-

Surgery
Transplantation *continued*

tion, percutaneous drainage, stents, or operative intervention, as indicated. A summary algorithm for the diagnosis of renal allograft dysfunction is presented below.

Figure 39.1
Algorithm for the workup of graft dysfunction (reduced urine output) after renal transplantation.

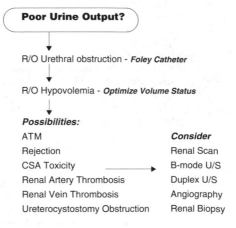

Poor Urine Output?

↓

R/O Urethral obstruction - *Foley Catheter*

↓

R/O Hypovolemia - *Optimize Volume Status*

↓

Possibilities:

ATM	*Consider*
Rejection	Renal Scan
CSA Toxicity	B-mode U/S
Renal Artery Thrombosis	Duplex U/S
Renal Vein Thrombosis	Angiography
Ureterocystostomy Obstruction	Renal Biopsy

Rejection

The most common complication of any transplant is **rejection**. Clinically, rejection manifests itself as decreasing renal function, with decreased urine output, increasing serum creatinine, acid/base and electrolyte abnormalities, temperature elevation, and leukocytosis. The anti-allograft response mounted by the transplant recipient can be classified, for ease of understanding, into four categories distinguished by their time of onset, clinical findings, and their response to anti rejection therapy.

Hyperacute rejection occurs minutes to hours after transplantation. Preformed anti-ABO, anti-Rh, or HLA antibodies target donor cells, specifically the vascular endothelium. Antigen-antibody complexes on vessel walls lead to complement deposition, neutrophil and platelet aggregation, and thrombus formation. Clinically, the patient exhibits acute anuria, hyperkalcmia, and metabolic acidosis, and the diagnosis should be suspected in any patients with anuria immediately following renal transplantation. If hyperacute rejection occurs the allograft usually must be removed. A positive cross match (indicating that such antibodies are present) is a contraindication to transplantation for this reason, as a result, hyperacute rejection is extraordinarily rare.

Accelerated acute rejection occurs due to antibody mediated graft destruction initiated by **newly** formed donor specific antibodies. It is hypothesized that the patient has been previously sensitized to Class I HLA antigens similar to donor antigens due to, for example, previous blood transfusions or transplants. It is often indistinguishable clinically and pathologically from hyperacute rejection, but differs in an absence of preformed donor specific antibodies, and onset is usually later (days to weeks). Again, treatment is usually removal of the graft.

Acute cellular rejection is the most common form of rejection. It is most prevalent during the first 3 months post transplant and accounts for 85% of rejection episodes. This form of rejection is primarily mediated by T-cells, although some humoral B-cell mechanisms play a role. Histologically, a dense perivascular, mononuclear cell infiltrate is the predominant finding. Clinically, patients will exhibit low grade fever, malaise, weight gain, oliguria, hypertension, graft tenderness, and edema. Definitive diagnosis is by biopsy, and treatment consists of increased or additional immunosuppression as discussed above.

Although improvements in immunosuppression have increased short-term graft survival to approximately 80% (at one year) and reduced the incidence of acute rejection, longterm graft survival rates (50% at six years) remain unchanged. Most late losses are due to the poorly understood entity of **chronic rejection**, which produces a slow decline in graft function. The main histologic findings are of arteriolar, intimal hyperplasia, tubular atrophy, glomerular sclerosis, and fibrosis. Both immunologic (cellular and humoral mechanisms) and nonimmunologic (ischemia and surgical manipulation) factors appear to be important. Currently there is no treatment other than prevention with ongoing immunosuppression.

Infections

Infections are the leading cause of death and one of the most common problems faced by transplant recipients. The immunosuppression necessary to prevent rejection increases the risk of infections; striking a balance between the twin problems of rejection and infection remains one of the "arts" a good transplant surgeon must develop. Treatment consists, in general, of reducing the level of immunosuppression in conjunction with specific pharmacologic therapy. *(continued)*

Bacterial infections are common in the immediate post-operative period. Staphylococci, Streptococci, and gram negative rods are the most frequently encountered organisms while opportunistic organisms (Aspergillus, Nocardia, Pseudomonas) are rare during this period. Empiric broad spectrum antibiotic therapy is initiated and should be modified once culture results and sensitivities are known.

Viral infections are a direct result of impaired cell mediated immunity secondary to immunosuppression. Cytomegalovirus (CMV) is the most common infection in transplant recipients after the first post transplant month. Patients can develop CMV as a primary infection, via superinfection from a seropositive organ transplanted into a seronegative patient, or by reactivation of latent virus within the recipient. CMV may cause a spectrum of syndromes from mild to life threatening disease, and is diagnosed by cytomegalic inclusion bodies, positive tissue culture, or increased serum antibody titers. Gancyclovir is usually used as therapy. Herpes simplex virus reactivation is common after transplantation, and prophylaxis with acyclovir during the immediate post transplant period is helpful. Other viruses that can be detrimental in transplant patients include Epstein-Barr virus, adenovirus, and varicella-zoster.

Protozoan or **parasitic agents** are also sources of infection in these patients. Pneumocystis carinii can lead to fatal pneumonia, usually in the first 6 months post-transplantation. Patients are given prophylactic Trimethoprim/Sulfamethoxizole (Bactrim) or aerosolized pentamidine. Other organisms of importance include Toxoplasma gondii and Strongyloides stercoralis.

Fungi are the final pathogens of note in the immunosuppressed. Candida and Aspergillus account for over 80% of fungal infections, and usually occur in the first two months post transplantation. Oral candidiasis is very common and prophylaxis with clotrimoxazol troches or nystatin is effective prevention. Aspergillus occurs most often in the lungs and commonly spreads to the central nervous system. Other fungi include Cryptococcus, Mucor, Rizopus, and Histoplasma capsulatum. The mortality of systemic fungal infections in transplant patients ranges from 30% to 100%. ∎

40   Gastrointestinal Bleeding

Gastrointestinal (GI) bleeding is one of the most common causes of hospital admission. The goals of therapy have remained essentially unchanged over the past few decades: hemodynamic stabilization, cessation of active bleeding, and prevention of recurrence. Other than the rapidity and amount of bleeding at presentation, the best predictor of adverse outcome is the presence of other illness. Well over half the episodes of acute GI bleeding will spontaneously resolve without surgical intervention. Unfortunately, the longer the delay, the sicker the patient.

Presentation

GI bleeding is manifest in one of four ways: hematemesis, melena, hematochezia, or occult blood loss. **Hematemesis** is bloody vomit, and almost always indicates an upper GI source. The color of the vomit suggests the rapidity of bleeding: bright red blood suggests "real-time", ongoing bleeding, while "coffee ground" emesis is seen after the blood has had a chance to sit in the stomach and be exposed to acid. **Melena** refers to the passage of black, tarry stools, with a very characteristic foul odor. This, again, suggests an upper GI source, with the black color and odor resulting from bacterial digestion during passage through the GI tract, although slow lower GI bleeding can produce melena as well. **Hematochezia** is the passage of bright red blood or clots from the rectum, and usually indicates a lower GI source if the patient is stable (a rule of thumb is that an upper GI bleed that is rapid enough to result in bright red blood per rectum invariably results in shock). Finally, **occult** blood loss is, by definition, hidden. This is usually identified by a positive guaiac exam (caused by as little as 10cc of blood), but those patients who are found to be anemic on routine exam also fall into this category. The rapidity and location of bleeding are the most useful factors guiding treatment, and can often be reliably inferred from the issues presented above.

It cannot be overstressed that before any diagnostic evaluation is begun, resuscitation must be performed. In any

Surgery
Gastrointestinal *continued*

sick patient the initial priorities are the establishment of an adequate airway, ensuring oxygenation and ventilation, and restoring circulatory status to normal. The first two are seldom problematic in an isolated GI bleeder. **Circulatory status**, obviously though, is critical.

Resuscitation

The basic pathophysiologic problem in bleeding from any source is isotonic volume loss, leading to decreased pre-load and cardiac output. **Volume replacement** is the mainstay of treatment for hemorrhage, and in the uncom-plicated bleeding patient inotropic or vasoconstrictive agents are unhelpful and actively detrimental due to peripheral vasoconstriction and cellular hypoxia (see Chapters 5 and 6, "Shock" and "Basic Hemodynamics"). Because loss is isotonic, volume replacement should be initiated with lactated Ringer's solution, with blood (packed red blood cells) given as needed for oxygen-car-rying capacity. **Adequate IV access** is critical; at least 2 large bore intravenous catheters are required in any unsta-ble patient. The most useful initial measurement of intravascular volume is adequacy of urine output, thus a **Foley catheter** to accurately measure urine output in "real time" is also required. Laboratory values to be obtained routinely include the hematocrit, type and cross matching, and baseline coagulation studies (prothrombin time, activated partial thromboplastin time, and a platelet count). Any tests needed for general anesthesia (such as an EKG) should be obtained early so that there will be no delay if surgery is required. Plain x-rays are of very little value in GI bleeders.

Workup Once resuscitation has been initiated and volume status improved or normalized as evidenced by adequate urine output, blood pressure, and pulse, detailed evaluation and diagnostic workup can begin. The most important piece of information to obtain is whether the source of bleeding is from the upper or lower GI tract, because workup, treatment, and prognosis fundamentally differ. **Upper GI bleeding** originates proximal to the ligament of Treitz (usually esophagus, stomach, or duodenum), while **lower GI bleeding** originates distally (usually colon or rectum). The easiest way to make this distinction is by passage of a **nasogastric tube**. This is required early in the evaluation of any GI bleeder. Return of blood or coffee-ground material virtually assures an upper GI source, while the return of bile-stained normal gastric juice strongly suggests a lower GI source. If no bile is seen, however, the division is not yet clear, because the lack of bile implies no reflux (including blood from a bleeding duodenal ulcer) through the pylorus. Unfortunately, clinical judgment of whether bile is present is inaccurate, and thus these findings can only suggest, not confirm, the location. The nasogastric tube can also be used for gastric lavage with room temperature fluids in preparation for endoscopy, although an Ewald (very large) tube may be necessary to remove clots.

The **history** is unusually important. Previous episodes of GI bleeding and their causes, medication use such as aspirin, non-steroidal inflammatory agents, anticoagulants, or steroids, previous symptoms of typical causative lesions, ethanol intake, vomiting, or previous abdominal or aortic surgery are all clues as to the cause. The presence of possible coagulopathies should be sought. Likewise, family history (such as the presence of a coagulopathy or colon cancer) may be helpful. **Physical exam**, however, is not often as useful. Pain is not characteristically associated with GI bleeding. It is very important to look for stigmata of cirrhosis, such as ascites, spider angiomata, jaundice, or facial changes associated with alcohol abuse. Rectal exam is likewise required to rule out hemorrhoids or rectal carcinoma, and sometimes an abdominal mass can be palpated (suggesting a tumor). Any patient with bright red blood per rectum should undergo bedside anoscopy to rule out an anal source. *(continued)*

Once a judgment has been made whether the source is proximal or distal to the ligament of Treitz, workup and treatment strategies diverge.

Figure 40.1

Workup of gastrointestinal bleeding. The most critical move to guide such workup is to pass an NG tube as soon as possible because it will usually tell you whether the bleeding is due to an "upper" (proximal to the ligament of Treitz) or "lower" source. This distinction is critical because workup and treatment fundamentally differ.

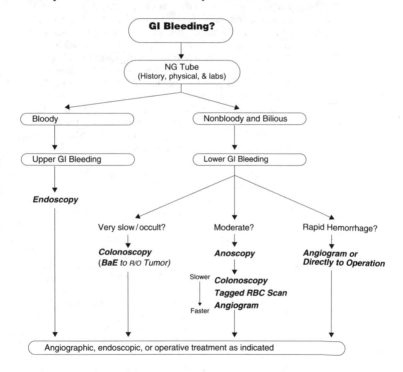

Upper GI Bleeding

Upper GI bleeding is suggested by hematemesis or blood via the NG tube. The darker the blood, the longer it has been sitting in the stomach, exposed to acid. Melena usually indicates an upper GI source, while true bright red blood from the rectum from an upper GI source indicates an extremely rapid and massive bleed, and the patient in this case will almost always be unstable.

Endoscopy

The initial and universal test of choice for an upper GI bleed is **endoscopy**. This allows accurate identification of the source, and often is therapeutic as well. The most common causes of upper GI bleeding are duodenal or gastric ulcers, gastritis or esophagitis, and esophageal varices.

Duodenal ulcer

Peptic ulcer disease is the most common cause of upper GI bleeding, and commonly recurs—thus a past history of an ulcer strongly suggests that this is the diagnosis. Their incidence has declined over the past few decades, originally antedating the widespread use of antacids and H_2 blockers—an unsolved mystery of medicine! **Duodenal ulcers** occur more frequently than do **gastric** (2:1). Characteristically, posterior duodenal ulcers present with bleeding, because they erode into the gastroduodenal artery as it passes behind the first portion of the duodenum. Anterior ulcers, on the other hand, characteristically present with perforation (but not bleeding), because there is no protective retroperitoneum (see Chapter 34, "Peptic Ulcers"). Gastric ulcers anywhere can bleed, although often more slowly. Endoscopy can be therapeutic, allowing cauterization or vasoconstriction of the ulcer's vasculature by injection. Most ulcers stop bleeding without surgery. Finding a visible blood vessel (bleeding or not) or clot or active bleeding at initial endoscopy, as well as hemodynamic instability at presentation, empirically predict a high likelihood of failure of endoscopic management and subsequent need for surgery—so be prepared. Ulcers are caused by excessive acid production (peptic ulcer) or deficient mucosal defenses (many gastric ulcers), thus reducing acid output by means of H_2 receptor or Na^+/K^+ pump blockade, neutralizing gastric acid directly, or augmentation of mucosal defense directly (e.g., with sucralfate) are helpful. Helicobacter pylori bacterial colonization is found in many patients with peptic ulcers, and pharmacologic eradication of this organism may be of benefit.

If medical management fails, surgery is required. There are no hard or fast rules regarding transfusion requirements, but, in general, a patient who rebleeds while receiving optimal medical management should be operated on. One should have a **lower** threshold to explore elderly or sick patients, because delay will make them disproportionately sicker. Operative treatment consists of opening the proximal duodenum with oversewing of the bleeding point (with cephalad and caudad sutures to control the gastroduodenal artery itself). A decision should be made about the need for an "acid-reducing procedure" such as a vagotomy, taking into account the stability of the patient and evidence that surgical acid reduction will actually help. Bleeding gastric ulcers can be resected or oversewn, keeping in mind that the risk of cancer is higher. Ulcers on the lesser curve are not associated with acid hypersecretion, and acid-reducing procedures are thus not indicated.

Esophagitis gastritis

Esophagitis and **gastritis** can produce surprisingly major bleeding. Both are caused by irritation of the mucosa, often in patients with severe gastroesophageal or pyloric reflux (bile may be as important as acid in its erosive ability). Both are more common in severely ill inpatients; alcoholics are prone to gastritis, and immunocompromised patients can develop esophageal ulcers. Both usually stop with conservative nonoperative treatment, although rarely total gastrectomy may be required for refractory hemorrhagic gastritis.

Stress ulcer

Patients who are very sick or who require ICU care are at risk for **stress ulcers** or **gastritis**. A Curling's ulcer is a stress ulcer in a burned patient, while a Cushing's ulcer is one occurring in neurosurgical patients, but, in practice, the root cause (acid hypersecretion with reduced mucosal blood flow and hence defense) is probably the same. All significantly stressed patients should receive stress ulcer prophylaxis via acid-reduction or mechanical mucosal protectants. Patients who are anticoagulated or on a ventilator are at particular risk. There is debate whether or not prophylaxis increases the risk of iatrogenic pneumonia due to bacterial overgrowth in the stomach resulting from increased gastric pH and subsequent subclinical aspiration, but there has clearly been a dramatic decline in the incidence and mortality of bleeding stress ulcers in hospitalized patients over the past few decades.

Esophageal varices

Patients with alcoholic cirrhosis develop dilated collateral venous pathways for portal blood to bypass the obstructed liver, the most important of which are **esophageal varices**. Importantly, a significant minority (possibly even half) of acutely bleeding alcoholics with known varices are bleeding from non-variceal sources, making endoscopy mandatory even in these patients. Initial therapy consists of endoscopic sclerosis (by injection) of the bleeding veins, which can be repeated several times. Unfortunately, there is often a significant gastric variceal component, and these are very hard to reach. Systemic vasopressin is used to constrict the varices; nitroglycerin can be added to protect coronary perfusion and perhaps lower portal pressure if the patient can tolerate it. If sclerotherapy fails, management is complex. Traditionally, management of an acute variceal bleed has been to surgically reduce portal venous pressure by providing outflow into the low-pressure systemic venous circulation by means of a portacaval shunt. With the exception of a few centers with vast experience and continued practice, however, results of emergent shunts for acute variceal bleeding have been poor. The varices can be surgically interrupted by means of esophageal transection and reanastomosis, but again, morbidity and mortality are high. Recently, a technique has been developed for performing a transjugular intrahepatic portacaval shunt (TIPS) that offers the same physiologic benefit of a reduction in portal pressure without the need for laparotomy. Initial results show good short-term success. The definitive "cure" of the problem is liver transplantation; a TIPS can buy time and allow resuscitation, evaluation, and elective transplantation. Obviously, the underlying cause of liver failure needs to be corrected (i.e., the alcoholic patient needs to stop drinking—an often significant hurdle). A

Surgery
Gastrointestinal *continued*

TIPS seems to make subsequent liver transplantation easier and may be associated with better graft survival. Patients who are literally bleeding to death can be helped by the **temporary** placement of a nasogastric Sengstaken-Blakemore tube that physically tamponades the bleeding vessels. This produces significant associated morbidity, however, and rebleeding rates are high, so it should be thought of and used as a temporary bridge to definitive therapy (TIPS, shunt, or transplant).

Prophylactic shunts

Patients with known varices who have never bled fall into a unique class. Prophylactic shunts (that is, before any bleeding has occurred) have not been shown to be of value. The decrease in portal pressure is offset by the high incidence of encephalopathy, due in part to loss of the liver's detoxification function from bypassing the portal flow. Shunts after a documented bleeding episode are beneficial at avoiding recurrent bleeding, but there is increasing evidence that serial endoscopic sclerotherapy may yield a much lower complication rate with excellent control of bleeding.

Other causes

Other causes of upper GI bleeding are less common. Patients who give a history of forceful retching or vomiting followed by hematemesis may have a **Mallory-Weiss tear**, or partial-thickness tear of the mucosa of the distal esophagus and stomach. These usually heal without surgery (Boerhaave's syndrome, or full-thickness rupture of the esophagus after retching, is a separate entity and usually leads to sepsis and critical illness, not major bleeding). **Arteriovenous malformations** of the stomach can occur, and often must be oversewn for control. Although spontaneous fistulae are rare, a person who has had a previous aortic procedure (aneurysm repair or aortofemoral bypass) and is bleeding from the upper GI tract should be suspected of having an **aortoduodenal fistula** due to erosion of the proximal suture line into the third or fourth portion of the duodenum. This problem is difficult to diagnose (usually by deep endoscopy or direct surgical exploration) and is highly lethal. Patients with **isolated** gastric varices should be suspected of having **splenic vein thrombosis**, resulting in sinistral ("left-sided") portal hypertension. Splenectomy is curative.

Lower GI Bleeding

In general, evaluation of lower GI bleeding is harder, but treatment is easier. There is no one test that is applicable in all situations. Three options are available, appropriate roughly according to the amount of bleeding that is felt to be present. If bleeding is very slow or occult, **colonoscopy** may be best. Colonoscopy allows direct visualization of the source, but cannot be performed if too much blood is present within the lumen. Luckily, blood acts as a cathartic, producing an "auto-prep" by removing most of the stool. If bleeding is moderate, technetium-tagged red blood cell scan can be done. This is quite sensitive for the presence of bleeding, but is not very specific, i.e., the picture is very fuzzy and anatomic location is poor. If bleeding is massive, an angiogram can be done, with visible extravasation precisely marking the bleeding vessel. There is poor correlation between actual, "real-time" bleeding and bowel movements or vital signs. Thus, many radiologists will request a tagged scan to document that bleeding is occurring before subjecting the patient to the much more invasive angiogram (for all but the most massive of bleeding episodes). Any patient with a lower GI bleed should routinely undergo bedside anoscopy; frequently a source can be identified (hemorrhoid or rectal ulcer) that is treatable at the bedside. Frequent, small episodes of bright red bleeding without stool suggest an anorectal source.

Diverticulosis and AVM

Diverticulosis is one of the most common causes of lower GI bleeding. Note that diverticulitis (active infection) itself is rarely associated with significant bleeding. Although diverticular disease is more prevalent in the sigmoid colon, right-sided diverticula seem to have a relatively greater propensity to bleed. This may be due, in part, to improvements in diagnosis. Many bleeding episodes that may have in the past been ascribed to right-sided diverticular disease are now felt to be due to **angiodysplasia** (or localized arteriovenous malformations). These tend to occur in the right colon, and diagnosis is usually made by endoscopy or angiography. Both of these lesions tend to resolve with nonoperative therapy.

Colon Ca

Colon cancer is the third most common cause. Bleeding is almost always occult, but may require transfusion. Diagnosis is straightforward by endoscopy. Especially in

Surgery
Gastrointestinal *continued*

younger patients, **inflammatory bowel disease** (Crohn's disease and ulcerative colitis) can cause lower GI bleeding, as can **hemorrhoids** or acute **colitis**. In older patients, **bowel ischemia** should be considered, particularly if there are risk factors for emboli (atrial fibrillation), atherosclerosis, or unexplained acidosis or leukocytosis. If no source can be found after adequate workup, **small bowel lesions** (such as tumors or vascular malformations) should be considered. Bleeding from the small bowel is very uncommon and is notoriously difficult to manage, often requiring intraoperative pan-endoscopy.

Luckily, most lower GI bleeding stops spontaneously. When it does not, there are few therapeutic options available other than surgery. Angiography can sometimes be used to inject thrombotic substances into specific arteries, and occasionally colonoscopic cautery or sclerotherapy can be successful. Again, there is really no specific number of transfused units of blood that should be thought of as an automatic trigger for operation, but bleeding that recurs during optimal medical management usually will not stop by itself. Ideally, treatment is by resection of the specific segment of colon that is bleeding. Be very cautious of doing a partial resection based on a tagged scan alone—it is notoriously inaccurate, and rebleeding is common. If bleeding is ongoing and workup cannot localize the source, subtotal colectomy is required. In this situation (nonlocalized lower GI bleeding) subtotal colectomy has been shown to produce lower overall morbidity, mortality, and rebleeding rates than localized resection, even with attempts at intraoperative localization. Be very careful that a small bowel or rectal source is not the culprit. ■

41 Bowel Obstruction

Bowel obstruction, or blockage of the intestine at any point, accounts for more than 20% of all urgent general surgical admissions and is one of the most common indications for nonelective surgery. Although most common in adults over 50, obstruction can occur at any age. Approximately three quarters of such episodes occur in the small intestine, and the remaining are colonic.

"Obstruction" of either the small or large intestine results from one of two general causes: mechanical blockage or paralytic ileus. **Mechanical obstruction** can result from an intraluminal (e.g., gallstones or tumor), extraluminal (e.g., adhesions or herniation), or intramural (e.g., Crohn's disease) process. Obstruction can be **partial** or **complete**, based on the degree of occlusion. **Paralytic ileus**, not a true obstruction, is the result of intestinal paralysis where intestinal contents are not able to pass through the intestine due to a loss of organized peristalsis.

Etiology

Small bowel

The majority of **mechanical small bowel obstructions** (**SBO**) are due to **postoperative adhesions** (most common) or an incarcerated inguinal **hernia**. Postoperative adhesions obviously are not present unless previous surgery has occurred, and thus are more common in older patients. If the patient is younger, a hernia, either inguinal, femoral, or ventral, becomes increasingly likely. Intra-abdominal **tumors** (primary small bowel tumors are rare) are the third most common causative factor. Rarer causes include inflammatory bowel disease, ischemic or post-irradiation strictures, or intussusception (particularly in children). An uncommon but important cause of SBO in the elderly is gallstone "ileus" (really obstruction): a large gallstone erodes through the wall of the gallbladder into the duodenum, producing intraluminal obstruction typically at the ileocecal valve. The classic scenario is that of an elderly female with intermittent ("tumbling") SBO and air in the biliary tree (from the cholecystoenteric fistula).
(continued)

Surgery
Bowel Obstruction *continued*

Large bowel

Large bowel obstruction (LBO) is due most commonly to **colon cancer** or **diverticular disease**. Both are prevalent in the elderly, and differentiation can be difficult on clinical grounds alone. Less common in the western world (but the most common cause of LBO in developing countries, probably due to dietary differences) is **volvulus**. A loose, floppy sigmoid colon is usually present, but the cecum, if mobile enough, can also twist. Rarer causes of LBO include inflammatory bowel disease, fecal impaction (severe constipation), gallstone ileus with the stone impacted in the sigmoid colon, and strictures due to irradiation or inflammatory bowel disease.

Ileus

Ileus is a normal part of the "fight or flight" response, and is thus normal and expected after any significant stress (such as trauma or sepsis). The bowel can react quite variably to insult, and judgment of the magnitude of ileus expected in various situations can be obtained only through clinical experience. In general, actual handling of the intestines produces the most ileus, non-bowel intra-abdominal procedures produce less, and laparoscopy and non-abdominal procedures produce the least. The small bowel is often relatively spared from ileus occurring after trauma or sepsis, making it a good choice for early enteral feedings in very sick patients (see Chapters 27 and 3, "Postoperative Care" and "Nutrition"). Ileus can also be produced by electrolyte imbalances, uremia, or a variety of general insults to the body as a whole. Narcotics are a common and often overlooked cause of ileus, particularly in hospitalized or institutionalized elderly patients. **Ogilvie's Syndrome** is a unique form of ileus of the colon, typically occurring in elderly, stressed, hospitalized patients. The proximal colon is dilated, with a "cut-off" at the splenic flexure, closely mimicking a tumor in this location. Characteristically, the patient has minimal subjective discomfort. It is the distal, nondilated colon that is abnormal; sacral parasympathetic malfunction with left colonic ileus has been postulated to be the cause. Finally, **intestinal pseudo-obstruction** is a poorly understood but increasingly recognized entity. Here, the bowel just doesn't work, and no mechanical or physiologic cause can be found. This can be a very frustrating problem to deal with.

Pathophysiology

Mechanical obstruction

Simple mechanical obstruction implies blockage of the intestinal lumen **without** vascular compromise. If obstruction is complete, ingested fluid and food, gas, and native secretions accumulate orad to the point of obstruction, causing distention of the proximal bowel. As the bowel wall becomes edematous and congested, the normal secretory and absorptive functions of the mucosa are lost, and as proximal intraluminal pressure rises, blood flow is compromised.

Strangulated obstruction

Strangulated obstruction occurs when arterial inflow stops, and the bowel becomes ischemic. This can result from increased intraluminal pressure alone, a constricting external band, volvulus of the vascular pedicle, or edema of a portion of bowel herniated through a fascial defect (see Chapter 30, "Hernia"). It is very important to remember that increased intraluminal pressure alone can eliminate blood flow–actual proximal arterial interruption is not needed. In this situation, venous occlusion usually occurs first, causing arterial blockage and thrombosis due to increasing resistance.

Closed-Loop obstruction

Closed-loop obstruction occurs when a loop of bowel is obstructed both proximally and distally, for example after torsion of a loop of small bowel or with an obstructing left colon cancer in the setting of a competent (i.e., closed) ileocecal valve. The intraluminal pressure within the loop rises quickly, leading to bowel wall edema and early vascular occlusion and perforation. Paralytic ileus alone very rarely leads to strangulation and infarction.

Diagnosis

Clinical symptoms vary depending on the site, cause, and duration of obstruction. **Vomiting**, crampy abdominal pain, and abdominal **distension** are the most common presenting symptoms. In general, the more proximal the obstruction, the closer together are the episodes of pain and emesis, and the less the distention. Hypovolemia and electrolyte disturbances are common due to both emesis and to accumulation of fluid in the lumen of the bowel proximal to the obstruction, within the bowel wall, and within the peritoneal cavity. Unchecked, progressive fluid losses can lead to hemoconcentration, hypovolemia, acute renal insufficiency, and shock.

H&P

Intermittent crampy abdominal pain usually accompanies vomiting. Pain is visceral and is usually referred to the midline. Small amounts of feces, usually loose, may be passed early, but **failure to pass flatus** is virtually universal if the obstruction is complete. Initially bowel sounds are hyperactive, high-pitched, and tinkling, but later become decreased, indicating the presence of a component of paralytic ileus. Patients can have nonspecific abdominal **tenderness** due to distention, but peritonitis is not evident until the bowel wall becomes gangrenous. True peritonitis, suggested by consistent absence of bowel sounds, abdominal rigidity, severe tenderness, and shock, suggests strangulation (infarcted bowel) or even frank perforation. Partial mechanical obstruction generally leads to milder symptomatology, with ongoing passage of stool and gas.

Labs

Several laboratory tests, including determination of complete blood count, serum electrolytes, and acid-base status, should be obtained. The white blood cell count can initially be normal, although a leukocytosis is usually present both from stress demargination and progressive local ischemia and resultant systemic inflammation. The hematocrit can be elevated due to hemoconcentration. Electrolyte abnormalities occur as a result of the loss of gastrointestinal fluid, with an elevated blood urea nitrogen being common due to the prerenal azotemia of dehydration. Acidosis implies tissue ischemia, i.e., strangulated bowel.

X-rays

X-rays of the abdomen are very helpful and should be obtained early, including supine, upright, and lateral decubitus views along with an upright chest x-ray (a "free air series"). The classic findings in obstruction are gas-filled, **distended** loops of bowel with **air-fluid levels** as the partially fluid-filled loops layer out under the influence of gravity. Differentiation of small and large bowel can be surprisingly difficult. The presence of distended small bowel is suggested by visualization of plicae circulares that traverse the **complete width** of the bowel shadow and occur at regular intervals, while distended large bowel is identified by haustral markings that do **not** completely traverse the width of the bowel. X-rays are very poor at differentiating paralytic ileus from mechanical obstruction—clinical events and patient status are much more important. A common mistake is to misinterpret a large bowel obstruction with an incompetent (i.e, open) ileocecal valve as a small bowel obstruction, due to the refluxed air into the small bowel.

The x-ray can, however, identify certain discrete events. Air in the biliary tree due to a cholecystoenteric fistula is the hallmark of gallstone ileus. Sigmoid volvulus presents as a large bowel obstruction with a tremendously distended sigmoid ("omega loop") in the pelvis. Ogilvie's syndrome presents with a dilated proximal and transverse colon, "cut-off" at the splenic flexure. Finally, some air in the colon (but not just the rectum after a digital rectal exam!) implies that a small bowel obstruction is partial.

Contrast studies

Contrast studies are of variable value. If obstruction is complete, administering anything from above (e.g., barium) is counterproductive, usually will not alter management, and thus should be avoided. An upper GI series can, however, sometimes help to identify rarer causes of partial SBO, or differentiate pseudo-obstruction or atypical ileus from mechanical blockage. Barium enemas are somewhat more useful in LBO, because they can safely confirm the colonic position of the blockage and sometimes can identify the cause (especially if volvulus is expected, because initial management may differ). If a complete LBO exists, early surgery is almost always required, and decisions can be made intraoperatively. Further, barium can trickle past (proximal to) a physiologically complete LBO, thus such passage is not an indication that operation can be deferred. Therefore, barium enemas also are not usually helpful.
(continued)

Surgery
Bowel Obstruction *continued*

Ultimately, diagnosis rests on the clinical scenario combined with judicious radiologic studies (always plain films, occasionally contrast studies). Ask yourself four questions in an orderly fashion: first, is the diagnosis a paralytic ileus or mechanical obstruction? Second, is the obstruction in the small or large bowel? Third, what is the cause? And, finally, does the patient need surgery or medical management, and, if surgery, how soon?

Treatment

Three basic principles apply to the treatment of bowel obstruction: initial fluid and electrolyte **resuscitation**, **decompression** of the gastrointestinal tract, and **definitive correction of the problem**.

Fluids and electrolytes are lost by vomiting, by sequestration of fluid within the bowel wall and lumen, and by transudation of fluid into the peritoneal cavity. Third-spaced fluids produce isotonic losses, while emesis tends to deplete acid, sodium, and chloride. Hypokalemia is common, but potassium can be elevated if renal failure occurs. Large volumes of crystalloid such as lactated Ringer's solution or normal saline with added potassium are most physiologic. Resuscitation should be guided by the general principles put forth in other chapters; in the majority of cases restoration of adequate intravascular volume reestablishes renal perfusion and urine output. In complicated or severe cases, or in patients with renal or cardiac disease, more invasive monitoring such as a central venous catheter or Swan-Ganz catheter may be needed. It cannot be stressed enough that a **Foley catheter** (to reliably monitor urine flow in real time) is an absolute requirement in this situation. Initial estimates are made about fluid and electrolyte deficits, and ongoing assessment is used to guide further therapy. In this situation (and in any situation short of uncontrolled hemorrhage), the patient cannot be brought to the operating room until he or she is making urine (more precisely, cannot safely be put under general anesthesia until he or she is euvolemic).

NG tube

Initial gastrointestinal **decompression** can be accomplished by the insertion of an 18 Fr nasogastric tube (NG). Most surgeons consider anything smaller to be of little value. An NG tube does not decompress the bowel much beyond the pylorus, but merely acts to prevent further secretions and gas from accumulating. Even so, it is surprisingly helpful, and many episodes of obstruction resolve without surgery. Colonoscopic decompression of dilated large bowel is helpful in two major situations: sigmoid volvulus and Ogilvie's Syndrome. In the former, decompression can relieve the acute problem, allowing time for resuscitation and elective definitive correction (by resecting or "tacking down" the floppy sigmoid), while in the latter, decompression may be the only treatment required.

Treatment

Definitive correction of the problem is the ultimate goal, and management differs in different situations.

Many small bowel obstructions resolve with conservative care only. Each operation creates more adhesions, thus the goal is to avoid surgery if possible. Patients with **localized**, **constant** pain or peritonitis (suggesting necrosis or perforation) or an obvious cause that will not resolve (such as an incarcerated hernia or an intraluminal gallstone) require early surgery. Patients with partial mechanical obstruction or even complete adhesive obstruction without evidence of compromised bowel can usually safely undergo a trial of conservative management (nasogastric suction and intravenous fluids). It is important to set clear time limits, and to plan on surgical exploration if resolution does not occur within 24-48 hours or so. Obviously, any clinical decline strongly suggests the need for earlier exploration. Many such patients, even with an apparent "complete" obstruction by x-ray, will resolve without surgery (illustrating the low predictive power of x-rays in this situation). The old dictum of "never let the sun rise or set on an SBO" does not really apply anymore. Interestingly, x-ray findings often lag about 24 hours behind clinical events, also supporting the concept of basing decisions on the clinical scenario rather than on the x-ray itself.

Urgency of operative intervention is often greater if the large bowel is obstructed. There are two reasons: the most

Surgery
Bowel Obstruction *continued*

common causes (tumor, diverticular disease, and volvulus) are less likely to spontaneously resolve, and closed-loop obstructions (due to the ileocecal valve) with their greater morbidity are more common. If a sigmoid volvulus is suspected, initial colonoscopic decompression can "cure" the acute problem. Recurrence is likely, however, and usually the redundant sigmoid must be resected or fixed into position semi-electively. In most other causes of LBO, operation is usually required when the diagnosis is made. As discussed above, usually a tumor or obstructing diverticular mass will be found (and sometimes cannot be differentiated intraoperatively). Many options exist. The old "three-stage procedure" (initial proximal colostomy, later resection and reanastomosis, and final colostomy closure) requires 3 operations and leaves the disease in place for a while, and is thus seldom performed today. The most conservative approach is to resect the diseased colon, leaving a proximal colostomy ("Hartmann's procedure"), and electively closing the colostomy at a later date. Under certain circumstances, however (a right colon obstruction, early diagnosis and intervention, a healthy patient, or a bowel preparation performed intraoperatively), resection and primary repair can be considered (weighing the advantages of only one operation versus the risks of an anastomotic leak). ■

Pediatrics

Jeffrey M Kaczorowski
and
Laura Jean Shipley
Section Editors

42   The Pediatric Patient and Well-Child Care

The joy of pediatrics lies not only in the variety of ages and diagnostic possibilities of each encounter, but also in the diversity, resilience, and personality of each child. Your humor, your willingness to play as you talk with and examine the child, and your ability to communicate and explain your thoughts will often make the difference between a stressful or successful visit. Although the pediatrician's primary responsibility lies in caring for the child, caregiving must extend to the family as well. Involvement of both patient and parent in the history, physical examination, and planned therapeutic intervention is essential to an effective encounter.

History

Flexibility with different ages of children and sensitivity to individual family dynamics will allow for optimal **history** taking. Judgment should be used, and each encounter is different. For example, while the caregiver's historical account is crucial in caring for the infant with fever, a 7 year-old should be allowed to relate her own symptoms of abdominal pain before additional information is elicited from the parent. Likewise, the confidentiality and independence of an adolescent should be respected by allowing private conversation with the physician whenever possible.

The outline followed for the pediatric history naturally includes questions relevant to the history of present illness, past medical, family, and social history, and a pertinent review of systems. A pediatric history also includes questions regarding immunization status, development (see Chapter 46, "Growth and Development"), and birth history. The birth history should include information about any complications of pregnancy, delivery, or neonatal course. Birthweight, gestational age, prolonged hospitalization, and need for intervention (such as oxygen or medications) are particularly relevant.

Physical Exam

The **physical examination** in pediatrics begins with your observation of the child as you first enter the room. In well-child care visits, a good assessment of the child's developmental status can often be obtained by just watching. For an illness or emergency visit, it is important to make a rapid assessment of whether the child is "sick," that is, requiring immediate intervention, or "not sick," allowing a more thorough history and physical exam before any intervention. Respiratory distress (fast and/or labored breathing) and altered levels of consciousness are two of the more obvious signs that urgent intervention (the ABCs) may be needed, but ultimately this is a skill that can be acquired only with experience.

The vast majority of children seen in the outpatient or office setting do not require urgent treatment. A thorough history (as described above) is obtained and a physical exam completed. Growth parameters (height, weight, and head circumference) should be measured and plotted on growth curves. Infants and toddlers are often best examined in the parent's lap where they are comfortable and more likely to be cooperative. In general, the exam is most easily conducted in a progression from less invasive to more invasive components. After observation, many pediatricians will next listen to the heart and lungs because the child is most likely to be quiet prior to parts of the exam that require manipulation. Interacting with the child by talking, smiling, joking, making noises or "baby talk" can often be reassuring. Allowing a 2 or 3 year-old to hold the otoscope or pretend to look in your mouth is helpful in relieving the anxiety associated with examination of the ears or oropharynx.

Adolescents

In the adolescent patient, the examination can be modified to be more like the exam you would conduct in an adult. It is important to always respect the privacy of adolescent patients by allowing them to change into a gown in private, by conducting the rectal, genital, and breast examinations last (when the adolescent is most comfortable), and by employing a chaperone for these latter portions of the exam.
(continued)

Pediatrics
The Pediatric Patient and
Well-Child Care *continued*

Well-Child Care

The goals of health promotion or "well-child care" are ambitious and difficult to define narrowly. The establishment of a schedule of visits at specific stages of a child's life allows for the monitoring of physical, cognitive, and emotional growth and development so that abnormalities can be recognized when intervention is most likely to be successful. The physician takes an active role in the prevention of disease and injury through immunization, health screening, and anticipatory guidance. It is the primary care physician's responsibility to prepare families for the events ahead by offering appropriate education without dictating an inflexible outline for parenting. By establishing a long-term, trusting relationship with the patient and family, the physician encourages confidential and open discussion of sensitive issues when necessary. In all of these interactions, support and positive reinforcement are given to patient and parent.

Immunizations

The **schedule** of well-child visits varies with the age of the child. Recommended visits are as frequent as every 2-3 months during the first year of life, and every 3-6 months during the second year. Visits continue on an annual basis through late adolescence.

The **immunization** schedule continues to evolve with advances in medical technology. At present, childhood vaccines are available against polio, diphtheria, pertussis, tetanus, Haemophilus influenzae type B, measles, mumps, and rubella, and hepatitis B. Most recently, varicella (chickenpox) vaccine has been licensed and approved. Detailed immunization schedules are available through the American Academy of Pediatrics Red Book (Report of the Committee on Infectious Diseases). Appropriate information on the benefits and risks of immunization should be communicated prior to administration of any vaccine.

Health screening

The term **health screening** is broad and refers to the history and physical examination as well as to specific procedures and laboratory tests. Screening by history is often used to determine the need for laboratory studies. For example, exposure to tuberculosis or contact with a recently incarcerated or HIV-positive person requires tuberculin skin testing. The physical examination is modified for different ages to screen for specific abnormalities such as developmental dysplasia of the hip in the infant and scoliosis in the adolescent. Other screening procedures and laboratory studies vary with the age of the child. The American Academy of Pediatrics recommends blood pressure measurement, vision and hearing assessment, hematocrit measurement for anemia, lead testing, and urinalysis. Sexually active adolescent females should have an annual pelvic examination, including Pap smear and testing for sexually transmitted diseases; this procedure can be deferred until after the age of 18 in those not sexually active.

Guidance and education

Anticipatory guidance and education provide both challenge and reward to the primary care physician. Because an inexhaustible amount of information can be communicated, most physicians tailor advice to suit the needs of the particular patient and family. Nearly every encounter includes some discussion of safety. Accident prevention includes use of seat belts and bicycle helmets, fire safety measures, and home childproofing.

In addition to matters of safety, pediatricians advise young families about providing proper nutrition, environmental stimulation, and age-appropriate play. Questions regarding behavior, school readiness and school problems are likely to be anticipated and addressed. As the patient matures, the physician's role as counselor to the parents is modified by the need for a confidential relationship with the adolescent; sensitive topics such as substance use and sexuality must be discussed. Anticipatory guidance for the adolescent includes discussion of school performance and career goals, counseling for HIV risk, and instruction in techniques of breast and testicular self-examination.

Despite the goals of well-child and adolescent care, a significant number of children in our country remain underimmunized and live in environments for which appropriate anticipatory guidance centers around daily survival skills rather than sleep disturbance or bicycle safety. These children are a reminder that advocacy for children's health must extend beyond office and clinic encounters. Every child deserves the benefits of well child care: prevention of disease, early detection of illness, and promotion of health. ■

Pediatrics

A pediatrician should be present in the delivery room if complications with the baby are expected (or arise), otherwise the pediatrician's first encounter with a newborn will generally occur in the nursery.

Newborn Resuscitation and Delivery Room Evaluation

When a newborn is handed to a health care provider in the delivery room, the immediate goal is to assess the need for assistance in making the transition to the new environment. The baby should be immediately dried and placed under a warmer (to reduce heat loss) and stimulated. Mucus should be removed from the oropharynx and nares with a bulb syringe (suctioning beyond the distal nares with a catheter can trigger bradycardia during this transition period). The Apgar score is used to easily and reproducibly assess a newborn's status; assessments are made at 1 and 5 minutes of age. Respiratory effort, heart rate, color, tone, and reflex irritability are assessed, with scores of 0, 1, or 2 assigned to each category. A score of less than 5 indicates severe physiologic depression. One **should not** wait to assign Apgar scores prior to the initiation of resuscitation.

Resuscitation

Following drying, stimulation, and bulb aspiration of mucus, most infants will initiate and maintain sufficient respiratory function so that no further resuscitation is necessary. Six percent of infants born in the US, however, and 80% of those weighing less than 1500gm require some form of resuscitation. Infants with gasping, apnea, or heart rates below 100 require positive pressure ventilation. Hand ventilation with a bag and mask device will provide adequate respiratory support in most situations; endotracheal intubation, however, should be performed for delivery of medications if no intravenous access is present, if prolonged ventilation is required, if a diaphragmatic hernia is present, or if hand ventilation is inadequate. Chest compressions are rarely required, but should be instituted if the heart rate is less than 80 and not increasing after 30 seconds of positive pressure ventilation. Epinephrine is used for persistent bradycardia or asystole. Naloxone will rapidly reverse respiratory depression in neonates born to mothers given narcotics within the 4 hours prior to delivery. Caution should be exercised in infants born to mothers who abuse street drugs, because naloxone can precipitate acute opiate withdrawal and result in intractable seizures.Hypovolemia is treated with volume expansion (normal saline, 5% albumin, or blood). Neonates with prolonged arrest unresponsive to other therapy should receive sodium bicarbonate to reverse metabolic acidosis. Atropine has no clear role in neonatal resuscitation at this time.

Meconium

The treatment of infants born with meconium-stained amniotic fluids is controversial. All infants with meconium staining should undergo suctioning of the oro- and nasopharynx prior to delivery of the shoulders. Infants born through thick or particulate meconium or who are physiologically depressed at birth, should further undergo immediate intubation and suctioning via the endotracheal tube until clear. Vigorous infants born through thin meconium can generally be observed, although their management is controversial.

Delivery room exam

Once stability is assured, the delivery room examination, a brief inspection for birth trauma and any gross deformities, is performed. Infants at risk for hypoglycemia (e.g., infants born to diabetic mothers) should have blood glucose levels checked; the administration of oral or IV 10% dextrose solution is considered in infants with glucose levels less than 40mg/dL. Erythromycin ointment should be applied to the eyes to prevent conjunctivitis secondary to gonorrhea or chlamydia exposure during the delivery process, and vitamin K should be administered to prevent hemorrhagic disease of the newborn secondary to vitamin K deficiency.

The initial delivery room evaluation of an infant allows the examiner to "introduce" the infant to the family, to reassure parents about normal physiologic changes, and to provide the parents with an initial assessment of any problems. Including the parents in the initial evaluation and communicating honestly and directly with them begins to build an important therapeutic alliance.

Nursery Evaluation

A second, more comprehensive examination is done in the nursery on the first day of life. Whenever possible, this examination should occur in the presence of the parents. Less invasive aspects of the exam should be done first, beginning with vital signs and observation of the infant's general behavior.

Skin

The **skin** is assessed for color. Peripheral cyanosis (acrocyanosis) is a normal finding in neonates, but central cyanosis (often seen in the intraoral mucus membranes) is abnormal and indicates hypoxemia. Jaundice can be normal at 3-4 days, but raises concern about ABO incompatibility, other causes of hemolysis, or sepsis if present during the first 24 hours (see Chapter 44, "Neonatal Jaundice"). Plethora is due to polycythemia (hematocrit greater than 65%). Any evidence of ecchymosis, abrasions, or lacerations resulting from birth trauma is identified. Mongolian spots, hyperpigmented melanin collections commonly found in the lumbosacral region or lower extremities of neonates of African, Asian, or Hispanic origin, should be identified for the parents so that they are not mistaken for bruises.

Lungs

The **lungs** and **chest wall** are next. Respiratory distress is suggested by tachypnea, cyanosis, grunting, flaring, or retractions. Auscultation of the lungs should specifically rule out respiratory distress syndrome (crackles), pneumothorax (decreased breath sounds), or congenital diaphragmatic hernia (bowel sounds in the chest). Both male and female infants can have hypertrophied breast tissue secondary to intrauterine estrogen exposure.

Heart

Heart sounds of a newborn can be difficult to differentiate from breath sounds because of similarities in pitch. Watching the rise and fall of the abdomen during respirations as well as feeling a peripheral pulse will help. Note the intensity of the heart sounds, whether or not the second heart sound is split, and whether murmurs are present. Be sure to check femoral or distal leg pulses (see Chapter 52, "Pediatric Cardiology").

Abdomen

Inspection of the **abdomen** may reveal abdominal wall defects (see Chapter 38, "Pediatric Surgery"), or a diaphragmatic hernia (scaphoid abdomen). A normal umbilicus should have 3 vessels present (2 thick-walled arteries and 1 thin-walled vein)—the presence of only 2 suggesting the possibility of associated genitourinary tract anomalies. The liver can normally be palpated 1-2cm below the costal margin, but flank masses are abnormal and can be due to renal enlargement secondary to hydronephrosis or polycystic kidney disease. Hypertrophy of the urinary bladder secondary to outlet obstruction may present as a suprapubic mass or failure to void within the first 24 hours, while intestinal obstruction is suggested by bilious emesis, abdominal distension, or failure to pass meconium within the first 48 hours.

Genitalia

The appearance of the **external genitalia** can provide clues about gestational age. In males the testes are undescended at the 30th week of gestation and completely descended by the 40th week. Scrotal ruggae typically progress inferiorly to superiorly from the 30th to the 40th week. In females, the labia majora are widely separated and the clitoris is prominent until the 36th week, while the labia majora completely cover the minora and clitoris by the 40th week. Females can have a white or bloody vaginal discharge due to withdrawal of maternal estrogen. Inspection of the penis for evidence of hypospadius or epispadias (opening of the urethral meatus anywhere between the base of the penis and the tip of the glands) is important because both contraindicate early circumcision. Inguinal hernias often appear after straining or crying and are reducible, while hydroceles present as constant, nonreducible masses (see Chapter 38, "Pediatric Surgery").

Reflexes

Multiple **primitive reflexes** can be elicited in the newborn infant (see Chapter 46, "Growth and Development"). The palmar and planter grasps allow you to assess symmetry in tone and strength. By placing a finger in the infant's mouth, the strength, duration, and frequency of the sucking reflex is assessed.

Musculo-skeletal system

When examining the **musculoskeletal system**, the limbs and spine are evaluated. Asymmetry of extremity movement suggests brachial plexus injury (Erb's palsy) or clavicular fracture during delivery. Gross deformities such as extra (polydactly) or fused (syndactly) digits or short or absent limbs should be obvious. The entire length of the vertebral column should be inspected for bony and skin defects. A "clunk" (as the femoral head passes back into the acetabulum; Ortolani sign) or posterior dislocation of the hip (Barlow sign) with hip adduction and downward pressure suggest the presence of a congenitally unstable or dislocated femoral head. The most severe deformity of the foot in the newborn is the equinovarus deformity (clubfoot), which consists of fixed forefoot adduction, inversion of the hind foot, internal tibial torsion, and small calf muscles.

HEENT

The **head and neck** examination should be performed last because it is the most invasive. A bulging anterior fontanelle signals the presence of increased intracranial pressure. Edema that crosses the suture lines of the skull is most likely located in the subcutaneous tissue (caput succedaneum), while swelling that follows the suture lines is due to hemorrhage in the subperiosteal region (cephalohematoma). Facial palsy, caused by injury to the facial nerve after forceps delivery, is manifest by asymmetric mouth movement with crying. Scleral or subconjunctival hemorrhage are common after birth and will resolve with time. It is important to visualize the retinal red reflex bilaterally, ensuring the absence of obstructing lesions (such as cataracts, corneal opacities, or retinal tumors) between the cornea and the retina. The presence of a cleft lip or palate is usually obvious, but a submucosal cleft palate may be detected only by palpation. An asymmetrical neck tilt may be caused by torticollis (due to sternocleidomastoid hematoma).

Common Neonatal Issues

The anticipatory guidance offered to the family should be tailored toward issues of concern over the first 2-3 weeks of life. Parents should be told that it is common for newborns to lose up to 10% of their birthweight during the first week, due to fluid re-equilibration as the infant makes the transition from the moist environment of the womb to the relatively dry outside environment. If breastfeeding (see Chapter 45, "Infant Fluids, Electrolytes, and Nutrition"), the mother should feed her new infant in a relaxed state, away from other distractions, to best allow the milk let-down reflex to be stimulated. The baby should be fed on demand; frequent feedings (10-12 daily) will ensure adequate hydration and weight gain. A breastfeeding mother should eat well and drink plenty of fluids to supply the extra nutrients and calories required for lactation.

The **umbilical stump** should be inspected and cleaned several times throughout the day, conveniently during diaper changes. A call should be made to the primary care provider if erythema or pus are noted. The umbilical stump typically falls off within the first 2 weeks of life; once this has occurred, the baby can be bathed.

Each infant will establish her or his own **stooling pattern**. Normal newborn stools are initially dark and tarry due to meconium, but become soft, seedy, and yellow over the first few days. Newborns can stool as frequently as 10 times per day or as infrequently as a few times per week. Constipation is present when the stools become hard and pellet-like, and can be treated with glycerin suppositories or dilute fruit juice until the stools are soft. A newborn should have a wet diaper 6-8 times per day. If urine output is less than this, dehydration may be present.

Many **dermatologic changes** occur during the first few weeks. Cradle cap (dry, scaly patches of skin localized to the scalp) is common; gentle shampoo once a week will assist in resolution. Milia (sebaceous retention cysts) are fine white papules on the nose, chin, forehead, or cheeks. Acne neonatorum consists of comedones and papules that are seen on the cheeks, forehead, and chin, while pustular melanoses are generalized skin lesions that present as pustules, ruptured pustules with scale, and hyperpigmented macules. All are benign and self-limited.

Newborns can develop **jaundice** (see Chapter 44, "Neonatal Jaundice"). Jaundice (yellowing of the skin) is caused by increased levels of bilirubin. Neonatal jaundice typically progresses from head to toe; the primary care provider should be contacted if this yellow hue is present below the umbilicus (signifying higher bilirubin levels).

The **sleeping** infant should be placed on the side or back to decrease the risk of **sudden infant death syndrome** (**SIDS**; see Chapter 51, "Pediatric Respiratory Diseases"). Most infants will sleep through the night by the first 3-4 months.

Parents should be instructed about the signs and symptoms of **illness** in a **neonate**. If the baby is irritable and difficult to console, uninterested in feeding, or has a rectal temperature greater than 38°C, the primary care provider should be contacted. ■

44   Neonatal Jaundice

Jaundice is a common finding in the newborn; almost 50% of infants develop visible jaundice during the first week of life. When clinically apparent jaundice is present, the serum bilirubin level is usually in excess of 5mg/dL. Jaundice typically progresses from head to toe; jaundice present on the lower extremities signals high bilirubin concentrations. Jaundice occurring in the first 24 hours of life is **abnormal** and usually signals the presence of a hemolytic process. Indirect (unconjugated) hyperbilirubinemia is far more common than is direct (conjugated; see below). Hyperbilirubinemia is a problem because of the increased risk of **encephalopathy** due to **kernicterus**. At high levels, unconjugated bilirubin can cross the blood brain barrier. Once in the CNS, it causes neuronal death and pigment deposition, particularly in the region of the basal ganglia and the cerebellum, potentially leading to opisthotonos, seizures, and death.

Bilirubin Metabolism

Hyperbilirubinemia can result from the disruption of normal bilirubin metabolism at any of 6 stages: synthesis, plasma transport, hepatic uptake, hepatic conjugation, hepatic excretion, and enteric reabsorption (see also Chapter 24, "Jaundice"). Bilirubin **synthesis** (bilirubin is the breakdown product of heme) occurs in the reticuloendothelial cells of all organs; in the newborn synthesis is increased due to the short red cell life span. The synthesized, unconjugated bilirubin is bound to albumin for **transport** to the liver. After hepatocellular **uptake**, it is next **conjugated** by the hepatic enzyme glucuronyl transferase (present in relatively low levels in the newborn). In the adult, conjugated bilirubin is **excreted** into the intestinal tract where it is converted to urobilinogen or stercobilin by intestinal bacteria; the newborn gut is initially sterile, however, and conversion is limited. In the newborn gut, conjugated bilirubin is instead hydrolyzed by beta-glucuronidase; the reformed unconjugated bilirubin is **resorbed** and returned to the liver via the portal vein (enterohepatic circulation).

Jaundice in the newborn can be broken down into conditions causing either **indirect**, **direct**, or **mixed** hyperbilirubinemia. Indirect (unconjugated) hyperbilirubinemia generally results from increased bilirubin synthesis (overwhelming the low levels of glucuronyl transferase), but can occur with disorders of hepatic uptake and/or conjugation or increased enteric resorption. Direct hyperbilirubinemia generally results from problems with hepatic excretion, and implies that all steps up to and including conjugation are normal.

Indirect Hyperbilirubinemia

Conditions that cause increased red cell breakdown include **hemolytic disorders** (Rh, ABO, and other blood group incompatibilities), **inherited red cell disorders** (spherocytosis), **red cell enzyme deficiencies** (G6PD or pyruvate kinase deficiency), and **resorption of blood** (cephalohematoma, ecchymoses). Exaggerated enterohepatic circulation can occur if **mechanical gastrointestinal obstruction** (atresia/stenosis and meconium ileus/plug) or **reduced peristalsis** is present. Increased bilirubin synthesis, deficient hepatic transport and conjugation, and increased enteric reabsorption in the newborn all contribute to the development of **physiologic jaundice**, the most common cause of neonatal indirect hyperbilirubinemia. Whereas the severe hemolytic anemias are more likely to present with rapidly progressive jaundice during the first 24 hours of life and often require intervention, physiologic jaundice typically presents on the third or fourth day of life. The bilirubin levels decline to insignificant levels by the tenth or twelfth day, and often no intervention is required.

Physiologic jaundice is more common in infants who are breastfed, and is thought to be related to the period of relative dehydration experienced in the few days before nursing is well established. **Breastmilk jaundice**, in contrast, is the term used to describe a normal continuation of physiologic jaundice that begins after the fifth day and can continue for several weeks or months. Apparently related to enhanced enteric absorption of unconjugated bilirubin due to an unidentified factor in human milk, breastmilk jaundice is considered benign and does not require intervention.

In cases of prolonged indirect hyperbilirubinemia (beyond 1-2 weeks), **hypothyroidism** or enzymatic **disorders of**

bilirubin uptake (Gilbert's syndrome) or **impaired conjugation** (glucuronyl transferase deficiency) should be considered.

Direct Hyperbilirubinemia

Conditions that can inhibit hepatic excretion of conjugated bilirubin include **anatomic obstructions** (biliary atresia, choledochal cyst, and intestinal obstructions) or hepatocellular damage such as that seen in **neonatal hepatitis**, **cirrhosis**, reactions to certain **medications**, and **infection.**

Mixed Hyperbilirubinemia

Other problems can produce a mixed direct and indirect hyperbilirubinemia. These include **congenital infections**, **postnatal infections** or **sepsis**, and **metabolic disorders** such as galactosemia.

Treatment

When jaundice is discovered in a newborn, specific attention should be given to the time of onset, rate of progression, and hydration status of the infant (as reflected by the feeding history and voiding and stooling pattern). Family history may reveal siblings or relatives who have had unexplained jaundice, and is particularly significant if an exchange transfusion was required. Physical exam should rule out hepatomegaly, splenomegaly, or any finding suggestive of infection. Hemolytic disease is more likely if the mother's blood type is O or her Rh status is negative (because she will produce A, B, and Rh antibodies that can react against the relevant fetal antigens, if present). If jaundice develops during the first 24 hours of life, a blood smear, hematocrit, Coombs test, ABO and Rh status, and total bilirubin should be obtained to rule out a hemolytic process. If the rate of rise of the bilirubin level is rapid (0.5mg/dL per hour) and hemolytic disease is suspected, phototherapy should be started immediately because infants in this group appear to be at increased risk for bilirubin encephalopathy.

If the newborn is more than 24 hours old, the extent of cutaneous jaundice should be assessed. If jaundice has reached the level of the groin or progression is evident on serial exams, then a total bilirubin level should be obtained and followed until the bilirubin level has begun to fall. In cases where the family history is significant for hemolytic jaundice (e.g., G6PD deficiency or spherocytosis) or non-hemolytic disease (Gilbert's syndrome), a repeat bilirubin, hematocrit, blood smear, and specific enzyme measurements should be obtained in 3-6 months.

Photo-therapy

Current consensus is that the minimal bilirubin level for risk of bilirubin encephalopathy in normal healthy newborns without hemolytic disease is 25mg/dL, but this recommendation does not apply to infants who are ill, have hemolytic disease, or are preterm. Treatment strategies are geared towards the elimination of bilirubin from the body. **Phototherapy**, the direct exposure of the newborn to blue and green visible light, converts the bilirubin molecule to a water-soluble form which can be excreted by the liver and kidney. Frequent feedings (of breastmilk or formula) are necessary in a jaundiced infant with or without the use of phototherapy. Infants who require phototherapy should have appropriate eye protection and careful monitoring of their hydration status because of increased insensible water losses. Intravenous fluids are rarely required. Regardless of the time of onset or severity of jaundice, **exchange transfusion** should be considered in infants showing signs of bilirubin encephalopathy such as seizure activity or changes in the level of consciousness, tone, or cry.

Exchange transfusion

Term infants who are visibly jaundiced at less than 24 hours of age are not considered healthy, require further evaluation, and will likely require phototherapy (and possibly exchange transfusion). Asymptomatic infants who become jaundiced after the first 24 hours are considered candidates for phototherapy at bilirubin levels that vary based on the age of the infant and presence or absence of underlying disease. Exchange transfusion should be implemented if phototherapy fails and the bilirubin level is greater than 25 mg/dL, and immediate exchange transfusion is recommended if the presenting bilirubin level is greater than 30 mg/dL. ■

45   Infant Fluids, Electrolytes, and Nutrition

Children come in different sizes, and therefore fluids, medications, and nutritional support must be calculated for each child. Most such calculations, however, are based on a simple parameter-weight.

Fluids and Electrolytes

Maintenance

Calculation of **maintenance fluids**, those needed to maintain resting equilibrium in the absence of stress, is based on energy expenditure. For every kilocalorie (kcal) of energy expended, 1mL of water is required. Children burn calories and require fluid at different rates that vary according to size: for the first 10kg, they require 100kcal/kg/day and 100mL/kg/day, for the next 10kg, 50kcal/kg/day and 50mL/kg/day, and for every additional kg, 20kcal/kg/day and 20mL/kg/day. Fluid orders are generally written in mL/hour. Since a day consists of 24 hours, the corresponding rates per hour are 4mL/kg for the first 10kg, 2mL/kg for the next 10kg, and 1mL/kg for every kg thereafter.

Empirically, about 30meq/L of sodium and 20meq/L of potassium are necessary maintain normal electrolyte homeostasis. This translates into roughly 1/4 normal saline (NS) with 20meq of potassium added per liter. Some carbohydrate (generally 5gm of dextrose per 100mL of fluid; D5) is usually added to the electrolyte solution to prevent hypoglycemia and give it some caloric value (supplying approximately 20% of caloric needs).

Dehydration

These calculations assume the child does not have a fluid deficit. **Pre-existing fluid deficits**, however, are relatively common in pediatrics, often because of gastroenteritis; in third-world countries diarrhea and resultant dehydration are a major cause of mortality in children. Just as in adults, short-term changes in body weight directly reflect fluid (rather than caloric) status. The best means of assessing the degree of dehydration of a child, therefore, is to measure changes in body weight occurring over a limited period of time. A child who has lost weight during an acute diarrheal illness is assumed to have lost that weight in body fluid; unfortunately, a child's true weight just before illness is not often known. In practice, estimation of the degree of dehydration is frequently made on the basis of clinical judgment. In general, a child who has lost more than 5% of fluid volume will exhibit dry mucus membranes, reduced tearing, mild tachycardia, and decreased urine output; losses greater than 10% lead to pronounced tachycardia, little or no urine output, lethargy, decreased blood pressure and perfusion, weak pulses, and decreased skin turgor (i.e., shock).

Fluid replacement for significant dehydration should initially consist of the **rapid** infusion of **isotonic** fluid such as normal saline or lactated Ringer's solutions (see Chapter 7, "Fluids and Electrolytes," and Chapter 27, "Postoperative Care") administered in 20mL/kg boluses until a response is seen. Serum electrolytes should be measured, however, to determine whether dehydration is isotonic (serum sodium 130-150meq/L, most common), hypotonic (sodium less than 130meq/L), or hypertonic (sodium greater than 150meq/L). Dehydrated children are generally hypokalemic, and require additional potassium, although potassium should not be administered until the child has voided to ensure the kidneys are functioning. Rehydration with isotonic solutions is generally safe, although overzealous correction of hypertonic dehydration can result in central nervous system dysfunction and seizures due to cerebral edema. The basic technique of rehydration should be familiar: an initial, educated guess should be made, with therapy then modified (typically to 1/2 NS with 5% dextrose) based on laboratory results and the patient's response.

Nutrition

Adults require about 35kcal/kg/day to maintain homeostasis. Children, however, can require as much as 150kcal/kg/day, depending on size, stress, and growth requirements. Maintenance needs (as discussed above, about 100kcal/kg/day for the first 10kg, 50kcal/kg/day for the next 10kg, and 20kcal/kg/day for every kg thereafter) are calculated the same way as are fluids. Most infant formulas when mixed properly have a caloric density of 20kcal/ounce (1 ounce equals about 30cc). Thus, a 3kg baby who requires 300kcal per day will need to consume 15oz or 450cc of formula to meet its needs.
(continued)

Pediatrics
Infant Fluids, Electrolytes, and Nutrition *continued*

Breast-feeding

How do infants receive nutrition? **Breast-feeding** is clearly best. Unfortunately, however, only about half the infants in the US are initially breast-fed, and less than 20% are still being breast-fed at 6 months, despite clear evidence of its superiority. Breast milk is readily available and requires no preparation. Breast milk contains maternal IgA and may enhance IgA production by the infant. There is an unequivocally decreased incidence of diarrheal illnesses, lower respiratory tract infections, otitis media, bacteremia, dental caries, and sepsis in infants who are breast-fed.

Most mothers who desire to breast-feed can successfully do so. Rarely, primary lactation failure (inability to produce adequate milk), insufficient glandular tissue, or neurohumoral deficiencies can result in inability to breast-feed. Surgical procedures that sever breast ducts or nerves can also make breast-feeding impossible. There are few situations where breast-feeding is contraindicated. Mothers who have HIV disease (except those in third-world countries), use illicit drugs, or are undergoing chemotherapy should not breast-feed. Breast-feeding should be at least temporarily suspended in women with herpes or syphilis lesions of the breast, chicken pox, pertussis, non-B-hepatitis, or active tuberculosis. Infants with galactosemia should not be breast-fed because breast milk contains lactose as its major carbohydrate. Mastitis is not a contraindication to breast-feeding nor is maternal hepatitis B if the infant has received hepatitis B immunoglobulin and hepatitis B vaccine.

It is recommended that all breast-fed infants (as well as those who are bottle-fed) receive vitamin K at birth as prophylaxis against hemorrhagic disease of the newborn. This is especially important in breast-fed infants because of the low levels of vitamin K in breast milk. The American Academy of Pediatrics does not recommend fluoride supplementation for breast-fed infants in areas where water is fluorinated, but in the second 6 months of life iron-fortified cereal should be introduced into the child's diet because neonatal stores have been depleted and iron is present in low (but very bioavailable) levels in breast milk. If maternal nutrition is inadequate or exposure to sunlight is minimal, vitamin D supplementation may also be necessary for breast-fed infants.

Formula-feeding

Parents choose to feed their infant with formula for a variety of reasons. Bottle-feeding with commercial formulas is a safe and nutritionally sound method of infant feeding. The use of whole cow milk in the first 12 months of life does not provide adequate nutrition for infants. Different preparations of commercial formulas including cow milk-based (Similac, Enfamil), soy-based (Isomil, Nursoy, Prosobee), and elemental (Pregestimil, Alimentum, Nutramigen) are widely available. Low iron formulas should not be used for the term infant; studies have not demonstrated any detrimental effects of iron, and iron is important for infant neurologic development. Infants are not normally lactose intolerant (excepting those rare infants with galactosemia). Some infants have adverse reactions to proteins in cow milk-based formulas (estimates vary from 1%-8%), soy formulas (less commonly), or even to elemental diets.

Most infants tolerate commercial formula. These formulas are packaged as ready-to-feed, concentrated liquid, and powder forms. Ready-to-feed formula needs no preparation but is expensive and contains no fluoride. Concentrated liquid formula is diluted 1:1 with water and is intermediate in cost, while powdered formula is prepared by mixing one scoop (enclosed in the can) with 2oz of water, and is least expensive.

Sterilization is not necessary if sanitary tap water is available. Formula can be warmed under a hot tap, in a bottle warmer, or on the stove. Microwaves should not be used because they can result in extreme heating of the formula and resultant burns. Vitamin and mineral supplementation is not necessary in formula-fed infants, providing that the water used to reconstitute the formula is fluoridated. If using a ready-to-feed formula, fluoride supplement is necessary.

Frequency

Infants will generally breast-feed every 2 hours in the weeks immediately after birth, but by 1 month of age the number of feedings decreases to approximately 6-8 per day. Most mothers let their baby suckle about 10-15 minutes on one breast, burp the baby, then charge to the second breast and allow the infant to suckle as long as he or she desires. The first 4 minutes of sucking on each breast accounts for about 85% of total milk intake. The milk that is released after the initial minutes of feeding ("hind-

Pediatrics
Infant Fluids, Electrolytes, and Nutrition *continued*

milk"), however, contains about 5 times the fat content of the early milk and is very important for adequate nutrition. If intake is adequate, breast fed infants will urinate 8 or more times per day (this can be very difficult to assess in these days of super-absorbent diapers) and will stool with virtually every feed.

Most bottle-fed infants take 1oz of formula per feed the first day. This increases to 1-3oz per feed in the first week, and to 3-5oz per feed by 1 month. Feeding frequency decreases from 6-10 per day initially to 5-7 per day at 1 month. As discussed above, most formulas have a caloric density of 20kcal/oz (1oz = 30mL). If all is well, the baby will surpass birthweight by 2 weeks and thereafter gain about an ounce per day ("an ounce a day with time off for weekends"). Weight should double by 4-5 months of age.

Infants should receive breast milk or formula with iron through the first year of life. The current recommendation is to introduce solid food at 4-6 months. Typically, cereal is begun first and high protein food (meat) introduced last. Cup feeding can begin at 5-6 months of age. ■

46   Growth and Development

Growth is measured by changes in size of the body, while development refers to the differentiation and evolution of form and function. In the course of normal growth and development there is a natural tendency for periods of rapid progress to alternate with periods of consolidation. In general, the **rate** of development for each individual varies, but the **sequence** of events will be similar. The pediatrician needs to identify the points where growth and development fall outside normal values. Genetic endowment, acute or chronic illness, physical handicaps, the quality of the child's environment, nutritional status, cultural exposure, and emotional or psychologic maltreatment all can affect the rate of growth and development.

Newborn Infants

Bodily proportions at this stage are unique: the head is relatively large, the face is round, and the extremities relatively short. There is a high body surface area to mass ratio. Most full-term infants regain their birth weight by 10 days of age; this doubles by 4-5 months and triples by one year.

Neurologic development at this stage is characterized by the **primitive reflexes**. The **rooting reflex** is demonstrated when a touch to the cheek causes the mouth and tongue to move toward the stimulus. If the baby's head is dipped while supine, the arms will abduct and extend with hands open and fingers slightly curved; the **moro reflex**. If an object is introduced into the palm or sole, the fingers or toes will flex and grip the object; the **grasp** and **plantar reflexes**. With passive head rotation, there is an increase in the tone of the ipsilateral upper limb with flexion of the contralateral side; the **asymmetric tonic neck reflex** (demonstrating how strongly the newborn's limb motions are influenced by head position). The **placing reflex** is elicited by placing the anterior aspect of the tibia or ulna against the edge of a table; infants will lift their legs up to step onto the table, or elevate their arms to place their hands on the table. If the sole of the foot is pressed against the table while the baby is held upright, flexion and extension of the legs occur; the **walking reflex**. The primitive reflexes persist for a variable time period during the first months of life and are considered abnormal if present in the older infant or child. Newborns are capable of brief periods of eye contact and preferentially gaze at a human face.

The First Year

Physical development is marked by rapid growth, fusion of the fontanelles, and eruption of teeth. The anterior fontanelle generally diminishes in size after 6 months and becomes effectively closed by 9-18 months of age, while the posterior fontanelle generally is closed to palpation by 4 months. The first deciduous teeth generally erupt between 5-9 months. First to appear are the lower central incisors, then the upper central and upper lateral incisors.

When evaluating the **developmental progress** of a child, pediatricians commonly refer to screening tools such as the Denver Developmental Screen. By **1-3 months,** there is relaxation of the normal newborn flexed position at rest. If prone, infants will be able to hold the chin up, turn the head, and lift the head to the plane of the body, and if supine, the head lags behind when pulled to a sitting position. At this stage the infant can visually track an object through 180? By 3-5 weeks the first social smile occurs.

By age **3-6 months** infants demonstrate increased awareness of and interaction with their surroundings. They raise their head and chest with arms extended, and by 4-6 months can roll from supine to prone. Head lag will disappear. By 4 months they can laugh out loud, make vowel sounds, and begin to articulate consonants and guttural sounds such as "ah" and "goo." They bring objects to their mouth and support weight on their extended extremities.

By **6-8 months** children can roll both ways, creep, sit, and extend the arms appropriately to prevent falling if tilted while sitting. They will bounce actively when held and support most of their own weight, and can transfer objects from hand to hand. Babbling, the use of polysyllabic vowel sounds, begins.

By **8-10 months**, a time of assisted mobility and increased socialization, children assume a sitting position without help, sit alone without support, pull themselves to

a standing position, and walk holding on to furniture.
They begin to demonstrate a pincer grasp. They respond
to their names, wave bye-bye, and play peek-a-boo or
pat-a-cake

Near independence of locomotion is achieved by **10-12
months.** The child walks with one hand held, rises independently, and take several steps. Vocabulary consists of a
few single words. Cognitively, the child begins to learn
through activity, exploration, and manipulation of the
environment. This is the beginning of awareness of self
and of object permanence.

The Second Year

After the first year, growth begins to decelerate somewhat; the average gain is about 2.5kg and 12cm per year.
Subcutaneous tissue ("baby fat") begins to decrease and a
decreased appetite is also common. The first deciduous
molars and cuspids erupt.

The developmental gains during the second year of life
allow for increasing control over the child's environment.
By **12-15 months,** children walk alone and crawl up
stairs. They scribble with a crayon and stack 3 cubes.
Social skills advance as the child indicates needs, often
by pointing and vocalizing. They follow simple commands and may name familiar objects.

By **15-18 months** children can run stiffly, sit on small
chairs, and walk up stairs with one hand held. Imitation
begins. They speak about 10 words, name pictures, and
identify body parts. Children begin to feed themselves
and seek help when in trouble.

At **18-24 months** they run well, walk up and down stairs
one step at a time, open doors, and jump. They stack multiple cubes, scribble, and handle a spoon well. By this
stage they will first put 3 words together (subject, verb,
object) in a sentence, and begin to relate their experiences
and listen to stories.

Often labeled as the "terrible twos", this period is characterized by an increasing sense of self as separate from
others, and by the ability to take initiative and make
choices. Increasing concerns with the expectations of

adults, standards of behavior, and daily routines develop. Play is generally solitary and consists of active manipulation of available objects. There are often contests over control or possession. Children may start to show increasing frustration and anger; temper-tantrums, breath-holding, and other outbursts are common. These developmentally expected clashes of will, however, are accompanied by the emergence of the child's unique personality.

Ages 3-5 (Preschool)

Physical development is marked by a relatively steady weight and height gain of 2kg and 6-8cm per year, respectively. An average of 20 deciduous teeth have erupted.

During the preschool years, the child continues to exercise independence and make choices, but begins to learn self-control. **Three year olds** ride a tricycle, stand momentarily on one foot, and alternate feet up the stairs. They stack multiple cubes, copy circles, and draw stick figures. They know their age and sex, count to 3, and sustain brief conversations. They help dress themselves and wash their hands. Toilet training is typically in progress and may be nearly complete.

Four year olds hop on one foot, throw a ball overhand, use scissors, and alternate feet when descending stairs. They copy a cross and a square, count objects, and tell stories. At this age reciprocal play ("give-and-take") and role-playing begin.

Five year olds skip, walk on tiptoes, and balance on one foot. They draw shapes and name opposites and colors. They begin domestic role-playing, dress and undress well, and ask about the meaning of words.

Cognitively, preschool children become capable of symbolic representations of the world ("make-believe"), although they are not capable of sustained, systematic thought. There is some decline in egocentricity. The search for independence needs to be encouraged for the child to develop self-confidence.

Ages 6-12 (School Years)

Physical development is characterized by relatively steady growth ending in a preadolescent growth spurt at age 10 (girls) to 12 (boys). The first permanent teeth appear around age 6-7, and shedding of deciduous teeth follows in the same sequence as acquisition. Gross motor development is essentially complete; fine motor abilities continue to be refined.

The school-aged child becomes capable of some logical thought processes. Awareness of the principles of conservation, reversibility, and classification is achieved. Children learn to initiate activities, enjoy accomplishments, and acquire direction and purpose in tasks. They typically enjoy school and are eager to learn. They should be allowed to explore and assert independence, but limits must be clear in order to avoid conflict.

With the development of self-esteem, children become increasingly independent and able to look outside the home for goals and standards of behavior. There is the initiation of independence from the family, a wish for privacy, and increased distance from open physical affection. Friendships are typically with members of the same sex and tend to center on joint activity. There is a very high degree of conformity among this age group.
(continued)

Ages 12-18 (Adolescence)

Adolescence is more fully discussed in Chapter 47, "Adolescent Medicine." Physical and sexual maturation of adolescents can be described by Tanner stages I through V:

Females:	Pubic hair	Breast
I	None	Preadolescent
II (10-13 yrs)	Sparse, slightly pigmented, straight	Breast and papilla elevated as a smalmound
III	Darker, beginning to curl	Breast and areola enlarge, no contourseparation
IV	Coarse, curly, abundant	Areola and papilla form secondary mound
V (14-17 yrs)	Adult feminine triangle, spread to medial surface of thighs	Mature, nipple projects, areola part of general breast contour

Males:	Pubic hair	Genitalia
I	None	Preadolescent
II (10 -1 4 yrs)	Scant, long slightly pigmented	Slight enlargement of scrotum and testes
III	Darker, starts to curl	Lengthening of penis, enlargement of scrotum and testes
IV	Coarse and curly, abundant	Glans and breadth of penis increase in size
V	Adult in quantity and type, extends onto thighs	Adult in size and shape

In females, puberty generally occurs between the ages of 11-15, with menarche in mid-to-late puberty (the average age being about 12.5). The female growth spurt occurs during Tanner stage III, with peak growth velocity normally preceding the onset of menstruation just prior to Tanner stage IV. The age range for pubertal changes in males is 11.5-15.5 years with the growth spurt a relatively late event, generally peaking at stages IV-V. An increase in height by 8-10cm/year is expected. Proportionate growth between the sexes diverges: fat deposition is greater in females, while muscle mass is greater in males;

the androgen-dependent wider shoulder width in males is in contrast to the estrogen-dependent increase in hip width for females.

Cognitively, adolescents progress to logical and abstract reasoning and can formulate and test hypotheses. School and peer groups become more important and sex differences in peer relationships become apparent. A time for self-definition, adolescence is also the time when sexual identity becomes solidified and a sense of sexual adequacy is developed.

Abnormalities of Growth and Development

Acquisition of developmental skills may not be smooth, but rather can occur in intermittent bursts. Screening tools with guidelines and average age limits are useful for identifying the outer limits of acceptable delay so that further investigation, close followup, and intervention, if possible, can be initiated. **Loss of previously acquired milestones** is particularly concerning and suggests a neurologic or neuromuscular abnormality.

It is necessary to follow patterns of growth over time. **Failure to thrive** is a term used to describe a child less than 2 who is consistently below the third percentile for height or weight parameters or whose height or weight curve "plateaus" over a period of time. Growth failure will first manifest as weight loss. Subsequently, height and head circumference may be affected; this degree of growth arrest carries a more worrisome developmental prognosis. The differential diagnosis for failure to thrive is extensive but usually can be divided into one of three categories: **organic**, which may be due to dysfunction of any organ system; **inorganic** (the majority of cases), which is caused by various degrees of psychosocial disturbance; or a **combination** of the two.

Along with identifying developmental and growth abnormalities, the pediatrician must also educate parents as to the course of normal development and foster appropriate expectations. ■

47 Adolescent Medicine

Adolescent medicine is a part of pediatrics but includes treatment of problems familiar to internal medicine, gynecology, and psychiatry. Adolescence is the developmental time frame that encompasses the cognitive, emotional, and physical transition from childhood to adulthood. The term **adolescence** is much broader in scope than **puberty**, which refers to the physical changes leading to reproductive capacity (see Chapter 46, "Growth and Development").

General Overview

Adolescent health care focuses on prevention, education, and health promotion. When interviewing an adolescent, the mnemonic **PACES** can be used as an outline for discussing relevant issues: peers and parents (interactions and relationships), accidents, alcohol and other substances of abuse, cigarettes, emotions, eating habits, and exercise, school, sexually transmitted diseases, and suicide. An alternative mnemonic is **HEADS**, suggesting discussion of home (issues relating to parents and siblings), education and emotions, ambitions and accident prevention, drugs (including tobacco and alcohol), sexually transmitted diseases, and suicide.

Consent and emancipation

In certain circumstances, minors have the right to consent for health care without parental consent or knowledge. These conditions vary based on state laws and health care institution policies, but usually include emancipation (physical and financial independence, marriage, pregnancy, or service in the armed forces), minors requiring emergency care, or minors seeking care related to sexuality, substance abuse, or mental health. There is a legal concept that defines the "mature minor" as an adolescent who can understand the risks and benefits of treatment and give consent for care, generally considered to be at approximately age 14-15. The issue of confidentiality, especially as it relates to parents, should be stressed. Although confidentiality is always an integral part of the relationship with the adolescent, it must be made clear to the adolescent that if imminent danger exists for either the patient or others, confidentiality may have to be breached.

Disorders of Menstruation

Amenorrhea, dysfunctional uterine bleeding, and dysmenorrhea, discussed in general in Chapters 63, "Ambulatory Care Gynecology," and 67, "Reproductive Endocrinology and Infertility," are the most common menstrual disorders in adolescents. **Primary amenorrhea** is defined as the absence of menstruation by age 16 in patients with breast development, and by age 14 in those without. **Secondary amenorrhea** is the cessation of previously regular menstruation for greater than 3 months; it is considered pathologic only if it occurs more than a year after menarche.

Amenorrhea can be caused by functional or structural abnormalities of the hypothalamus, pituitary, ovary, uterus, or vagina; differential diagnosis is broad. Primary amenorrhea can be physiologic, chromosomal (e.g., Turner's syndrome), structural (imperforate hymen or congenital absence of the uterus), or hormonal (e.g., hypothyroidism or polycystic ovary disease). Secondary amenorrhea is often due to stress, exercise, or abnormal dietary patterns, but **pregnancy must always be considered**. Hormonal, metabolic, and structural abnormalities are also possible.

Evaluation for amenorrhea consists of a thorough history and physical examination, including pelvic examination, pregnancy test, and thyroid stimulating hormone and prolactin levels. Progestin challenge, either by injection or oral administration, should result in withdrawal bleeding within 1-7 days if appropriate estrogen priming and an intact hypothalamic-pituitary-ovarian axis exist (see Chapter 67, "Reproductive Endocrinology and Infertility"). If the progestin challenge is negative (no bleeding), LH and FSH levels will help differentiate between primary ovarian failure (high levels caused by lack of negative feedback) and hypothalamic-pituitary abnormalities (low levels due to primary failure of production).
(continued)

Dysfunctional uterine bleeding is defined as excessive or heavy menstrual flow, generally in excess of 8 days. It is a diagnosis of exclusion, and most often secondary to anovulatory cycles. In the absence of other abnormalities, treatment consists of hormonal therapy. Iron supplementation should be provided for those with ongoing blood loss.

Dysmenorrhea is a common problem that can lead to school absenteeism and interference with daily activities. Most cases are primary (no structural problem). Secondary dysmenorrhea occurs in patients with pelvic pathology such as endometriosis, pelvic inflammatory disease, benign tumors, or anatomic abnormalities. Nonsteroidal antiinflammatory drugs (NSAIDs) are usually sufficient treatment for primary dysmenorrhea; hormonal therapy with oral contraceptives is reserved for those with moderate to severe symptoms that limit daily activities.

Recognition and treatment of **sexually transmitted diseases**, unfortunately common in adolescents, are fully addressed in Chapter 64, "ED Gynecology."

Adolescent Pregnancy

Adolescent pregnancy is a concern because of the problems with which it is frequently associated: premature birth, low birth weight, increased infant mortality, and poor subsequent maternal employment and educational advancement. Early recognition and diagnosis of teenage pregnancy is essential to allow informed choice and optimize outcome. **Secondary amenorrhea always suggests pregnancy even if there is no history of sexual activity reported**. The history should address possibilities of rape or incest, particularly in younger patients. Dating the pregnancy and counseling about options for continuation, adoption or termination are necessary subsequent to a positive pregnancy test. Confidentiality must be preserved, but adolescents should be encouraged to involve their parents in this decision process whenever possible. Prevention remains the primary goal: discussion of sexuality and counseling about contraception are critical.

Eating Disorders

The prevalence of eating disorders in adolescents is estimated at approximately 1%-5% with an overwhelming female preponderance. **Anorexia nervosa** is characterized by severe weight loss (defined as body weight 15% below that expected or more than a 15% discrepancy between expected weight gain and growth), disturbances of body image with fear of obesity, secondary amenorrhea, and the absence of a physical illness that would otherwise explain these symptoms. **Bulimia** is the syndrome of recurrent episodes of binge eating accompanied by a desire to purge (self-induced vomiting); excessive concern with body image and weight are also present. Adolescents can have symptoms of both bulimia and anorexia nervosa, and either disorder can be associated with laxative use or other weight control methods such as compulsive exercise. Both disorders are accompanied by a high proportion of psychiatric problems, notably depression. Multidisciplinary treatment is required, and includes a feeding program, therapy for the patient and family, and close monitoring. Hospitalization may be required for patients who have severe weight loss, constitutional problems such as bradycardia, dysrhythmias, or hypokalemia, and for those in whom outpatient management has failed.

High Risk Behaviors

Factors that increase the likelihood of high-risk behavior in adolescents include persistent concrete thinking, feelings of invulnerability, and peer pressure. **More than three-quarters of adolescent deaths are due to injuries and violence.** The leading causes of death are accidents (80% motor vehicle accidents), homicides, and suicides, all preventable to some degree. Social problems such as truancy, dropping out of school, running away, and gang-related activities correlate with increasing morbidity and mortality.

By age 18 approximately 80% of all adolescents have initiated **sexual activity**. Decreasing age of sexual initiation, multiple partners, and inconsistent use of contraceptives place adolescents at high risk for pregnancy and sexually transmitted diseases.
(continued)

Pediatrics
Adolescent Medicine *continued*

The most commonly abused substance is **alcohol**. More than 90% of adolescents report trying alcohol by age 18. Alcohol contributes greatly to the morbidity and mortality associated with motor vehicle accidents.

Adolescent use of **cigarettes** and smokeless tobacco is increasing. Patterns of lifelong tobacco use correlate strongly with use in adolescence; persons rarely begin smoking after 20. Both alcohol and tobacco use can be accompanied by experimentation with other drugs leading to physical and psychologic addiction. ■

48 TORCH Infections

The developing fetus is vulnerable to a number of congenitally acquired infectious problems that may lead to severe, long-term sequelae. The classic mnemonic that identifies these organisms is "**TORCH**." **toxoplasma, other, rubella, cytomegalovirus,** and **herpes**. Since the time of its original institution, the "other" category has been extended to include not only **syphilis, varicella,** and **enterovirus,** but also **hepatitis B** and **HIV**. All of these are initially acquired by the mother and transferred to the fetus through the placenta or at birth. Unfortunately, treatment options are few, so prevention is critically important.

Toxoplasmosis

Toxoplasma, an intracellular parasite whose primary hosts are domestic and wild cats, is acquired through consumption of undercooked, infected meat, or by direct ingestion of infectious oocysts. The greatest risk for transmission is during a primary active maternal infection acquired in the third trimester, although outcome for the infant in this case usually is benign. In contrast, primary maternal infection during the first trimester carries a low rate of transmission, but transmission at this time often results in spontaneous abortion or fetal death. The majority of congenitally infected infants are asymptomatic at birth.

If clinical infection does occur, the classic triad consists of **obstructive hydrocephalus, chorioretinitis,** and **periventricular calcification**. A small proportion of infected infants will also develop hepatosplenomegaly, jaundice, and a maculopapular rash. Common laboratory abnormalities include thrombocytopenia, hyperbilirubinemia, anemia, and abnormal liver function tests. Diagnosis is suggested by serologic studies and confirmed by detecting parasites in tissues, blood or cerebrospinal fluid (CSF). Therapeutic options are limited and largely experimental. Mortality rates for affected infants range from 1%-6%, and the majority of survivors with neurologic symptoms at birth have substantial long-term disabilities. In order to prevent this, control measures should be encouraged for pregnant women. One of the most important is to avoid handling cats' feces. Gardens frequented by cats are also potential sources of infection. Pregnant women should also eat meat cooked to a minimum of 66 degrees C (freezing to -20 degrees C is also effective, but this level is not reached in home freezers).

Rubella

Rubella infection in children (and adults) is characterized by a generalized maculopapular exanthem, a low-grade fever, and posterior auricular and suboccipital lymphadenopathy. The greatest risk of transmission from a primarily infected mother to a fetus occurs in the first trimester and leads to significant late problems. As the pregnancy progresses, the risk of transmission decreases, and transmission leads to fewer consequences. Sequelae of first trimester infection include premature delivery, fetal loss, stillbirth, or the **congenital rubella syndrome** (**CRS**). Manifestations of CRS include growth retardation, ocular abnormalities (cataracts and microophthalmia), congenital heart disease, hepatosplenomegaly, jaundice, hearing loss, and meningoencephalitis. Affected infants can develop hyperbilirubinemia, thrombocytopenia, and elevated serum transaminases. Long-bone radiographs demonstrate metaphyseal lucencies, and CSF analysis may show lymphocytic pleocytosis and elevated protein. Central nervous system (CNS) abnormalities include intracranial calcifications, delayed myelination, and ventriculitis. The diagnosis is confirmed by isolating the virus from urine, CSF, nasopharyngeal secretions, or blood; excretion of virus may persist in the infected child for as long as a year.

Currently, treatment is largely supportive. Infants with proved infection should remain on respiratory isolation while hospitalized and be considered infective for approximately a year unless negative viral cultures are obtained. Emphasis should be placed on longitudinal assessment and early intervention for problems that develop (especially hearing and visual disorders). Infants that survive have a high rate of neurodevelopmental sequelae including mental retardation, sensorineural deafness, motor delay, and behavioral abnormalities. The best prevention is maternal immunization. Every mother (of unknown status) should be checked early in pregnancy; awareness and immunization has decreased the incidence of congenital rubella syndrome to near zero.

Cytomegalovirus

Cytomegalovirus (CMV), a large, enveloped DNA virus of the herpes virus family, is ubiquitous and causes the most common congenital viral infection in the world. Infected persons can excrete CMV in urine, saliva, semen, cervical secretions or breast milk. Transmission can occur in utero across the placenta or postnatally via breast-feeding. Infants infected early in gestation have more severe problems, although the majority of those with congenital infection are asymptomatic at birth. When present, clinical manifestations include jaundice, hepatosplenomegaly, intrauterine growth retardation (IUGR), petechial or purpuric rash, and pneumonitis. CNS problems include microcephaly, chorioretinitis, seizures, meningoencephalitis, and intracerebral calcifications (most characteristically in the subependymal area). About 20% of affected children have progressive sensorineural hearing loss. Laboratory abnormalities include thrombocytopenia, elevated liver enzymes, anemia, hyperbilirubinemia, and elevated protein or pleocytosis in the CSF. CT can reveal a variety of abnormalities including subependymal intracranial calcifications. Definitive diagnosis is made by isolating the virus from urine or saliva within the first 3 weeks of life; detection after this may reflect perinatal acquisition.

Treatment with gancyclovir will not reverse intrauterine damage, but may diminish the adverse effects of persistent postnatal virus replication in the CNS or inner ear. Symptomatic infants have a mortality rate of 20%-30%, and 90% or more of surviving infants have substantial long term sequelae including visual deficits, motor and intellectual retardation, seizure disorders, and hearing loss.

Herpes Simplex Virus

Herpes simplex virus (HSV) types 1 and 2 are ubiquitous DNA viruses. HSV-1, usually transmitted nonsexually, causes stomatitis, keratitis, skin lesions, and encephalitis, while HSV-2 is typically transmitted by sharing of bodily fluids and causes genital lesions. Both can infect the neonate, although approximately two-thirds of congenital infections are caused by HSV-2. Neonatal disease most often occurs with primary maternal infection (but can occur with recurrent disease). HSV can be acquired in utero (rarely), at delivery, or postnatally. Unfortunately, 50%-80% of mothers delivering infected infants have no history, signs, or symptoms of genital herpes at the time of delivery.

Congenital HSV presents in one of four ways. **Local infection** usually affects the skin, eyes, and/or mucous membranes. This is generally a mild disease characterized by vesicular or bullous skin lesions or keratoconjunctivitis that become evident after the first 24 hours of life. **Disseminated disease** generally causes multiorgan system involvement with fever, lethargy, poor oral intake, hepatic dysfunction, pneumonitis, disseminated intravascular coagulation (DIC), or shock. Onset is within 7-10 days after birth, and it can be caused by both HSV-1 and -2. **Encephalitis** is generally caused by HSV-2 and leads to fever, poor feeding, irritability, and lethargy, typically before the third week of life. A skin rash develops in two-thirds of affected patients, and seizures can occur, often within 24-48 hours of presentation. Finally, **in utero infection** occurs in approximately 5% of those with HSV infection; all known cases have been due to HSV-2. These infants generally present with skin lesions at birth, chorioretinitis, microopthalmia, and severe CNS damage (microcephaly, hydrocephaly, or intracranial calcifications).

Laboratory abnormalities are nonspecific and include anemia, thrombocytopenia, and elevation of liver enzymes. CT scan or MRI may reveal cerebral edema or focal hypodensities in infections acquired perinatally. Definitive diagnosis is made by isolating the virus from the oropharynx, CSF, skin vesicles, conjunctiva, or rectum; HSV antibody titers in cord blood or infant serum are generally not helpful.

HSV infection should always be considered as part of the differential diagnosis of late-onset neonatal sepsis. Overall mortality from untreated infection is approximately 50%. Infants with suspected HSV infections should be treated with IV acyclovir for a minimum of

10-14 days. With prompt initiation of treatment, those with local disease have virtually no mortality and minimal late sequelae, although infants with disseminated disease do poorly. Infants with CNS disease, unfortunately, have significant long-term neurologic problems.

Other

Syphillis

Syphilis is caused by the spirochete Treponema pallidum. Although all stages of maternal disease (see Chapter 64, "Emergency Department Gynecology) pose a threat to the fetus, the risk of transmission is greatest during secondary syphilis when the high maternal load of spirochetes facilitates hematogenous dissemination to the placenta and fetus. About a third of infected live-born infants have physical stigmata of syphilis at birth. Early problems consist of low birth weight, hepatosplenomegaly, jaundice, a maculopapular skin rash (including the palms and soles), persistent rhinitis, lymphadenopathy, meningitis, and periostitis or osteochondritis of long bones, while late manifestations (generally appearing after 2) include "saddle nose," peg-shaped upper incisors (Hutchinson teeth), mulberry molars, perioral fissures (rhagades), interstitial keratitis, sensorineural hearing loss, hydrocephalus, and mental retardation. Workup includes serologic testing (venereal disease research laboratory test; VDRL, and the fluorescent treponemal antibody absorption test; FTA-ABS), radiography of long bones, CSF analysis, and histopathologic examination of the placenta, umbilical cord, or skin lesions. VDRL analysis of CSF should be done to exclude neurosyphilis.

Congenital syphilis is presumed to be present in any infant whose mother had untreated or inadequately treated syphilis at delivery, or any infant with a positive VDRL and physical signs of congenital syphilis, compatible long-bone abnormalities, a positive CSF VDRL, or elevated CSF cell count or protein (without other explanation). As many as 40% of congenitally infected infants die in the perinatal period. Infants identified and treated appropriately (parenteral penicillin G for 10-14 days) have a low risk of long term sequelae. Untreated or inadequately treated infants are at substantial risk for physical deformities and late neurologic problems.
(continued)

Pediatrics
TORCH Infections *continued*

Varicella zoster

Fetuses are at risk for infection with **varicella zoster** if a primary maternal infection occurs early in pregnancy (shingles poses no risk). Most infants will have few or no effects. One to five percent of exposed infants, however, will develop the congenital varicella syndrome (caused by an in utero infection during the first trimester), which includes dermatomally-distributed skin lesions, chorioretinitis, limb hypoplasia, and neurologic abnormalities. Many of these infants die in the perinatal period; most survivors have substantial late morbidity.

Viruses

Congenital infection with **enterovirus** can mimic bacterial sepsis or disseminated HSV. Most infants survive without long-term sequelae if appropriate general supportive care is delivered. **Human parvovirus B19** can cause spontaneous abortion, stillbirth, or hydrops fetalis with primary maternal infection. Infants who survive appear to have no long-term problems.

HIV

Infection with the **human immunodeficiency virus** (**HIV**) can occur transplacentally or, more commonly, perinatally. Current data indicate that about a third of infants born to infected mothers will acquire the infection, but treatment of infected mothers with AZT seems to lower transmission to less than 10% (see Chapter 19, "HIV and AIDS").

Hepatitis B

While the vast majority of neonates that acquire **hepatitis B** have subclinical infection, 60%-95% will become asymptomatic chronic carriers. Administration of hepatitis B immune globulin to infants of Hepatitis B surface antigen-positive mothers within twelve hours of birth (with concurrent vaccination) significantly reduces the risk of developing a chronic carrier state. ■

Most of the problems that develop in otherwise healthy children are related to infection. This chapter covers **neonatal sepsis**, **occult bacteremia**, **meningitis**, **osteomyelitis**, and **septic arthritis**; common minor infections usually managed without hospitalization are covered in the following chapter. See Chapter 18, "Infectious Diseases" for a discussion of general principles related to infectious diseases, fever, and antibiotic selection.

Neonatal Sepsis

Pathogenesis

Neonatal sepsis is defined as serious bacterial infection in the first 2 months of life. Distinguishing the "sick" from the "well" infant based on clinical findings can be difficult; a truly septic infant can present with nothing more than poor feeding or a low-grade fever. **Fever or abnormal behavior in an infant under 2 months suggests sepsis**. Incidence of neonatal sepsis in the US varies from 1-10 per 1,000 live births, with a mortality rate of about 10%-15% in full-term infants. Substantial morbidity can occur in surviving infants, including lifelong cognitive deficits or frank mental retardation, deafness, and seizures. **Morbidity and mortality are significantly reduced if bacterial illness is treated within the first 24 hours**.

Bacterial infections acquired in the perinatal period are usually the result of infection with group B Streptococcus, Escherichia coli, or enterococcus (Streptococcus faecalis); infection with Listeria monocytogenes is rare but can be seen in infants under 4 weeks. Perinatal transmission can occur through transplacental transmission of maternal bacteremia, from the vagina and cervix through the ruptured membranes, or by contamination during passage through the birth canal. Infection with "community-acquired" bacteria such as Streptococcus pneumonia and Neisseria meningitidis is more common after 1-2 months. The incidence of sepsis secondary to Haemophilus influenza type B has declined rapidly because of vaccination.
(continued)

Fever

Fever in the neonate is defined as a rectal temperature greater than or equal to **38.0°C. A febrile neonate should be evaluated promptly**. In addition to fever or abnormal behavior, a septic neonate can exhibit hypothermia, lethargy, irritability, respiratory distress, apnea and bradycardia, vomiting, diarrhea, skin rash or petechiae, jaundice, or convulsions. **Risk factors** for sepsis should be addressed in the history: prematurity, prolonged rupture of membranes (greater than 24 hours prior to delivery), maternal illness, fever, or antibiotic treatment near delivery, and the need for neonatal treatment of infection or hyperbilirubinemia.

Conservative management

"Conservative" management of febrile infants under 2 months of age is to culture blood, urine, and cerebrospinal fluid (CSF), hospitalize, and treat with IV antibiotics until cultures are negative 48 or more hours after treatment begins. Initial antibiotic coverage typically is with ampicillin in combination with an aminoglycoside or third-generation cephalosporin. Controversy has arisen over such conservative medical management, given that many febrile infants without serious bacterial infection (SBI) are needlessly admitted.

Rochester criteria

Several institutions have established protocols based on research studies designed to identify infants **unlikely** to have SBI. The goal is to be sure to include everyone **with** the disease (at the expense of including some without), ensuring that everyone you send home definitely does **not** have sepsis. The **Rochester criteria** for evaluation and management of **febrile infants under 2 months of age** demonstrates such a screening protocol. Any infant who appears subjectively sick, has evidence on exam of a focal bacterial infection, or has any risk factors by history (discussed above) for sepsis is fully cultured, admitted to the hospital, and given IV antibiotics. Febrile infants who appear well, have a normal examination, and have no historical risk factors undergo laboratory evaluation, including white blood cell count (WBC) and differential, blood culture, urinalysis and sterile urine culture (obtained via catheterization or suprapubic bladder tap), stool smear for leukocytes if diarrhea is present, and other testing as clinically indicated.

Infants are classified as "low risk" for SBI if they have no risk factors and a normal physical exam, a WBC of 5,000-15,000 cells/mcL with fewer than 1,500 bands, a sterilely-obtained urinalysis showing less than 10 WBCs per high power field, and, if diarrhea is present, a stool smear with less than 5 WBCs per high power field. These "low risk" infants are considered for close outpatient monitoring without treatment if a physician is available to assume responsibility for outpatient care and the parents have reliable observation skills, a phone in the home, and access to medical care within 30 minutes. These patients have a followup evaluation by phone in 12 hours, and re-examination within 24. Any patient who does not meet **all** of these "low risk" criteria must be managed conservatively, as discussed above. If the physician elects to treat a "low risk" patient with antibiotics, a lumbar puncture for CSF analysis and culture must be obtained prior to starting antibiotics.

Occult Bacteremia

Occult bacteremia refers to the presence of bacteria in the bloodstream of a febrile child without an obvious source. Fever is the presenting complaint in greater than 10% of all pediatric outpatient visits for children between 3-36 months. The great majority of such children appear well and many will have no evident focus of bacterial infection on exam, but between 3%-5% of children in this age group with temperature greater than 39°C will have bacteremia. Complications caused by bacteremia include pneumonia, osteomyelitis, meningitis, and other focal bacterial infections.

Risk factors

Several historical factors are helpful in assessing the likelihood that a febrile child is bacteremic. The age of the child is clearly important—the highest incidence occurs in children less than 24 months of age. Poor feeding, irritability, lethargy, and disrupted sleeping patterns also increase the likelihood of bacteremia. Examination should include a search for common infections such as otitis media, pharyngitis, pneumonia, osteomyelitis, cellulitis, and meningitis. General appearance, although subjective, is important; a sick or toxic-appearing child is more likely to have bacteria in the blood, but **a well-appearing child still can be bacteremic**. Numerous studies have demonstrated a correlation between temperature and the incidence of bacteremia; the incidence ranges from less than 1% in children with a temperature less than 39°C to as high as 20% in children with temperatures greater than 41°C.

In many studies, the utility of laboratory data to determine which febrile children are bacteremic has been evaluated. WBC count and differential, erythrocyte sedimentation rate, and antigen detection tests all have been advocated as such in the literature. The WBC count correlates with the incidence of bacteremia, varying from approximately 1% in children with a WBC count less than 15,000 to 10%-15% in children with WBC counts greater than 15,000, but other tests have not been shown to be predictive.

Pathogenesis

Currently, the organisms primarily responsible for bacteremia are Streptococcus pneumoniae and Neisseria meningitidis; the advent of the Hemophilus influenza type B (HIB) vaccine has markedly reduced the incidence of bacteremia from this organism. Persistent bacteremia, the development of focal bacterial complications, and mortality are more common with infections caused by H. influenza and N. meningitidis. Treatment of children with positive blood cultures is individualized according to organism and clinical scenario.

Treatment

Current guidelines suggest that children between the ages of 3-36 months with a temperature of greater than 39°C and no obvious focus of infection should undergo determination of WBC and differential. Some believe children with a WBC count greater than 15,000/mcL or more than 1,500 bands should receive empiric antibiotic therapy after obtaining blood, urine, and possibly cerebrospinal fluid cultures. Careful observation without antibiotic treatment is a reasonable alternative in this situation. **There is no substitute for close followup**.

Meningitis

Meningitis is one of the more serious diseases seen in children. Early symptoms can be subtle, nonspecific, and similar to those of benign viral infections; thus, a high index of suspicion must be present to avoid delay in diagnosis and treatment.

The most common cause of meningeal inflammation is **viral** or **aseptic meningitis**, in which there is clinical and laboratory evidence of meningitis but no bacteria on Gram stain or culture. **Nonpolio enteroviruses** cause most cases of aseptic meningitis in the US.

Pathogenesis

Incidence of **bacterial meningitis** is related to age. Nearly 100 cases per 100,000 live births occur in the first month of life, 45 per 100,000 during the second month, and nearly 80 per 100,000 at 6-8 months; 90% of cases occur between 1 month and 5 years of age. Before 1 month of age, two-thirds of cases are caused by group B Strep or Gram negative enteric organisms, primarily E. coli; Listeria monocytogenes is third on the list, but is very uncommon. After 1 month, most bacterial meningitis is caused by Neisseria meningitidis or Streptococcus pneumoniae; Haemophilus influenzae infection is now fairly rare because of immunization. All can be isolated from the throat or nasopharynx of healthy individuals, and there is evidence to suggest that children colonized with these organisms are at highest risk.

The immediate cause of meningitis is believed to be hematogenous spread during bacteremia from a remote infection, such as otitis media, sinusitis, pharyngitis, cellulitis, pneumonia, septic arthritis, or osteomyelitis. Any break in the integrity of the brain's protective cover increases the risk of meningitis. Meningitis can occur after head trauma, particularly if fractures of the paranasal sinuses occur. A persistent CSF leak after trauma is a known risk factor, and meningitis can follow an operation to drain ventricular fluid or other neurosurgical procedure.

History and exam

Typical symptoms of meningitis include headache, fever, lethargy, confusion, nausea, vomiting, stiff neck, and photophobia. Neonates and young infants may have only nonspecific findings such as temperature instability, poor feeding, irritability, or lethargy. Children with meningitis are usually febrile, but the absence of fever does not eliminate the diagnosis. Nuchal rigidity, focal neurologic signs, seizures, or coma can also occur, and infants can have full or bulging fontanelles. Papilledema is rare, and if present, raises the suspicion of a space occupying lesion such as an abscess. Petechiae and purpura can be seen with meningococcal meningitis, and indicate a high risk of imminent septic shock. Clinical presentation in any age group is highly variable, and **the diagnosis of meningitis should be considered in any febrile patient with any neurologic signs or symptoms, no matter how subtle**.

LP

When meningitis is suspected in a patient who does not have papilledema, a **lumbar puncture** should be performed for measurement of opening pressure and examination of CSF; if the fluid is turbid or purulent, antibiotics should be started immediately. A normal CSF WBC count in an infant greater than 1 month is less than 6 cells/mL, and 95% of healthy individuals have no polymorphonuclear cells (PMNs) in their CSF; a high WBC or the finding of PMNs in the CSF suggests meningitis. A Gram stain and culture are crucial, as are measurement of glucose and protein levels—glucose can be low and protein high in bacterial meningitis.

Treatment

Blood cultures should be obtained in all children with suspected bacterial meningitis; they yield the responsible organism up to 90% of the time. As soon as bacterial meningitis is diagnosed or strongly suspected, broad-spectrum IV antibiotics should be started. Cultures should be obtained before antibiotics are begun, but, in an emergency, antibiotic administration takes priority. Antibiotic coverage should be tailored to the sensitivities of the organism cultured; therapy is typically continued for 7-10 days.

Steroids have been found to decrease subsequent hearing loss and other neurologic sequelae in patients with Hemophilus influenza type B meningitis and should be strongly considered; the American Academy of Pediatrics Committee on Infectious Diseases currently recommends that dexamethasone be given at the time of the first dose of antimicrobial agents to children 2 months of age or older. **Prophylaxis** with rifampin or sulfisoxazole should be offered to household, day-care center, and nursery school contacts of patients with confirmed bacterial meningitis caused by N. meningitidis and (in certain cases) H. influenza type B.

Osteomyelitis

Osteomyelitis is infection of bone. It occurs in 1 of every 5,000 children under the age of 13, and is more frequent in males and children under 5. The most common causative organism is Staphylococcus aureus; others include Streptococci (especially group A; group B in neonates), Pseudomonas, Enterobacteriaceae, Salmonella (in patients with sickle cell disease), and Hemophilus influenza. Rarer causes include viruses, fungi, rickettsia, and some species of mycobacteria. Infection occurs by hematogenous spread, local invasion from a nearby focus of infection, or direct inoculation during trauma or operation.

Greater than 90% of cases involve tubular bones, usually those of the lower extremity; physical findings vary according to the age-related changes in bone structure. The neonatal skeleton has a thin cortex with loosely attached periosteum. Infection in this age group may extend through into the surrounding soft tissues, and the risk of associated septic arthritis is quite high; with increasing age, the periosteum is tighter and the risks of associated soft tissue infection and septic arthritis are less. Neonates are generally irritable with palpation or movement of the affected extremity, while older infants and children usually experience pain, display an obvious limp, or refuse to use the affected extremity. Point tenderness is common. Systemic symptoms are variable, not age-related, and not correlated with the severity of damage to the bone.

Diagnosis

Evaluation requires attempted isolation of bacteria from the bone itself by needle aspiration; blood cultures should be obtained but are often negative. WBC and erythrocyte sedimentation rate (ESR) are often elevated. A firm radiologic diagnosis via a plain film is often made in neonates, because decreased bone density is easily detected and an extended duration of disease is not required for changes to be present in this age group. In older patients, the characteristic findings of bone destruction and periosteal elevation due to new bone formation are generally not evident until 10-21 days after the onset of symptoms. Radionuclide imaging with Technetium 99m polyphosphate compounds is more than 90% accurate. Most institutions use a 3-phase bone scan: any condition causing increased blood flow to the area being examined will cause increased uptake in the first 2 phases, whereas only osteomyelitis causes focal uptake in the third. Bone scans are generally positive within the first few days after the onset of symptoms in older children, although can be unreliable in neonates. When Tc99m scans are nondiagnostic, Gallium 67 scans can be used. Gallium has slower elimination from the blood, and uptake in inflammatory foci is less dependent on blood flow.

Treatment

Treatment consists of IV antibiotics directed against the most likely organisms. Once culture results are obtained (bone or blood), coverage can be appropriately tailored, and transition to oral therapy is often considered once the patient is afebrile and local signs or symptoms are improved. Oral therapy is usually used only if a specific agent has been isolated and serum bactericidal concentrations of the drug can be monitored. Duration of therapy is generally 4-6 weeks, the first 2-3 of which are almost always parenteral; shorter courses have repeatedly been shown to be associated with poor outcome. Treatment is frequently continued until the ESR and WBC have returned to normal. Drainage is required if a soft tissue or periosteal abscess occurs.

Septic Arthritis

Septic arthritis, acute bacterial infection of a joint, is more common in children than adults; between one-half and two-thirds of affected patients are younger than 20. Lower extremity joints are the sites of 80% of cases. Bacterial entry into the joint occurs by the same mechanisms seen in osteomyelitis: hematogenous spread, local invasion, and direct inoculation.

Diagnosis

Staphylococcus aureus (the single most common cause), group A Streptococci, and Pneumococci are most commonly isolated. There has been a decrease in the number of cases caused by Hemophilus influenza type B because of immunization. Less common causative organisms include enteric Gram negative rods such as Enterobacteriaceae and Salmonella, group B Streptococcus in neonates, Neisseria gonorrhea in sexually active adolescents, and Pseudomonas in patients with a history of IV drug use.

Neonates with septic joints frequently do not develop fever or appear toxic, although older children with septic joints almost always experience **fever** and **malaise** in addition to focal pain, swelling, warmth, and erythema. A patient with a septic hip usually keeps the joint abducted and externally rotated, because this is the position of lowest intracapsular pressure and greatest comfort, but may not have other focal signs.

The diagnosis is made by isolation of the offending organism from joint fluid via needle aspiration. Fluid should be cultured, and a Gram stain is essential. Up to 30% of joint fluid samples from patients with clinical and laboratory findings consistent with septic arthritis are sterile. Fluid should be examined for clotting ability, number and type of leukocytes, and glucose content. Fluid from a septic joint generally has more than 50,000 WBC/mcL with more than 90% PMNs and a glucose concentration that is only 30% of the serum value, while joint fluid from patients with an inflammatory process such as juvenile rheumatoid arthritis typically has fewer leukocytes (15-20,000/mcL) and a glucose concentration close to that of the blood.

Treatment   Initial treatment is the same as that for osteomyelitis; once an organism is isolated, coverage is narrowed. Oral antibiotics can be used to complete the treatment course because antibiotic penetration into the joint capsule is generally good. Duration of therapy is typically 2-4 weeks; efficacy can be determined by re-examination and/or serial aspiration and assessment of joint fluid. Operative drainage is needed when there is sufficient fibrous material within the joint to prevent good drainage via needle aspiration. In certain special cases, such as hip or shoulder infections in infants, immediate operative drainage is usually indicated. ∎

50   Common Outpatient Infections

Infectious diseases are by far the most common complaint of children visiting their pediatrician. Most problems are viral and consequently self-limited, and nearly all can be managed on an outpatient basis.

Otitis

Otitis externa

There are two common inflammatory conditions of the ear in children: otitis externa and media. **Otitis externa** ("swimmer's ear") is irritation of the ear canal secondary to frequent swimming or bathing, impacted cerumen, or a foreign body. Although normally a sterile inflammation, superinfection with pseudomonas, Staphylococcus, or fungi may supervene. Examination reveals an erythematous canal with scaling or purulent drainage; pain with manipulation of the pinna is pathognomonic. Treatment consists of simply keeping the canal clean and dry; topical antibiotics and corticosteroid ear drops are sometimes helpful.

Otitis media

Otitis media (OM) is an infection of the middle ear. About three-quarters of children will have at least one episode during their childhood (highest frequency 6 months to 2 years); a quarter experience repeated infections. About a third of episodes are viral infections, with respiratory syncytial virus (RSV) being most common, while the rest are bacterial, usually due to Streptococcus pneumoniae, nontypable Haemophilus influenzae, or Moraxella catarrhalis. Older children usually complain of ear pain, while infants usually display only irritability, crying and difficulty sleeping; fever is present in fewer than half the cases, and tugging at ears is an unreliable sign. Diagnosis is based on the presence of a red, bulging tympanic membrane (TM) with fluid, generally cloudy or yellow, behind the drum, although a red TM in a screaming child can be normal. Obscured landmarks and a splayed light reflex, as well as decreased tympanic mobility noted on insufflation, are helpful. Definitive diagnosis can be made by tympanocentesis for culture; this procedure is not generally necessary but should be considered for persistent OM despite apparently adequate therapy.

Treatment for acute OM often begins with amoxicillin, although it is not effective against beta-lactamase positive organisms (some Hemophilus and Moraxella). Trimethoprim-sulfamethoxazole (TMP/SMX) or Augmentin (amoxicillin and clavulanate) are used if amoxicillin is not working or if OM occurs within 2 months of the last infection with no proved resolution. Ceftriaxone is effective, and since it is given only once (by injection) it is useful if poor compliance is anticipated. New broad spectrum antibiotics are being introduced regularly and may end up offering better results. Improvement should occur after 48 hours—if not, resistant organisms might be present. This condition can be extremely painful: acetaminophen or ibuprofen, topical analgesic drops, and local heat are helpful. Prophylaxis should be considered if there are more than 3 episodes in 6 months or 4 in a year; after full treatment of the current infection the child should begin daily antibiotics for 3-6 months, particularly during the winter (frequent colds block the Eustachian tubes). Parental smoking and day care attendance have been shown to increase the incidence of OM, while breast feeding decreases it. Surgical pressure equalizing (PE) tubes are indicated if recurrent infections persist despite adequate prophylaxis. Ruptured TMs can occur (with prompt resolution of pain) but generally heal without sequelae. Hearing loss and subsequent speech delay are the most concerning complications of recurrent OM. Rarely, cholesteatoma, labyrinthitis, mastoiditis, osteomyelitis of the temporal bone or facial nerve paralysis can occur.

Sinusitis

Not nearly as frequent as otitis media, **sinusitis** complicates about 0.5%-5% of upper respiratory infections (URIs) in early childhood. Mucosal swelling (viral URI, allergic inflammation, facial trauma) or mechanical obstruction (choanal atresia, deviated septum, nasal polyps, foreign body, tumor) produce sinus ostial obstruction and resulting infection. Bacteria (Streptococcus pneumoniae, nontypable Hemophilus influenzae, Moraxella catarrhalis) account for about 90% of cases; viral causes (adenovirus, parainfluenzae, influenza, rhinovirus) make up the rest. Symptoms include persistent nasal discharge (longer than 10 days), persistent daytime cough, and malodorous breath. Facial pain and headache are uncommon, while nasal discharge can be of any quality; a cough is frequently present during the day but worse at night due to post-nasal drip. The combination of fever and purulent nasal discharge is highly suggestive of sinusitis.

Physical examination generally is not very helpful in children under 10. Periorbital swelling or tenderness over the sinuses is helpful but rare, and transillumination is hard to perform in small children. The benefit of imaging is somewhat controversial; diffuse sinus opacification, mucosal thickening of at least 4mm, or air-fluid levels present on plain radiographs are suggestive of the diagnosis. CT scans are not needed for uncomplicated sinusitis, but can be of use in complicated or chronic situations.

Treatment is identical to that of OM. If there is no improvement in 48 hours, the patient should be re-evaluated. Treatment is continued for 10-14 days. Recurrent sinusitis suggests the possibility of cystic fibrosis or an underlying immunodeficiency.

Conjunctivitis

Conjunctivitis

While sinusitis may make the child feel miserable, **conjunctivitis**, typically painless, is more likely to get him or her sent home from school! Commonly referred to as "pinkeye," conjunctivitis is caused by bacteria or viruses. It is impossible to tell the difference between bacterial and viral conjunctivitis on clinical grounds alone. Symptoms include marked conjunctival hyperemia and moderate to copious purulent drainage; the eyelids are frequently stuck together upon wakening by dried discharge. Inflammation at lid margins is common. Nontypable Haemophilus influenzae and Strep pneumoniae are most common, followed by adenovirus and other viruses. Treatment consists of ophthalmic "polytrim" (polymixin and trimethoprim), polymixin bacitracin, or erythromycin drops (or ointment) placed in both eyes. Sodium sulamyd drops, gentamicin, or tetracycline are also used but can burn. Warm damp washcloths facilitate the removal of the dried discharge. Conjunctivitis is highly contagious, and it is important to wash hands and avoid sharing of towels and linen. The infection should resolve in less than a week; children are not infectious after 48 hours of treatment and thus can return to school or day care after that time.

Allergic conjunctivitis

Allergic conjunctivitis can mimic infectious conjunctivitis, but the former is particularly itchy, produces a stringy, mucoid discharge, and is often seasonal or associated with hay fever. In neonates with conjunctivitis, the presence of Chlamydia trachomatis and Neisseria gonorrhea should be considered. The nasopharynx (as well as the eyes) should be cultured, and the infant should be treated based on culture results. Nasolacrimal duct obstruction (seen in up to 6% of newborns) is another cause of early conjunctivitis. The combination of conjunctivitis and pharyngitis suggests adenovirus, and the combination of OM and conjunctivitis suggests nontypable Haemophilus influenzae (oral antibiotic treatment without the ophthalmic antimicrobials is sufficient in this situation).

Upper Respiratory Tract Infections

Sore throat

Next to OM, the presence of a sore throat and fever may prompt the most office visits in the pediatric age group. **Pharyngitis** is almost always viral; only about 10% are due to Group A beta-hemolytic Streptococci although the latter are much more important to diagnose and treat. **Strep throat** is most frequently seen in school-age children during the school year (due to close person-to-person contact). Cervical adenitis, palatal petechiae, a beefy-red uvula and a tonsillar exudate are typical, although this classic presentation is uncommon in children under 3. Vomiting, anorexia, and headache can be present. Throat culture is the gold standard; rapid tests are specific, but sensitivity varies. Strep throat must always be treated, because of the possible complication of acute rheumatic fever. Penicillin is the treatment of choice, but if the child can't (or won't) swallow pills, liquid amoxicillin is better tasting than liquid penicillin (although amoxicillin use in a child with mononucleosis can cause a rash). Erythromycin or first-generation cephalosporins are used in penicillin-allergic patients.

Adenovirus is the most likely pathogen in viral pharyngitis. Others include influenza, parainfluenza, infectious mononucleosis (Epstein-Barr virus, EBV), herpes simplex virus, and various coxsackie viruses. Children under the age of 3 generally have viral pharyngitis. Symptoms are similar to those of strep pharyngitis. Adenovirus can cause an exudative pharyngitis similar to strep, and conjunctivitis is sometimes present. EBV infections can lead to generalized lymphadenopathy and splenomegaly; a positive mononucleosis spot test (Monospot) is common in older children (but is not as sensitive in younger ones). Coxsackie A infections usually produce vesicles or ulcers. Treatment for viral pharyngitis consists of supportive measures only. The maintenance of adequate hydration is most important; liquids (popsicles are useful) should be taken in sufficient amounts.

Common cold

A sore throat is one of the hallmark symptoms of the **common cold**; children average 6-8 colds per year. Transmission is by aerosolization (sneezing). Rhinoviruses, parainfluenza viruses, and respiratory syncytial virus (RSV) are the three most common causes, but more than 200 viruses can cause the common cold. Rhinoviruses are most common in fall and spring, RSV and influenza in winter, and adenoviruses in summer. Symptoms include throat irritation, sneezing, and nasal congestion at first, followed (in a couple of days) by rhinitis and watery eyes. Hoarseness and cough secondary to post-nasal drip can develop. Fever is usually low-grade, if present at all. Young infants are likely to be irritable and restless, and more likely to have fever. Treatment remains only symptomatic because no effective antiviral agent exists. Cold remedies have little benefit and can be harmful in younger children (by masking more serious infections and by producing sedation), although acetaminophen will help with fever or discomfort. Humidification and the use of nasal saline drops are both helpful. Parental smoking will aggravate and prolong symptoms—the frequency of colds in households where a member smokes is increased.

Gastroenteritis

Diarrhea

Another frequent cause for parental concern is diarrhea. **Gastroenteritis** can also be due to bacterial or viral agents. Bacterial gastroenteritis often presents with bloody stool (differentiating it from viral gastroenteritis). Salmonella presents with fever, abdominal pain, and liquid, foul-smelling stool with leukocytes and gross or occult blood. Bacteremia is present in 5%-10% of cases.

Patients with Shigella have fever, tenesmus, abdominal pain, and emesis, and can develop neurologic symptoms. Stool is typically grossly bloody. Other bacterial agents include Yersinia, Campylobacter (which can closely mimic appendicitis) and E. coli (invasive, enterotoxic, enteropathogenic and hemorrhagic 0157:H7). Diagnosis is made by stool culture for Salmonella, Shigella, Yersinia, and Campylobacter. Specialized tests for strains of E. coli are generally not performed routinely, but one can culture E. coli 0157:H7 using sorbitol McConky plates. Treatment varies. Mild Salmonella infections do not require therapy, but ampicillin or TMP/SMX should be used if the infection is severe or the patient is bacteremic or very young. Shigella and invasive E. coli are usually treated with TMP/SMX for 5 days. Campylobacter is also generally treated with erythromycin for 5-7 days, while infection with Yersinia and the others are usually self-limited and do not require treatment.

The most common viral agent is rotavirus, accounting for roughly half the diarrheal illnesses in children. Occurring in all age groups, it is especially common in children from 6-24 months of age, and is most often seen in late winter or early spring. Diarrhea is explosive and watery, and infection often produces emesis. A low-grade fever and concurrent URI are common. Other viral agents include enteric adenovirus and Norwalk-like viruses. These pathogens can be cultured, although this can take weeks. Rotavirus is diagnosed by an enzyme immunoassay that is quick, reliable, and sensitive. There is no cure for viral gastroenteritis. Fluid and electrolyte replacement should be administered as needed; oral rehydration is preferred to parenteral if emesis is not a significant problem.

Chicken Pox

Chicken pox

A discussion of outpatient childhood diseases would not be complete without **chicken pox**. This viral disease, caused by the varicella-zoster virus (VZV) is extremely contagious; it is spread by respiratory secretions or by direct contact with freshly erupted vesicles. The disease is communicable from 1-2 days before the rash or any other symptoms occur, and afterward until all the vesicles have crusted over (6-8 days). The incubation period is 10-21 days. Therefore, the absence of vesicles does not imply lack of communicability! About 90% of people acquire chicken pox during childhood, then have lifelong immunity. Chicken pox is much less severe in children than in adults. It begins with a mild prodrome of malaise and low-grade fever, followed in a couple of days by the eruption of vesicles, appearing in crops. These usually start on the scalp and mucosal surfaces, followed by the trunk and extremities. A reddish macule first appears that becomes a papule, then develops into a vesicle on an erythematous base (referred to as "a dewdrop on a rose petal"). This gradually becomes a crusted vesicle and finally a scab. Pruritus can become severe when the vesicles are crusting. Diagnosis is obvious, especially in the setting of crops of lesions in various stages of development. Herpes zoster (shingles) can occur later in patients who have already had chicken pox (due to reactivation of viruses dormant in sensory nerve ganglia) and can present first with pain at the site where the vesicles will appear a few days later—a classic puzzler for the first few days when it occurs in adults.

Treatment of chicken pox is generally supportive. Antivirals such as acyclovir are usually reserved for complicated cases, although some studies have shown the use of acyclovir early on in the course of the disease can shorten the time course and lessen the severity. VZIG (varicella-zoster immune globulin) should be given immediately to immunocompromised patients exposed to the virus; they are at risk for severe infection. Treatment of pruritus with topical agents or Benadryl is helpful: scarring occurs if the scabs are picked, therefore the elimination of scratching is important. Complications from chicken pox are rare, but pneumonia can occur in adults and the immunocompromised. The most common complication in children is bacterial superinfection of the vesicles. A live attenuated VZV vaccine has recently been approved in the USA, so chicken pox may one day become as uncommon as measles and mumps are now. ■

51   **Pediatric Respiratory Diseases**

Respiratory diseases that children face include **asthma,
pneumonia, bronchiolitis, foreign bodies** in the trachea
and lungs, **croup**, and **epiglottitis**. **Sudden infant death
syndrome (SIDS)** is hypothesized to be due to respiratory problems and is also discussed below.

Clinical manifestations of respiratory distress in children
include hyperpnea, cyanosis, use of accessory muscles,
head-bobbing, grunting, and mental status changes. If the
PCO_2 is greater than 40mmHg in a child not known to
chronically hypoventilate (e.g., with bronchopulmonary
dysplasia), respiratory failure **may be** imminent; if
greater than 50, respiratory failure **is** imminent.

Asthma

Asthma is the leading cause of hospital admissions and
affects 10%-15% of boys and 7%-10% of girls at some
time during childhood; incidence and associated morbidity and mortality have **increased** dramatically in the last
20 years. There is no universally accepted definition, but
asthma, in general, is a diffuse obstructive lung disease
caused by hyperreactivity of the large and small airways
leading to inflammation, smooth muscle contraction, and
mucus secretion. The stimuli for airway constriction
include viruses, fumes and smoke, exercise, cold air, and
various allergens such as dust mites, pollen, and vegetable
proteins. Age of onset is variable, with 30% of those who
have asthma exhibiting symptoms by age 1, and 80%-
90% by age 5. Only about 5% of those with asthma are
severely affected; these patients often have a strong family history of asthma or atopy and usually experience the
onset of symptoms before 1 year of age.

**Signs and
symptoms**

The combination of edema, smooth muscle contraction,
and increased mucus production leads to diffuse airway
obstruction, primarily during exhalation (which is prolonged). This leads to air trapping, causing increased
work of breathing. Onset of symptoms can be rapid, upon
exposure to an irritating agent, or insidious, arising after a
viral infection or prolonged exposure to a less noxious
stimulus. The usual symptoms are cough, wheezing (**not**
always present), tachypnea, dyspnea, or even frank

respiratory arrest; wheezing may not occur if obstruction is severe enough because air movement may not be adequate to produce audible sounds.

CXR

Chest x-ray (CXR) usually shows hyperinflation only. Most physicians obtain a CXR on any child with a first episode of wheezing to rule out other causes; a CXR is not generally useful during subsequent episodes unless the child is febrile. Oxygen saturation should be checked; treatment can transiently decrease arterial oxygen tension by increasing ventilation-perfusion mismatch as airways to underperfused areas are opened. Arterial blood gases should be checked in those who are showing signs of fatigue or other signs of respiratory failure or are not responding to therapy.

PFTs

Once a child is old enough to cooperate, pulmonary function testing (see Chapter 35, "Thoracic Surgery") is useful. Functional vital capacity (FVC) and forced expiratory volume in one second (FEV_1) are usually decreased, and total lung capacity (TLC), functional residual capacity (FRC), and residual volume (RV) are usually increased. The presence of obstruction (FEV_1 less than 80% of predicted) with more than 10% improvement after administration of bronchodilators is diagnostic of asthma.

The diagnosis of asthma, however, is usually clinical and is based on recurrent episodes of wheezing and dyspnea. Occasional patients with asthma have only a cough (without wheezing). Unless the child is old enough to have pulmonary function testing, the diagnosis of asthma may need to be assumed. This entity, termed **cough-variant asthma**, is not uncommon. The differential diagnosis of asthma is important to consider during the first episode of wheezing as well as during subsequent episodes. Other diseases to consider include foreign body aspiration, congenital malformations, bronchiolitis, pneumonia, gastroesophageal reflux, and cystic fibrosis: "all that wheezes is not asthma."

Treatment

The goals of treatment of an **acute** asthma attack are to relax the airway smooth muscle, reduce inflammation and edema, and, if possible, decrease mucus production. The **beta-2 receptor agonists** are rapid-acting smooth muscle relaxants. To reduce the beta-1-mediated side effects such as tachycardia and tremor, beta-2 selective agents such as

albuterol are preferable. **Epinephrine**, historically the most commonly used medication, is beta-nonselective. **Corticosteroids** are used to reduce inflammation; because they take a few hours to work, it is preferable to give the first dose soon after the onset of an asthma exacerbation. A short course (5 days) of treatment has been shown to be safe and effective. **Theophylline** has many effects including bronchodilation and stimulation of the diaphragm; multiple studies, however, have shown that it provides no additional benefit in children when used in conjunction with standard therapy. Finally, **acetylcholine-receptor inhibitors** prevent smooth muscle contraction; recent studies demonstrate benefit in the treatment of acute bronchospasm when used in conjunction with the beta-2 agonists.

Long-term management

Long-term management of patients with asthma has changed considerably in recent years. All patients with asthma should be considered candidates for chronic treatment with an agent that reduces airway inflammation and/or reactivity, both to reduce the frequency and severity of exacerbations, and to reduce damage from chronic inflammation. The two agents used for this purpose are **cromolyn** and **inhaled corticosteroids**. Cromolyn stabilizes mast cell membranes, and is effective in approximately 80% of children with asthma. Inhaled corticosteroids are more likely to be beneficial, but are less well tolerated due to taste and the possibility of oral candidiasis with chronic use. Modification of the patient's environment to reduce the exposure to irritants is also important; cessation of smoking (by the patient and household members) is required. Yearly influenza immunization should be offered to these patients because this disease, if acquired, often affects patients with asthma severely.

Pneumonia

Pneumonia can be caused by bacteria, viruses, or mycoplasma. **Bacterial pneumonia** in children is often secondary to a primary viral upper respiratory infection with aspiration of oral flora; less commonly, hematogenous spread can occur. Recurrent pneumonia is rare and raises the possibility of underlying disease such as cystic fibrosis, bronchiectasis, or an aspirated foreign body. *(continued)*

Pediatrics
Pediatric Respiratory Diseases *continued*

The most common causative agent in children is Streptococcus pneumoniae (pneumococcus). Staphylococcus aureus, group A Streptococcus, and, now less commonly, Haemophilus influenzae type B can also cause pneumonia. Pneumonia in the neonatal period is caused by the same organisms responsible for generalized neonatal sepsis (see Chapter 49, "Pediatric Infectious Diseases").

Signs and symptoms

Signs and symptoms referable to the lower respiratory tract are often absent in younger children. In infants, illness usually begins with 2-3 days of upper respiratory symptoms, followed by the sudden onset of high fever, irritability, and respiratory distress. Cough is unusual. Presentation in children and teenagers is similar to that in adults; a brief upper respiratory infection is followed by shaking chills and fever, often accompanied by splinting and a dry cough. Physical exam usually shows signs of consolidation such as decreased breath sounds, dullness to percussion, and possibly rales. Laboratory studies reveal a leukocytosis with a left shift. CXR findings are variable: pneumococcus usually causes lobar consolidation, although other bacteria can produce an interstitial infiltrate. Blood and sputum cultures should be obtained in all hospitalized children in an attempt to determine the organism responsible but are not always helpful.

Management

Management depends on the severity of illness. Most children can be treated on an outpatient basis with oral antibiotics, but hospitalization is recommended for infants and is required for any child who is hypoxic or appears toxic. Since isolating the causative organism is often difficult, therapy should be selected to cover the most common organisms (as well as Mycoplasma in older children and teenagers).

Viral pneumonia

Respiratory syncytial virus (RSV) is the most common cause of **viral pneumonia** in children. It causes pneumonia in pre-school children and bronchiolitis (see below) in infants younger than 2 years. Parainfluenza, adenovirus, and enterovirus are also common. Clinical manifestations are similar to those of bacterial pneumonia, and wheezing is often present, especially with RSV. CXR most often demonstrates a diffuse, perihilar infiltrate, but lobar infiltrates and focal atelectasis can occur. Few effective antiviral therapies exist; ribavirin is helpful. Most clinicians will treat the patients for presumed bacterial pneumonia when infiltrates in association with fever are present.

Mycoplasma pneumonia

Mycoplasma (walking or atypical) pneumonia is rare before age 3; peak incidence is in school-aged children. It causes one third of pneumonias in 5-9 year-olds, and two-thirds in 9-15 year-olds. Illness progresses gradually. Symptoms typically include headache, malaise, fever, dry cough, and often a sore throat; substernal chest pain can occur. The cough often worsens and becomes more productive of sputum. The WBC and differential are usually normal, and CXR often shows a bilateral interstitial infiltrate or lobar pattern. The diagnosis is usually made on clinical grounds; a positive cold agglutinin test is helpful. A macrolide such as erythromycin, azithromycin, or clarithromycin is the antibiotic of choice.

Bronchiolitis

Bronchiolitis is an acute respiratory viral infection seen in children under age 2; respiratory syncytial virus (RSV) is the cause in the vast majority of cases. While the prognosis is good for healthy infants with bronchiolitis, infants with underlying cardiac or pulmonary disease (preterm infants or those with bronchopulmonary dysplasia) are at increased risk for complications and death. Clinical features include tachypnea and wheezing. Apnea can occur, more commonly in very young or preterm infants. CXR typically reveals hyperinflation and atelectasis. Fluorescent antibody techniques, ELISA assays, and viral cultures of nasopharyngeal secretions can identify the responsible organism.

Most infants can be managed with close outpatient monitoring and careful attention to hydration. Hospitalization is required for those requiring oxygen or IV fluids and for those with underlying cardiopulmonary disease. Antiviral treatment with aerosolized ribavirin may be used for RSV bronchiolitis. Bronchodilator therapy is generally not effective, and there is no role for antimicrobial agents or steroids.
(continued)

Foreign Bodies

Children have a tendency to put anything in their mouths, and any **foreign body** can enter the respiratory tract. Respiratory foreign bodies are most frequently seen in 6 month- to 2 year-olds, but can be seen in younger children if an older child is around to put objects in the infant's mouth. Symptoms are usually of abrupt onset, but a symptom-free period followed by infection can occur. Symptoms depend on where the object lodges. If in the nose, sneezing, cough, mild discomfort, and bloody sputum are usual; if in the larynx, respiratory distress, hoarseness, croupy cough, aphonia, hemoptysis, and dyspnea with wheezing all are possible. Tracheal foreign bodies generally cause wheezing and, less commonly, cough, hoarseness, dyspnea, and cyanosis. A unilateral wheeze, right-sided more commonly than left, may occur in the setting of a bronchial foreign body. Most foreign bodies are radiolucent, but inspiratory and expiratory chest films or fluoroscopy can reveal differential overdistention due to air trapping. X-rays can be deferred if suspicion is high.

Treatment

Removal of most nasal foreign bodies can be readily accomplished in the ED. If the presence of a bronchial or tracheal foreign body is established or highly suspected, either fiberoptic bronchoscopy or direct laryngoscopy **in the operating room** is undertaken; rigid bronchoscopy is usually required to remove the object. Large tracheal and laryngeal foreign bodies can produce sudden, lethal airway obstruction, usually before the patient has the chance to reach the hospital. The Heimlich maneuver is recommended for children over the age of 1, while back blows and abdominal thrusts should be used in younger children.

Croup

Croup is a general term used to describe inspiratory stridor, cough, and hoarseness resulting from airway obstruction in the region of the larynx; in common usage, "croup" refers to a disease of viral origin. Parainfluenza viruses types 1 or 3 are the cause in two-thirds of cases, but influenza A and B, respiratory syncytial virus (RSV), adenoviruses, rhinoviruses, and enteroviruses also cause croup. Croup typically occurs in children ranging from about 3 months to 5 years of age, and peak incidence is from October to December, although croup may occur at any time of the year. The differential diagnosis of croup includes foreign body aspiration, tracheal compression by masses or aberrant vessels (e.g., vascular ring), laryngomalacia, bacterial tracheitis, and epiglottitis.

The clinical course is characterized by upper respiratory symptoms, low grade fever, and the gradual onset of hoarseness, a barky cough, and stridor, typically worse at night. There is generally a narrow subglottic airway, the so-called "steeple sign," on neck x-ray.

Treatment

Treatment of croup is symptomatic. A cool mist vaporizer or warm steam from the shower is often helpful; children frequently improve on the car ride to the hospital, presumably because of the cool, moist night air. Crying makes croup worse, so minimizing agitation is important. Treatment strategies include mist (in a tent, with or without supplemental oxygen), corticosteroids, and racemic epinephrine in children with significant stridor; use of epinephrine mandates either hospitalization or observation for a minimum of 6 hours because its effect may only be temporary. Rarely, intubation can be required for patients with severe upper airway obstruction and respiratory distress.

Epiglottitis

Epiglottitis is a rapidly progressive infection of the epiglottis and surrounding airway structures which can produce sudden, catastrophic airway obstruction. The cause in nearly all cases is Haemophilus influenzae type B, although rarely other organisms, such as Staphylococcus aureus, have been documented. Incidence has markedly decreased with the advent of the Hemophilus influenzae type B (HIB) vaccine. Epiglottitis is usually seen in children ranging in age from 1-7, and there is no seasonal variation. Patients typically develop the abrupt onset of high fever and rapidly worsen over the next 8-12 hours. The patient looks toxic and assumes the characteristic position of **sitting forward with the neck extended and mouth open**. This is accompanied by drooling, a sore throat, and a muffled voice or aphonia secondary to pain. In contrast to croup, cough, hoarseness, and stridor are rare. When a child presents

with these classic signs and symptoms, the diagnosis of
epiglottitis is apparent. If the diagnosis is unclear,
a lateral neck x-ray should be obtained; the characteristic
"thumb print" sign of a swollen epiglottis is
pathognomonic.

Management

Epiglottitis is an emergent, life-threatening problem. **A
patient suspected of having epiglottitis should not be
left unattended**. Every effort should be made to keep the
patient calm. Manipulations should be avoided; the child
should not be placed in the supine position and **the pharynx should not be examined**. A child with epiglottitis
must be taken to the operating room quickly for controlled intubation; an endotracheal tube one size smaller
than estimated for age is generally used. Once the airway
is secured, parenteral antibiotics should then be given.

SIDS/ALTE

SIDS

Sudden infant death syndrome (**SIDS**) is defined as the
sudden death of a child under 1 that remains unexplained
after thorough investigation including post-mortem examination, examination of the death scene, and review of the
history. SIDS, therefore, is a diagnosis of exclusion. SIDS
occurs throughout the world. In the US, SIDS is the leading cause of post-neonatal (28 days-1 year) death; the
incidence ranges from 1.6-2.3 /1,000 live births. SIDS
deaths peak at 2 months, and 90% of deaths occur prior
to 6 months of age. Most SIDS deaths occur between
midnight and 9:00 am.

Risk factors

Risk for SIDS can be divided into maternal, infant, and
environmental factors. **Maternal** risk factors include
smoking, young maternal age (less than 20), lack of prenatal care, poor socioeconomic status, increased parity
and short interpregnancy intervals, and a family history
of SIDS. **Infant** risk factors include low birth weight,
prematurity, multiple births, male sex (approximately a
3:2 predominance in most series), prone sleeping position, and soft sleeping surfaces. **Environmental** risk factors include winter and hyperthermia. **Possible** risk factors for which there are conflicting data include lack of
breastfeeding and maternal use of illegal drugs such as
cocaine and narcotics during pregnancy. There is **no**
evidence that the DPT or any other immunization
increases risk.

Patho-physiology	The cause(s) of SIDS are unknown. Proposed mechanisms include apnea, asphyxia from rebreathing carbon dioxide, a blunted arousal mechanism, cardiac conduction abnormalities, metabolic disorders, abnormal thermoregulation, infection (mild infections precede death in many SIDS victims), and chronic hypoxia. In 1992 the American Academy of Pediatrics (AAP) recommended that healthy infants, when being put down for sleep, be positioned on their **side or back** ("back to sleep"). The AAP acknowledged that there were still good reasons to place certain infants in the prone position, including infants with gastroesophageal reflux, those with certain upper airway anomalies, and premature infants with respiratory distress. **Countries that have recommended avoidance of the prone sleeping position have experienced significantly decreased SIDS rates.** Unfortunately, despite current knowledge, the US has been slow to adopt this practice. There is also evidence that soft, "gas-trapping" sleeping surfaces play a role; the AAP recommended in 1994 that soft surfaces and gas-trapping objects be avoided in an infant's sleeping environment.
ALTE	An **apparent life-threatening event** (**ALTE**) is defined as an episode involving an infant that is frightening to the observer and that involves some combination of apnea, color change (most often cyanotic or pallid but occasionally plethoric), hypo- or hypertonia, bradycardia, and/or choking, often leading to vigorous stimulation or resuscitation attempts. The relationship between ALTEs and SIDS is unclear. In the past such episodes were called "near-miss SIDS" or "aborted SIDS." These terms should be abandoned because they imply a relationship which probably does not exist: most infants with an ALTE do not die of SIDS, most infants who die of SIDS have not had an ALTE (a history of a prior ALTE is present in less than 7% of SIDS victims), and home monitoring programs for infants who have experienced an ALTE have not lowered the SIDS death rate.
Workup	The differential diagnosis of an ALTE is very broad and includes infectious (sepsis, RSV), respiratory (airway abnormality, vascular ring, breath holding spell), gastrointestinal (gastroesophageal reflux), neurologic (seizure disorder, meningitis), cardiovascular (congenital malformation, arrhythmia, cardiomyopathy), metabolic (inborn

error of metabolism, hypoglycemia), and traumatic (abuse, drug overdose) entities. History is especially important, and should cover the time course of the last 24 hours, becoming increasingly "microscopic" as the time of the event gets closer. A second-by-second description of the event, any interventions needed or performed, and subsequent appearance of the child is warranted. A serum bicarbonate level should be obtained to look for evidence of acidosis or chronic hypoventilation.

Management

A child who has experienced an ALTE should be hospitalized for evaluation and monitoring, observation of subsequent spells, and counseling and teaching for the parents (as well as for any specific treatment needed). A possible cause for the ALTE is identified only about half the time. The decision whether to institute home apnea monitoring is complicated; if home monitoring is instituted, the parents must be taught infant CPR. ■

52   Pediatric Cardiology

Pediatric cardiology is the study of heart problems in children, the cause of which is overwhelmingly congenital. The prevalence of congenital heart defects is 8 per 1,000 live births, and cardiac malformations are the leading cause of death due to congenital problems.

Approach to the Pediatric Heart Patient[1]

Children with heart disease present in a variety of ways; the recognition that a problem exists is the first step, and is not as straightforward as it is in adults. Although peripheral cyanosis, the result of sluggish blood flow in the extremities, is a frequent finding in the normal newborn, the presence of **central cyanosis** is always abnormal and often is the earliest marker of heart disease. Central cyanosis is best identified by looking at the tongue or mucous membranes (which should be pink). **Gray pallor** indicates shock from any cause. **Clubbing**, a thickening of tissues at the bases of the nails, is a consequence of chronic hypoxemia and is rare in infants under 3 months. **Peaceful tachypnea**, or more than 60 breaths per minute (in newborns) without noticeable effort, is seen in 90% of infants with serious heart disease. With increasing pulmonary congestion or hypoxemia, true **dyspnea** can be seen, which can be especially prominent with feeding, crying, or exercise (in older children). The clinical hallmarks of **congestive heart failure (CHF)** in children are "too (2) fast and too (2) big:" tachypnea and tachycardia; hepatomegaly and cardiomegaly. While **syncope** can occur due to an arrhythmia or an obstructive heart lesion, **chest pain** in children is rarely of cardiac etiology. Recognition (or suspicion) that a defined syndrome (such as Down's or Turner's) exists increases the likelihood that a congenital heart defect is present. Similarly, because about 25% of children with heart disease have extracardiac anomalies, the presence of a noncardiac congenital malformation increases the chance of a congenital heart defect. **Failure to thrive**, **diffuse diaphoresis**, or **unexplained persistent lethargy** or **irritability**, although nonspecific, should also prompt a search for a cardiac lesion.
(continued)

[1] With thanks to J. Peter Harris, MD, consummate clinical pediatric cardiologist, for his "pearls," especially regarding peaceful tachypnea and the second heart sound.

Physical examination

Examination can be difficult in children—like anything else, it takes practice. **Failure of the second heart sound (S_2) to split** usually indicates congenital heart disease, but **murmurs** are most often benign, and almost every child at one time or another will have one. In general, murmurs that are loud (more than grade 3/6 or so), pan- or late systolic, diastolic, or continuous are pathologic. Of course, the absence of a murmur does not indicate the absence of heart disease. **Ejection** or **midsystolic clicks** and the presence of a **fourth heart sound (S_4)** also suggest cardiac pathology. **Poor pulses** suggest reduced cardiac output, and **decreased lower extremity pulses and blood pressure**, especially with upper extremity hypertension, are the classic signs of coarctation of the aorta.

Other diagnostic tests

Echocardiography is a valuable investigative tool in the child with suspected cardiac disease. It is very accurate, and physiologic data (such as pressure gradients and direction of flow) in addition to anatomic information can be collected. If more information is needed, **cardiac catheterization** will demonstrate the relevant anatomy, and can provide useful information in the form of pressures and oxygen content of the various chambers.

Congenital heart problems are most conveniently divided into three categories: left-to-right shunts ("acyanotic" defects), obstructive lesions, and complex defects (often "cyanotic").

Left-to-Right Shunts

Conditions where an opening exists between the two sides of the circulation result in flow of blood from the left to the right side of the heart if pulmonary resistance is less than systemic resistance (**left-to-right shunt**). Because the shunted blood is fully oxygenated, these are also called **acyanotic defects**. The major problems these defects pose are a reduction in systemic output and increased pulmonary blood flow with the risk of eventual pulmonary hypertension (see below).

VSD

Ventricular septal defects (VSD) constitute 20%-25% of congenital heart defects (most common, if bicuspid aortic valves are excluded). Most (80%) occur in the perimembranous portion of the septum, while muscular VSDs occur in the trabecular septum below. Subarterial (supracristal) VSDs are defects in the infundibular or outlet septum, and since part of the defect involves the aortic valve annulus, aortic insufficiency can occur. Small defects are asymptomatic, producing a harsh, holosystolic or regurgitant murmur at the left lower sternal border. EKG and chest x-ray (CXR) are normal. Moderate to large defects, in contrast, are associated with decreased exercise tolerance, frequent respiratory infections, delayed growth and development, and congestive heart failure (CHF). These defects produce a loud P_2 with holosystolic or ejection murmurs depending on the size of the defect. EKG may exhibit left and possibly right ventricular hypertrophy (LVH and RVH, respectively); CXR demonstrates cardiomegaly and increased pulmonary blood flow. Spontaneous closure occurs in 30%-40% of cases and is more likely in small defects during the first year of life. Direct surgical closure with a patch is performed if the defect fails to close and a moderate to large shunt persists.

ASD

Atrial septal defects (ASD) represent 7%-10% of congenital heart lesions. Secundum defects are in the region of the fossa ovalis, while sinus venosus defects, often associated with partial anomalous pulmonary venous return, occur in the superior atrial septum near the superior vena cava. Isolated ASDs usually are asymptomatic. Patients typically exhibit a widely split second heart sound (S_2) and a soft systolic ejection murmur at the upper left sternal border. EKG shows an rsR' pattern in V1 and CXR usually depicts cardiomegaly, a prominent right atrium and ventricle, and increased pulmonary blood flow. Spontaneous closure occurs in 40% of patients by 2 years; after age 2, open surgical repair by suture or patch is performed if the ratio of pulmonic to systemic blood flow exceeds 2:1.

PDA

A **patent ductus arteriosus (PDA)** is the persistent patency of the normal fetal ductus beyond the neonatal period and represents 5%-10% of congenital defects. This lesion is asymptomatic when small, but can cause CHF, if large. The magnitude of the shunt is determined by the diameter and length of the ductus and the relative systemic and pulmonic resistances. Usually a continuous "machinery" murmur is present at the upper left sternal border. Bounding peripheral pulses are present with a large shunt. Findings on EKG and CXR are similar to those with a VSD; closure is accomplished by ligation (with or without division).

AV canal defect

Endocardial cushion defect (ECD) or **atrioventricular (AV) canal defect** represents 2% of congenital heart defects, but is present in a third of those with trisomy 21 (Down's syndrome). ECD represents the failure of the primitive AV canal to "septate" into mitral and tricuspid valves; both AV valves are attached to the ventricular septum at the same level and can thus be insufficient. Partial ECDs have only an atrial component whereas complete ECDs have a ventricular defect in addition to the opening in the inferior atrial septum. Presenting symptoms in patients with complete ECDs include failure to thrive, recurrent respiratory infections, and CHF 1-2 months after birth. A hyperactive precordium, holosystolic regurgitant murmur, and loud S_2 can be seen. EKG reveals an axis between -40° and -150°, RVH and possibly LVH, and a prolonged PR interval, while the CXR shows cardiomegaly and increased pulmonary blood flow. Repair is required.

If uncorrected, complete ECDs, large VSDs, and occasionally other left-to-right shunts can cause pulmonary hypertension due to chronically increased pulmonary blood flow and pressure. As pulmonary resistance increases, the magnitude of the shunt decreases. Eventually, if pulmonary resistance exceeds systemic resistance, the shunt will reverse, becoming right-to-left (cyanotic). Called **Eisenmenger's syndrome**, this event is usually irreversible and signals end-stage, preterminal disease.

Obstructive Lesions

Obstructive lesions force the heart to do too much work, producing symptoms of decreased cardiac output and cardiac failure.

PS

Pulmonic stenosis (PS), or stenosis of the right ventricular outflow tract, accounts for 5%-10% of congenital heart defects. Symptoms range widely from none (if small to moderate) to those simulating pulmonary atresia (if severe or critical). Most PS (90%) are valvular; the others are subvalvular (infundibular) or supravalvular. In valvular PS the valve is typically dome-shaped with fusion of the leaflets producing a central orifice. Post-stenotic dilatation is frequent. Obstruction causes right ventricular hypertrophy (that itself can lead to dynamic infundibular obstruction). Patients may have dyspnea on exertion or early fatigue, and often exhibit a systolic ejection click, systolic murmur at the upper left sternal border, and a widely split S_2. EKG is normal, if mild, but shows right atrial and ventricular hypertrophy with strain, if obstruction is severe; CXR shows a prominent main pulmonary artery. The key prognostic indicator (as in any valvular lesion) is the pressure gradient across the lesion (measured by Doppler ultrasound). Balloon valvuloplasty or surgical repair is recommended when the gradient excceds 40mmHg or severe symptoms occur.

AS

Aortic stenosis (AS), stenosis of the left ventricular outflow tract, can be valvular (75%), subaortic (20%), or supravalvular. Patients with valvular AS usually have a **bicuspid valve** with partially fused commissures and an eccentric, "fish mouth" orifice. Variable leaflet thickening and post-stenotic dilatation of the ascending aorta are often seen. Children with mild to moderate AS are usually asymptomatic. Critical neonatal AS can produce low output cardiac failure, while older children can develop the classic symptoms of chest pain, syncope, or sudden death (see Chapter 36, "Cardiac Surgery"). A systolic thrill, ejection click, and a harsh systolic ejection murmur at the right base are common. Critical AS in infants results in thready pulses and a faint murmur that often intensifies with improvement of cardiac output. EKG demonstrates LVH with strain. Valvular AS tends to be progressive, and is a major cause of adult aortic stenosis. Initial surgical valvulotomy is palliative (balloon valvuloplasty is not as helpful as it is for PS). With progressive restenosis or severe regurgitation, valve replacement is indicated.

Coarctation

Coarctation of the aorta is relatively common (8% of congenital heart defects) and is frequently associated with a bicuspid aortic valve. Coarctation is usually caused by a discrete shelf arising from the posterolateral wall of the descending thoracic aorta opposite the orifice of the ductus arteriosus, although tubular hypoplasia of the aorta just proximal to the ductus can occur in the absence of a discrete shelf. Infants can present with CHF at 1-4 weeks of age. A loud S_3 and poor lower extremity pulses are typical, but pulses can be initially normal in the newborn nursery until the ductus closes. EKG demonstrates RVH;

CXR reveals cardiomegaly and pulmonary edema. Prostaglandins (PGE_1) keep the ductus open to maintain distal perfusion prior to surgical repair. Coarctation may not present immediately in the newborn period, and is then a classic cause of hypertension in older children who also present with claudication, decreased femoral pulses, and decreased lower extremity blood pressure. The classic late CXR finding is rib notching caused by enlarged, collateral intercostal vessels, but this is rarely seen today.

Complex Congenital Cardiovascular Malformations

Complex congenital cardiovascular malformations often produce cyanosis. Cyanosis can be due to decreased pulmonary blood flow (frequently described as a right-to-left shunt) or to improper mixing of oxygenated and deoxygenated blood.

Tetralogy of Fallot

Tetralogy of Fallot (TOF) represents 10% of congenital heart defects and is the most common cyanotic defect seen beyond infancy. TOF may be associated with chromosome 22q11 microdeletion ("CATCH 22") that results in a spectrum of conotruncal abnormalities. TOF consists of four problems: a VSD, right ventricular outflow tract obstruction, resultant RVH, and an overriding aorta caused by anterior and cephalad deviation of the outlet. The VSD is always large enough to equalize systolic pressures in both ventricles. Outflow obstruction is usually caused by an infundibular stenosis, and a quarter of these patients have a right-sided aortic arch. Symptoms include cyanosis, clubbing, dyspnea on exertion, squatting (rarely), and hypoxic or "tet" spells. Infants are often asymptomatic ("pink tets"). Patients have a loud, single S_2 and a systolic ejection murmur at the mid-left sternal border. EKG shows right axis deviation and RVH; CXR shows a "boot-shaped" heart caused by the upturned apex and concave main pulmonary artery.

Hypoxic ("tet") spells frequently first occur at 2-4 months. Spells are often brought on by defecation, crying, and feeding, and are characterized by marked cyanosis with paroxysms of rapid and deep respirations, loss of muscle tone, and, at times, syncope. Immediate improvement is produced by increasing pulmonary blood flow, usually by augmenting venous return and increasing peripheral resistance. Symptomatic infants should be placed in a knee-chest position; older children may learn to squat. Morphine and oxygen are beneficial, phenylephrine or volume can be given to increase peripheral resistance and venous return, respectively . Cardiac catheterization is usually necessary to delineate pulmonary and coronary arterial anatomy. Creation of a systemic to pulmonary shunt (subclavian to pulmonary connection; Blalock-Taussig shunt) is a temporizing measure to preserve pulmonary blood flow while the child matures. Definitive repair includes closure of the VSD and relief of the right-sided outflow tract obstruction.

TGA

Transposition of the great arteries (d-TGA) is the most common cyanotic defect in neonates. In this condition the pulmonary artery arises (posteriorly) from the left ventricle and the aorta arises (anteriorly) from the right ventricle, resulting in parallel rather than series circulation. Survival requires mixing at the atrial, ventricular, or ductal level to allow oxygenated blood to reach the systemic circulation. Patients are often deeply cyanotic with a loud, single S_2 and usually no audible murmur. EKG usually demonstrates right axis deviation and RVH; CXR shows cardiomegaly, increased pulmonary blood flow, and a cardiac shadow with a narrowed mediastinum or "egg-on-string" appearance. PGE_1 and, if necessary, a balloon atrial septostomy (Rashkind procedure) increase the magnitude of mixing between the pulmonary and systemic circulations. Repair is complex and involves transection and switching of the great arteries above their respective valves and sinuses with transfer of the coronary ostia; surgery must be performed during the neonatal period when the left ventricle is still "primed" to become the systemic ventricle. Intra-atrial repair by the Mustard or Senning procedure are options.

TA

Tricuspid atresia is rare; in 25% of patients associated TGA is found. Tricuspid atresia is the absence of the right AV orifice with a hypoplastic right ventricle and pulmonary artery; an ASD and VSD or PDA are necessary for survival. Variable cyanosis, poor feeding, and tachypnea are seen. CXR shows a "boot-shaped" heart due to the concave main pulmonary artery. Surgical repair is complex.

PA

Pulmonary atresia (PA) consists of an imperforate membrane of variable thickness at the hypoplastic pul-

monary valve annulus, and obviously requires a shunt to
supply blood to the lungs. Pulmonary blood flow usually
originates from a narrow, tortuous ductus, and systemic
venous return crosses the atrial septum. PA is often associated with a severely hypoplastic right ventricle and tricuspid valve, and there is severe and progressive cyanosis
from birth. Initial management consists of PGE_1 to keep
the PDA open to maintain pulmonary flow, and occasionally a Rashkind procedure if the atrial communication is
too small. Initial surgery consists of pulmonary valvo-
tomy and, if necessary, a Blalock-Taussig shunt. If the
right ventricle grows, the outflow tract is reconstructed; if
not, other options are available.

Truncus
arteriosus

Truncus arteriosus is characterized by a single great
artery arising from the base of the heart: the aorta, pulmonary arteries, and coronary arteries originate from this
single great vessel, and the truncal valve serves as a roof
for a large, malaligned VSD. There is high morbidity and
mortality associated with this lesion, and early treatment
is necessary to decrease the torrential pulmonary flow.
Repair is undertaken in early infancy and consists, in
essence, of an attempt to create two separate (pulmonary
and systemic) outflow sources.

Hypoplastic
left heart

Hypoplastic left heart syndrome (HLHS) accounts for
only 1%-2% of congenital heart defects, but is the most
common cause of cardiogenic shock and death in early
infancy due to congenital heart disease. It is really a
"gray pallor" defect, producing profoundly diminished
cardiac output. A spectrum of problems is seen, all having
in common hypoplasia (to varying degrees) of the left
side of the heart. Initial survival depends upon an ASD
and a patent ductus, and systemic cardiac output, including retrograde perfusion of the coronaries, is maintained
through retrograde ductal flow. Closure of the ductus thus
leads to severe low output cardiac failure. The majority of
infants with HLHS die within the first week without intervention, and these children are often critically ill with low
output failure in the first 1-3 days of life. Management
options include compassionate care without intervention,
cardiac transplantation (currently performed infrequently), or a Norwood procedure. The Norwood procedure involves an extensive atrial septectomy, separation of
the branch pulmonary arteries from the MPA, anastomosis of the MPA to the hypoplastic aortic arch, relief of the

frequently associated coarctation, and reestablishment of pulmonary blood flow via a Blalock-Taussig shunt. If the infant survives the initial Stage 1 Norwood, a bidirectional Glenn and then a modified Fontan are performed. Results of this three-staged approach are fair, although long term prognosis is currently unknown.

Acquired Pediatric Heart Disease

Although the vast majority of pediatric heart problems are congenital, acquired problems can occur. **Kawasaki's syndrome** is an acute febrile vasculitis, associated with an elevated ESR and thrombocytosis, most frequently seen in children under 4. The vasculitis can result in the development of coronary artery aneurysms. Diagnosis is made by the presence of a non-exudative conjunctival injection, oral and/or buccal hyperemia (strawberry tongue and erythema and fissuring of the lips), erythema of palms and soles with induration, a polymorphous erythematous rash, and cervical lymphadenopathy in the setting of prolonged fever (greater than 5 days). Therapy consists of IV gamma globulin and high-dose aspirin. Serial echocardiograms are performed to monitor the coronary arteries.

Rheumatic fever

Acute rheumatic fever (ARF) is a nonsuppurative sequela of Group A streptococcal pharyngitis. Its major hazard lies in the development of carditis with the attendant risk of late valvular dysfunction (see Chapter 36, "Cardiac Surgery"). Prompt treatment of "strep throat" with penicillin (or a substitute) reduces this risk, underscoring the importance of throat cultures in children with pharyngitis. Diagnosis is according to the Revised Jones criteria. ARF is diagnosed by the presence of 2 major or 1 major and 2 minor criteria plus evidence of a preceding streptococcal infection. Major criteria include polyarthritis, carditis (pericarditis, myocarditis, or endocarditis), chorea, erythema marginatum, and subcutaneous nodules; minor criteria include fever, arthralgias, a history of rheumatic fever or rheumatic heart disease, elevated ESR, positive C-reactive protein, and a prolonged PR interval. Treatment includes bedrest, penicillin, and aspirin (and corticosteroids with moderate to severe carditis), with further therapy directed toward alleviation of specific symptoms. ■

53   Pediatric Endocrinology

This chapter deals with insulin-dependent diabetes mellitus, diabetic ketoacidosis, hypothyroidism, and disorders of growth. See also Chapter 9, "Endocrinology," for a general discussion of the endocrine system.

Diabetes Mellitus

Diabetes mellitus is divided into **type I** and **type II**, based on the underlying cause. Type I diabetes is caused by destruction of the pancreatic beta cells (see below), always requires insulin, and is associated with the risk of **ketosis**. Type II diabetes, on the other hand, is caused by peripheral insulin resistance, is usually associated with obesity, and is not associated with ketosis; type II diabetics can require insulin or be treated with dietary modification or oral hypoglycemics alone. Diabetes can also be classified according to treatment or age at onset. Thus, **insulin-dependent diabetes mellitus (IDDM)** simply means insulin is required (all type I diabetics and some type II diabetics), while **non-insulin-dependent diabetes (NIDDM)** means that it is not (type II diabetics only); similarly, **juvenile-onset diabetes** means onset was during childhood, while **adult-onset diabetes** means onset was in adulthood.

Patho-physiology

The cause of type I diabetes is not completely clear. The underlying problem is the presence of autoantibodies against the insulin-producing pancreatic islet beta cells, and onset of type I diabetes may follow a viral infection. The autoimmune process eventually leads to cellular destruction of the beta cells; approximately 90% of the beta cell mass must be destroyed before symptoms appear. There is a strong genetic susceptibility to the disease, and affected patients have a high prevalence of other autoimmune diseases, including thyroiditis, autoimmune adrenal problems, and rheumatoid arthritis; susceptibility is linked to human leukocyte antigens (HLA) DR3 and DR4. Incidence and prevalence vary worldwide; increased risk is seen in colder countries, farther from the equator. Incidence increases with age and peaks around the time of puberty; males and females are equally affected.

Presentation   Although the destruction of beta cells can take several
years, the majority of patients present with symptoms of
less than a month's duration, frequently after a precipitant
such as a viral illness. Classic symptoms include polydipsia, polyuria, bed wetting, an increased appetite, and,
often, recent weight loss; fasting blood glucose levels of
greater than 140mg/dL on two or more occasions are
diagnostic. Provocative glucose tolerance testing is rarely
needed. If symptoms are ignored, the patient can present
in diabetic ketoacidosis (DKA).

Treatment   Initial treatment (for the patient not in DKA) consists of
subcutaneous (SQ) insulin, monitoring of blood glucose
levels (BGs), and education. Most patients will be hospitalized for several days to achieve glucose control and
ensure proper insulin dosing. Because it is a complex protein, insulin must be given parenterally. Lifestyle changes
or adjustments are required to incorporate insulin administration, blood glucose determination, institution of diabetic meal planning, and exercise planning. For many
children and their families these changes represent a
daunting task.

Most patients with newly-diagnosed diabetes are started
on a combination of short- and intermediate-acting
insulin administered twice daily. Human recombinant
insulin has become the most frequently prescribed form
of insulin, although pork and beef preparation are still
available:

Type	Name	Onset	Peak	Duration
Short-acting	Regular Semi-lente Humulin R	30 minutes	2-4 hours	6-8 hours
Intermediate	NPH Lente Humulin N	1.5-2 hours	6-12 hours	18-24 hours
Long-acting	Ultralente	6-10 hours	18-24 hours	36 (or more) hours

A common initial daily regimen consists of 0.5-0.7 units (U) of insulin per kilogram, with two-thirds of the total given in the morning and one-third in the evening. Typically, two-thirds of the morning dose consists of intermediate (i.e., NPH), and the rest short-acting (Regular); the evening dose is usually divided equally between NPH and Regular. For example, an 8 year old weighing 30kg would be initially prescribed 15U a day (30kg x 0.5U/kg); two-thirds (10U) would be given in the morning, and one-third (5U) in the evening. The morning dose, taken 30 minutes before breakfast, would consist of 6U NPH and 4U regular, and the evening, taken 30 minutes before the evening meal, of 2.5U NPH and 2.5U Regular.

Dosage and formulation must be adjusted based on individual response. Fingerstick BGs should be monitored at least 5 times a day in the beginning, before each meal, at bedtime, and at 2:00 am; the ideal BG is 80-180mg/dL before meals. Once stable BGs and insulin dosages have been achieved, levels should be checked before each meal and at bedtime. Both patient and family need to be educated about the management of diabetes, including insulin injections, BG monitoring, nutrition, and recognition of emergencies.

Diabetic Ketoacidosis

Diabetic ketoacidosis (DKA) is a complication resulting from an absolute or relative lack of insulin combined with glucagon excess. It is most commonly seen in new-onset diabetics whose diagnosis is delayed, and in known diabetics who are noncompliant or ill; physiologic stress suppresses insulin secretion. Impaired cellular uptake and overproduction of glucose contribute to hyperglycemia and utilization of lipids for energy. The former produces **dehydration** due to osmotic diuresis, the latter, **ketoacidosis**; dehydration, if severe, markedly worsens acidosis. Marked **electrolyte disturbances** will occur as the result of vomiting, dehydration, acidosis, hyperlipidemia, and hyperglycemia. DKA occurs only rarely in type II diabetics.

Characteristic signs include polydipsia, polyuria, nausea, vomiting, abdominal pain, and, in severe cases, mental status changes. Physical exam is usually significant for evidence of dehydration, "fruity" breath (caused by ketonemia), and Küssmaul respirations. Glucose levels are usually greater than 250 mg/dL but **can be near normal**. There will always be marked **ketonuria** and an **anion-gap metabolic acidosis** (see Chapter 2, "Acid-Base Disorders"); if absent, another diagnosis should be considered.

Treatment

Treatment revolves around the correction of acidosis, rehydration, and insulin administration. These patients can be very ill; admission to an ICU is indicated for most patients with moderate-to-severe DKA. BGs, electrolytes, and acid-base status should be monitored frequently until the acidosis resolves. Continuous cardiac monitoring is needed if the patient is unstable, the acidosis severe, or electrolytes (especially potassium; see Chapter 7, "Basic Fluids and Electrolytes") are markedly abnormal. Acidosis will correct with a combination of **rehydration** and insulin. Whether to use bicarbonate remains controversial, but it is usually not indicated in the absence of cardiac toxicity.

In general terms, half the volume deficit should be replaced over the first 12 hours with a crystalloid such as 1/2 normal saline. Dextrose (D_5) is added when the BG is less than 300mg/dL. Because whole body potassium is always depleted, potassium should be added. The remainder of the fluid deficit should be replaced more slowly, usually over the next 24-36 hours, along with ongoing maintenance needs.

Insulin should be started in conjunction with rehydration. Only regular insulin should be used. Because SQ blood flow is often reduced or abnormal during illness, insulin should be given intravenously to ensure reliable absorption. The patient should be given an initial IV bolus of 0.1U/kg, followed by a continuous IV infusion of 0.1U/kg/hour. Hyperglycemia should be corrected fairly slowly (no greater than 100mg/dL/hour) to reduce the risk of cerebral edema. Insulin administration can be switched to the SQ route when acidosis and hyperglycemia are corrected; the first SQ injection should be given at least 30 minutes before IV insulin is discontinued.

The most dangerous complication of DKA is **cerebral edema** leading to brainstem herniation and death. Coma and herniation are rare (1%) but deadly (95% fatal), and may be caused by overly vigorous rehydration and/or correction of hyperglycemia. Mannitol should be given if mental status deteriorates after initial improvement was seen.

Hypothyroidism

The incidence of **congenital hypothyroidism** is about 1 in 4000; clinical signs and symptoms are not apparent for weeks or months, so screening at 2 days of age is performed in all 50 states. **Hypothyroidism in the newborn should be considered a medical emergency, because early treatment can prevent devastating and irreversible mental retardation (cretinism).**

Congenital hypo-thyroidism

Primary congenital hypothyroidism is a condition whereby the thyroid gland is unable to produce thyroxine (T_4). It is characterized by low T_4 and high thyroid-stimulating hormone (TSH) levels, and is most commonly due to dys- or agenesis of the thyroid gland. Less commonly (10% of the time), primary congenital hypothyroidism is caused by inborn errors of thyroid metabolism. This condition can be accompanied by the presence of goiter (enlargement of the thyroid gland) due to stimulation by TSH; although TSH levels are also high with thyroid agenesis, there is no thyroid tissue to become enlarged. **Secondary congenital hypothyroidism** refers to the condition of inadequate or absent production of TSH or thyrotropin releasing hormone (TRH) by the pituitary or hypothalamus, respectively, leading to low T_4 and TSH levels. It is rare, occurring only once in 100,000 live births, and usually in conjunction with other pituitary problems.

Transient hypothyroxinemia is commonly seen in preterm infants. There is normally a linear rise in T_4 and TSH beginning at midterm and continuing through delivery. Low T_4 and TSH levels seen in premature babies thus do not represent a pathologic condition, but, rather, lack of maturation. The overall prevalence in preterm infants is 25%, higher with increasing prematurity. Treatment is not necessary.

Transient primary hypothyroidism can be due to low maternal perinatal iodine intake (rare in the US), exposure to maternal goitrogenic substances such as propylth-iouracil, cobalt, or radiographic contrast agents, or placental transfer of TSH receptor-blocking antibodies in women with autoimmune thyroiditis. Though transient, hypothyroidism can be prolonged, and treatment is often warranted.

Acquired hypo-thyroidism

Hashimoto's (chronic lymphocytic) thyroiditis is the most common cause of acquired hypothyroidism in children and adolescents. It occurs in genetically predisposed individuals (30%-40% of patients have a positive family history), and usually presents with goiter, low T_4, and high TSH levels. It is characterized by the presence of antithyroglobulin and antimicrosomal antibodies, and lymphoid and plasma cell infiltration of the thyroid gland. There is a strong association with other autoimmune diseases, particularly type I diabetes. **Acquired secondary hypothyroidism** can be seen after an insult to the pituitary or hypothalamus caused by trauma, tumor, meningitis, or a vascular accident. It usually occurs in conjunction with global pituitary hypofunction. Hypothyroidism can also be **iatrogenic**, due to surgical resection or radioactive ablation (much more common in adults) or cranial irradiation for treatment of malignancy.

Treatment consists of the administration of L-thyroxine. Patients need 10micrograms/kg/day during the first year of life; 2-6micrograms/kg/day thereafter. The aim of therapy is to normalize TSH while maintaining the T_4 level within the age-appropriate normal range. T_4 levels are normally higher in infancy than in older children or adults. A trial period without replacement therapy is reasonable in all children in whom hypothyroidism is believed to be transient, but this should be delayed until the child is older than 3 to avoid the risk of mental retardation.

Abnormal Growth

Growth is a dynamic process resulting in an increase in length or height over time. Birth size correlates poorly with adult height, and two-thirds of infants will cross at least 2 percentile lines (up or down) by 18 months of age. Height at 2 years of age has an 80% correlation with final adult height, and, after this age, growth normally occurs at a rate of at least 5cm/year until puberty. Normal growth is accompanied by bone maturation, and skeletal maturation, as assessed by **bone age**, is more closely associated with growth potential, final adult height, and onset of puberty than are height or chronologic age. Bone age is determined by obtaining an x-ray of the left hand and wrist and comparing it to standards published in the Greulich and Pyle Atlas. All pathologic conditions that interfere with overall growth do so by interfering with bone growth.

Growth hormone (GH) is a pituitary peptide produced in response to growth hormone releasing factor from the hypothalamus that is necessary, but not sufficient, for normal growth. It is secreted in a pulsatile fashion, peaking at night, and is low throughout most of the day. Therefore, a single, random assessment of the GH level is rarely useful if GH deficiency is suspected. Instead, provocative testing using vigorous exercise or administration of L-dopa, clonidine, or arginine is used to determine endogenous GH reserve; a rise of less than 10ng/mL is generally considered subnormal. **Insulin-like growth factor-1 (IGF-1)** is produced in the liver and related tissues, and mediates GH-dependent growth through mitogenic effects on most cells in the body, particularly cartilage. In short stature due to GH deficiency, IGF-1 levels are low. IGF-1 concentrations are often used as screening tests for GH function, but should be interpreted with caution; poor nutrition can depress levels even when GH is normal. IGF-1 levels are more closely associated with bone age than chronological age. **Thyroid hormone** is also essential for normal growth and for the normal secretion of growth hormone. **Sex steroids** promote growth and are largely responsible for the pubertal growth spurt and the fusion of epiphyseal growth plates. Excess **glucocorticoids** are a powerful suppressor of growth.

Short stature is the most common complaint that causes referral to the pediatric endocrinologist. Generally, abnormal growth can be classified as intrinsic shortness, delayed growth, or arrested (attenuated) growth. Growth rate is a sensitive indicator of overall health, and most cases of short stature are due to problems other than endocrinopathy; a full endocrine workup is justified only when more common causes have been eliminated. When taken together, the combination of bone age, chronologic age, growth rate, and height age (apparent age of the child, read off the growth chart, when current height is plotted at the 50th percentile) offer clues to the etiology of short stature.

Children with **intrinsic shortness** are short (height age is reduced), but bone age is appropriate for chronologic age, and growth rate is normal; puberty and epiphyseal closure generally occur at a normal age. This is also referred to as **genetic short stature**. In primordial dwarfism, intrauterine growth retardation, children with chromosomal abnormalities such as Turner's or Down's syndromes, and in some bone dysplasias, short stature is also intrinsic and is not due to GH deficiency. In children with **delayed growth**, shortness is accompanied by a proportional delay in bone age (greater than 2 standard deviations), although growth rate is generally normal. Puberty is delayed, and growth can continue well into the late teens or early adulthood. Final adult height is usually normal. This constitutional delay in growth and puberty is often familial; mild chronic illness or malnutrition may also result in delay. Children with **arrested (attenuated) growth** have a true decrease in their growth **rate** (less than 5cm/year); they "fall off the curve." Bone age is delayed but is usually proportional to height. Arrested growth is most indicative of true pathology (not necessarily endocrine), and always warrants attention. Causes include chronic diseases such as renal problems, malabsorptive syndromes, or metabolic abnormalities. Abnormal growth is characteristic of endocrine abnormalities such as hypothyroidism, growth hormone deficiency, and glucocorticoid excess (Cushing's syndrome). It can also be caused by chronic psychologic or emotional trauma.

Short stature is **not** usually caused by endocrine abnormalities, and only in well-defined instances is hormonal intervention warranted. Little can be done to alter genetic short stature or delayed growth. In the latter situation, reassurance that puberty will proceed normally and that full adult height will be achieved is usually sufficient. Low-dose testosterone can sometimes be tried in boys (in whom the condition is most prevalent) and will often bring about gratifying pubertal changes without advancing bone age or reducing final adult height. In children with arrested growth, treatment should be directed at the underlying cause.

(continued)

GH deficiency is treated with recombinant human GH, which often results in dramatic increases in growth velocity. GH is given parenterally and results in resumption of normal growth. In children with chronic renal failure or Turner's syndrome, who do not usually have GH deficiency, increases in height velocity can be achieved with exogenous GH. Current evidence suggests that increases in final adult height can be achieved, although the degree of increase remains to be established. ■

Pediatric hematology/oncology is the study and treatment of hematologic disorders and malignancies that occur during childhood. The most common hematologic problems are the anemias, including sickle cell disease, and childhood leukemias; solid organ tumors (see Chapter 38, "Pediatric Surgery") are relatively less common. See Chapter 17, "Hematology" for discussion of leukemias and bleeding disorders.

Anemia

Anemia, the most common hematologic disorder seen in pediatrics, is often detected by routine screening, but can be detected by physical exam. Although practices vary widely, the American Academy of Pediatrics recommends obtaining a screening hematocrit between 6 and 14 months in otherwise healthy children; normal values vary based on age, sex, and race. The cause of an anemia can range from an easily treatable dietary deficiency to a life-threatening disorder. There are three underlying mechanisms for anemia (in any patient at any age): blood loss, decreased production of red blood cells (RBCs), or increased destruction.

History

Workup starts with a thorough clinical **history**. Dietary habits are important; excess milk intake in toddlers is associated with iron deficiency anemia, as is pica (ingestion of non-food items such as dirt or paint chips). History of blood loss, including the presence of heavy menses, nosebleeds, or bleeding from the gums is important both to identify loss and because it signals the need to look for coagulation abnormalities. Drug exposure history is likewise useful because certain drugs cause marrow suppression or hemolysis. Various illnesses can cause anemia, and certain congenital anemias are associated with specific ethnic backgrounds. Family history of anemia, blood transfusion, cholecystectomy at a young age, or splenectomy (for reasons other than trauma) suggests the possibility of a hereditary disease.

Physical exam

Physical exam is helpful. Skin, mucous membranes, and nailbeds show pallor; visible jaundice and scleral icterus suggest hemolysis. Some anemias can be associated with

Pediatrics
Pediatric Hematology and Oncology

continued

distinctive skeletal abnormalities, such as frontal "boss-ing" or maxillary prominence caused by the extramedullary hematopoesis occurring in response to certain congenital hemolytic anemias. Severe anemia may result in cardiac failure resulting in a murmur, gallop, or pulmonary edema. Lymphadenopathy and hepatosplenomegaly are suggestive of an underlying infection or malignancy, and bleeding and bruising can occur secondary to thrombocytopenia.

Laboratory workup

Laboratory studies are essential to determine the cause of an anemia. If the hematocrit is abnormal, a complete blood count including red cell indices, blood smear, and a reticulocyte count should be obtained. Reviewing the peripheral smear provides a direct view of RBC size and morphology, provides evidence of hemolysis, and allows evaluation of the other cell lines. Additional laboratory testing is directed by the history and physical findings. *(continued)*

The most common approach to the workup of anemia is based on RBC size, measured as **mean corpuscular volume** (**MCV**):

Figure 54.1
Algorithm for classification of pediatric anemias based on mean corpuscular volume.

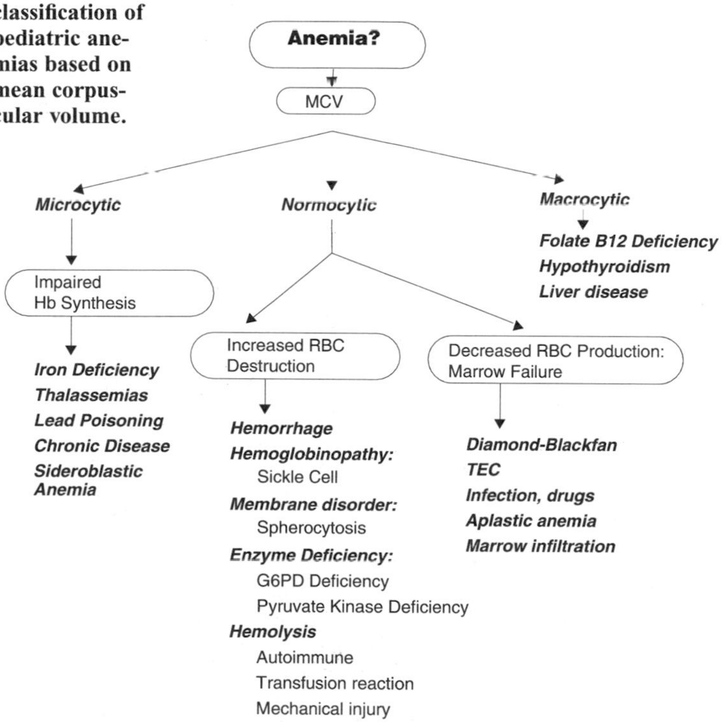

Microcytic Anemia

Patients with **microcytic anemia** have decreased amounts of hemoglobin (Hb) in their cells, suggesting that **an underlying problem with hemoglobin synthesis exists**. The most common causes of microcytic anemia are iron deficiency and thalassemia trait.

Iron deficiency   **Iron deficiency** can be due to decreased intake, impaired absorption, or blood loss, and has been shown to adversely affect longterm development and intellectual

performance (see Chapter 57, "Poisoning"). In infants
and toddlers (under 2 years old) the most common cause
is poor dietary intake, often due to drinking too much
cow's milk at the expense of sources of iron; the most
common causes in adolescents are poor diet and blood
loss. Laboratory evidence that supports this diagnosis
includes decreased serum ferritin, iron, and iron saturation, and increased total iron binding capacity. Iron supplementation for approximately 1 month after the hematocrit is corrected usually reestablishes iron stores. Dietary
modification, if applicable, and evaluation for the possibility of chronic blood loss are required.

Thalassemias

The **thalassemias** are a group of inherited disorders of
globin chain synthesis. Beta-thalassemia is found in people of Mediterranean heritage. **Homozygous beta-thalassemia (thalassemia major)** results in a severe, transfusion-dependent anemia, while heterozygotes (**beta-thalassemia trait**) have 1 normal beta-globin gene and 1
deficient gene, leading to a mild, microcytic anemia that
usually does not require specific treatment. The MCV in
those with beta-thalassemia trait is lower than expected
for the degree of anemia. The Mentzer index
(MCV/RBC) can help differentiate between iron deficiency and thalassemia: a value less than 11.5 suggests
iron deficiency, while a value of 13.5 or more suggests
beta-thalassemia trait. The diagnosis of beta-thalassemia
is confirmed by hemoglobin electrophoresis, which will
show an elevated hemoglobin A2 level. **Alpha-thalassemia** is seen in the Southeast Asian and African-
American population, and is caused by mutations within
1 or more of the genes coding for alpha-globin. There are
4 alpha-globin genes, and the severity of the disease
depends on the number of functional genes. **Hydrops
fetalis** (all 4 genes nonfunctional) is not compatible with
life. **Hemoglobin H disease** (3 nonfunctional genes)
results in a chronic microcytic anemia, often associated
with splenomegaly, requiring folic acid supplementation.
Alpha-thalassemia trait (2 nonfunctional genes) is a
mild anemia that does not require treatment, and **silent
carriers** (only 1 nonfunctional gene) are completely
asymptomatic.

Less common causes of microcytic anemia include lead
poisoning, anemia of chronic disease, and sideroblastic
anemia.

Normocytic Anemia

Normocytic anemias can be divided into disorders associated with decreased RBC production and those associated with increased destruction. If production is decreased, the reticulocyte count will be low; if RBC destruction is taking place, the reticulocyte count will be elevated as the marrow responds appropriately to make up the loss.

Deficient RBC production

Decreased RBC production is synonymous with **bone marrow failure**. **Diamond-Blackfan syndrome** is a congenital failure of RBC production that presents with severe anemia in the first year of life; treatment with corticosteroids often leads to improvement, but occasional patients are transfusion-dependent. **Transient erythroblastopenia of childhood** (**TEC**) is a self-limited suppression of RBC production seen in children aged 1-3, often associated with a preceding viral infection. It may be severe enough to require transfusion. Marrow suppression can also be caused by drugs or **infection**; parvovirus, Epstein-Barr virus, and sometimes nonspecific viral infections can cause temporary marrow suppression. Suppression is not usually clinically evident in the absence of an underlying red cell abnormality, and other cell lines may also be affected. **Aplastic anemia** (pancytopenia) can be caused by drug exposure or infection, but most commonly is idiopathic. Supportive treatment for severe aplastic anemia includes transfusion and antibiotics for infections; definitive treatment consists of bone marrow transplantation. **Marrow-infiltrative processes** such as leukemia, metastatic malignancy, or myelodysplastic processes rarely present as isolated anemia, but more commonly with pancytopenia, lymphadenopathy, hepatosplenomegaly, or weight loss.

Increased RBC destruction

Normocytic anemias due to **increased RBC destruction** may be caused by hemorrhage or hemolysis. **Hemorrhage** severe enough to cause anemia should be obvious; sources include heavy menses and GI bleeding. **Hemolysis** is suggested by the blood smear, an elevated reticulocyte count (indicating appropriately increased production by the marrow), elevated indirect bilirubin levels as the RBCs are metabolized, and decreased haptoglobin. Many conditions leading to increased RBC destruction are inherited as either a **hemoglobinopathy, membrane disorder,** or **enzyme deficiency**.

Sickle cell disease

The most serious hemoglobinopathy is **sickle cell anemia** (and related syndromes). Patients with sickle cell anemia have defective hemoglobin (Hb-S) which, when subjected to stressors such as hypoxia, infection, cold, or dehydration, undergoes a conformational change, causing an irreversible change in the shape of the RBCs (sickling), rendering them unable to carry oxygen. The sickled cells become trapped in the microcirculation, leading to capillary occlusion with resultant decreased oxygen delivery.

The most common clinical problem resulting from sickling is a **painful crisis**, typically caused by bone marrow ischemia and/or infarction. Patients present with local or generalized pain, often in the back or extremities. Treatment is directed toward pain control and hydration; patients often require admission for narcotics and IV fluids. Vaso-occlusion at the capillary level can occur in any organ; common problems include priapism and cerebral or splenic infarction. Both vaso-occlusion and infection can occur in the lungs of patients with sickle cell disease, and are difficult to differentiate. The clinical presentation of chest pain, respiratory distress, hypoxia, and pulmonary infiltrates in a patient with sickle cell disease is termed **acute chest syndrome**. Treatment is supportive, but exchange transfusion can be necessary. **Splenic sequestration** is a sudden, spontaneous sequestration of blood in the spleen leading to a rapid fall in the hematocrit; it is rarely seen in children older than 3. Patients with sickle cell anemia have an increased risk of infection due to **autosplenectomy** from repeated splenic microinfarction resulting in functional asplenism, and to poorly-defined, nonspecific immunologic deficiencies. Routine care for asymptomatic patients includes daily folic acid supplementation, penicillin prophylaxis, and immunization against the encapsulated organisms (such as Pneumococcus and Hemophilus influenza type B) that the spleen normally filters out. **Sickle trait** is clinically asymptomatic, but genetic counseling is important for carriers. The "maladaptive" sickle cell gene has persisted throughout evolution because heterozygotes have an increased resistance to malaria.

Other RBC disorders

The most common **membrane disorder** is **hereditary spherocytosis**. An inherited defect in spectrin, a structural protein within RBC membranes, causes abnormally spherical RBCs that are functionally normal but undergo excessively rapid hemolysis in the spleen. The severity of the anemia varies, and affected patients are at risk for episodes of virally-induced RBC aplasia or increased hemolysis. Splenomegaly is usually present. The diagnosis is suspected based on family history and the presence of spherocytes on the smear; confirmation is by means of the osmotic fragility test. Splenectomy is beneficial and results in markedly reduced hemolysis and symptom control, although the spherocytes are still present.
Hereditary elliptocytosis and **stomatocytosis** are similar but less common diseases.

An enzyme deficiency caused by a defect in one of the two major enzyme pathways for glucose metabolism can also result in a normocytic hemolytic anemia. **Glucose-6-phosphate dehydrogenase (G6PD) deficiency** is an inherited condition leading to impairment of the hexose-monophosphate shunt and subsequent low levels of NADPH, an antioxidant; exposure to sulfa drugs, certain foods, or other oxidants leads to hemolysis and subsequent anemia. G6PD deficiency is fairly common, existing in 10% of African-American males; G6PD levels can be directly measured to confirm the diagnosis. The other major defect in the RBC glycolytic pathway is **pyruvate kinase deficiency**, an inherited disorder causing a severe, often transfusion-dependent hemolytic anemia due to inadequate ATP production by the RBCs.

Hemolysis

The most common acquired cause of hemolysis is **autoimmune hemolytic anemia**, which can be caused by infection (often viral), underlying collagen vascular disease, lymphoma, or certain medications; it can also be idiopathic. An **Rh** or **ABO incompatibility** results in an isoimmune hemolytic anemia with hyperbilirubinemia in neonates (see Chapter 44, "Neonatal Jaundice"). Spherocytes, caused by an antibody-mediated decrease in membrane size and surface area, are often present on the blood smear. The Coombs test for antibody is diagnostic; steroids are the first line of treatment, but transfusion may be needed if the anemia is severe. Hemolysis can be caused by **mechanical injury** to the RBCs due to a mechanical heart valve, renal disease, the hemolytic ure-

Pediatrics
Pediatric Hematology and Oncology

continued

mic syndrome (see Chapter 56, "Pediatric Nephrology"), or a vascular malformation such as a hemangioma.

Macrocytic Anemia

Macrocytosis is normal in certain populations, including neonates and children with trisomy 21 (Down's syndrome). True pathologic macrocytic anemia is rare in children. The main causes include **folate, vitamin B-12 deficiency**, **hypothyroidism**, **liver disease**, **bone marrow disorders**, and certain **drugs**.

Leukemia

Acute leukemia is the most common malignancy of childhood, accounting for approximately a third of childhood cancers. It results from the malignant transformation of a single undifferentiated progenitor cell that reproduces uncontrollably within the bone marrow (see also Chapter 17, "Hematology"). The cause of transformation is unknown; almost certainly multiple causes exist. Certain risk factors associated with leukemia have been identified, including exposure to ionizing radiation, exposure to certain chemicals (benzene), prior chemotherapy, genetic defects (Down's syndrome), and certain familial disorders (Fanconi's anemia).

Signs and symptoms

Presenting signs and symptoms are caused by the suppression of normal hematopoesis by overgrowth of the malignant clone of cells within the marrow and organ infiltration by malignant cells. Patients commonly present with fatigue and pallor due to **anemia**, bleeding, bruising, and petechiae due to **thrombocytopenia**, or fever and infection due to **neutropenia**. Increased cellular activity within the marrow can cause bony pain and limping. Leukemic cells released from the marrow infiltrate various organs causing hepatomegaly, splenomegaly, lymphadenopathy, and testicular enlargement; patients can present emergently with severe respiratory distress caused by enlarging mediastinal lymphatic tissue. Collections of leukemic cells can form solid masses in the retina and skin, called chloromas. Increased intracranial pressure, causing headache, neck pain, or a decreased level of consciousness can be caused by infiltration of the central nervous system (CNS).

Laboratory data are reflective of the underlying bone marrow "failure," revealing anemia, thrombocytopenia, and an elevated or decreased white blood cell count, depending on the specific disease. Blasts (immature white cell precursors normally found only in the marrow) can be seen in the peripheral blood, and lactate dehydrogenase (LDH) and urate, reflecting abnormally high cellular turnover, are often elevated. A chest x-ray should be obtained to evaluate the mediastinum for lymphadenopathy. Definitive diagnosis is made by direct examination of the bone marrow.

Leukemias are classified by the progenitor cell. In **acute lymphocytic leukemia** (**ALL**) the progenitor cell is of lymphoid origin, while the malignant cell in **acute non-lymphocytic leukemia** (**ANLL**) is of myeloid, erythroid, or megakaryocytic lineage. Morphologic criteria, specific stains, cell marker studies, and cytogenetic testing are used to make this distinction.

ALL

ALL is one of the most curable pediatric malignancies; overall survival is approximately 75%. Factors associated with poor prognosis include age under 2 or greater than 10 years, and CNS disease or prominent leukocytosis at diagnosis. Further cytogenetic risk factors are under investigation. Conventional treatment for ALL is multidrug chemotherapy; commonly including steroids, methotrexate, adriamycin, asparaginase, vincristine, and 6-MP. Treatment of the CNS by means of intrathecal chemotherapy or cranial radiation is also usually employed.

ANLL

Treatment and outcome of **ANLL** is not as successful; cure rates are approximately 25%-50%. Chemotherapy regimens are based on the specific subtype. Supportive care includes transfusions, treatment of infection (usually related to neutropenia), and prophylaxis for Pneumocystis carinii pneumonia. Bone marrow transplantation is increasingly used for treatment of leukemias. ■

55 Pediatric Gastroenterology

Gastrointestinal (GI) complaints are common in children, and include symptoms of constipation, soiling, diarrhea, abdominal pain, vomiting, and gastroesophageal reflux. The majority of these problems are the result of functional disorders (those without an obvious structural cause) of the GI tract, due either to intrinsic abnormalities of the gut or to the gastrointestinal "side effects" of extraintestinal conditions. True structural defects of the GI tract itself, other intra-abdominal pathology, and most of the problems usually seen in adults (see Chapters 22, "Gastroenterology," and 38, "Pediatric Surgery") can also occur in children.

Stooling

Constipation

Constipation is defined as excessively infrequent stooling or the passage of unusually hard stools. Stool frequency is variable in children, ranging from 3-4 stools per day to one stool every 3-4 days; the prevalence of constipation is estimated to be as high as 3%-5% in the outpatient pediatric setting. Age of presentation varies according to the etiology. Less common causes of constipation include the side effects of many medications (such as narcotics), neurologic disorders that affect intestinal motility, metabolic problems such as hypothyroidism, hypokalemia, and hypercalcemia, and true structural abnormalities of GI tract such as colonic aganglionosis (Hirschsprung's Disease; see Chapter 38, "Pediatric Surgery"), anorectal malformations, and colonic strictures. Most cases of constipation seen in pediatric practice, however, are due to dietary factors such as excessive cow's milk, inadequate fiber, or poor fluid intake, or to functional chronic retentive constipation (**encopresis**).

The evaluation of the child with constipation starts with a thorough history, including age of onset, stooling, medical, and dietary histories, and assessment of toileting practices. Physical exam should be directed toward the elimination of underlying neurologic disorders, structural abnormalities, and extraintestinal disease. Laboratory investigation and radiologic studies should be reserved for situations in which a structural abnormality or mechanical obstruction is suspected. For example, if constipation has been present since birth and is associated with abdominal distention, a barium enema should be obtained to exclude Hirschsprung's disease (without bowel preparation, because enemas can dilate the rectum and lead to a false negative result).

Treatment of functional constipation should start with education about normal stooling patterns and the role of diet. Simple dietary changes such as increasing fruit, vegetable, and fluid intake and decreasing the amount of cow's milk ingested are often effective. Measures to soften (malt extract, metamucil, or docusate) or lubricate (mineral oil) the stool are next. Laxatives are often necessary in the treatment of children with retentive constipation, while treatment of constipation due to a specific structural condition is individualized.

Encopresis

Encopresis (soiling) is defined as repeated, involuntary defecation into clothing in children 4 and older. Prevalence ranges between 0.5%-2%, decreases with age, and is three times more common in boys. Causes are multifactoral; both physiologic and psychologic factors contribute. Chronic retention of stool due to painful bowel movements, inattention to the need to defecate, oppositional behavior, or toilet phobias during toilet training lead to rectal hyposensitivity and subsequent rectal overfilling.

Evaluation of children with encopresis is similar to that of children with constipation. It is important to rule out **fecal impaction** and **anal problems** such as an anal fissure that can contribute to painful defecation. Plain x-rays of the abdomen, by revealing the amount of stool within the colon, can be of help in deciding in which direction intervention should proceed.

Treatment must emphasize education and behavioral management. A structured toileting program with scheduled toileting times and positive reinforcement should be initiated. Medication use is similar to that in uncomplicated constipation, but early medication use may be necessary more often to improve the chances for a successful behavior program. Enemas or cathartics are occasionally necessary in children with excessive amounts of stool on exam or x-ray. Minor "relapses" are common and usually due to deviation from the treatment plan after initial success is achieved. Followup visits are important because resistant encopresis may necessitate referral to a pediatric gastroenterologist or behavioral specialist.

Diarrhea

Diarrhea can present in an acute or chronic fashion. Infection is most often the cause of acute diarrhea, covered in Chapter 50, "Common Outpatient Infections." **Chronic diarrhea** is defined as excessive stool output that persists more than 21 days. Causes are multiple, and include infection, inflammatory disorders, functional problems, certain foods, and intestinal malabsorption.

The history should specifically assess growth, diet, and medication use, and should characterize stool pattern and consistency. Essential components of the physical examination include measurement of growth, a search for abnormal skin or pulmonary lesions commonly seen with certain problems, and checking whether or not occult blood is present on rectal exam. Assay for bacteria and parasites in the stool is usually performed before further workup, unless the cause is obvious after the history and physical examination. If infection is not the cause, an initial trial of lactose avoidance is a practical first step. Further evaluation, including examination of the stool for reducing substances and fat (present in malabsorptive syndromes), sweat chloride testing (abnormal if cystic fibrosis is present), more complex nutritional assessment, workup for celiac sprue, and endoscopy may be necessary.

Recurrent Abdominal Pain

Recurrent Abdominal Pain (RAP) is defined as episodic abdominal pain, with or without other symptoms, occurring more than once a month for 3 consecutive months, severe enough to interfere with daily activities, and clearly separated by asymptomatic periods. Prevalence in children ranges from 8%-30% with a slight female preponderance. Typical age at presentation is between 5-12; presentation before this is rare.

Causes of RAP can be classified as functional, psychogenic, or organic. The majority are **functional** (that is, without definable cause); the most frequently identified causes are nonulcer dyspepsia, irritable bowel syndrome, carbohydrate intolerance, and constipation. **Psychogenic**

RAP is hard to define, but is more likely to be present in patients with personality disorders, depression, or other psychiatric problems. RAP caused by **organic** conditions is less common in the pediatric population; possibilities include cholelithiasis, peptic ulcer disease, inflammatory bowel disease, dysmenorrhea, and nephrolithiasis.

Evaluation

Evaluation of a child with RAP should be directed toward eliciting information that can differentiate organic from functional or psychogenic causes. **Nonorganic pain** is usually periumbilical in location, does not radiate, is not temporally related to meals or bowel movements, and is frequently coupled with vague, nonabdominal complaints, while **organic pain** is more likely to present away from the umbilicus, awaken the child from sleep, and be associated with specific constitutional symptoms (see Chapter 25, "Abdominal Pain"). The presence of organomegaly, perianal abnormalities, a rash, arthritis, evidence of weight loss, or occult GI blood loss on examination indicates a high probability of organic disease. Extensive laboratory testing, radiologic workup, or specialist referral are not warranted unless suspicion for organic disease is strong.

Treatment

Treatment obviously depends on the etiology of the pain. Organic problems require specific medical or surgical treatment or correction. Treatment of functional pain is focused on education about the benign nature of the pain and the need to prevent the pain from interfering with important activities such as school or family functions. Specific dietary modifications may be helpful if lactose intolerance or constipation is thought to be the cause. The discontinuation of NSAIDS or the addition of antacids can be of benefit in patients with nonulcer dyspepsia. Followup visits for reassurance are an important part of the treatment plan.

Vomiting

Most **vomiting** in children is due to viral gastrointestinal infections and, as such, is self limited. Structural and functional abnormalities of the GI tract, extraintestinal infections, diabetic ketoacidosis, metabolic diseases, and central nervous system (CNS) lesions can also be responsible. The presence or absence of diarrhea is helpful: vomiting **plus** diarrhea makes the diagnosis of viral gastroenteritis far more certain. Age is important, too: vomiting presenting in the first 2 months of life is less likely to be the result of infection and can be due to formula intolerance, inborn errors of metabolism, gastroesophageal reflux, or a structural abnormality of the GI tract (see Chapter 38, "Pediatric Surgery"). Vomiting without nausea in association with a headache raises suspicion that an intracranial lesion is present. In general, vomiting that persists more than 7-10 days, presents in early infancy, or that is associated with respiratory or CNS complaints requires further evaluation; such evaluation is individualized according to the specific clinical circumstances.

Gastroesophageal Reflux

Gastroesophageal reflux disease (GERD) is common in infants, frequently presenting as recurrent vomiting or "spitting." Since virtually all children have some degree of reflux, the diagnosis of GERD should be reserved for children who have demonstrated an **abnormal quantity** of reflux (either frequency or duration) or who have **developed complications related directly to the reflux**. GERD is defined as the retrograde movement of stomach contents into the esophagus. In most children the cause is likely multifactorial, but the essential problem is dysfunction or incoordination of upper GI motility including abnormalities of the lower esophageal sphincter (LES), distal esophageal motility, and gastric emptying (although abnormal LES **position** does **not** seem to be the problem as it is in adults; see Chapter 22, "Gastroenterology"). The great majority of infants with GERD present with vomiting or frequent spitting, but clinically relevant GERD can be present in children without these symptoms. Other presenting problems include failure to thrive, irritability, apnea, recurrent wheezing or pulmonary infections, and apparent seizures.

Evaluation

Evaluation of the patient with suspected GERD begins with the exclusion of partial upper intestinal obstruction (pyloric stenosis, gastric antral web, duodenal stenosis, and malrotation, for example) and the causes of vomiting discussed above. **Contrast studies** of the upper GI tract with the child drinking the barium rather than having it administered through an NG tube can be done to confirm normal anatomy and motility. Esophageal pH monitoring is very sensitive for defining the frequency and duration of reflux; low pH indicates acid in the esophagus, hence reflux.

Treatment

Treatment of GERD should be undertaken with the understanding that the condition will resolve by one year of age or so without specific therapy in most children. If treatment is initiated, it should focus first on conservative, nonpharmacologic measures designed to reduce reflux, including thickened feeds, smaller, more frequent feedings, frequent burping, the maintenance of an upright, sitting position after meals and the prone position while lying down, and the avoidance of medications that lower LES tone. Pharmacologic therapy should be reserved for children with complications related to the GERD. Prokinetic agents such as cisapride (Propulsid) are the first line of therapy; antacids or H_2-blockers are generally only used if there is evidence of esophagitis. Only in severe cases or in special situations (patients with severe mental retardation often have refractory GERD; see Chapter 38, "Pediatric Surgery") is surgical intervention warranted. ■

56   Pediatric Nephrology

Pediatric nephrology is the study of disorders of the kidney during childhood. Renal failure is discussed in general in Chapter 21, "Nephrology," and Wilms' tumor in Chapter 38, "Pediatric Surgery." This chapter focuses on hematuria, proteinuria, and infections of the urinary tract in the pediatric population.

Hematuria and Proteinuria

Hematuria

Neither red blood cells (RBCs) nor protein are normally filtered at the glomerulus, and, thus, do not normally appear in the urine. Hematuria on a single urinalysis (UA) occurs at some point in approximately 5% of school-aged children, but only 0.5%-1% have persistent hematuria. Clinically significant **hematuria** is defined as the presence of greater than 2-5 RBCs per high power field (hpf) on at least 2 of 3 consecutive spun urine specimens obtained over a 2 month period. Hematuria can originate anywhere along the genitourinary (GU) tract. Conditions disrupting the architecture of the glomerular basement membrane result in **glomerular** bleeding. Hematuria may also be **nonglomerular**, resulting from structural damage, anoxic injury, trauma, toxins, or irritation.

Proteinuria

The prevalence of asymptomatic, transient **proteinuria** in children is 2%-12%, but only 0.6%-5% have persistent proteinuria. Urinary protein excretion is considered abnormal if it exceeds $4mg/m^2/hour$. Like hematuria, proteinuria can be of **glomerular** or **nonglomerular** origin. Proteinuria occurs in conditions where the normal size and charge selectivity of the glomerular basement membrane is damaged, or where glomerular hyperfiltration or decreased tubular resorption occur.

Nephritis is a general term for the clinical syndrome of hematuria and proteinuria usually combined with hypertension, oliguria, azotemia, and edema, while **nephrosis** refers to syndromes marked by heavy proteinuria (greater than or equal to $40mg/m^2/hr$) and resultant hypoalbuminemia and edema. The differential diagnosis for disorders of the kidneys in children is complex. In general, **the various conditions are best approached according to whether the child has hematuria, proteinuria, or both**:

Hematuria

Benign familial hematuria

Renal calculi

Idiopathic hypercalcuria

Urinary tract infection

Glomerulonephritis:
APSGN
IgA nephropathy

Sickle cell disease

Trauma

Cystic kidneys

Nephrocalcinosis

Renal vessel thrombosis

Proteinuria

Orthostatic proteinuria

Persistent benign proteinuria

Chronic glomerular disease:
Minimal change nephrotic syndrome
Focal segmental glomerulosclerosis

Combined Hematuria & Proteinuria

Glomerulonephritis:
APSGN
Membranoproliferative
Henoch Schonlein purpura
IgA nephropathy
Alport's nephritis

Systemic lupus erythematosis

Hemolytic-uremic syndrome

Acute tubular necrosis

Isolated Hematuria

Benign familial hematuria is an inherited glomerular disease characterized by thin glomerular basement membranes and preservation of renal function; as the name implies, prognosis is very good. **Renal calculi**, although more common in adults, occur in children. Stones can be congenital, related to infection or an underlying metabolic disorder, or idiopathic. **Idiopathic hypercalciuria** is fairly common and is the cause of bleeding in about a third of children with persistent, isolated hematuria. Bleeding can be microscopic (no grossly visible blood in the urine) or gross. Idiopathic hypercalciuria is a diagnosis of exclusion, and is defined by a urine calcium-to-creatinine ratio of 0.2 or greater or a 24 hour urinary calcium excretion greater than 4mg/kg/day in the absence of a discernible cause for hypercalciuria.
(continued)

Glomerulonephritis (discussed below) can present with isolated hematuria. **Sickle cell disease** and **trauma** also cause hematuria; in general, posttraumatic microscopic hematuria is not significant unless associated with penetrating injury or hypotension. The most common causes of hematuria in neonates are **urinary tract infection** (discussed below), **nephrocalcinosis** (often the result of chronic diuretic therapy), and **renal vessel thrombosis**.

Isolated Proteinuria

Isolated **transient** proteinuria can occur with fever or dehydration. Isolated **persistent** proteinuria can be benign or pathologic. **Orthostatic proteinuria** and **persistent benign proteinuria** typically occur in teenagers and carry a good prognosis. Orthostatic proteinuria characteristically causes proteinuria with upright posture; the first morning void is protein-free. Persistent benign proteinuria is characterized by a fixed, low-level of protein excretion.

The chronic glomerular diseases can present with isolated proteinuria or proteinuria combined with hematuria, with or without a full-blown nephrotic syndrome. **Minimal change nephrotic syndrome** (**MCNS**) classically occurs in 2-8 year-olds and is the most common cause of nephrotic syndrome in this age group. It is steroid-responsive and generally carries a good prognosis. **Focal segmental glomerulosclerosis** (**FSGS**) can be primary (idiopathic) or secondary to conditions such as ureteral reflux or AIDS. The prognosis varies; approximately 30%-50% of patients will eventually progress to end-stage renal disease (ESRD). Membranous nephropathy, the most common cause of nephrotic syndrome in adults, is rare in children.

Combined Hematuria and Proteinuria

The coexistence of hematuria and proteinuria suggests glomerulonephritis (GN). Acute post-Streptococcal GN (APSGN) is the most common acute GN in childhood and generally presents 7-21 days after a sore throat or skin infection. Immune complexes form and are deposited in the glomerular basement membrane, resulting in glomerular inflammation. Hematuria and proteinuria are usually both present; hematuria alone is sometimes seen early in the course of the disease or during the resolution phase. APSGN is associated with elevated anti-streptolysin O (ASO) titers and decreased C3 levels. C3 should normalize within 6-8 weeks; otherwise, membranoproliferative GN or lupus may be present. Proteinuria typically resolves over 1-2 months, but microhematuria can persist for 1-2 years. Prognosis is generally excellent. **Membranoproliferative GN (MPGN)** presents either as an acute nephritis or as asymptomatic hematuria and proteinuria. Three-quarters of patients have low C3 levels, but, in contrast to ASPGN, C3 levels remain persistently depressed. **Henoch Schonlein purpura (HSP)** is associated with purpura, abdominal pain, and arthritis. Nephritis can be present at the onset of illness or may develop up to several years later; prognosis is generally good. HSP is closely related to **IgA nephropathy**, which often presents as gross or microscopic hematuria following an upper respiratory tract infection. Proteinuria may or may not initially coexist, but patients require longterm followup; proteinuria indicates more significant renal injury and worsens prognosis. **Alport's hereditary nephritis** is an X-linked disorder that is associated with sensorineural hearing loss. Again, while Alport's nephritis often presents with isolated hematuria, proteinuria often develops later. Males usually progress to ESRF in early adulthood.

Other causes

Systemic lupus erythematosis (SLE) is a vasculitis that may be associated with photosensitivity, a malar rash, arthritis, pleural effusions, pericarditis, and cerebritis (in addition to nephritis). Characteristic laboratory studies include low C3 and C4 levels and positive anti-nuclear antibody (ANA) and anti-ds DNA titers. Prognosis for renal function depends on the type and degree of renal involvement, which is variable. **Hemolytic-uremic syndrome (HUS)**, the most common cause of acute renal failure in children in this country, is a microangiopathic hemolytic anemia associated with thrombocytopenia, uremia, and swelling of renal microvascular endothelial cells. It typically follows a diarrheal illness (often due to to E. coli 0157:H7); prognosis is generally good, although some patients may be left with significantly impaired renal function. **Acute tubular necrosis (ATN)** refers to the syndrome of tubular damage caused by renal hypoperfusion, hypoxia, or nephrotoxins. Because the tubular cells have the capacity to regenerate, full recovery can occur. Infections, particularly **pyelonephritis**, can cause hematuria, proteinuria, or both, and are discussed below.

Pediatrics
Pediatric Nephrology*continued*

Evaluation and Treatment

In patients who present with hematuria or proteinuria, important clues include whether or not a preceding or prodromal illness (including sore throat, skin infection, upper respiratory infection, or diarrhea), constitutional symptoms (fever, malaise, or weight loss), or symptoms suggesting a systemic inflammatory condition (rash, arthralgias or arthritis) are present. The use of potentially nephrotoxic drugs (such as nonsteroidal anti-inflammatory agents, aminoglycosides, or diuretics), episodes of hypotension or hypoxia, and recent trauma should be specifically excluded. A history of either an umbilical vessel catheter or maternal gestational diabetes increases the risk for renal vessel thrombosis. Relevant family history includes the presence of kidney stones, hypertension, arthritis, early hearing loss, hematuria, dialysis, and kidney transplant. Edema, headache, blurry vision, chest pain, and palpitations all indicate the need for unusually urgent evaluation.

On examination, evidence of fluid overload, edema, or rashes should be noted. Fundoscopic exam will identify hypertensive changes such as arteriovenous nicking, hemorrhage, or papilledema. Abnormal shape and position of the ears suggest a possible underlying renal anomaly since both organs develop at approximately the same gestational age. A sacral dimple can be seen with a neurogenic bladder.

Laboratory evaluation

Laboratory evaluation of hematuria and proteinuria begins with a complete **urinalysis (UA)**. The "dipstick" detects heme by a peroxidase reaction; it is sensitive but not specific. If the urine is discolored but heme-negative, dyes, drugs, or Serratia infection may be present. If the dipstick is heme-positive, microscopic analysis to confirm the presence of red blood cells (RBCs) must be done; absence of RBCs suggests hemoglobinuria or myoglobinuria. Up to 2-5 RBCs/hpf on a spun urine is normal. **Casts** are clumps of cells and debris in the shape of renal tubules; their presence indicates renal (as opposed to ureteral or cystic) pathology. RBC casts signify GN, but their absence does not exclude it.

The dipstick detects albumin only, thus, a false-negative result or underestimation of the degree of proteinuria can occur if non-albumin protein is being lost. False-positive results can occur in the presence of alkaline urine, Gram negative bacterial contamination, or certain skin cleansers. "Dipstick" proteinuria is confirmed by precipitation with **sulfasalicylic acid (SSA)** which detects all proteins. The degree of proteinuria can be estimated by checking a spot urine protein-to-creatinine ratio (normally less than 0.2), but for precise quantitation, a 24-hour urine collection is required.

Workup

Patients presenting with **hematuria** should also be evaluated for proteinuria by SSA testing. The evaluation of patients with persistent isolated hematuria should include determination of the urine calcium-to-creatinine ratio, blood chemistries, and complete blood count. C3 and C4 levels, ASO and ANA titers, IgA levels, urine culture, and renal ultrasound, as well as screening of family members, should also be performed. Consideration should be given to intravenous pyleography (IVP), specialized audiology and ophthalmology exams, and screening for sickle cell disease as indicated by history and physical findings. Patients with **hematuria and persistent proteinuria** should undergo 24 hour urine collection for determination of total protein and creatinine in addition to the workup above. If **proteinuria** is isolated and persistent, collection of the first morning and evening voids for 3 days is done to exclude orthostatic proteinuria. Additional workup includes a 24 hour urine collection for total protein and creatinine, chemistries, CBC, C3 and C4 levels, urine culture, renal ultrasound, and possibly IVP. Renal biopsy should be considered in situations where knowledge of the degree or type of renal involvement will help guide therapy. **Hematuria associated with hypertension, edema, oliguria, proteinuria, or RBC casts should be evaluated promptly**.

Specialty referral

Referral to a pediatric nephrologist for hematuria or proteinuria is indicated if signs of systemic disease are present, hematuria and proteinuria coexist, kidney function is abnormal, non-orthostatic proteinuria persists, or a family history of kidney disease exists. Therapy depends on the disease process. Some conditions, such as APSGN, resolve spontaneously, whereas others, such as MCNS, respond to steroids and/or other immunosuppressive agents. For many conditions, there is no specific therapy. Management of patients with these conditions is supportive, including diuresis, control of hypertension, and diet modification. Dialysis or renal transplant (see Chapter 39, "Transplantation") are required for those who progress to ESRF.

Urinary Tract Infections and Pyelonephritis

Urinary tract infections (**UTIs**) are common during childhood. In infancy, incidence is greater in males, but later in childhood, the "adult" female preponderance takes over. Diagnosis is based on the presence of significant bacteriuria (see below) in the context of appropriate symptoms; the characteristic symptom complex varies with age. In the neonatal period (birth-1 month), symptoms are nonspecific and include fever or hypothermia, poor feeding, jaundice, vomiting, irritability, and failure to thrive. During infancy (1-24 months) the patient may also have cloudy or foul-smelling urine, hematuria, dysuria, or frequency. The preschool child can present with abdominal or suprapubic pain, frequency, dysuria, fever, urgency, or enuresis, while the older child can complain of flank or abdominal pain and have costovertebral angle (CVA) tenderness. It has traditionally been taught that systemic symptoms (such as fever) indicate the presence of **pyelonephritis** (infection of the kidney parenchyma), whereas localized symptoms or asymptomatic bacteriuria indicate the presence of **cystitis** (infection localized to the bladder). This distinction between upper and lower tract UTIs, however, **cannot** reliably be made on the basis of presenting symptoms in **children**.

UA

The UA is used as a screening test for UTIs in older children and adults, but may be unreliable in young children. The dipstick method of identifying UTIs is based on a colorimetric assays for **leukocyte esterase** and **nitrites.** These assays depend on urine concentration and hence can be falsely negative in neonates and young children with dilute urine. Infants with fever and no obvious source of infection (including a "negative" UA by dipstick) should undergo urine culture and Gram staining. Leukocyte esterase indicates the presence of white blood cells in the urine, but does not necessarily mean that infection is present; sterile pyuria can occur with renal tubular acidosis, dehydration, glomerulonephritis, kidney stones, fever, or appendicitis (see Chapter 25, "Abdominal Pain"). Urinary **nitrites**, in contrast, are much more specific (99.7%) for the presence of a UTI, although also insensitive—like leukocyte esterase, when negative do not rule out a UTI.

Urine culture

The presence of a UTI is confirmed when a **significant number** of bacteria of a **single colony type** (2 different colony types can be present in newborns) are present in a **clean** urine specimen. Criteria for determining what constitutes a significant number vary depending on the method used to obtain the urine culture. In general, the presence of greater than 100,000 colonies indicates infection regardless of how the specimen was obtained. Lower counts (1,000-100,000) after catheterization are highly suspicious; essentially any growth after sterile suprapubic aspiration is considered significant.

Pathogenesis

Pathogenesis of UTIs varies with age. In the infant under 3 months, infection usually results from hematogenous spread; about one-fifth of patients have positive blood cultures. The organisms responsible are the same as those that cause neonatal sepsis (see Chapter 49, "Pediatric Infectious Diseases"). In patients older than 3 months, infection generally ascends from the periurethral tissues into the bladder. Therefore, the most common organisms seen are those normally present in the patient's own bowel flora: E. coli accounts for 90% of community-acquired UTIs; Klebsiella is the second most common organism. Patients with genitourinary tract anomalies have a higher frequency of infections with Proteus, Enterococcus, and Pseudomonas. Conditions that are associated with a higher frequency of UTIs include vesicoureteral reflux, congenital abnormalities, obstruction secondary to posterior urethral valves or ureteropelvic junction obstruction, renal calculi, neurogenic bladder, and infrequent voiding.

VUR

Although the incidence of **vesicoureteral reflux (VUR)** is less than 1% in normal children, it can be documented in as many as 40% of children with UTIs. VUR is a congenital anomaly in which the ureteral orifice is displaced laterally. The intracystic course of the ureter is shortened, producing an incompetent "valve." During micturition, high pressures are generated within the bladder. Urine is thus forced back into the ureters; after voiding, this urine then drains from the ureters back into the bladder, where it remains stagnant, promoting bacterial overgrowth. If significant reflux is present, bacteria can be introduced into the renal parenchyma in a retrograde fashion through the ureters.

Treatment

Infants under 3 months or any patient who is ill-appearing or dehydrated with a UTI should be admitted to the hospital, hydrated, and given parenteral broad spectrum antibiotics, typically a synthetic penicillin and an aminoglycoside to cover Gram positive and negative organisms, respectively. Urine cultures must be obtained before antibiotics are given; coverage is narrowed when identification and susceptibilities are available. There is controversy about the optimal duration of parenteral therapy for these patients, but, in general, intravenous antibiotics should be continued until the urine culture is sterile and the patient has been afebrile for 24-48 hours. Some physicians advocate at least 1 week of parenteral therapy in infants under 2 months. Oral antibiotics are used to complete a total of 10-14 days of coverage.

Patients who are not admitted to the hospital can be managed with a 7-10 day course of oral antibiotics tailored to organism susceptibility. Cultures to assure adequate coverage should be obtained before treatment, several days after starting antibiotics, and again after therapy is complete.

Further workup

The chance that an underlying structural abnormality exists is significant in young children who have had a UTI; many pediatricians will keep children who have had UTIs on oral antibiotic prophylaxis pending workup. In general, an **ultrasound** and **voiding cystourethrogram (VCUG)** should be obtained after the first UTI in boys regardless of age and in girls under 5; older girls should be evaluated if there is suspicion for pyelonephritis or if they have a second UTI. Ultrasound and VCUG are usually obtained 4-6 weeks after resolution of infection, but if the child is not improving after 2 days of therapy, the tests should be done at this point to rule out an anatomic problem requiring immediate attention. If there is no reflux, prophylaxis is discontinued. If reflux is present, prophylaxis should continue and an intravenous pyelogram (IVP) or nuclear medicine scan should be considered in order to evaluate function. Referral to a urologist is indicated in cases of significant reflux or other structural abnormalities. ■

57   Poisoning

Ingestion of a toxic substance (either accidentally or intentionally) by a child or adolescent is a problem frequently faced by pediatricians. Poison control centers receive roughly 1.5 million calls per year in the United States, 60% of which involve children under 6. Two peak age groups are at risk: **toddlers**, because of increasing mobility, oral behavior and curiosity, coupled with a lack of awareness of what is harmful and what is not, and **adolescents**, both because drug ingestion is frequently a means of attempted suicide, and because recreational drug use and experimentation are common.

Agents commonly involved in poisoning are those readily available in the child's environment, and include medications (frequently analgesics, antidepressants, cardiovascular agents, and salicylates), household products (cleaning agents, detergents, and caustics), plant and plant products, lead, iron supplements, and carbon monoxide.

Management

First, be aware of your **resources**. The PDR contains photographs of medications for easy identification as well as information on basic pharmacology and toxicology, but information regarding treatment of overdose is limited. Many emergency departments have a POISINDEX computer system, which contains information about virtually every known agent to which an ingestion or exposure has been reported; treatment and management guidelines are provided. The local poison control center is an essential resource and can be contacted by phone. The poison specialists (usually nurses or pharmacists) who staff the center can be most helpful in identifying products and providing basic information on the evaluation and management of the poisoned patient, and can get you in touch with a medical toxicologist, if needed.

H&P

As always, a detailed **history** is crucial for appropriate patient care. Patients who have been poisoned often present with the acute onset of an unknown illness, thus, a high index of suspicion is warranted. Several key historical points are important. The route of exposure must be ascertained; poisons can be ingested, inhaled, or contacted

Pediatrics
Poisoning *continued*

topically (skin and eyes). The time from exposure is important, because management often varies based on the time elapsed since ingestion. The exact ingredients of the agent must be elucidated. This is most easily accomplished if the container is brought by the family or EMS crew to the site of care. The maximal possible exposure must be estimated based upon the number of pills not accounted for; for children, calculate the per kilogram dose (mg/kg). Do not assume that adolescents will provide a reliable history since they may be attempting suicide. Documentation of events is important and should include any interventions (ipecac administration, emesis) occurring prior to your care.

The initial **physical evaluation** should be an assessment of the patient's ABCs. The airway and breathing can be compromised by excessive secretions, caustic airway burns, pharmacologic respiratory depression, or seizures. Hypotension and malignant cardiac dysrhythmias are hazards of many drug overdoses. Elective endotracheal intubation should be seriously considered for any patient with decreased mental status, and IV access and monitoring of oxygenation should be routine. Two drugs are critical in an unstable patient suspected of toxic ingestion: a comatose or seizing patient should be given **glucose** to treat potential hypoglycemia, and the opiate antagonist **naloxone** should be administered empirically if mental status is depressed (because children have access to narcotics in a multitude of analgesic, antidiarrheal, and cough preparations).

Toxidromes

Once immediate resuscitation issues have been addressed, the potentially poisoned patient should be carefully examined for signs of drug exposure. **Toxidromes** are syndromes (changes in vital signs, symptoms and signs) associated with specific toxins:

Organophosphates—Miosis, salivation, diarrhea, lacrimation, seizures, respiratory failure, bradycardia.

Salicylates—Fever, tachypnea, hyperpnea, lethargy, acidosis, tinnitus.

Anticholinergics—Dry mouth, flushed appearance, mydriasis (big pupils), fever, ileus, urinary retention, disorientation. "Dry as a bone, mad as a hatter, red as a beet..."

Sympathomimetics (cocaine, amphetamines)—Fever, tachycardia, hypertension, delirium, tremor, seizures, mydriasis, sweaty skin.

Phenothiazines—Oculogyric crisis, dystonia, opisthotonos.

Methanol—Severe metabolic acidosis, blurred vision, hyperemic retina.

Ethanol—Hypoglycemia, lethargy, ataxia, seizures, breath odor.

Ethylene glycol—Lethargy, coma, metabolic acidosis, crystalluria, hematuria.

Opiates—Pinpoint pupil, coma, respiratory depression.

Carbon Monoxide—Headache, "flu like" symptoms, dizziness, coma, redness of skin and nails.

Tricyclic Antidepressants—Prolonged QRS interval, coma, seizures, mydriasis, malignant ventricular dysrhythmias, metabolic acidosis.

Cyanide—Bitter almond odor, sense of doom, coma, metabolic acidosis, hypotension.

Clonidine—Coma, bradycardia, hypotension, pinpoint pupils.

Often the vital signs and physical exam narrow the possibilities in cases of possible ingestion of an unknown substance. In a child the amount actually swallowed is often unclear—the physical findings may be the only marker to guide patient management.

Laboratory evaluation should consist of electrolyte and arterial blood gas determinations and acetaminophen and salicylate levels (because they are so commonly ingested). The presence of an increased anion gap or frank acidosis are important to identify. Serum and urine toxicology screens may be obtained when the diagnosis is unclear; these take time, however, and therefore may not be immediately helpful. In almost every patient, gastrointestinal decontamination should be considered.

Gastrointestinal Decontamination

The goal of gastric decontamination is to minimize absorption from the GI tract. This can be done by inducing emesis, by lavaging the stomach, by the administration of activated charcoal, and/or by whole-bowel irrigation.

Emesis

Syrup of ipecac, an **emetic**, is widely distributed by pediatricians as part of routine preventive care. Ipecac generally induces vomiting within 30 minutes, and administration can be repeated once if ineffective. Ipecac can be used at home if the patient is alert, although parents should only administer ipecac under the guidance of a physician or poison control center. Patients who have ingested hydrocarbons or caustics should **not** have emesis induced due to the risk of further esophageal, pharyngeal, or pulmonary injury. Induction of emesis is also contraindicated if the use of activated charcoal is imminent or after ingestion of any agent that might produce coma or seizures, because of the risk of aspiration.

Gastric lavage

Gastric lavage through a large bore tube is a time-honored and fairly efficient method to empty the stomach (as well as to sample its contents). If the child does not have an intact gag reflex, prophylactic endotracheal intubation must be performed prior to lavage. If performed within an hour or so of ingestion, lavage may be helpful, especially after ingestion of a severely toxic substance, but activated charcoal alone may be satisfactory in many cases.

Charcoal

Activated charcoal is the mainstay of modern poison treatment and is indicated for almost any patient. There are few contraindications for charcoal administration, but adsorption is poor for caustics, heavy metals, iron, ethanol, methanol, and ethylene glycol. Younger patients may require an NG tube for administration. The initial dose is usually given concurrently with a cathartic agent (sorbitol) to speed elimination. Because cathartics can exacerbate electrolyte disturbances, repeat dosing should be with plain (sorbitol-free) solutions.

Irrigation

Whole-bowel irrigation refers to the use of osmotically active agents usually used for preoperative bowel preparation. Typically, polyethylene glycol is given orally or by nasogastric tube. It is an attractive therapy for the treatment of ingestion of iron, lithium, lead, batteries, and other substances that are not appropriately treated with activated charcoal.

Management of Specific Agents

Tylenol

Acetaminophen (Tylenol) is ubiquitous in American households, and, as such, is commonly encountered in accidental poisonings and suicide attempts. Doses of 140mg/kg are in the toxic range. Toxicity results from hepatic accumulation of a toxic metabolite which must be detoxified by glutathione. If glutathione is depleted, fatal hepatic failure can occur. Initial manifestations are vague and include nausea, pallor, and weakness. These resolve by 12-24 hours. The patient may appear symptom free for the next 1-4 days, but jaundice, liver tenderness, and LFT elevations follow. Treatment with **N-acetyl-cysteine (NAC)** replenishes hepatic glutathione activity and is therefore protective. Serum acetaminophen levels should be obtained and interpreted using the widely available nomogram (Rumak et al). A level of 150mcg/mL or 75mcg/mL at 4 or 8 hours after ingestion, respectively, is an indication for treatment with NAC. NAC is given orally, and because charcoal adsorbs NAC, their dosing should be staggered, if possible. Close surveillance of hepatic function is important, and recovery is usually complete by day eight.

Lead

Chronic **lead** exposure is a major public health problem affecting millions of children across all socioeconomic levels. Most children are exposed to environmental sources such as lead paint chips (window frames) and dust (when remodeling a home). The removal from the market of leaded gasoline and paint has done much to lower the environmental burden and limit continued exposure, but millions of children still continue to have high levels. In 1991 the CDC issued new guidelines regarding lead poisoning. The current definition of an elevated lead level is now 10mcg/dL, and therefore approximately 20%

Pediatrics
Poisoning *continued*

of American children have an unacceptably high amount of lead in their bodies. Population-based testing shows decremental reductions in IQ when the lead level is above 10mcg/dL—roughly, 1-3 IQ points are lost for every 10mcg/dL increase in blood lead levels.

Children with blood lead levels less than 75mcg/dL are usually asymptomatic. Most children with elevated levels show evidence of a microcytic anemia due to concurrent dietary iron deficiency as well as a direct, lead-induced marrow toxicity. Increased levels of free erythrocyte protoporphyrin (FEP) result; this is a good screening test for lead exposure. Iron replacement is indicated to treat the underlying deficiency and to decrease the rate of gut lead absorption.

The best treatment is prevention. Universal lead education and funding for removal of lead from the homes of children with elevated screening tests are provided by most states. High lead levels (greater than 75mcg/dL) can lead to an acute encephalopathy. Pharmacologic treatment (chelation therapy) is indicated when the blood level is approaching 40mcg/dL. Intravenous EDTA chelation therapy is most commonly used, while BAL (British anti-Lewis agent), given by IM injection, is reserved for children with very high levels. Two oral agents, DMSA and d-penicillamine, have been advocated by some for outpatient chelation therapy.

Iron

Iron poisoning usually occurs by accidental consumption of adult iron preparations. X-rays will sometimes show iron pills in the stomach. Iron is an essential enzyme cofactor, but in high doses causes gastric irritation, hypotension, hepatic dysfunction, mitochondrial failure, and acidosis. A characteristic sequence of events occurs with toxic ingestion: first, local GI irritation and possible hemorrhage occur (Stage I). This may be followed by a quiescent period, the onset of systemic symptoms, including acidosis and lethargy (Stage II), and finally by potentially fatal multiple organ failure (Stage III). Stage IV consists of late sequelae such as GI strictures or gastric outlet obstruction in survivors. Ingestion of 20mg/kg or less of elemental iron is probably not harmful. Initial treatment (for exposures greater than this) includes gastric lavage for recent ingestions—ipecac is not recommended because persistent emesis could be confused with stage I illness, and activated charcoal does not adsorb iron and is not useful. Case reports have shown that whole-bowel irrigation with polyethylene glycol is effective, although controlled trials have not been done. Chelation therapy should be instituted if any signs of toxicity occur. Treatment generally lasts until the patient is asymptomatic or the iron is eliminated.

TCAs

A single dose of a **tricyclic antidepressant (imipramine, amitriptyline**, etc), can be fatal to a toddler. The tricyclics' therapeutic effects stem from blocking norepinephrine reuptake, thus increasing brain levels. They also have anticholinergic effects that are greatly exaggerated after an overdose. Early signs of toxicity include tachycardia and mydriasis, with QRS complex prolongation after higher dosages. A prolonged QRS complex is the hallmark of tricyclic antidepressant toxicity and indicates that further problems such as ventricular dysrhythmia or hypotension may be at hand. CNS manifestations are usually present and range from mild lethargy to coma and seizure.

Tricyclic poisoning is quite serious. If the history is unclear and the patient is asymptomatic, a 6 hour observation period is prudent. If no symptoms have occurred during this period the patient can be safely discharged. Patients with documented ingestion (or in whom a high level of suspicion is present) should receive charcoal (and gastric lavage if seen soon after ingestion). Ipecac is not recommended due to the danger of aspiration if mental status deterioration occurs. An EKG should be obtained. Cardiac toxicity is treated by alkalinization of the blood with bicarbonate infusion. Tricyclic overdose remains the most common cause of death from prescription drugs.

Caustics and corrosives

Caustics and **corrosives** include a wide variety of household chemicals capable of causing mucosal burns and irritation. Sodium hydroxide, ammonia salts, and acids are often tasted by inquisitive toddlers. **Alkalis** combine with proteins and fats to cause deep liquefaction necrosis. The most commonly encountered agent in this category is sodium hydroxide, found in drain cleaners, lye, and some industrial products. Solid dishwashing detergent contains sodium carbonate, also an alkali. Ingestion can produce deep tissue necrosis of oral and esophageal mucosa, progressing at times to perforation and mediastinitis. The first treatment priority is airway assessment, since glottic edema can cause obstruction. Affected skin should be washed with copious amounts of water, and eyes should be irrigated for at least 15 minutes. If ingested, dilution with water or milk is carried out if the patient can swallow. After large ingestions early endoscopy should be performed to assess the degree of injury; corticosteroids can limit esophageal inflammation and reduce later stricture formation. A pediatric surgeon should be involved. Topical **acid** exposure should be treated with dilution; ingestion is rare. Vapor inhalation can occur and may cause respiratory compromise, thus, careful evaluation of the victim's respiratory status is mandatory. No attempt should be made to neutralize an acid or a base, either exposed topically or ingested, because the resulting heat will do more harm than good. Water is the most useful dilutant.

Hydocarbons

Hydrocarbons such as kerosene, gasoline, or mineral oil are also commonly ingested. These agents rarely cause systemic toxicity; the major clinical problems stem from aspiration and resulting pulmonary injury. Less viscous agents are more easily aspirated. Minor ingestions with no prolonged cough can be managed with careful observation at home, but if any prolonged cough or evidence of respiratory compromise is present, hospital evaluation is required. Fever, intercostal retractions, respiratory distress, and CXR changes may begin within 30 minutes after aspiration. After severe aspiration, symptoms generally progress for the first 24 hours, with gradual resolution over the next few days.

Salicylates

Salicylate ingestions are becoming less common. In addition to aspirin, liniments containing methyl salicylate are potential sources. Aspirin is also found in combination in multiple pharmaceutical products. Salicylates are gastric irritants. They interfere with platelet aggregation, cause uncoupling of oxidative phosphorylation, are central respiratory stimulants, and can be directly hepatotoxic. Signs and symptoms of salicylate poisoning include tinnitus due to direct ototoxicity, profuse sweating and flushing, fever, hyperpnea, seizures, coma, and both hyperglycemia (early) and hypoglycemia (late). Treatment should include emesis or lavage and the administration of activated charcoal. A salicylate level should be obtained upon presentation and repeated in 2 hours. Initial ingestion of more than 150mg/kg is the average toxic dose, and a 6-hour level of greater than 100mg/dL indicates severe poisoning. Alkalinization of the urine speeds elimination, and hemodialysis has been used in severe cases.

Severe toxins

Recent analysis has identified several agents that can be fatal to a toddler in a single dosing unit (single pill or mouthful). This short list of medications is responsible for approximately 50% of fatal ingestions in children just under 2: **camphor**, **chloroquine**, **tricyclic antidepressants**, **phenothiazines**, **quinine**, **methyl salicylate (oil of wintergreen)**, and **theophylline**. Any exposure to these agents by a young child should be considered a medical emergency.

Final Considerations

Accidental or intentional ingestions are serious events for victims and their families. A toddler's folly may expose a family in desperate need of social service support. All intentional ingestions of any product, no matter how benign, should be regarded as serious suicide attempts —patients do not know what is deadly and what isn't. No such patient should be discharged from your care without a thorough psychiatric evaluation and risk assessment (see Chapter 70, "Psychiatric Emergencies") ■

58 Child Abuse

Child abuse and neglect are underrecognized and under-reported. Both the clandestine nature of intentional injury and the subtlety of signs and symptoms make diagnosis difficult. Teachers, doctors, nurses, social workers, day care providers, and all those whose jobs include interactions with children are required by law to report suspected maltreatment.

Definitions

The maltreatment of children is divided into four categories: neglect, physical abuse, sexual abuse, and emotional abuse. The most common form of maltreatment, **neglect**, is defined as failure of a custodian to provide support, shelter, food, clothes, supervision, or medical care for the child. Inflicting bodily harm constitutes **physical abuse**. Improper exposure of a child to sexual acts or materials as well as frank intimate contact between adults and children constitutes **sexual abuse**, while pathologic criticism or aloofness that disrupts the social and psychologic development of the child constitutes **emotional abuse**.

Screening and Diagnosis

Pediatricians and other primary care physicians are in the position to routinely screen their patients for abuse and neglect. The presence of other forms of violence within the family increases the chance of child abuse; early detection of family dysfunction can prompt a life-saving referral. Once any such problem is suspected, investigation of family dynamics is imperative. Familial "risk factors" for abuse or neglect include parents with a history of having been abused themselves, children who are the products of unwanted and/or adolescent pregnancies, illegitimate children, substance abuse within the family, families without extended family or support groups, and families lacking strong social skills or financial resources.

History and physical

Worrisome **historical** findings include a story that is inconsistent with the injuries sustained, different caretakers offering differing explanations for the same injury, delay in seeking medical attention, multiple visits to different hospitals, and an inappropriate reaction by the parents to the severity of injury. Children and parents should be interviewed separately at some point in the process of evaluation. Findings on the **physical exam** that raise the suspicion of child abuse include bruises or burns in the shape of objects, well-demarcated burns in a "stocking-glove" distribution (suggesting immersion injury), soft tissue swelling in normally protected areas such as the stomach, thighs, or upper arms, human bites, bruises of various colors indicating varying ages, perineal or genital injury, gross deformity of an extremity, otherwise unexplained seizures, altered consciousness, or coma. More subtle signs include growth retardation, poor hygiene and appearance, irritability, flat affect, and repressed, age-inappropriate behavior. Look for signs of injuries that are not normally encountered in a child's day-to-day life, and for evidence that ongoing emotional and/or physical stress has been applied to the patient.

Specific Injuries

Head trauma is the leading cause of fatalities due to child abuse; infants less than 1 year of age are most commonly affected. Abused infants often have no external injuries or skull fractures; retinal hemorrhages and long bone or rib fractures, however, are common and suggest the victim has been vigorously shaken and/or thrown. Retinal hemorrhages are present in 50%-80% of infants with **shaken baby syndrome** as opposed to only 3% or so of accidentally injured children.

Abdominal trauma is the second most common cause of fatalities from abuse. Symptoms are no different from those of abdominal injury from any cause (see Chapter 28, "Trauma"); the task is to distinguish whether abuse has taken place or not. In general, significant abdominal injury in a child from causes other than a motor vehicle or bicycle accident, major fall, or deceleration injury (sledding, for example) is fairly rare.

Bruises are common during childhood. As the heme in the ecchymosis is metabolized to bilirubin, the bruise changes color; the coloring of the lesion gives an estimated date of injury. A newly inflicted bruise is red, tender and swollen; over the next few days, the bruise becomes black and blue. Between the fifth and seventh day, the bruise is green; between the first and second weeks, yellow; and, finally it turns brown before disappearing. The hallmark of abuse is the finding of multiple bruises of different colors, suggesting that repetitive injury has occurred.

Bites have a characteristic appearance and can, in fact, be used (by a forensic dentist) to specifically identify the abuser. If the distance between the marks of the canine teeth is greater than 3-4cm, the bite was made by an adult.

Although **fractures** are fairly common during childhood, some are more suspicious than others, primarily because of the amount and direction of force needed to break certain bones. **Femur** and **spiral fractures** in children under 3 are uncommon; likewise, **metaphyseal fragmentation** and **epiphyseal separations** are rarely caused by accidental trauma. **Fractures in various stages of healing**, like bruises of different ages, suggest that a pattern of repetitive injury has occurred; total-body x-ray (skeletal survey) must be obtained when abuse is suspected. Several rare childhood diseases such as osteogenesis imperfecta, congenital syphilis, and rickets can present with multiple or unusual fractures, and these must be considered in the differential diagnosis of abuse.

Sexual abuse of children occurs in every community and at all socioeconomic levels. After sexual abuse, a child's errors of memory tend to involve omission rather than commission. That is, the child may have problems recalling specific details, but is unlikely to fabricate events that did not occur. Like adults, however, children may be susceptible to suggestion and therefore must be questioned very carefully; a thorough history of the alleged event is particularly important for the purpose of criminal investigation and prosecution.

It has been shown repeatedly that physical exam is usually normal or inconclusive, even after proven cases of sexual abuse: a **normal** exam does **not** exclude abuse. Even if no physical trauma is believed to have occurred, however, examination is important to identify any medical problems requiring treatment, to document normal findings, to screen for pregnancy and sexually transmitted diseases, and to collect forensic evidence. The examiner must be aware of the range of normal female genital findings. Contour, configuration, orifice size, and color of the hymen can vary depending on the age of the child, pubertal development stage, and position during examination. Findings suggesting abuse in a girl include vaginal discharge, notches in the lower half of the hymen, jagged and/or irregular hymenal margins, and absence of the hymen.

Perianal erythema, lacerations, and/or ecchymoses are common acute sequelae of **sodomy**; these typically resolve within days after the abuse has stopped. Signs of chronic anal penetration include hypertrophy and/or hyperpigmentation of anal tissue, an oddly shaped anal orifice, and lax rectal tone.

Sexually transmitted diseases (STDs) are rarely seen in sexually abused children, but any prepubertal child with an STD must be presumed to have been abused. Treatment of STDs (see Chapter 64, "Emergency Department Gynecology"), prevention of pregnancy, treatment of traumatic injuries, and assurance of the child's safety after sexual abuse are often best accomplished by hospital admission.

All children who are abused suffer significant consequences. Frequent sequelae include delayed social, language, or emotional development, poor interpersonal skills, and behavioral dysfunction. The major challenge for those working with abused children is **rehabilitation** of the child and family. The evaluation and management of child abuse is always a multidisciplinary effort. In every case of suspected abuse or neglect, a compassionate but **thorough evaluation** with **meticulous documentation** is essential. ■

OB-Gyn

Men-Jean Lee
and
Giuseppe Del Priore
Section Editors

59   Prenatal Care

The goal of prenatal care is to optimize the health of two patients: mother and fetus. Lack of adequate prenatal care is one of the most significant risk factors for poor pregnancy outcome.

Diagnosis of Pregnancy

The diagnosis of pregnancy is not always straightforward. There are presumptive, probable, and positive diagnostic criteria. **Presumptive signs** include amenorrhea, breast fullness, skin changes, nausea, vomiting, urinary frequency, and fatigue. Fetal movements (quickening) are not usually noted by the mother until 18-20 weeks into the pregnancy. **Probable signs** include uterine enlargement, softening of the uterine isthmus (Hegar's sign), vaginal and cervical cyanosis (Chadwick's sign), and positive urine or blood pregnancy tests (beta subunit of the human chorionic gonadotropin molecule; beta-hCG). Note that none of these excludes a molar pregnancy (see Chapter 66, "Gynecologic Malignancies"). **Positive diagnostic signs** are the detection of fetal heart sounds or palpable fetal movements. Fetal heart tones can be detected 10-12 weeks from the last menstrual period (LMP) by Doppler. An abdominal ultrasound (US) can identify a gestational sac 42 days after LMP (or with a beta-hCG of 5000); transvaginal US is even more sensitive.

Due date

The next question to answer is when the baby is due, termed EDC (estimated date of confinement) or EDD (estimated due date). The mean duration of pregnancy is 40 weeks (280 days) from the **first day of the LMP** (note this is **not** the true age of the fetus, but a convention). Nagele's rule is useful: add 7 days to the first day of the LMP, then subtract 3 months to obtain the EDC. In the first trimester the crown-rump length of the fetus by US is the most accurate determinant of fetal age, within 3-5 days.

Prenatal Care

Prenatal care begins with the initial office visit and continues until birth. A detailed but directed history and physical examination is the first step. In addition to her overall health, the **history** should cover the woman's menstrual history and history of contraceptive use, previous laparotomies (particularly operations on the uterus such as myomectomy), and whether or not she has had any abnormal Pap smears and how they were treated (because cervical procedures can weaken the cervix and result in cervical incompetence).

The first task of the obstetrician is to establish the woman's EDC. If the patient's LMP was regular, normal, and reliable, her EDC can be easily calculated. If the patient cannot recall her LMP, however, has irregular menses, or has been on hormonal contraception within the previous 6 months, US should be performed to date the pregnancy. Prompt and correct establishment of the EDC provides for properly timed prenatal care.

Terminology

Gravidity (total number of pregnancies) and **parity** (total number of pregnancies delivered) should be ascertained. Parity is typically recorded as 4 numbers: term deliveries, preterm deliveries, abortions (spontaneous and elective prior to 20 weeks estimated gestational age; EGA) and living offspring. For example, a woman pregnant for the fourth time whose 3 previous pregnancies ended up as miscarriage (prior to 20 weeks), preterm delivery, and full-term delivery, with 2 living children, would be recorded as a "$G_4 P_{1112}$." The terms "nulligravida," "primigravida," and "multigravida," respectively, refer to women who have never been pregnant, who have been pregnant once, and who have been pregnant more than once. In a similar fashion, the terms "nullipara," "primipara," and "multipara," respectively, refer to women who have never delivered, who have delivered once, and who have delivered more than 1 pregnancy at more than 20 weeks gestational age.

History

The **details of past pregnancies** (length of labor, type of delivery, and complications) are important, as are details of environmental exposure, medications taken while possibly pregnant, and DES exposure (while her mother was pregnant with the patient herself). Information from pre-

OB-Gyn
Prenatal Care *continued*

vious pregnancies is useful for counseling during the current pregnancy. For example, a woman who has delivered 9 and 10 pound babies vaginally in the past should have no trouble delivering a 7 pound baby this pregnancy, but needs to be screened early for diabetes (see section on prenatal labs below); a woman who underwent a classic Caesarean section in the past would not be offered a vaginal delivery this pregnancy.

Review of the woman's **medical problems** helps determine the level of care needed along the spectrum from midwife to a high-risk specialist (perinatologist). Social issues such as tobacco, alcohol, and illicit drug use are addressed with respect to their effect on the developing fetus. A history of any genetic disease, if present, should be obtained. Postpartum family planning and contraceptive counseling should be initiated at the first prenatal visit, and postpartum tubal ligation can also be considered. Most patients are started on vitamins and iron at their first visit.

Exam

A complete general **physical exam** is performed. The abdominal exam includes assessment of fundal height and the presence of fetal heart sounds. A pelvic exam is done to assess cervical appearance and dilatation, and to perform a Pap smear and cultures for Neisseria gonorrhea and Chlamydia (see Chapters 48, "TORCH Infections," and 64, "ED Gynecology"). The gestational age can be estimated by the size of the uterus:

Gestational age

- 8 weeks-twice normal size
- 12 weeks-top of uterus just palpable above the symphysis
- 16 weeks-uterine fundus midway between symphysis and umbilicus
- 20 weeks-fundus at umbilicus
- 20 weeks to term-age of fetus is equal to the fundal height in cm (±3cm).

Uterine size exceeding the estimated gestational age by 3cm or more suggests the presence of a molar pregnancy (see Chapter 66, "Gynecologic Malignancies"), multiple fetuses, leiomyomas, polyhydramnios (excess amniotic fluid), or an inaccurate LMP; an US will clarify the situation. The adnexa are difficult to evaluate in a pregnant woman.

Pelvimetry

Clinical **pelvimetry** is the evaluation of the bony pelvis by exam to predict its adequacy for delivery, although it is fairly unreliable. X-ray or CT pelvimetry are rarely used, never in early pregnancy. The gynecoid pelvis (hollow and roomy) is most common in females and is best suited for vaginal delivery. The anthropoid pelvis is more often associated with fetuses that go through labor in an occiput posterior position; true android pelves are narrow and associated with cephalopelvic disproportion. Platypelloid pelves (flat pelvis) are risk factors for transverse arrest during labor and delivery.

Ultrasound

Ultrasound is often performed in the United States, often at 16-20 weeks when the fetal anatomy is clearest. There is controversy whether routine sonography for all pregnant women is truly indicated for all pregnancies because the rate of unexpected, correctable anomalies is fairly low and the costs of mass screening are high. The utility of US is that if an abnormality (such as renal, cardiovascular, spinal, or abdominal wall defects) is found, the appropriate specialists (neonatologists or pediatric surgeons, for example) can be consulted prior to delivery; it also produces a great deal of patient satisfaction.

Laboratory

Routine initial laboratory screen for all pregnant women includes a complete blood count (CBC), blood type and antibody screen, rubella antibody screen, urinalysis and culture, screening tests for syphilis, a Pap smear, gonorrhea and chlamydia genital cultures, and a hepatitis screen; sickle cell screening is recommended in the African-American population. Specialized tests, such as carrier screening for Tay-Sachs disease and cystic fibrosis, can be offered to those couples who are at risk by demographics or family history. Urine toxicology testing can be performed at the physician's discretion. HIV testing should also be offered, regardless of professed risk factors, because prophylactic zidovudine (AZT) can now be given during pregnancy to decrease perinatal HIV transmission from 26% to 8%.
(continued)

AFP

A **maternal serum alpha-fetoprotein (MSAFP)** test is offered at 15-20 weeks, originally to identify possible neural tube defects (which affect 1 in 1000 pregnancies). If the MSAFP is elevated, detailed US to look for such defects or other anomalies can be performed, as can an amniocentesis to measure **amniotic** AFP and cholinesterase (released from the malformed neural tube). A fetus with a NTD requires special care during delivery and can grow up to have mild to severe paraplegia. Some laboratories add an hCG level (known as a "double screen") to increase the chance of detection of Down's syndrome or other syndromes associated with aneuploidy. A woman with low MSAFP but a high hCG is at risk for carrying a fetus with chromosomal abnormalities; amniocentesis for karyotyping and genetic counseling are recommended in this situation.

Gestational diabetes screening

Other tests recommended during pregnancy include a Glucola test (a 1-hour screening test for hyperglycemia utilizing 50g of oral glucose) to rule out gestational diabetes at 24-28 weeks, and followup hematocrit and syphilis screening. The cutoff for an abnormal Glucola test ranges from 130-140mg/dL, depending on the institution. If the patient has an abnormal Glucola screening test, a confirmatory 3-hour glucose tolerance test (3-hour GTT) should be done to rule out gestational diabetes mellitus (GDM). The 3-hour GTT is performed after 3 days of carbohydrate loading (with fasting the night before the test). In the morning, a fasting blood glucose is obtained and the patient is given a 100g glucose load. Blood glucoses are then drawn at 1, 2, and 3 hour intervals; normal cutoff values are 190, 165, and 145mg/dL, respectively. A patient with 2 or more out of 4 abnormal values (including fasting) is diagnosed as having GDM.

The frequency of office visits varies. In general, women less than 28 weeks are seen every 4 weeks. Between 28-36 weeks they are seen every 2 weeks, and from 36 weeks to delivery, weekly. At all office visits, the patient is weighed and the fundal height and fetal heart rate are measured. Routine pelvic exams are not needed unless the patient is at risk for preterm labor. At every visit the patient is screened for hypertension, edema, and proteinuria to rule out preeclampsia (see Chapter 61, "Obstetric

Complications"), and glucosuria to rule out gestational or previously undiagnosed pregestational diabetes (i.e., chronic diabetes mellitus).

Medications

Certain medications should be avoided in a pregnant woman. It is important for the physician to weigh the risk/benefit ratio of each drug, as well as to consider whether or not the fetus is sensitive to the drug at that particular gestational age. For example, lithium has been associated with cardiac defects. If the patient presents to the physician at 20 weeks, however, stopping the lithium at that point does not make sense, because the fetal heart has already formed.

Coumadin is a known teratogen that causes nail hypoplasia, scoliosis, and skeletal deformities, but the maternal benefits can outweigh the fetal risks in women with prosthetic heart valves requiring full anticoagulation.

Tetracycline is a known teratogen that causes staining of the teeth and bones (although this is not life threatening).

Thalidomide is a known teratogen that causes limb reduction defects (phocomelia); it is **absolutely** contraindicated during pregnancy.

Methotrexate, a cancer chemotherapeutic agent, is a known human teratogen that causes skeletal and cardiac defects, and is a folic acid antagonist that targets rapidly dividing trophoblastic tissue; it is **absolutely** contraindicated during pregnancy (in fact, trials are underway studying its usefulness for elective abortion).

Retinoic acid, used to treat acne, is a known teratogen that causes cardiac, CNS, and skeletal defects; it is **absolutely** contraindicated during pregnancy.

Antiseizure medications such as **phenytoin**, **carbamazapine**, and **valproic acid** have been associated with congenital anomalies; but the risks of stopping these medications during pregnancy, however, include increasing the chances of a seizure with the potential for hypoxia and fetal death.
(continued)

Angiotensin converting enzyme (ACE) inhibitors have been found to cause oligohydramnios, permanent renal damage, and fetal death.

Most medications are safe to use during pregnancy, including many antibiotics (penicillins, erythromycin, macrodantin, gentamicin, clindamycin, and metronidazole), acetaminophen, heparin (which is too large to cross the placenta), narcotics (pain is not good for either the mother or the fetus), Benadryl, pseudoephedrine, and Robitussin. Although aspirin has traditionally been believed to be contraindicated during pregnancy, it is now commonly used in low doses to treat immunologic disorders under close supervision.

Common Minor Problems

Pregnant women can develop the same gynecologic problems as can nonpregnant (see Chapter 64, "ED Gynecology"). Some are more common, more troublesome, or pose a risk to the fetus.

A **Bartholin's gland abscess** is an infection of a cystic Bartholin's gland or duct. It presents as a painful, erythematous cystic enlargement on either side of the lateral vaginal introitus. Treatment options are the same as for any abscess in a can nonpregnant patient; sitz baths, antibiotics, and analgesics are adequate if small, while incision and drainage is needed, if large. **Condyloma acuminata** (genital warts) are hyperkeratotic, flat, or polypoid lesions in the vulvar or perineal areas, caused by infection with human papilloma virus. Pregnancy can stimulate proliferation of the lesion. Treatment is problematic; trichloroacetic acid (TCA) application, cryotherapy, cautery or laser ablation can all be attempted during pregnancy, but podophyllin or 5-FU should be avoided due to possible fetal side effects. Treatment is usually deferred until after delivery.

Herpes lesions, due to infection with the herpes simplex virus (HSV), are small, painful, erythematous ulcerations. Acyclovir, sometimes beneficial, can be used under physician supervision during pregnancy. This infection can be transmitted to the fetus (see Chapter 48, "TORCH infections"): if active lesions are present in the birth canal when labor begins, Caesarean delivery is indicated.

Several benign infections are common during pregnancy. **Monilial vulvovaginitis** can be treated with nystatin or miconazole cream. **Trichomonas vaginitis** presents as vulvar itching with a frothy, malodorous discharge. Clotrimazole can be used during the first trimester; metronidazole can be used in the second and third trimesters. **Bacterial vaginosis** presents as an asymptomatic, white or gray malodorous discharge, and can be treated with clindamycin during the first trimester and with metronidazole in the second and third trimesters.

Chlamydia infection can be treated with erythromycin or azithromycin during pregnancy because of concern about tetracycline's effects on the fetus. **Gonorrhea** infection is treated with penicillins or cephalosporins. **Syphilis** infection during pregnancy is so difficult to treat, however, that penicillin is the ONLY drug recommended by the CDC. A woman with a history of penicillin allergy will require skin testing and desensitization in a monitored setting to receive her penicillin treatment. ■

60　Medical Complications and Pregnancy

When taking care of pregnant women with preexisting medical conditions or those who develop medical complications diagnosed during pregnancy, there are several basic questions:

– How does the disease affect the pregnancy?
– How does pregnancy affect the disease?
– How does the pregnancy affect diagnosis of the disease?
– How does the pregnancy affect treatment of the disease?

Cardiac Disease

Pregnant women with pre-existing cardiac disease pose special problems. Maternal mortality depends on the particular condition; pregnancy is rarely ever totally contraindicated unless Eisenmenger syndrome with pulmonary hypertension is present (see Chapter 52, "Pediatric Cardiology").

Cardiac lesions, particularly valvular abnormalities, necessitate antibiotic prophylaxis during labor and delivery, particularly if manual removal of a retained placenta is necessary. Prophylaxis typically consists of IV ampicillin and gentamycin every 8 hours starting at the beginning of labor; one postpartum dose is adequate. Patients who are chronically anticoagulated must be so identified. Warfarin (Coumadin) carries with it the risk of fetal anomalies, so, during pregnancy, subcutaneous heparin is used because it does not cross the placenta. Some women with severe cardiac disease may require intrapartum invasive cardiac monitoring; others may need a shortened second stage of labor or a scheduled Caesarean section (CS; see Chapter 62, "Labor and Delivery"). Obviously, the risk of transmission of a congenital heart defect from the mother to the child is possible. Most congenital heart defects are transmitted in a multifactoral inheritance pattern; the risk of transmission to the fetus ranges from 2%-5%.

Small ventricular septal defects (**VSD**) are usually well tolerated. Large VSDs may allow enough left-to-right shunting during late pregnancy and delivery to decrease cardiac output or cause congestive heart failure (CHF); invasive monitoring is recommended if the VSD is large. **Atrial septal defect** is the most common congenital anomaly in adults. Pregnancy is usually well-tolerated; supraventricular arrhythmias due to atrial stretching with physiologic hypervolemia of pregnancy may occur. Invasive cardiac monitoring is not usually necessary and the patient may undergo normal vaginal delivery. **Eisenmenger syndrome** exists when flow through a left-to-right shunt reverses due to longstanding pulmonary hypertension, and is a marker of end-stage heart disease. Maternal mortality is as high as 70% with pregnancy; termination is strongly recommended. **Mitral valve prolapse** is the most common congenital anomaly present in women of reproductive age and is often overdiagnosed. Pregnancies are usually uncomplicated; antibiotic prophylaxis is recommended only if true mitral regurgitation is documented.

Chronic Hypertension

Chronic hypertension during pregnancy leads to increased maternal and fetal morbidity and mortality. Chronic hypertension affects both large and small blood vessels, including uterine and placental arteries. The mother is at increased risk for myocardial infarction, acute congestive heart failure, stroke, renal insufficiency, and pre-eclampsia, and there is an increased risk of placental abruption, intrauterine growth retardation (IUGR), premature delivery, and fetal demise.

Essential hypertension is a diagnosis of exclusion. The possibility should be kept in mind that a treatable cause of hypertension exists, especially in young patients or those with new onset or newly worsened hypertension. Preeclampsia (see Chapter 61, "Obstetric Complications") must be ruled out.

Outcome has not been improved by treatment of mild to moderate hypertension (diastolic blood pressure less than

OB-Gyn
Medical Complications and Pregnancy
continued

105mmHg), although treatment of severe hypertension is beneficial. Various therapies are used to treat hypertension during pregnancy. Methyldopa, a postsynaptic alpha-2-blocker, is most frequently used. Clonidine is a second-line drug, as is nifedipine. Nifedipine is excellent for the management of acute hypertensive episodes and can be given sublingually, making it useful in patients who are NPO. Labetolol is becoming more popular, although it has been associated with neonatal bradycardia, hypo-glycemia, and IUGR, and can block the symptoms of hypoglycemia in diabetics. Hydralazine, nitroglycerine, and sodium nitroprusside are all used to treat acute hyper-tensive episodes. Diuretics and angiotensin-converting enzyme (ACE) inhibitors should be avoided: the former decreases plasma volume to the point that placental per-fusion can be compromised, and the latter have been asso-ciated with fetal anuria, renal failure, and stillbirth.

Hypertensive patients who are trying to conceive must not take diuretics or ACE inhibitors. Once pregnant, base-line renal function testing should be performed. Prophylactic aspirin prevents preeclampsia and IUGR; close surveillance of fetal growth by exam and ultrasound is wise. Epidural anesthesia during labor will help keep blood pressure down.

Pulmonary Disease

Tuberculosis (TB) is, unfortunately, not uncommon dur-ing pregnancy. Workup is the same as it is for any patient; PPDs and chest x-rays (CXR) are not contraindicated. A woman with a newly positive PPD screen and a negative CXR should receive daily TB prophylaxis with isoniazid (INH) beginning in the second trimester. If the patient has active TB (positive CXR and acid-fast bacilli in the spu-tum), she should immediately be treated with a multi-drug regimen (INH, rifampin, and ethambutol) whatever the gestational age. Congenital TB (via transplacental transmission) is extremely rare, but leads to infant mortal-ity rates of up to 50%. The risk of transmission of TB from a mother with active disease to a newborn, if untreated, is approximately 50%; INH prophylaxis should be given to the newborn in this setting.

Asthma, or reactive airway disease, is the most common lung disease seen during pregnancy (see Chapter 51, "Pediatric Respiratory Diseases"). Approximately a third of affected women improve during pregnancy, a third worsen, and a third remain stable. Yearly influenza vaccines are recommended for chronic asthmatics (the vaccine is safe to give in pregnancy). Therapy for acute attacks includes theophylline, beta-sympathomimetic drugs, and corticosteroids, all safe during pregnancy; prolonged maternal hypoxia, in contrast, can lead to fetal demise. Epinephrine is not contraindicated in status asthmaticus during pregnancy; although decreased uterine blood flow is theoretically possible, the benefits to the mother and hence the child strongly outweigh its risks. "Stress-dose" steroids should be given during labor and delivery if the mother has been on corticosteroids within the last year or so.

Untreated or improperly treated **pneumonia** during pregnancy yields a maternal mortality rate of up to 30%. Streptococcus pneumoniae is the most commonly isolated organism in pregnant women; empiric treatment with a penicillin antibiotic is useful. Mycoplasma and Chlamydial pneumonias are also common.

Chest x-rays are not contraindicated in pregnancy, especially if a misdiagnosis can be potentially unsafe to both mother and fetus. A standard CXR provides only 8mrads of radiation to the pelvis; the dosage is even less with proper abdominal shielding. There is no evidence of IUGR, fetal malformations, or miscarriage below 10 rads of radiation (more than a thousand-fold safety margin).

Renal Disease

Asymptomatic bacturia (greater than 100,000 colonies/mL) is commonly seen during pregnancy. Forty percent of such episodes become symptomatic urinary tract infections (UTI); 30% of these lead to **acute pyelonephritis**. Pyelonephritis is associated with stillbirth, preterm labor, and preterm delivery. The right kidney is affected more often, and E. coli is the most common organism isolated. Antibiotic prophylaxis (oral macrodantin) is recommended for the entire pregnancy for women with a his-tory of pyelonephritis in pregnancy

Medical Complications and Pregnancy

continued

or a history of frequent UTIs. Monthly surveillance urine cultures are a good idea in these patients.

Renal function in women with a baseline serum creatinine greater than 1.5mg/dL may irreversibly worsen during pregnancy. Pregnant women with renal disease have a higher risk of miscarriage, stillbirth, and preterm delivery; good blood pressure control is very important.

Successful pregnancy is possible in **chronic renal dialysis patients**, although more frequent dialysis and meticulous fluid management will be required. Successful pregnancy is also possible in **renal transplant patients**. Immunosuppressive medications such as azathioprine, cyclosporine, and prednisone are continued. Although possibly associated with IUGR, the benefits to the mother and fetus of these drugs outweighs the risks. Worsened renal function can occur during pregnancy, but this usually resolves after delivery.

Diabetes

The presence of poorly-controlled diabetes is associated with an increased rate of congenital anomalies and spontaneous miscarriage; these risks can be decreased with tight glucose control. Diabetics who are pregnant are managed with conventional insulin regimens. Screening for congenital malformations is important, and surveillance for evidence of macrosomia (associated with mild diabetes) or IUGR (more severe diabetes) is routine.

Insulin needs frequently change during pregnancy; some patients may need hospitalization for adjustment. The goal, in general, is maintenance of pre-meal blood glucose levels between 60-105mg/dL. An early US for dating and viability is performed, as are a baseline ophthalmologic exam and assessment of renal function. Neural tube and cardiac defects are commonly seen in children born to diabetics; an alpha-fetoprotein and fetal echocardiogram are both useful screening tests. Although sacral agenesis (caudal regression syndrome) is the "classic" anomaly associated with pregnancy in a diabetic, it is actually very rare.

During pregnancy, an US should be obtained every 4-6 weeks to assess growth. Daily monitoring of fetal "kick counts" is suggested after 28 weeks, and weekly non-stress tests (see Chapter 61, "Obstetric Complications") are obtained after the 32nd week. Insulin requirements drop dramatically in the postpartum period, and therefore the dosage is usually readjusted after delivery.

Gestational diabetes occurs in 4%-8% of pregnancies. Glucose levels can usually be controlled by diet alone, but insulin is occasionally required. Since it is usually a problem during the third trimester, the fetus is at risk for macrosomia but not congenital anomalies. Mothers with gestational diabetes are at significant risk of developing true diabetes later in life.

Thyroid Disease

Mild enlargement of the thyroid gland in pregnancy is normal. Thyroxine-binding globulin (TBG) levels are increased during pregnancy, but T_4, T_3, and TSH are not. While thyroxine and TSH do not cross the placenta, iodide does (and becomes concentrated in the fetal thyroid).

Grave's Disease is the most common cause of **hyperthyroidism** in pregnancy. Radioactive ablation is contraindicated due to the fetus's ability to absorb and concentrate iodide compounds. Propylthiouracil (PTU) can be used safely in pregnancy, but methimazole has been associated with aplasia of the fetal scalp and is therefore not recommended. Neonatal hyperthyroidism may result from maternal transfer of LATS (long-acting thyroid stimulator) -protein. Thyroid storm, though rare, can also occur. Treatment involves beta-blockade with propranolol and reduction in thyroxine production with IV sodium iodide and PTU.

Hypothyroidism during pregnancy has multiple etiologies including Hashimoto's thyroiditis and iatrogenic hypothyroidism as the result of radiotherapy, antithyroid medication, or thyroidectomy. Therapy consists of hormone replacement with L-thyroxine (Synthroid).

Hematologic Diseases

Most cases of **anemia** during pregnancy are due to iron deficiency. Pregnancy normally causes increased plasma volume leading to a dilutional fall in the hematocrit. The diagnosis of true iron deficiency anemia, however, is suggested by microcytic, hypochromic erythrocytes, a decreased ferritin level, and an increased total iron binding capacity. Daily iron prophylaxis is sufficient to prevent iron deficiency anemia.

Sickle trait (heterozygous for hemoglobin S) occurs in approximately 10% of the black population in the US (see Chapter 54, "Pediatric Hematology and Oncology"). These women usually have uneventful pregnancies. There is an increased risk of asymptomatic bactiuria and renal papillary necrosis, however, due to the risk of renal sickling; monthly urine cultures are recommended in these patients. Women with **sickle cell anemia** (homozygous for hemoglobin S) are at high risk for poor perinatal outcome (including miscarriage, preterm delivery, and IUGR). Maternal infections are common, including pyelonephritis and pneumococcal pneumonia, and painful sickle cell crises tend to occur more frequently during pregnancy. Patients should receive folate for anemia, but extra iron is not recommended because iron is released as the red cells sickle and are destroyed.

Neurologic Disorders

Preconceptual counseling for women with a pre-existing **seizure disorder** to address control is important. The issue of antiseizure medications is complex; almost all can be teratogenic to varying degrees. If the patient can be well-controlled on a less teratogenic agent before conception, medication can be adjusted, and some women who have been seizure-free for several years can stop medications under the supervision of a neurologist. Poor control is dangerous, however, because anoxia during a seizure can imperil the fetus—each case must be individually evaluated, keeping the risk-to-benefit ratio in mind.

Antiseizure medication dosing during pregnancy is difficult due to the mother's increased volume of distribution. Folic acid supplementation is recommended to reduce the chances of neural tube defects associated with several antiseizure medications.

Peripartum seizures may be due to eclampsia. Therefore, it is important to rule out correctable causes that do not require termination of the pregnancy, such as pre-existing epilepsy (check anticonvulsant levels), brain tumor, cerebral vascular malformation, subarachnoid hemorrhage, or electrolyte imbalance. If the seizure is due to eclampsia, the patient requires $MgSO_4$ and immediate delivery (see Chapter 61, "Obstetric Complications").

Cancer During Pregnancy

There is a basic dilemma involved in the management of a pregnant woman with a known malignancy—whether the mother or the baby should be "saved." Obviously for each situation the risks and benefits of each decision should be weighed individually.

Generally, chemotherapy (except methotrexate) is better tolerated by the fetus than most people presume, especially after the first trimester, although it is important to follow fetal growth closely for evidence of IUGR. Radiation for diagnostic purposes is generally acceptable, but exposure should be minimized with good shielding. In contrast, any therapeutic radiation with fetal exposure requires careful consultation with the mother, oncologist, radiation therapist, and obstetrician as to the advisability of termination of pregnancy.

Surgical procedures outside of the uterus and cervix may be performed (with caution) during pregnancy. Cancers of the uterine corpus and cervix may require termination of the pregnancy if the mother is to be saved. Pregnancy should not be an excuse for the misdiagnosis of cancer due to fear of fetal injury. ■

61   Obstetric Complications

A host of problems can occur, unfortunately, during pregnancy. Problems caused by preexisting (or new) medical conditions were discussed in the previous chapter ("Medical Complications and Pregnancy"); this chapter focuses on problems unique to the pregnancy itself.

Placental Problems

Placenta Previa

Placenta previa is the condition where implantation of the placenta occurs in a position completely or partially covering the cervix, preventing safe vaginal delivery. Placenta previa can cause hemorrhage before or during labor, potentially leading to death of the fetus and/or mother. Risk factors include prior uterine surgery or Caesarean section (CS), advanced maternal age, multifetal gestation, and multiparity. Fortunately, the condition is usually easily identified by ultrasound (US). "Placenta previas" are commonly seen on routine US examinations early in pregnancy, but as the uterus enlarges superiorly, the majority no longer overlie the cervical opening and are no longer considered placenta previas. Women with true placenta previa typically present with **painless** vaginal bleeding. **It is critical to avoid digital cervical examination of a patient in whom placenta previa is suspected because of the risk of perforation of the placenta with immediate, massive hemorrhage**. A patient with a complete placenta previa at term or in labor must be delivered by CS. Vaginal delivery may be possible for a fetus with a "borderline" placenta previa (often termed marginal placenta previa); a **double set-up** examination of the cervix in an operating room that is simultaneously prepared for an emergency CS if the placenta is encountered during digital palpation should be performed.

Placenta accreta

Placenta accreta is a condition where the placenta forms an abnormal attachment to the uterine cavity. There is no cleavage plane (Nitabuch's layer) for normal placental separation; the placenta can erode into the uterine muscle or even grow through the entire uterus, leading to a high risk of hemorrhage after delivery of the fetus. The incidence of accreta is as high as 25% in a patient with placenta previa who has had a prior CS. The diagnosis can sometimes be made by prenatal US, but accreta is more typically found on histologic examination of the hysterectomy specimen of a patient with uterine hemorrhage who failed conservative treatment.

Abruption

Placental abruption is the situation when the placenta separates prematurely, before delivery of the infant. Placental abruption usually presents with vaginal bleeding, abdominal pain, and uterine contractions, producing **painful vaginal bleeding** (differentiating it from placenta previa). Prior abruption, acute cocaine abuse, polyhydramnios, acute decompression of the uterus from premature rupture of membranes or delivery of a first twin, hypertension, and trauma have all been implicated as risk factors. Placental abruption is usually difficult to diagnose by US unless a large retroplacental clot is identified. Smaller abruptions are usually diagnosed clinically by physical examination and abnormal coagulation studies, while larger abruptions can cause disseminated intravascular coagulation (DIC). Separation of the placenta from the uterus results in decreased fetal perfusion, fetal hypoxia and bradycardia, and, eventually, fetal death if not delivered promptly.

Decreased Fetal Movement

The fetus is asleep most of the time. When awake, there are an average of 30 gross body movements per hour, and the mother feels about three-quarters of these. During active states, the fetal heart exhibits accelerations (an acute rise and fall in fetal heart rate) associated with fetal movement, cycling every 40 minutes or so. During quiet sleep, which usually lasts about 20 minutes at a time, the baseline heart rate is slower and exhibits less variability.

Decreased fetal movement can be real or due to perceptual errors. Factors associated with lessened perception of fetal movement include maternal drug ingestion (altered level of consciousness), polyhydramnios, or increased maternal activity. Actual causes of decreased fetal movement include a neurologically anomalous or hypoxic fetus, decreased or increased amniotic fluid volume, intrauterine growth restriction (IUGR), an anterior placenta, or intrauterine fetal death. If a woman complains of decreased fetal movement, a non-stress test (NST) should be performed to evaluate fetal status: fetal heart rate is recorded for 20-40 minutes while the patient simultaneously indicates perceived fetal movements with an event recorder. A normal or **reactive** NST means that fetal movements are associated with accelerations in fetal heart rate; there should be at least 2 accelerations of at least 15 beats per minute lasting 15 seconds in a 20 minute period:

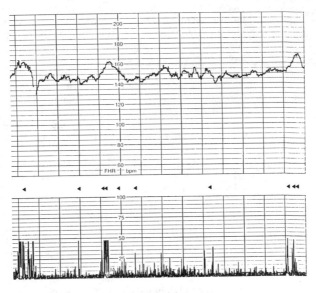

Figure 61.1
Reactive (normal) nonstress test. The baseline fetal heart rate is 145 with good short- and long-term variability.

If the NST is **non-reactive** (abnormal), an US can be performed to rule out fetal anomalies, growth restriction, or oligohydramnios. A **biophysical profile** (a special US examination to evaluate amniotic fluid volume, fetal tone, fetal breathing movements, and gross body movements) can be used to assess fetal status, and an **oxytocin challenge test** (**OCT**) used to evaluate placental reserve and fetal response to the "stress" of contractions. Fetuses with non-reassuring testing may need to be delivered prematurely. If the NST is reactive, the patient can be reassured of fetal well-being and taught self assessment of fetal kick counts to be performed at home. She should feel 3 or more movements an hour and at least 10 movements in a 12-hour period.

Pre-eclampsia/Eclampsia

Pre-eclampsia is the clinical syndrome of **hypertension**, **proteinuria**, and **edema** during pregnancy. A disorder of unknown etiology, it is unique to humans. Uncontrolled pre-eclampsia can ultimately lead to seizures (by definition, **eclampsia**), maternal intracranial hemorrhage, and/or fetal death. Recent evidence suggests either a systemic injury producing a diffuse capillary leak or altered hemostatic function as causative agents; other theories include abnormal trophoblastic implantation and immune dysfunction. **Severe pre-eclampsia** is defined by severe hypertension (diastolic blood pressure greater than or equal to 110 mmHg), proteinuria of greater than 5gm over a 24-hour period, oliguria, the presence of CNS complaints, pulmonary edema, impaired liver function, or thrombocytopenia (platelet count less than 100,000/mcL). Risk factors for preeclampsia/eclampsia include multiple gestations, nulliparity, extremes of age, molar pregnancy, chronic hypertension, family or personal history of pre-eclampsia, diabetes, non-immune hydrops, and collagen-vascular and autoimmune diseases.

Diagnosis

Most patients with pre-eclampsia are asymptomatic. Signs and symptoms vary widely, and include headache, visual disturbances, hyperreflexia, acute facial and finger edema, upper abdominal pain (due to liver capsule edema), and general malaise. Obviously, if pre-eclampsia is suspected, blood pressure and urine protein should be measured; a complete blood count, liver function tests, serum uric acid, BUN, and serum creatinine should also be measured. Fetal heart rate monitoring and US for fetal weight and fluid volume are also important. Non-reassuring maternal or fetal status may warrant urgent or emergent delivery or termination of pregnancy. Neonatology and anesthesiology consultations can be considered to optimize management.

Treatment

The only "cure" for pre-eclampsia is delivery of the fetus. Controversy exists over management when the fetus is premature; close observation with efforts to improve fetal maturity is a reasonable option if the situation is controlled. Most obstetricians will place the patient on a continuous infusion of intravenous **magnesium sulfate** for the 24 hours before and after delivery as protection against seizures. Antihypertensive medications do not alter the physiology and prognosis of preeclampsia, but are used to control dangerous hypertensive episodes that may lead to intracranial hemorrhage.

Preterm Labor and Birth

Preterm labor (PTL) is defined as the occurrence of 6-8 contractions per hour (or 4 in 20 minutes) associated with some cervical change occurring before 37 weeks gestation. **Cervical incompetence**, or painless cervical dilation without contractions, can also be associated with preterm delivery. **Premature rupture of the membranes (PROM)** is defined as rupture of the membranes at least one hour before the onset of labor, while **preterm PROM (PPROM)** is defined as ruptured membranes before 37 weeks gestation. Risk factors for preterm birth include uterine and cervical abnormalities (such as DES exposure, large leiomyomata, or previous cervical surgery/instrumentation), a history of PTL or PPROM, an underlying infection (especially of the GU tract), extremes of age, multiple gestation, placenta previa or abruption, poly- or oligohydramnios, coincident maternal medical illness, fetal anomalies, trauma, smoking, possibly sexual intercourse, low socioeconomic status, the use of illicit drugs, non-white race, and inadequate prenatal care. **Chorioamnionitis** is a clinical syndrome associated with PROM characterized by maternal fever, leukocytosis, tachycardia (maternal and/or fetal), and uterine tenderness from an inflammatory process involving the chorionic plate. Subacute chorioamnionitis may also be associated with PTL.

Premature labor can present with complaints of abdominal cramping or pain, backache, pelvic pressure, increased vaginal discharge, vaginal bleeding, nausea, vomiting, diarrhea, or any symptom of active labor (see Chapter 62, "Labor and Delivery"). A sterile speculum exam should be performed to rule out advanced cervical dilation and occult PROM, and to culture for pathogens. It is wise to avoid digital examination of the cervix until PROM is ruled out because of the increased risk of intrauterine infection associated with cervical examinations in women with ruptured membranes. Urinary tract infection should be ruled out, and a toxicology screen, to rule out cocaine-induced uterine contractions, should also be obtained. An US to confirm the gestational age of the fetus and to assess placental location, fluid volume, fetal anomalies, and fetal presentation is helpful.

Tocolysis

If premature labor occurs, **tocolysis** (an attempt to medicinally halt contractions), corticosteroids to accelerate fetal lung maturity, and bed rest are the mainstays of therapy; antibiotics are administered, if indicated. **Tocolytic drugs include magnesium sulfate** (often at higher doses than used for preeclamptic seizure prophylaxis) and beta-agonists (such as terbutaline or ritodrine) that cause smooth muscle relaxation. All must be used with care.

Uterine Rupture

Although rare, **uterine rupture** is a devastating complication. It most often occurs **before** the onset of labor. Risk factors include previous uterine surgery (e.g. myomectomy) or Caesarean section, abnormal fetal presentation and obstructed labor (see Chapter 62, "Labor and Delivery"), uterine hypertonus (either from acute cocaine use or iatrogenically from oxytocin use), aggressive intrauterine manipulations, and grand multiparity (greater than 4 deliveries). Patients can present with severe abdominal pain, hypotension secondary to blood loss, fetal bradycardia, extrusion of the fetus and placenta into the maternal abdominal cavity, and/or fetal death. During labor, uterine rupture is suspected if a patient at risk develops acute fetal bradycardia, a rise (more negative station) in the presenting part, and low intrauterine pressure. Rapid and prompt delivery of the fetus by emergency laparotomy will improve chances for fetal survival. Examination of the uterine wall after delivery confirms the diagnosis; the rupture site will most often be at the site of a previous uterine incision. Repair of the rupture site is usually performed without difficulty, but hysterectomy is necessary if the uterus is not salvageable.

Fetal Death

Intrauterine fetal demise (IUFD) before the onset of labor often occurs without a definable cause. Placental or cord accidents, intrauterine infections, erythroblastosis fetalis, fetal anomalies, fetomaternal hemorrhage, maternal antiphospholipid antibody syndromes, and maternal medical problems all are possible causes. Preterm labor or PROM, absence of fetal movement, vaginal bleeding, worsening coexistent maternal disease, prolapsed umbilical cord, uterine rupture, or DIC can all be associated with IUFD.

The diagnosis must obviously be established before treatment. If no fetal heart sounds are auscultated, a formal US should be performed to confirm the lack of fetal heart motion; features consistent with prolonged fetal death include overlapping skull bones and oligohydramnios. US will also give information about the position of the fetus, any gross anomalies present, and possible placental pathology. Methods for delivery depend on gestational age and maternal condition. At 12-16 weeks gestation, a dilation and evacuation (an outpatient operative procedure) is easily performed, while from 16-28 weeks, intravaginal prostaglandins can be used to induce spontaneous delivery. After 24-28 weeks gestation, oxytocin induction of labor is more successful because of an increase in uterine oxytocin receptors. Expectant management is appropriate if maternal condition allows. Many women enter spontaneous labor following fetal demise; 80% will spontaneously abort within 2-3 weeks.

After delivery, the products of conception should be examined to rule out a cause that can recur, be treated, or be prevented. Karyotyping should be performed on fetal or placental tissues. An autopsy and placental examination should be requested, and the placenta cultured for pathogens. Maternal blood can be examined for possible undiagnosed diabetes mellitus, isoimmunization, TORCH infections, and the antiphospholipid antibody syndrome. Parents should be allowed to see and hold the fetus if they desire, perinatal loss counselors should be consulted, if available, and close followup with the patient in 1-2 weeks should be arranged. ∎

62   **Labor and Delivery, Postpartum Care**

Labor is the progressive dilatation of the uterine cervix in association with repetitive uterine contractions. It is divided into three stages. The **first stage** begins with the onset of labor and ends when the cervix is fully dilated (10cm). The **second stage** begins when the cervix is fully dilated and ends with the birth of the infant, and the **third stage** begins after the delivery of the infant, and ends with the delivery of the placenta. Cervical dilatation over time is assessed by a graphic plot known as a **Friedman curve**. The average duration of the first stage of labor for a nullipara (a woman who has never given birth before) is 10 hours, while that for a multipara (woman with prior deliveries) is 8 hours; a woman whose labor is progressing too slowly ("off the curve") may require intervention.

Management of Labor (First Stage)

Patients are usually instructed to go to the hospital when they are having regular, painful contractions every 5 minutes for at least an hour that do not resolve with bedrest and hydration. If the cervix is dilated on presentation to Labor and Delivery, she will be admitted to the hospital. **False labor** is the presence of uterine contractions **without** cervical change; woman in false labor will often be sent home to rest until true labor begins.

Management of the first stage of labor consists essentially of waiting for the cervix to fully dilate while repetitive uterine contractions are occurring; the woman should not push at this stage to prevent cervical edema. While in labor, attention is paid to pain control and maintenance of maternal and fetal health.

OB-Gyn
Labor and Delivery and
Postpartum Care *continued*

On arrival to the labor and delivery suite, the diagnosis of labor is confirmed by cervical examination and fetal status is assessed. The prenatal record and pertinent past history are reviewed. Important questions include:

– What time did the contractions begin? How frequent are the contractions?
– Did your water break? When? What color is the fluid?
– Have you had "bloody show?" Is there any vaginal bleeding?
– Have you felt the baby moving?

Presentation

Leopold's maneuver is the identification of the baby's position by maternal abdominal palpation to determine what part is coming out first (**presentation**); usually the head, back, extremities, and buttocks can be identified. A gross estimation of the fetal weight (EFW) can be made as well, by comparing the abdominal size to bags of IV fluid. **Abnormal presentation** is identified by palpation of anything other than the fetal vertex on vaginal examination in addition to Leopold's maneuver. If a breech or transverse presentation is present, and membranes are intact, an **external version** (manually flipping the fetus to a cephalic presentation) can be attempted to allow normal delivery. Very select babies in breech presentation can be delivered vaginally, but a fetus in a transverse or shoulder presentation requires Caesarean delivery.

ROM

A sterile speculum exam can be performed to rule out rupture of the amniotic membranes (ROM), although often it will be obvious. Other than history of a sudden "gush" of water, rupture is suggested by a pool of fluid in the vagina that, because of its neutral pH, will turn nitrazine litmus paper dark blue (although cervical mucus and blood will also turn it blue). Amniotic fluid, when placed on a glass slide and allowed to dry, will produce a "ferning" pattern.

Cervical status

Serial **cervical exams** are performed to follow the progression of labor. Three attributes are used to describe findings. **Cervical dilatation** is measured in centimeters, ranging from a closed, nondilatated cervix to a 10cm, fully dilated cervix that is no longer palpable on vaginal exam. **Effacement** describes the length of the cervix, and can be expressed as an actual length or as an estimated percentage of normal. For example, a "full thickness" cervix that is 3-4cm long may be considered 0% effaced, while a cervix that is flush with the vagina is termed 100% effaced, implying that the cervix is completely thinned out. **Station** refers to the level of the presenting part in relation to the maternal ischial spines (0 station); stations above and below are described in 1cm intervals with a negative or positive sign depending on whether the head is above or below, respectively. By the time the baby is at +5 station, the fetal head is **crowning**.

Fetal monitoring

In most settings, fetal status is assessed by **fetal monitoring**, which can take many forms and vary widely as to degree of invasiveness. At the simplest level, continuous auscultation of the **fetal heart rate (FHR)** can be performed by means of a Doppler ultrasound probe attached externally to the maternal abdomen; FHR can also be measured by means of an internal fetal scalp electrode attached to the fetal scalp through the partially dilated cervix. Important FHR monitoring parameters include the **baseline**, which should be 120-160 beats per minute, the short-term variability, or how "squiggly" the tracing is, and the presence of **periodic changes**, or acute rises and falls in the FHR (**accelerations** and **decelerations**, respectively). Normal FHR variability is a good indicator of adequate oxygenation of the fetal heart and central nervous system (see Figure 61-1 in the previous chapter). Capillary blood can be obtained from the fetal scalp (via the vagina) to directly determine the pH of the infant as an indicator of fetal oxygenation.

Contractions

Uterine contractions are monitored during active labor for frequency, duration, and intensity. Contractions can be assessed by manual palpation, external tocodynamometer ("toco") recordings, or an intrauterine pressure catheter (IUPC). The external monitor aids in detection of frequency and duration, but only the IUPC quantifies the actual intensity of contractions. Contractions occurring every 3 minutes measuring 50-80mmHg above baseline uterine tonus are optimal. Both external FHR and contractility monitoring are relatively "invasive" because they require the mother remain in bed, making labor more difficult. For this reason, many centers will monitor in an intermittent fashion, allowing the mother long periods of freedom to walk, shower, change position, and so on.

If labor is progressing well and following the Friedman curve, the strength, duration, and frequency of contractions can be assumed to be adequate. If labor is not progressing well, however, re-evaluate the 3 P's:

– **Passenger**: How large is the fetus? is it too big to fit?
– **Passageway**: Is the maternal pelvis large enough for the fetus to be delivered through it?
– **Powers**: Are the uterine contractions strong enough to push the baby through the birth canal?

Pain management

Obstetrical anesthesia and **pain management** in labor is a field in itself. Modern techniques for pain management involve a combination of education, massage, focusing techniques such as breathing or even hypnotism, and pain medication and regional anesthesia. Narcotics are powerful analgesics, but have respiratory and central nervous system depressant effects on both the mother and baby. Narcotics are short-acting and can be used to "take the edge" off the pain. Regional anesthesia such as an **epidural** block (see Chapter 12, "Anesthesiology and Pain Management") are also utilized, particularly in women with particularly prolonged labor or those requiring more than narcotic analgesia.

Dysfunctional labor

In the setting of dysfunctional labor when the patient "falls off" the Friedman curve, several options are available. If membranes are still intact, an amniotomy or artificial rupture of membranes (AROM) can be performed, which theoretically releases prostaglandins that stimulate uterine contractions, or **Pitocin** (oxytocin) can be infused intravenously to stimulate myometrial contractions if labor is not progressing. Overstimulation of uterine contractions can impair placental blood flow and produce fetal bradycardia, and can lead to placental abruption or uterine rupture (see Chapter 61, "Obstetric Complications").

Induction

Induction of labor is indicated when the benefit of early delivery outweighs the potential problems that may occur if the pregnancy continues. Indications may be maternal or fetal, and include preeclampsia, chorioamnionitis, a "postdates" pregnancy (one that is over 42 weeks), and diabetes mellitus. Induction can be accomplished by cervical "ripening" agents such as prostaglandins or laminaria, an oxytocin infusion, and/or amniotomy. The

Bishop score is a prelabor scoring system used to predict inducibility. The cervix is evaluated and scored for dilatation, effacement, consistency, position, and fetal station; a score of 9 or more indicates that induction should be successful. An unsuccessful induction is an indication for Caesarean delivery (i.e., a vaginal delivery is the endpoint of a successful induction).

Delivery (Second Stage)

Women have obviously delivered for tens of thousands of years without the presence of obstetricians. The goals of an **assisted delivery** are to prevent precipitous, uncontrolled expulsion of the baby, to minimize trauma to the woman's genital tract and perineum, and to manage complications of delivery.

Once the cervix is fully dilated, the second stage of labor begins. The patient is encouraged to "push" or actively bear down (contract the abdominal muscles and diaphragm) to facilitate descent of the fetal head. Pushing before the cervix is fully dilated will be counterproductive; the cervix will become edematous and progression may be delayed. The second stage of labor typically lasts between 1-2 hours. If the fetus is not delivered by 2 hours (3 hours with an epidural) and is not descending further, delivery may be assisted with vacuum extraction, forceps, or Caesarean section (see below).

Delivery

The **cardinal movements** of labor are the changes in the position of the fetal head during its passage through the pelvis. There are seven: **engagement, descent, flexion, internal rotation, extension, external rotation (restitution),** and **expulsion.** During the first stage of labor, the fetal head enters the maternal pelvis (**engagement**) and starts its **descent** into the birth canal. The fetal head usually engages with the back of the head toward the left or right (occiput transverse). As the head descends, it becomes **flexed** and **internally rotates** so that the back of the head is anterior, against the pubic symphysis (occiput anterior). The fetal head is delivered during the final aspect of **extension**, and the fetal mouth and nares are suctioned of mucus while the woman is asked not to push. The attendant checks that the cord is not looped around the fetal neck (nuchal cord), **externally rotates** the fetal head (**restitution** to the occiput transverse position), and delivers the anterior and posterior shoulders. The remainder of the infant is delivered by maternal **expulsion** as the attendant supports the baby's neck and spine. The cord is clamped and cut, and the infant stimulated to provoke crying (respirations).

An **episiotomy** is an incision into the perineal body (the junction of the posterior aspect of the vagina to the perineum) made prior to delivery to allow more room for the delivery of the fetal head. Whether or not to perform an episiotomy requires judgment; the purpose is to create a controlled, shallow, easy to repair incision to prevent an uncontrolled, jagged tear. A midline episiotomy is generally preferred over a mediolateral episiotomy. Midline episiotomies are easier to repair, cause less blood loss, and are associated with less postpartum pain, although mediolateral episiotomies are less likely to cause a fourth degree tear.

An **operative vaginal delivery** is sometimes necessary to shorten the second stage. Indications include maternal exhaustion, contraindications to Valsalva or expulsive efforts, or worrisome fetal status. Instruments used to assist in vaginal deliveries include forceps and the vacuum extractor; neither should be used unless the fetal head is at least in a 0 station with the cervix fully dilated.

After delivery, the perineum is inspected for any damage. A **first degree laceration** is a superficial tear confined to the vaginal mucosa or perineal skin, a **second degree laceration** is a tear from the vaginal mucosa through the muscular tissue of the perineum (the level of most episiotomies), a **third degree laceration** is a tear from the vaginal surface through the rectal sphincter, and a **fourth degree laceration** is a tear from the vagina all the way through the rectal mucosa. Most tears (and episiotomies) are repaired in multiple layers.

Placental Delivery (Third Stage)

The placenta will generally deliver spontaneously within 30 minutes. Signs of the placenta being ready for delivery include a hard and globular uterus, a gush of fluid and blood from the vagina, and lengthening of the umbilical cord. Manual traction on the cord while awaiting these signs will not quicken this stage, and risks tearing the cord, bleeding, and uterine inversion. The placenta should be examined for any missing pieces, and the cord evaluated for true knots, number of vessels (anything other than two arteries and one vein suggest a risk for associated birth defects), and length.

Caesarean Section

A **Caesarean section (CS)** is the delivery of the fetus through a surgical incision of the anterior uterine wall. Currently the CS rate in the US is as high as 25% of all live births, but despite this high frequency, perinatal mortality and morbidity have not significantly changed over the years.

Indications can be fetal, maternal, or both, and generally fall into two classes: situations where vaginal delivery is contraindicated or failing, and situations where immediate delivery is mandatory. Examples of the contraindications to or failed vaginal delivery include failure to progress, cephalopelvic disproportion (CPD; the fetal head is too large for the pelvis), and placenta previa; the classic example of the need for immediate delivery is an unexplained, persistent fetal bradycardia of less than 80 beats per minute. A previous CS no longer absolutely rules out vaginal delivery.

Skin and uterine incisions can be parallel or perpendicular. The most frequent skin incision is the Pfannenstiel ("bikini cut") incision, which is cosmetic and believed to be less painful and to heal with fewer complications. A vertical skin incision allows more rapid access to the lower uterine segment, less blood loss, and exposure of the upper abdomen for examination, and thus is best in emergent situations. The most frequently used (90%) uterine incision is the **low transverse (LTCS)**, made where the tissue is relatively thin. Advantages of a LTCS include greater ease of entry, less blood loss, lesser magnitude of repair, and **less likelihood of uterine rupture in subsequent labors**. A vertical uterine incision is termed **classical** if it involves the upper uterine segment, and **low vertical** if it remains in the lower segment. The advantages of the classical uterine incision include the rapidity of entry into the uterus and the ability to make a large enough incision for delivery of a fetus when the lower uterine segment is too narrow to make an adequate

OB-Gyn
Labor and Delivery and
Postpartum Care *continued*

transverse incision. A classical uterine incision, however, is bloodier and more difficult to repair due to the increased thickness of the myometrial wall of the fundus, and **commits a woman to repeat CS for the remainder of her reproductive career** because of the increased risk of uterine rupture.

A trial of **vaginal birth after caesarean (VBAC)** is highly encouraged in women who have had previous LTCS. The prognosis for a successful vaginal delivery ranges between 70%-85% and depends on the indication for the prior CS; complications include uterine rupture (less than 0.5%) and the need for a repeat CS.

Postpartum Care

The duties of the obstetrician do not end with delivery of the infant, but continue until the mother recovers from her delivery (the first hour or so after delivery, when bleeding is the greatest concern, is sometimes called the fourth stage of labor). Patients usually remain on the postpartum ward for 1-2 days following an uncomplicated vaginal delivery and 4-5 days following a CS.

During hospitalization, early signs of infection and subtle hypertension that may suggest pre-eclampsia need to be assessed. Fevers due to atelectasis are normal the first few days after a CS (see Chapter 27, "Postoperative Care"). Breast engorgement can be associated with postpartum fever; warm compresses and a breast pump help if breast-feeding, ice-packs and a binder, if not. The uterus should be palpated daily for tenderness suggestive of endometritis, and its position relative to the umbilicus followed to ensure it is not filling with blood clots. Patients who have had a CS are treated like any other postoperative patient; ileus is routine. The perineum should be inspected daily to evaluate the episiotomy or tear site for a hematoma or signs of infection. The lochia (postpartum vaginal discharge) should be inspected for color and odor – a foul smell may indicate infection. Patients who have a third or fourth degree laceration generally benefit from a stool softener; rectal exams and suppositories are contraindicated because they may damage the repair and promote formation of a rectovaginal fistula. Pregnant women are relatively hypercoagulatable and are at risk for deep venous thrombosis; unfortunately, calf tenderness and leg swelling are highly insensitive and nonspecific signs. Women who have had a CS or a periurethral laceration generally benefit from a Foley catheter for the first 24 hours.

Rh-negative mothers have the capacity to produce anti-Rh antibodies if exposed to Rh-positive blood. If the woman becomes sensitized and carries another Rh-positive fetus, it is at risk for developing hemolysis, hydrops fetalis, and fetal death. Therefore, Rh-negative mothers are given anti-Rh antibodies (**Rhogam**) to neutralize any fetal Rh antigens released into her bloodstream and prevent her immune system from becoming sensitized.

Several complications should be anticipated in the postpartum period. **Postpartum hemorrhage** (**PPH**) is loosely defined as more than the usual amount of blood loss, generally 500cc or so, at or after delivery. Management initially includes fundal palpation to rule out uterine atony, manual exploration of the uterus to rule out retained placenta, and a thorough inspection of the vulva, vagina, and cervix for actively bleeding lacerations. Treatment for **uterine atony** initially includes bimanual uterine massage and oxytocin infusion/injection. Methylergonovine maleate (Methergine) and/or prostaglandin-F-2-alpha methyl analog (Hemabate) can be given to contract the uterus further. If pharmacologic treatment fails, operative methods such as uterine curettage, uterine or hypogastric artery ligation, or even hysterectomy may be required in order to save the woman's life.

Endometritis is an infection of the postpartum endometrium that presents with fever, uterine tenderness, foul smelling lochia, and an elevated white blood cell count. Infection is often polymicrobial, including anaerobes, and generally responds to intravenous clindamycin and gentamicin. Antibiotics are stopped when the patient has been afebrile for 24-48 hours; there is no benefit in continued oral antibiotics beyond this point.

Asymptomatic thrombi in the dilated veins of the pelvis are common and relatively innocuous. However, endometritis can extend into these pelvic thrombi (then called **septic thrombophlebitis**), resulting in minimal response to IV antibiotics. Diagnosis is difficult; if fevers

OB-Gyn
Labor and Delivery and
Postpartum Care *continued*

persist despite broad-spectrum antibiotics and no other source of infection is present, heparin may be added. Resolution of the fever within 48 hours of starting heparin defines the syndrome.

Mastitis typically occurs 2-3 weeks after delivery, typically presenting as a localized area of cellulitis on the breast of a breastfeeding mother with a high fever. Staphylococcus aureus is the causative organism in 95% of cases. Continued breast feeding and oral dicloxacillin usually resolve the problem, but a frank abscess usually requires surgical drainage. ■

63   Ambulatory Care Gynecology

The routine, annual gynecologic exam, or periodic health update, in the absence of active disease should focus on education, screening, and prophylaxis. If these are done effectively, the need for actual treatment will decrease. This chapter focuses on the routine, "well-patient" visit, contraception, and abnormal uterine bleeding. Other issues that arise commonly in routine gynecologic practice such as vulvovaginal infections and menopausal issues are covered in other chapters.

"Well-patient" History and Physical

History

The **gynecologic history** begins with the menstrual history, called the **catamenia**. The catamenia can be written in shorthand as 3 numbers: the age menses started, the length of the menstrual cycle, and the number of days of menstrual flow (e.g., 12 x 28 x 5). Significant premenstrual symptoms and heaviness of flow, stated as the number of pads or tampons used, should be recorded. The **obstetric history** is recorded in analogous fashion as the **gravidity** (total number of pregnancies) and **parity** (total number of deliveries); the latter typically recorded as 4 numbers: term deliveries, preterm deliveries, abortions (spontaneous and elective) and living offspring. Thus, a woman pregnant for the fourth time whose 3 previous pregnancies ended in miscarriage, preterm delivery, and full-term delivery, with 2 living children, would be recorded as a "$G_4 P_{1112}$." Note should be made of any abnormal Pap smears, contraception use, history of sexually transmitted diseases (STDs), and hormone use.

Exam

Physical exam is comprehensive but directed by the age of the patient. Note the stage of development of the **external genitalia** and the presence or absence of lesions. If the patient is postmenopausal and/or gravid and the vaginal walls look relaxed, pelvic floor weakness may be present; bulging of the anterior or posterior vaginal walls, especially with a Valsalva maneuver, is suggestive (see Chapter 65, "The Postmenopausal Patient"). On exam of the **cervix**, look for thin, watery mucous indicating follicular estrogen production, or thick, stretchy mucous indicating post-ovulation progesterone production. A friable, bleeding cervix can be the only sign of infection or neoplasm. The **bimanual exam** includes an assessment of the size and position of the uterus, evaluation for cervical motion tenderness, and assessment of adnexal tenderness or masses. It is difficult to feel normal ovaries in women, particularly if postmenopausal. A rectovaginal exam is part of the pelvic exam in patients over 30. Stool guaiac should be checked; change gloves after the bimanual to avoid false-positive results. A **Pap smear** (see Chapter 66, "Gynecologic Malignancies") is done at every annual exam in every woman, including those who have had a hysterectomy, and vaginal and cervical cultures and a wet prep are done if there is anything to suggest infection in the history or exam (see Chapter 64, "ED Gynecology").

Contraception

Many **contraceptive** methods are available. Selection clearly depends on predicted efficacy, but other health benefits such as STD and cervical cancer prevention should be considered. Despite considerable efforts, there are over two million unplanned pregnancies and one million abortions in the US annually. A problem common to all methods of contraception is that the actual failure rate (usually expressed as percent pregnant within 1 year of use) is much higher than the theoretic failure rate, mostly because contraceptives are not used correctly.

1-year Failure Rate

Method	Theoretic	Actual	STD Prevention
Rhythm	10%	20%	None
Male Condom	<2%	2%-12%	Good
Female Condom	<2%	10%-20%	Fair
Spermicides Alone	3%-9%	18%-28%	None
Diaphragm, Cervical Cap	2%	6%-18%	Poor
OCPs	<2%%	10%-50%	Poor
Depo-Provera	0.2%	0.3%-0.5%	Poor
Norplant	0.04%	< 0.1%	None
IUD	<2%	3%	None
Tubal Ligation	0	0.3%-0.5%	None
Vasectomy	0	0.3%-0.5%	None

Rhythm method	The "**rhythm method**" (**periodic abstinence**) requires tremendous commitment on the part of both partners. Morning basal body temperature measurement and assessment of cervical mucus are used to ascertain when ovulation occurs; the couple abstains from intercourse for approximately 10 days around this time. This technique is most effective in those with a regular menstrual cycle. Used by a monogamous, motivated couple, it has about the same failure rate as do the diaphragm and spermicides (20%). Periodic abstinence offers no STD or cancer protection.
Condoms	The **male condom** is a barrier contraceptive, usually made of latex. Non-latex condoms are less effective. Condoms offer the most reliable STD and cancer protection, and should be used concurrently with every other method of contraception in non-monogamous relationships for this reason. Although in theory 100% reliable, a host of factors makes this number unrealistic. Condoms break up to 10% of the time, with approximately 1 pregnancy resulting every 3 breakages or so. Vaseline weakens the condom and increases the breakage rate; water-based lubricants such as K-Y Jelly are safe. To be effective, a condom actually has to be worn before the penis touches the partner. If used absolutely correctly, only 2% of women will become pregnant the first year of use; a failure rate of 12% is more typical. Compliance may be enhanced by suggesting condom use become part of foreplay; the use of a spermicide will greatly decrease the failure rate.
	The **female condom** (Reality) has also been shown to be effective in preventing pregnancy and STDs. Initial reports indicate a high level of satisfaction. It is inserted the same as a diaphragm and should be used with a spermicide.
Spermicides	**Spermicides** damage the sperm membrane. They come in many forms, including foam, gel, cream, suppositories, foaming tablets, foaming suppositories, and soluble film. They are inexpensive, simple to use, and widely available. Spermicides need to be put in the vagina 10-30 minutes before intercourse. Although most preparations last up to 8 hours, tablets and suppositories are good for an hour or so only. Unless used with a condom there is no STD protection. When used alone, this method has a high actual

failure rate (18%-28%) although the theoretic rate is only 3%-9%. One to five percent of women have minor allergic reactions to the spermicide or the carrier; changing preparations is usually sufficient. **Each new coitus requires reapplication**.

Diaphragm

The **diaphragm** and the **cervical cap** are barrier contraceptives that offer minimal STD protection. Both are small and easy to carry around, should be used with spermicides, and their efficacy does not rely on the male. The diaphragm can be inserted up to 6 hours ahead of intercourse. Both must be kept in place for 8 hours after coitus to inactivate the sperm; the cervical cap can stay in place for up to 3 days (although removal as soon as possible is recommended). Both require fitting by a physician. Again, spermicide should be reapplied in the vagina after each act of coitus. Married women can experience a failure rate as low as 2%, although overall failure in the first year is 6-18%.

OCPs

Oral contraceptive pills (**OCPs**) became available in the US in the 1960s and were immediately embraced by women as an effective, neat, and reliable contraceptive method. The side effects seen in the first generation of OCPs have been largely eliminated by a combination of lower dosages and patient selection, although the legacy of high-dose pills is still with us. For example, approximately 35% of women perceive OCPs as increasing the risk of cancer (they almost certainly do not). All OCPs currently sold in the US contain only low-dose estrogen (ethinyl estradiol); the more active component is the progestational agent (of which there are many). OCPs work by inhibiting secretion of FSH and LH, by creating a thick cervical mucous, and by causing endometrial atrophy, all of which inhibit implantation of a fertilized ovum. The estrogen inhibits ovulation; the progestin affects the cervix and endometrium. The estrogen also stabilizes the endometrium to minimize breakthrough bleeding. Progestin-only contraception is also available and comes in four forms: pill, depo-medroxyprogesterone acetate (Depo-Provera; DMPA), Norplant, and the progesterone IUD (see below). The progestin-only pill works primarily by producing changes in the cervical mucous and the endometrium; 40% of women ovulate with this pill. These are good for women in whom estrogen is contraindicated and for women who experience significant side effects on combination OCPs. Non-contraceptive advantages of OCPs include a reduction in uterine leiomyomata and benign breast disease, fewer ovarian cysts, regular menses with less flow and less anemia, less dysmenorrhea, protection against PID, fewer ectopic pregnancies, and a reduction in endometrial and ovarian cancer. OCPs have little or no impact on the incidence of breast cancer, hypertension, migraine, or weight gain or loss. The theoretic first year failure rate is 0.1%, but poor compliance(mainly the result of intermittent use) increases this considerably. The first year failure rate in multiparous adolescents approaches 50%.

The few absolute contraindications to combination OCPs are a history of a thromboembolic disorder or hypercoagulatable state, markedly abnormal liver function, a hepatic adenoma, breast cancer (even low-dose estrogens can stimulate already cancerous cells), undiagnosed vaginal bleeding, pregnancy, and tobacco use in a patient over 35 (synergistically causing a hypercoagulatable state). OCPs can be used as a "morning-after pill:" 2 conventional pills taken 12 hours apart for 2 days are greater than 90% effective in preventing pregnancy if begun within 72 hours of intercourse.

DMPA

Medroxyprogesterone acetate (DMPA; Depo-Provera) is given IM four times a year. By inhibiting the LH surge, ovulation is prevented. Because FSH is not fully suppressed, however, there is enough ovarian follicular growth to keep estrogen levels in the early follicular range, and the patient is not hypo-estrogenic. DMPA is convenient and private. Non-contraceptive benefits include decreased menorrhagia and dysmenorrhea, and decreased risk of endometrial and ovarian cancer. Special medical benefits include a decrease in seizure frequency and a decrease in sickle cell disease crises in patients with these conditions. The failure rate of 0.3%-0.4% is equivalent to sterilization. The major complaint with DMPA is irregular bleeding that can occur in up to 30% of patients the first year. Other side effects, all reversible, include breast tenderness, weight gain, osteoporosis, and hair loss.

Norplant

Norplant is a subdermal implant consisting of 6 silastic rods containing the progestin levonorgestrel, inserted in the subcutaneous tissue of the upper inner aspect of the

OB-Gyn
Ambulatory Care Gynecology *continued*

non-dominant arm. The levonorgestrel diffuses through the capsules and is effective within 24 hours of insertion. The first year release rate produces a progestin dose that is approximately equivalent to that of the progestin-only pill, less than that of combination OCPs. Effective levels are maintained for at least 5 years, even in heavier women. Like the progestin-only pill, about a third of the cycles are ovulatory but the LH surge is suppressed. Additionally, cervical mucous is thick and the endometrium atrophic. Norplant requires essentially no compliance after implant, is highly effective, and is rapidly reversible. Like DMPA, Norplant users also have irregular bleeding, worst in the first year. Insertion and removal are both minor office procedures. Norplant has its disadvantages: initial cost is high, implants may be visible, and there is no STD or cervical cancer protection. Of all the reversible contraceptives, however, Norplant is most effective, with only 0.2 pregnancies per 100 woman-years.

IUD

The **intrauterine device (IUD)** originated more than a century ago. A combination of specific problems with the Dalkon shield and changing sexual practices during the 1960s produced a fairly high rate of pelvic infection and infertility, which continue to give IUDs a bad name. Current IUDs, however, do not have the same problems and continue to be used clinically with good results. Modern IUDs are of two types—copper-impregnated and progesterone-containing—and all have monofilament strings which reduce the risk of infection. Copper IUDs work by creating a sterile inflammation of the endometrium, are long-lasting, and are approved for 10 years' worth of use. Copper IUDs, however, have an initial one year expulsion rate of 5%-8%, and 10% -15% of women require removal at one year due to bleeding or pain. Progesterone-containing IUDs work similarly, but require replacement every year. Progesterone-containing IUDs significantly reduce dysmenorrhea and menorrhagia, but insertion and removal can cause discomfort. Make sure the patient feels the string and knows to check it frequently. The pregnancy rate for those using IUDs is only 3% the first year and decreases with duration of use and increasing age of the patient.

Dysfunctional Uterine Bleeding

The normal menstrual cycle is composed of a follicular, or proliferative, phase, and a luteal, or secretory, phase. These are separated by ovulation, and, at the opposite end of the cycle, menses, which results from withdrawal of estrogen and progesterone. The average menstrual cycle has a 28 ($\pm$ 7) day interval, a 4 day duration, and a 35 mL blood loss.

Many disorders of uterine bleeding can occur. **Oligomenorrhea** is defined as regular cycles with intervals greater than 35 days apart, while **polymenorrhea** occurs when regular cycle intervals are less than 21 days apart. **Menorrhagia** refers to cycles with prolonged (greater than 7 days) or heavy (greater than 80mL) bleeding, and **metrorrhagia** denotes any irregular episode of uterine bleeding. Thus **menometrorrhagia** refers to excessive or prolonged uterine bleeding occurring at frequent and irregular intervals. **Dysfunctional uterine bleeding (DUB)** is used to describe abnormal uterine bleeding in the absence of any identifiable pathology.

DUB is a diagnosis of exclusion. It usually is caused by exposure of the endometrium to estrogen alone without progesterone after an anovulatory cycle. The key is to determine the cause of anovulation. Pregnancy must always be ruled out. Other causes include medications, malignancy, myomata, polyps, cervicitis, vaginitis, bleeding disorders, pelvic trauma, IUDs, hypothyroidism, or uterine foreign bodies. Adolescent and premenopausal females are at the highest risk for anovulation. Patients with polycystic ovarian syndrome also do not always ovulate and at are higher risk for DUB. It is very important to rule out endometrial carcinoma in higher risk patients (see Chapter 66, "Gynecologic Malignancies").

Therapy depends, in part, on the patient's future plans for childbearing. If future fertility is desired, pharmacologic ovulatory induction is the therapy of choice. Conversely, the progesterone found in OCPs is useful to control bleeding in women who desire contraception. Acute therapy should begin with one pill twice a day for 5-7 days, after which a heavy withdrawal bleed will occur. The

OB-Gyn
Ambulatory Care Gynecology *continued*

patient can then drop down to a pill a day. Lower dose progesterones are useful to control bleeding in perimenopausal patients.

Therapy also depends on the rate of bleeding. Estrogen therapy is used to control an acute bleed that is troublesome but not extensive enough to require immediate dilation and curettage (D&C). High dose oral or intravenous conjugated estrogens should always be followed with progesterone supplementation. Non-steroidal anti-inflammatory agents can also be used and will decrease bleeding in some patients by 40%-50%.

Gonadotrophic releasing hormone (GnRH) agonists are seldom used because they are expensive and not immediately effective. Danazol is an androgenic steroid that significantly reduces blood loss and frequency of bleeding episodes. It provokes androgenic side effects, such as acne and weight gain, and is expensive, and thus is not recommended as initial therapy.

Surgical treatment is indicated when medical therapy is contraindicated or unsuccessful. A **D&C** refers to the technique of dilating the cervix and scraping the endometrial lining; it is useful for both therapy and diagnosis, and usually requires general or regional anesthesia. A therapeutic D&C is usually transiently effective if intractable bleeding severe enough to cause anemia is present. It is also useful in a diagnostic sense in older women with persistent abnormal uterine bleeding, because malignancy is relatively more common.
Endometrial ablation may be performed for those resistant to medical therapy if hysterectomy is otherwise not desirable, but if bleeding persists, **hysterectomy** is the final (and definitive) option. ∎

64   Emergency Department Gynecology

Some of the most common conditions seen in the emergency department are treated by the gynecologist. Sexually transmitted diseases (STDs), also known as venereal diseases (VD), are a group of diseases caused by organisms acquired by varying degrees of intimate sexual contact. Patients with one STD may (and often do) have another simultaneously, and their partners are often infected, as well. Compliance with treatment is low, and reinfection is common. Vaginal bleeding is also a common complaint, as are Bartholin's gland problems, pelvic pain, and, unfortunately, sexual assault.

Sexually Transmitted Diseases

Trichomonas

Trichomonas vaginalis is a flagellated protozoan. One out of four patients are asymptomatic. The infected patient typically complains of thin, frothy gray or pale green discharge, a foul odor, vulvovaginal pruritis, swelling, and erythema. Occasionally she will have symptoms of a bladder infection; a classic "strawberry cervix" with petechiae is present less than 10% of the time. Application of KOH to the sample will yield a foul odor (positive "whiff test"), and small balloon- or pear-shaped flagellated motile protozoans in a saline preparation can be seen under the microscope. The pH of the discharge is usually greater than 4.5. Treatment is with oral metronidazole; 2gm can be given as a one-time dose, or 500mg bid for 7 days can be prescribed. The single dose yields high compliance (an important issue in the treatment of STDs), while the longer course results in a greater cure rate. Metronidazole should be avoided in the first trimester of pregnancy, and adverse reactions can occur when mixed with alcohol.

Gonorrhea

Neisseria gonorrhea is a Gram negative diploccoci typically found inside polymorphonuclear leukocytes. Gonorrhea (GC) is a very common infection in 15-25-year-olds, and can cause a host of problems including pelvic inflammatory disease (see below), cervicitis, vaginitis, and endometritis, as well as pharyngitis, urethritis, ocular infections, and septic arthritis. Scarring of the fallopian tubes can cause infertility and increase the risk for ectopic pregnancy. It has been associated with an adhesive perihepatitis causing right upper abdominal pain (Fitz-Hugh Curtis syndrome). Pelvic scarring and adhesions may cause chronic pelvic pain. Although the Gram stain may show the organism, definitive diagnosis is by growth and identification in culture. Cultures of the endocervix, rectum, or oropharynx are taken as appropriate for the patient's history. GC is treated with ceftriaxone (250mg IM once), norfloxin (800mg PO once), or ciprofloxacin (500mg PO once); erythromycin can be used if the patient is pregnant. Because as many as a third of patients with GC also have Chlamydia, concomitant treatment for this parasite (with doxycycline) is recommended. Because of the host of late problems associated with GC, the patient should be recultured in a month or so to rule out reinfection or resistant organisms.

Chlamydia

Chlamydia trachomatis is an obligate intracellular parasite. Serologic types D through K are associated with transmission through sexual contact. It can cause urethritis, cervicitis, salpingitis, "urethral syndrome" (urinary tract infection symptoms with negative cultures), newborn conjunctivitis and pneumonia, tubal scarring with associated ectopic pregnancy, infertility, chronic pelvic pain, and acute and chronic PID. More common than GC, it is estimated that 4%-5% of sexually active women in the United States have Chlamydial infections. Chlamydia typically causes a mucopurulent cervicitis. There is an accurate and rapid direct antigen test which is cheaper, easier, and faster than culture. 100mg of oral doxycycline twice daily for 10 days is usually effective; erythromycin, azithromycin, ofloxacin, and tetracycline (the latter contraindicated during pregnancy) are effective as well. One should again test for reinfection after treatment.

Scabies

Pediculosis pubis, or the **crab louse**, is the most contagious STD (it is transmitted through nonsexual contact, as well). The lice live in hair and feed off human blood. Infected patients will complain of irritation and vulvovaginal pruritus. The diagnosis is obvious if a louse or its eggs, larva, or fecal pellets is found; treatment is Lindane shampoo (RID solution, if pregnant).

Syphilis

Treponema pallidum, a spirochete, causes **syphilis**. Syphilis infection is classically described as occurring in three phases, although tertiary syphilis is extremely rare today because of the efficacy of modern treatment.

Primary syphilis occurs 10-60 days after initial exposure. The patient develops a firm, painless lesion with
rolled edges (syphilitic chancre) on the affected area.
Secondary syphilis occurs three to five weeks later.
Patients develop a viral syndrome, characteristic maculopapular skin rashes on the palms of the hands and soles
of the feet, and multiple large exophytic flattened lesions
that can ulcerate (condylomata lata) in the vulvar and
perianal regions and upper thighs. This stage is very
infective. Most patients are diagnosed before the onset of
tertiary syphilis which consists of gumma formation and
neurologic damage ("neurosyphilis"). The RPR (rapid
plasma reagent) and VDRL (venereal disease research
laboratory) serology tests are sensitive but not specific.
They are good screening tests but have a high incidence
of false-positive results. The highly specific fluorescent-
labeled Treponema antibody test (FTA-ABS) is used for
confirmation. Optimal treatment is 2.4 million units of
benzathine penicillin (2 weeks of tetracycline, doxycycline, or erythromycin are alternative choices for allergic
patient). One dose of penicillin is usually sufficient for
primary and latent disease of less than a year's duration.
The RPR titer should be followed every 3 months for a
year after treatment. If the patient has latent disease
greater than a year's duration, or tertiary disease, the
same dose of penicillin should be administered every
week for 3 weeks and titers followed every 3 months for
2 years. Neurosyphilis or a positive spinal tap (indicating
asymptomatic neuro-syphilis) may be treated with 4 million units IV of penicillin G every 4 hours for 14 days
and then 2.4 million units of IM benzathine penicillin
weekly for 3 additional weeks.

Condylomata

Condylomata acuminata are genital warts caused by
human papiloma virus (HPV). They are commonly found
on the vagina, cervix, perineum, and perianal and rectal
mucosa (and penis in males). The warts are singular or
multiple fleshy, cauliflower-like raised lesions.
Transmission occurs by contact, and much of the general
population probably carries the virus without developing
lesions. 25% trichloracetic acid or podophyllin applied to
small lesions may burn them off, but if the lesions recur
after 12 weeks of treatment or become very large, 5-FU,

cryotherapy, skinning vulvectomy, laser therapy, or formal surgical excision using electrocautery can be tried. Recurrence is common.

Herpes

Herpes simplex virus (HSV) type II causes 90% of **genital herpes;** HSV type I accounts for the rest. Genital herpes typically begins with a viral prodromal phase (dysuria, myalgias, malaise and high fever) about a week (but up to decades) after initial genital contact. The patient will develop intermittent outbreaks of genital paresthesias, burning pain, and the characteristic herpes ulcers. Definitive diagnosis is made by culturing the debrided ulcer material or vesicle fluid. Acyclovir shortens the course of an outbreak and decreases the frequency of recurrence, but is not curative. If an active herpes lesion is present in the birth canal during labor, Caesarean section is recommended to decrease the chance of neonatal herpes transmission.

HIV

The **human immunodeficiency virus (HIV)** is a RNA retrovirus that can remain asymptomatic for years. It attacks helper T cells resulting in decreased immunity, and is the cause of **acquired immunodeficiency syndrome (AIDS,** see Chapter 19, "HIV and AIDS"). Patients at high risk for contracting HIV infection are those with a history of STDs, multiple sexual partners, IV drug use, transfusions (much less common today), or blood or body fluid exposure. Patients with HIV are believed to present with more severe forms of cervical dysplasia and proceed to malignancy at a higher rate; thus, any patient with cervical cancer at an unusually young age may benefit from testing.

Pelvic Inflammatory Disease

Pelvic inflammatory disease (PID) refers to the presence of a deep-seated infection within the pelvic reproductive organs (uterus, fallopian tubes, and ovaries). The presence of PID is suggested by the presence of fever, leukocytosis, pelvic pain, and purulent cervical discharge. The patient is usually in her teens or early twenties and has a history of several previous STDs or PID, numerous sexual partners, or a new partner within the last few months. The exam demonstrates extreme cervical motion tenderness ("chandelier sign"), abdominal pain, tender adnexa without masses, and purulent cervical discharge. If the right side is primarily involved, presentation is very similar to appendicitis (see Chapter 25, "Abdominal Pain"). Infection is often bacterial. Neisseria gonorrhoeae and Chlamydia trachomatis are found about half the time, and Bacteroides, Escherichia coli, and other commensuals are often present as well.

Diagnosis

Diagnosis is problematic and only correct (by clinical suspicion) about half the time—laparoscopy is much more accurate and should be considered if it will change management. **Cervical motion tenderness** in the setting of abdominal and adnexal tenderness and evidence of an inflammatory state (fever, high erythrocyte sedimentation rate, leukocytosis with left shift, or increased C-reactive protein) is the hallmark of PID. Pus from the cervix or obtained by culdocentesis is highly suggestive. A pregnancy test, urinalysis, and cervical culture should always be done, as should screening for syphilis. Because of its prevalence, HIV testing may also be suggested.

Treatment

Not every patient with PID requires hospitalization. Untreated or severe PID may progress to **tubo-ovarian complex** (**TOC**), a complex intrapelvic inflammatory lesion, or frank pelvic abscess. Clearly, a clinically septic patient needs admission for intravenous antibiotics. Since PID (and especially TOC) may result in an increased risk for ectopic pregnancy and infertility, nulliparous and adolescent patients are also usually admitted. Admission is also indicated if a patient is believed to be poorly compliant, fails outpatient treatment, if the diagnosis is uncertain (for example, if appendicitis cannot be ruled out), has potential TOC, or is HIV-positive (because the rate of TOC is high).

The combination of ceftriaxone (250mg IM once) and doxycycline (100mg PO bid for 2 weeks) is highly effective for outpatient treatment of mild infections. Outpatients should be reevaluated a few days after treatment is started to verify initial improvement. If inpatient treatment is needed, IV cefoxitin or cefotetan with oral doxycycline or clindamycin and gentamicin are given until the patient improves, then continued for an additional 48 hours. Patients are discharged on oral doxycycline as above.
(continued)

OB-Gyn
Emergency Department Gynecology

continued

Vaginal Bleeding

Vaginal bleeding can be benign or life threatening. In patients who are **not pregnant**, initial workup is directed toward quantification of the amount of bleeding. Assessment of the number of tampons or pads used is very helpful. A pelvic examination with a thorough inspection of the vagina with a speculum will help determine the source of bleeding. Cervical and vaginal bleeding may arise from intercourse (especially if there is a history of vaginitis or cervicitis), foreign body trauma, vulvovaginal warts, recent surgery, or cancer. Bleeding from the base of a cervical cone biopsy site may be controlled with Monsel's solution. Keep in mind that a patient may complain of vaginal bleeding but may truly have urethral (urethritis or cystitis) or gastrointestinal bleeding.

If the source is uterine, a detailed menstrual history is mandatory, including the use of hormones (oral contraceptives, post-menopausal replacement therapy, Depoprovera, or Norplant) or the presence of very heavy periods (menorrhagia) or bleeding between periods (metrorrhagia). Carcinoma is always a concern, and biopsy may be necessary (see Chapter 66, "Gynecologic Malignancies"). The diagnosis of **dysfunctional uterine bleeding** (see Chapter 63, "Ambulatory Care Gynecology") is made if other sources have been ruled out. Patients may be treated for dysfunctional uterine bleeding with medroxyprogesterone acetate (Provera) 10mg daily for 10 days. Heavy, active bleeding may require transfusion, IV Premarin, or **dilation and curettage (D & C)** to remove the dysfunctional tissue.

Abortion

If the patient claims to be **pregnant**, the diagnosis needs to be confirmed with a pregnancy test and the gestational age determined. Fetal heart sounds may be heard as early as 11 weeks. Causes of vaginal bleeding during pregnancy include **threatened abortion** (pregnancy less than 20 weeks with a closed cervix), **inevitable abortion** (dilated cervix), **missed abortion** (nonviable fetus retained in the uterus), or **incomplete abortion** (not all of the fetal tissue has been passed). A **blighted ovum** refers to the presence of a gestational sac without fetal tissue. In a **complete spontaneous abortion** all the tissue has been passed, bleeding is decreasing, and the cervix is closed.

Half of patients with a threatened abortion may eventually abort. If the cervix is closed and the patient is stable and not actively bleeding, she may be allowed to go home. If fetal heart tones cannot be detected, an ultrasound should be obtained to determine if there is a viable pregnancy in the uterus. If not, uterine evacuation may be offered, especially if the cervix is dilated or the patient is having severe cramps or bleeding (to reduce the blood loss and risk of infection from retained, nonviable tissue), or if the gestational age is greater than 6 weeks (because complete, spontaneous passage of nonviable tissue may not occur). Rh negative patients should receive Rhogam, just as with a term pregnancy.

Ectopic pregnancy

An **ectopic pregnancy** can present with vaginal bleeding. This diagnosis should always be suspected in a patient with pelvic pain and a positive pregnancy test (or amenorrhea), especially if anemia or hemodynamic instability is present. Anything that can cause tubal damage increases the risk of ectopic pregnancy, such as prior tubal surgery, history of a prior ectopic pregnancy, history of prior STD or PID, IUD use, or a history of DES exposure. Ectopic pregnancies usually become symptomatic at 6-9 weeks.

The most common abnormal implantation site is tubal, but it may be anywhere in the peritoneal cavity. In other words, the gestational sac is not in the uterus. Pelvic ultrasound is the most important test, primarily to determine whether or not there is an intrauterine pregnancy. If not, an ectopic pregnancy must be considered. Extrauterine masses are not always seen, but are not necessary to make the diagnosis. A pregnancy with a beta-HCG greater than 1,500 mIU/mL should have a normal gestational sac in the uterus demonstrable by vaginal ultrasound. In a normal pregnancy, the quantitative beta-HCG doubles every 1-1/2-2 days until about 9-10 weeks, when it peaks at 50,000-150,000 mIU/mL. If the level rises at a slower rate, levels off, or goes up and down, the pregnancy is probably abnormal.

A patient with an ectopic pregnancy may need laparotomy, laparoscopy, or medical management with methotrexate based on the degree of hemodynamic instability, among other factors.
(continued)

OB-Gyn
Emergency Department Gynecology
continued

Pelvic Pain

Patients with "acute" **pelvic pain** often end up in the emergency room, even though their pain is actually chronic. Common gynecologic causes of pelvic pain include Mittelschmerz (mid-cycle pain with otherwise normal ovulation), adhesions, uterine myoma with central degeneration, or a torsed, ruptured, or bleeding ovarian cyst. In the latter situation, culdocentesis may demonstrate blood or yellow fluid and may be curative due to removal of the irritating cyst fluid from the pelvis. A common condition to be considered in the differential diagnosis of pelvic pain, if localized to the right, is appendicitis (see Chapter 25, "Abdominal Pain").

Bartholin's Gland Problems

A **Bartholin's gland** or **duct abscess** should be suspected if a woman develops an acutely painful, swollen vulvar mass with the typical signs of infection (redness, heat, swelling, and tenderness). Trauma or inflammation leads to obstruction of the gland opening causing cyst formation, which then can become infected. Simple incision and drainage of the abscess is curative in the short term, but special techniques may be required to prevent recurrence.

Sexual Assault

Up to 1 in 6 women in the United States claim to have been sexually assaulted. Goals in the ED include **treatment of acute physical injury**, **protection from potential infection**, **prevention of pregnancy**, and **collection of evidence** that will be helpful to the patient in court.

Injuries (both genital and systemic) are treated as indicated, at times with the help of a surgeon. The patient may be given antibiotics to prevent potential GC and Chlamydia infections. Screening for syphilis and HIV disease should be performed at the time of assault and 6 weeks later. Condom use to protect her partner from STDs in the interim can be recommended (this should also prevent any intervening pregnancy if used until the next normal period). Post-coital contraception with 2 oral contraceptive pills every 12 hours for 2 days is greater than 90% effective. Finally, gathering as much evidence as possible (with the guidance of institutional and local protocols) is critical. The type of contact (oral, anal, or vaginal) needs to be noted so that semen can be recovered. Information regarding loss of consciousness, emesis, bathing, change of clothing, tooth brushing, or douching are important for interpretation of evidence.

Treatment of psychologic injury is vital; social work and/or rape crisis organization intervention may be helpful and should be offered. ■

OB-Gyn

65   The Postmenopausal Patient

Menopause in the US occurs, on the average, at 51, so more than a third of a woman's life is spent after menstruation ceases. Onset is genetically predetermined, and is largely unaffected by parity or the use of oral contraceptives (but may be hastened by cigarette smoking).

The basic underlying pathophysiologic cause for most of the changes seen with menopause is a **relative estrogen deficiency**.

Pathophysiology

The basic feature of menopause is a gradual depletion of ovarian follicles with degeneration of the granulosa and theca cells. **Granulosa** cells produce estrogen synthesized from **thecal cell** androgens in the developing follicle; as follicles deplete and estrogen levels drop, compensatory production of the pituitary gonadotropins FSH and LH increases in an attempt to stimulate the ovary. Characteristic hormonal laboratory values seen in the postmenopausal women include low estradiol (less than 20pg/mL), high FSH (greater than 40 mIU/mL), and high LH (greater than 40 mIU/mL) levels. **Stromal** cells of the ovary do not atrophy and continue to produce androgens in response to the high LH levels after menopause. There is therefore a decrease in the estrogen to androgen ratio; this relative androgen excess causes the increased facial hair commonly seen in postmenopausal women. Because androgens are converted to estrogens in fatty tissue, obese women often have higher postmenopausal circulating estrogen levels and are at less risk of developing osteoporosis, hot flashes, and other conditions related to hypoestrogenemia than are thin women.

Signs and symptoms

Physiologic changes and the symptoms that result from estrogen depletion are extremely variable. Some women experience debilitating symptoms, while others have none. Genitourinary changes contribute to incontinence and urgency, frequency, and dysuria. Atrophy of the vagina can occur and lead to atrophic vaginitis, which is manifest as itching, burning, dyspareunia, or vaginal bleeding, while decreased skin collagen content causes increased fragility and wrinkling. Hot flashes occur in 75% of patients. They consist of a sudden reddening of the skin of the head and chest, associated with perspiration. Frequency of flashes varies from rare to every 10 minutes, and they frequently occur at night, awakening the patient. Patients may complain of insomnia. Their cause is not well understood, but are associated with a sudden autonomic discharge at the central level. They occur less often in obese women, implicating estrogen deficiency.

Postmenopausal women can complain of fatigue, nervousness, headaches, depression, irritability, or dizziness. Multiple studies have failed to show a causal relationship between these symptoms and estrogen deprivation. The patient should be thoroughly evaluated and all other sources considered before attributing such a sign or symptom to the menopause. If other disorders are excluded, hormone replacement, including testosterone, may be helpful. There seems to be an effective and beneficial placebo effect with any treatment in this situation.

Osteoporosis

Osteoporosis is a disease that affects 20 million women in the US. It seems to be caused by an estrogen-dependent reduction in the quantity but (not composition) of bone, and, until a fracture occurs, is asymptomatic. Other than menopause itself, risk factors include race (white or oriental), reduced weight-to-height ratio, early menopause, a family history of osteoporosis, a diet low in calcium and vitamin D or high in caffeine and alcohol, cigarette smoking, a sedentary lifestyle, and endocrine disorders such as diabetes and hyperthyroidism. Problems caused by osteoporosis include back pain, decreased height and mobility, and fractures; by age 80, 20% of all white women break a hip.

Estrogen replacement therapy (ERT) clearly reduces the risk of osteoporosis and is the best treatment and prevention strategy. Osteoporosis prevention also includes calcium supplementation (approximately 1000-1500mg/day), exercise, and probably fluoride, although the latter does not seem to change the fracture rate.
(continued)

Cardiovascular Disease

Though osteoporosis produces significant morbidity, **heart disease** is the leading cause of death in women in the United States. Estrogen replacement therapy reduces the risk of coronary artery disease (CAD) and stroke in postmenopausal women. As documented in several large, prospective studies (including Framingham), the age-adjusted relative risk of death from myocardial infarction (MI) in women on ERT compared to nonusers is 0.34-0.5. In other words, death from an MI is a third to half as likely in those receiving ERT than in those not being supplemented.

Estrogen replacement

Estrogen seems to retard atherosclerosis by maintaining a favorable lipoprotein profile—high HDL and low LDL levels. There is no relationship between hypertension and estrogen use. Hypertension is not a contraindication for ERT; in fact, a patient with hypertension is at high risk for CAD and may thus benefit most from estrogen therapy. Some form of progestone is needed to prevent endometrial hyperplasia due to unopposed estrogen (see Chapter 66, "Gynecologic Malignancies"); this has little effect on the lipoprotein profile or cardiovascular mortality.

If estrogen replacement therapy is so beneficial, why are only 20% of women in the US currently using it? Opinion polls of public and professional groups reveal a great deal of misinformation that may, in part, be responsible. Even if prescribed, noncompliance due to side effects such as irregular bleeding can be a problem. Despite its clear advantages for most women, estrogen may be inadvisable in certain patients. Women with breast or endometrial cancer diagnosed within the past 5 years (to prevent stimulation of **already malignant** cells), undiagnosed abnormal vaginal bleeding, active liver disease, or those who are pregnant should not be given exogenous estrogens. Estrogen therapy is associated with an increased risk of gallstones. Many women have abnormal menstrual bleeding during the first 3 months of ERT; if it persists past 6 months an endometrial biopsy to rule out carcinoma should be done. The majority of physicians do not believe ERT increases the risk of developing breast cancer (i.e., does **not** promote malignant transformation of **normal** cells), but some conflicting data and continued controversy exist.

Disorders of Pelvic Support

The main structures involved in pelvic support include the **endopelvic fascia, cardinal** and **uterosacral ligaments**, and **levator ani muscles**. Weakening of these structures is very common in older women; childbirth, obesity, heavy lifting, smoking, and (rarely) congenital prolapse all play a role. Clinical problems result from prolapse of any of the pelvic structures, including the urethra (urethrocele), bladder (cystocele), rectum (rectocele), uterus and cervix, and cul-de-sacs (enterocele, because the sac often contains a loop of bowel). It is unusual to have only one of the above structures herniate in isolation; about three-quarters of patients have a combined prolapse (such as cystocele with rectocele). The degree of prolapse through the urogenital region is described as first, second, or third degree, depending on whether the prolapsed structure stops short of, stops at, or passes the introitus, respectively.

Medical therapy for prolapse include strategies to reduce intra-abdominal pressure such as weight reduction and the avoidance of heavy lifting, Kegel exercises to strengthen the perineal muscles, and estrogen replacement. A pessary can be tried to mechanically contain the prolapse. If conservative therapy is unsuccessful or the prolapse is associated with significant morbidity, surgical repair is required. Each of the particular defects present in a different fashion; treatment varies accordingly.

Urethrocele and **cystocele** often present simultaneously. Patients commonly complain of a sensation of fullness, pressure, and an inability to empty the bladder completely, sometimes to the point of overflow incontinence (discussed below; see also Chapter 23, "Geriatrics"). Exam reveals a bulge or a mass in the anterior vaginal wall which enlarges with Valsalva. Surgical treatment is by means of an "anterior repair," whereby the anterior supporting structures are reinforced.

Patients with a **rectocele** present with constipation and inability to completely empty their rectum; exam reveals a bulging rectum, again worse with Valsalva. Sometimes the rectovaginal septum is paper-thin. Surgical repair is analogous to that for a ureterocele but is accomplished by a "posterior repair." **Enteroceles** occasionally occur after hysterectomy. The enterocele sac usually contains small bowel or omentum; medical therapy is ineffectual and primary surgical repair is usually indicated. **Uterine prolapse** can be mild, often occurring in asymptomatic, multiparous women, or severe. Prolapse of the uterus and cervix outside the vagina is also called **complete procidentia**. Patients complain of vaginal pressure and pain; a common comment is "something is falling out." Severe prolapse can cause bilateral ureteral obstruction and hydronephrosis. Surgical repair usually means total vaginal hysterectomy with anterior and posterior repair. Colpocleisis (LeFort procedure) is an option in poor-risk elderly patients with complete procidentia, which consists of essentially sewing the anterior and posterior vaginal walls together to support the uterus. Vaginal vault prolapse may occur after abdominal or vaginal hysterectomy. Symptoms are similar to uterine prolapse; the best treatment is surgical, consisting of sacrospinous ligament suspension.

Incontinence

Urinary incontinence affects approximately a quarter of women in the reproductive age group, and 30%-40% of postmenopausal women. Affected women are often embarrassed and believe that incontinence is a normal part of aging, so it is notoriously underreported to physicians. All women over 30 should be specifically asked whether or not such problems are present.

Incontinence occurs when pressure within the bladder (expulsive force) exceeds pressure within the urethra (retentive force). Incontinence can be broken down into two broad categories: **detrusor instability (DI)** and **stress incontinence (SUI)**. DI results from uninhibited detrusor contractions, causing bladder pressure to exceed urethral pressure. The cause of the bladder contraction is usually unknown. SUI usually results from inadequate support of the urethra and urethrovesical junction (UVJ) due to an anatomic defect. Normally the junction of the urethra and bladder is located within the abdominal cavity. If support structures weaken and UVJ support is lost, the UVJ falls into the pelvis. If abdominal pressure then increases (for example, during coughing, laughing, or straining), the increase is not transmitted to the urethra, and bladder pressure becomes greater than urethral pressure, causing incontinence. Approximately three-quarters of affected women have **mixed incontinence**, a combination of the two. Occasionally women have incontinence due to a urinary fistula, ectopic ureter, urinary diverticuli, or infection.

Diagnosis

Accurate differentiation between DI and SUI is critical because treatment differs. In terms of overall evaluation, a history of neurologic disorders such as stroke, diabetes, or back injury, potential (for example, a large baby) or actual obstetrical injuries, and history of diuretic or antihistamine use is particularly significant. Document the onset and duration of symptoms with a voiding diary, in which the patient is asked to record the time and volume of all voids, fluids ingested, and medications taken for 24-48 hours. The type of urine loss is usually helpful in distinguishing the two: nocturia, urge incontinence, and frequency are often seen with DI, while urine loss after coughing, laughing, sneezing, or physical activity is fairly classic for SUI.

Physical examination begins with a screening neurologic exam. The T10-S4 nerve roots control urination; they can be quickly assessed by checking ankle, knee, and hip flexion and extension, and the "anal wink" reflex. Pelvic exam is done to determine the estrogen status of the tissues, the presence or absence of cystocele or rectocele, and the status of the UVJ. A simple way of assessing the UVJ is the "Q-tip test": a sterile Q-tip is placed in the urethra to the level of the UVJ and the patient is asked to cough or strain. If the Q-tip swivels more than 30 degrees, hypermobility of the UVJ, consistent with SUI, is present.

Diagnostic testing

Although an accurate history and exam are important, they are often inadequate to distinguish DI from SUI, and interventional diagnostic studies are needed. Multichannel urodynamic testing, currently the most reliable test to differentiate the two, is accomplished by means of microtransducers within small catheters placed simultaneously in the bladder, vagina, and rectum to record simultaneous relative pressures. Urodynamics are especially important in women whose diagnosis is unclear after history and exam and women who have had prior incontinence surgery. Endoscopic cystourethroscopy is an alternative test, although it is rarely helpful unless a tumor, diverticula, or fistula is suspected.

Treatment

The primary treatment for DI is medical. Since the principal stimulatory nerves to the bladder are parasympathetic, anticholinergics such as oxybutynin or propenthine are usually effective in inhibiting spontaneous detrusor muscle contraction. Calcium channel blockers, tricyclic antidepressants, and smooth muscle relaxants can also be helpful. Behavior modification and bladder training exercises such as timed voids and Kegel exercises are beneficial in some patients.

SUI can also be treated medically. Estrogen therapy and alpha-adrenergics work synergistically to increase urethral smooth muscle tone. A pessary supports the bladder neck, partially occluding the UVJ, and thus increases the proximal urethral pressure. Surgical therapy is needed, however, if these measures fail and the morbidity (including the psychosocial distress of incontinence) is significant. All procedures seek to restore proper anatomy by lifting the UVJ, restoring it to an intra-abdominal position. The Burch procedure, transabdominal attachment of the pubocervical endopelvic fascia to Cooper's ligament, is currently believed to provide the best results; other commonly used variations include the Marshall-Marchetti-Krantz and Pereyra operations. ■

66   Gynecologic Malignancies

Gynecologic oncology is the subspecialty dealing with diagnosis and treatment of tumors of the female reproductive tract. The three major tumors that can arise are **endometrial**, **ovarian**, and **cervical carcinoma**; tumors of the **placenta** and **external genitalia** also occur.

Endometrial Hyperplasia and Carcinoma

Endometrial cancer, at approximately 37,000 new cases per year, is the most common gynecologic malignancy. Estrogens stimulate the endometrium, potentially causing hyperplasia. Endometrial hyperplasia, especially if atypia is present, is a risk factor and precursor for endometrial carcinoma.

Endometrial hyperplasia is common in situations where prolonged estrogen stimulation has occurred, such as anovulation, polycystic ovary syndrome, estrogen-producing tumors, obesity (due to the peripheral conversion of androstenedione to estrone) and unopposed estrogen replacement therapy. The term denotes a spectrum of histologic variants, from simple exaggeration of the normal proliferative state to carcinoma in situ. More important to remember than all the variants is the concept that the greater the degree of **atypia**, the greater the risk of frank carcinoma.

Presentation

The most common presenting symptom of endometrial hyperplasia is irregular menstrual bleeding or postmenopausal bleeding; all such patients and those with endometrial cells seen on Pap smear of the cervix need to have an endometrial biopsy. If biopsy is negative but suspicion is high, or the patient cannot tolerate outpatient biopsy, a **dilatation and curettage (D&C)** must be performed. Treatment depends on several factors, including age, desire for future childbearing, and the presence of atypia. Conservative management consists of a 3-4 month trial of a progestational agent such as medroxyprogesterone acetate (MPA) or megestrol. After treatment, repeat endometrial biopsy is done. If hyperplasia persists, a high-dose trial can be tried, but if hyperplasia persists after high-dose progestins, hysterectomy is recommended. The older the patient and the more atypical the hyperplasia, the higher the chance of cancer.

Risk factors

Risk factors for **endometrial cancer** are similar to those for endometrial hyperplasia; the use of oral contraceptives has been shown to be protective. Patients usually also present at age 60 or so with abnormal vaginal bleeding; 20% of patients evaluated for postmenopausal bleeding will have a gynecologic malignancy. Again, cancer can be excluded only by adequate endometrial sampling, and a negative endometrial biopsy in a symptomatic or older patient, in whom suspicion is high, must be followed by repeat biopsy or a formal D&C under anesthesia.

Histology

The endometrium is composed of a glandular and a stromal element, and either or both of these may undergo malignant transformation. **Adenocarcinoma** comprises 80%-90% of all endometrial cancers; the others (**papillary serous adenocarcinoma**, **clear cell carcinoma**, and **sarcoma**) tend to be more aggressive. Tumors are divided into pure (only mesenchymal malignant tissue) or mixed (both malignant mesenchymal and epithelial tissue) and homologous (the malignant tissue is normally present in the uterus) and heterologous (the malignant tissue is not normally present in the uterus). Endometrial cancer is staged at the time of surgery. Before operation, specialized testing is indicated only when history, physical, or preoperative labs suggest a problem. While an abdominopelvic CT scan is sometimes helpful in determining the presence and degree of metastatic disease, results do not affect staging unless CT-guided biopsy confirms cancer. Staging (I-IV) depends on the degree of spread, while grade (1-3) is determined by the degree of histologic abnormality of the glands.

Treatment

Primary treatment for nonmetastatic endometrial carcinoma is surgical, consisting of exploration and peritoneal washings to detect occult disease, and total abdominal hysterectomy with bilateral salpingo-oophorectomy (**TAH-BSO**). Periaortic and pelvic lymph node sampling is done if poor prognostic indicators are present. Adjuvant postoperative radiation therapy is added if the tumor is high-grade, deep myometrial invasion is present, or peritoneal cytology or lymph nodes are positive. Those unable or unwilling to tolerate an operation are treated with radiation only, and treatment of stage IV disease is individualized. Recurrent tumors are treated with local irradiation; chemotherapy can be tried in patients with maximal prior irradiation, but has not been shown to be very effective. Progestational hormone therapy can also be tried in this situation. Survival depends on multiple factors; the 5-year survival rates of women with surgical stage I and II disease are about 90% and 50%, respectively.

Ovarian Carcinoma

Ovarian cancer is the second most common gynecologic malignancy but the leading cause of gynecologic cancer deaths. Median age at presentation is 60; women who have a strong family history of ovarian cancer seem to develop their tumors at an earlier age. Ovarian cancer can be inherited in an autosomal dominant pattern, and in combination with increased risk for hereditary nonpolyposis colorectal cancer and cancer of the breast, endometrium, and stomach (Lynch Syndrome II). Risk factors include nulliparity, early menarche, late menopause, prior breast cancer, and a family history of ovarian cancer and infertility. Exposure to talcum powder and a diet high in animal fat may also be contributory. The use of oral contraceptives has been shown to significantly reduce risk; after stopping, the protective effect persists for at least 15 years.

Diagnosis

Because most patients present with nonspecific complaints, diagnosis frequently is delayed. Patients will usually complain of abdominal pain and swelling as well as vague gastrointestinal symptoms such as nausea, vomiting, anorexia, early satiety, constipation, and bloating. Many patients believe they are just gaining weight. Vaginal bleeding or abnormal discharge are not as common as they are with other gynecologic malignancies, and pelvic examination is not usually helpful unless the disease is advanced. A palpable ovary in a postmenopausal woman or a solid, fixed mass at any age is abnormal and should prompt further workup. Pelvic ultrasound may be helpful; predominately solid or multilocular masses are more likely to be neoplastic. A CT of the abdomen will identify enlarged retroperitoneal lymph nodes or other evidence of spread; chest x-ray will identify pulmonary metastases. Levels of the tumor-associated antigen CA-125 are helpful in following the patient's progress and response to therapy. Many ovarian tumors are first found at laparotomy done for other reasons, often by the general surgeon.

Histology

80%-85% of ovarian neoplasms are derived from coelomic epithelium and are thus called **epithelial tumors**, and are classified "behaviorally" as benign, malignant, or borderline (low malignant potential; LMP), and histologically as serous, mucinous, endometrioid, and clear cell (mesonephroid). Serous epithelial tumors are most common. Mucinous tumors can produce a thick, mucinous ascites that can cause bowel obstruction (**pseudomyxomatous peritonei**). The second most common ovarian cancer is the **germ cell tumor**, derived from primitive germ cells. These occur in younger patients, often teenagers, and frequently express tumor markers as human chorionic gonadotropin (hCG) or alpha fetoprotein (AFP). Histologic subtypes include dysgerminoma, endodermal sinus (yolk sac) tumor, teratoma, embryonal tumor, choriocarcinoma, polyembryona, and gonadoblastoma. The **sex cord-stromal tumors**, derived from specialized gonadal stroma, are least common, and often produce gonadal or adrenal steroid hormones. Subtypes include granulosa cell tumor (associated with endometrial cancer and isosexual precocious puberty), thecoma, and Sertoli-Leydig cell tumor (arrhenoblastoma, androblastoma). 4%-8% of ovarian cancers are metastatic. A **Krukenberg tumor** is a metastasis, usually bilateral, from a tumor of the GI tract that usually contains signet-ring cells; breast cancer also metastasizes to the ovaries.

Staging

Ovarian cancer is also surgically staged. At the time of exploratory laparotomy, peritoneal washings should be done or free ascitic fluid obtained for cytologic evaluation, and biopsy of any suspicious implants, adhesions, and lymph nodes should be performed. Stage I disease is tumor confined to one or both ovaries, while stages II, III, and IV denote disease limited to the pelvis, spread to the upper abdomen and inguinal nodes, or that with distant metastases, respectively. Ascites, probably due to obstruction of lymphatic drainage, is a prominent feature of ovarian cancer, as is gradual encasement and obstruction of the abdominal organs. Bowel obstruction is usually the preterminal event in these patients.

Treatment Epithelial tumors usually are treated with TAH-BSO and omentectomy, usually followed by chemotherapy. An important part of the initial operation is **cytoreduction** in order to attempt to remove as much intraabdominal tumor burden as possible; the degree of debulking has been shown to correlate with outcome. After chemotherapy, a **second-look** laparotomy or laparoscopy can be performed to evaluate response. If no gross disease is found, the patient can be closely followed or given consolidation chemotherapy; if microscopic or progressive disease is found after the initial treatment, the patient is usually offered enrollment in an experimental protocol, because second-line agents are rarely effective. If the initial attempt at cytoreductive debulking was suboptimal, an interval attempt after 3 courses of chemotherapy can be helpful.

For early stage germ cell tumors, conservative surgery in an attempt to preserve a clearly normal, uninvolved ovary may be possible. Recurrent dysgerminoma may be treated by irradiation, but, like all other advanced germ cell tumors, is usually treated with combination chemotherapy. Sex cord-stromal tumors usually require a TAH-BSO, although ovarian preservation can occasionally be attempted in a young women with early disease. Survival for epithelial tumors is poor overall; patients with germ cell tumors fare the best.

Cervical Carcinoma and the Papanicolaou Smear

Cervical cancer is the leading cause of cancer death in women worldwide, although screening based on the **Papanicolaou ("Pap")** smear has made cervical cancer mortality relatively rare in the United States. Unfortunately, approximately 15,000 new cases still occur each year.

Etiology The human cervix contains a **transformation zone** where the squamous and columnar epithelium merge. This area undergoes squamous metaplasia after puberty and is susceptible to neoplastic transformation, especially if induced by gene products of the human papilloma virus (HPV). Early age at first intercourse, high number of partners, tobacco use, and HIV infection all increase risk, while barrier contraception is protective. Oral contraceptives probably are not causally related to cervical neoplasms; although users do have a higher prevalence of cervical disease, it is probably related to confounding demographic factors. Cervical neoplasms progress in an orderly fashion, from mild to severe. The median time from preinvasive disease to cancer is approximately 7 years, although progression from mild dysplasia to invasive cancer in less than 2 years has been reported.

All women should have a Pap smear every year after age 18 or first coitus; women at low risk (monogamous, non-HIV positive, and non-smoking) may have Pap smear frequency reduced to every 1-3 years after 3 normal annual Pap smears. Pap smears have a false negative rate of about 20%, which can be reduced by careful specimen acquisition and computer-aided analysis of the smear itself. There is no contraindication to a Pap smear. It is safe during pregnancy, and patients should be examined regardless of the presence of vaginal bleeding.

Colposcopy, examination and biopsy of the cervix using a colposcope for magnification, is performed if an abnormal Pap smear is found. Colposcopy is useful to determine the severity of the lesion and is good at excluding invasive disease.

CIN

Cervical intraepithelial neoplasms (CIN) are usually discovered by Pap smear. The Bethesda classification system for reporting Pap smear results was introduced in 1989 in an attempt to improve accuracy. Results are reported as adequate or limited, and the smear is reported as normal, low grade squamous intraepithelial lesion, or high grade squamous intraepithelial lesion. Reliable patients with early histologic lesions can be observed; up to 90% of such lesions regress or remain the same.

Patients at greatest risk for disease progression, however, are the same people who are least likely to comply with necessary followup. Most patients today, therefore, with **any** grade of CIN are treated. The principle of treatment of CIN is to physically destroy the entire lesion. The first step is delineation of the margins of the lesion using colposcopy. **Cryotherapy** safely destroys the lesion with little discomfort. Many physicians, however, prefer an **excisional cone biopsy**, because it provides a tissue sample for examination. Excisional cone biopsy requires general anesthesia when performed with a scalpel, but excision using either a CO_2 laser or wire loop electrode (loop electrical excision procedure; LEEP, or loop excision of the transformation zone; LETZ) can be performed using local anesthetic in the outpatient setting. Cure rates for all techniques are about 90%, and are better if colposcopy is repeated at the time of treatment. Followup requires a Pap smear every 4 months for a year, followed by smears at less frequent intervals.

Occasionally the deep margin of the excised specimen will still be dysplastic. Repeat excision is an option, but if this is not technically possible, a hysterectomy may be considered. In patients wanting children, "observation" alone, including frequent Pap smears and colposcopy, is reasonable as long as invasive disease can be excluded because these lesions often remain static or spontaneously regress.

Invasive Ca

Even actual **invasive cervical cancer**, if detected early enough, has a 90% cure rate. Cervical cancer is divided into stages according to size and degree of invasion. Treatment of invasive cervical cancer is consistent with the general principles that apply to most malignant diseases. Disease confined to the cervix is best treated by hysterectomy; patients with positive lymph nodes or resection margins receive postoperative pelvic irradiation. Radiation therapy is used as primary therapy for those with inoperable tumors, and those with an extremely poor prognosis may benefit from concomitant radiation and chemotherapy.

Gestational Trophoblastic Disease

Gestational trophoblastic disease (GTD) refers to a group of neoplasms representing different levels of abnormal placental proliferation. Important characteristics of these tumors are their sensitivity to chemotherapy and expression of hCG. **Hydatidiform mole, invasive mole, choriocarcinoma**, and **placental site trophoblastic disease** arise from abnormal haploid germ cells, either maternal or paternal, and affect women of reproductive age.

The most common GTD is the **hydatidiform mole**. It most commonly follows another molar pregnancy, but can follow any type of conception including abortion, miscarriage, or term delivery. Partial moles, usually triploid, contain some fetal tissue and have a low potential for persistence after evacuation, while complete moles, usually diploid, contain no fetal tissue and have approximately a 10% chance of persistence. Though most moles resolve without additional therapy (beyond D&C), about 15% of patients have a persistently elevated hCG and eventually will develop signs of a postmolar trophoblastic neoplasm such as vaginal bleeding or metastases; these patients usually turn out to have an **invasive mole**. Both metastatic and nonmetastatic GTD respond well to methotrexate or actinomycin. A subset of patients with metastatic disease, however, fail this initial therapy and must be retreated with multi-agent chemotherapy. Surgery is rarely indicated in the treatment of GTD except for initial evacuation or eradication of a resistant focus of disease. Most women should be able to conceive again after a year without evidence of recurrence.

Vulvar Carcinoma

Vulvar cancer is the least common gynecologic malignancy, occurring in only 1 per 100,000 women. The overwhelming majority are **squamous cell lesions**; **melanoma** and **basal cell cancer** also occur. It is a disease of older women, although age at presentation seems to be decreasing. There appear to be two separate etiologies based on age: vulvar carcinoma in older women may be caused by cumulative genetic errors and environmental factors, while disease in younger patients appears to be related to infection with human papilloma virus,

Like cervical dysplasia, **vulvar intraepithelial neoplasms (VIN)** are found in patients 10-20 years younger than those with invasive tumors. VIN is treatable, and its eradication should decrease the chances of the development of invasive disease. Unfortunately, VIN is difficult to diagnose, possibly because of patient and physician hesitancy to examine and biopsy the vulva; the typical delay between first symptoms and the diagnosis of vulvar cancer is a year. These neoplasms are easily treated with either skinning vulvectomy or laser ablation; topical chemotherapy with 5-fluorouracil is useful in the immunosuppressed.

Most malignant vulvar lesions are treated with radical surgery, including inguinal and femoral lymphadenectomy. Adjuvant radiation is used for higher stages, and patients with distant metastases are treated with palliative chemotherapy. ■

67 Reproductive Endocrinology and Infertility

Endocrinologic issues are obviously of paramount importance to the gynecologist; it is perhaps surprising that disorders of this complex system don't occur more frequently. The field of reproductive endocrinology deals primarily with amenorrhea, hyperandrogenism, and infertility.

Amenorrhea

Amenorrhea is the absence of menses. **Primary amenorrhea** is defined as the absence of menses by age 14; **secondary amenorrhea**, the absence of menses for 6 months in a previously menstruating female. Amenorrhea can be classified by the anatomic area or "compartment" of the defect. **Compartment I** refers to outflow tract disorders of the uterus and vagina, **compartment II** to disorders of the ovary, **compartment III** to disorders of the anterior pituitary, and **compartment IV** to hypothalamic or other central nervous system (CNS) disorders. Primary amenorrhea can also be chromosomal, associated with an abnormal karyotype, as seen in 45X (Turner's syndrome), mosaicism, and pure gonadal dysgenesis.

Gonadal failure   The first "disorder" to rule out in any woman who presents with amenorrhea, obviously, is a normal pregnancy. A common group of patients with primary amenorrhea are those adolescents with no breast development but normal female genitalia, resulting from a lack of follicle development and estrogen production. Individuals with a primary ovarian defect have **gonadal failure**. There is no estrogen to exert its negative feedback on the hypothalamus, so gonadotropin levels are **elevated**. Because Müllerian development is estrogen-independent, the "default" mode of sexual development, a normal uterus and external female genitalia are present. In this situation (primary amenorrhea with elevated FSH levels) karyotyping is indicated because abnormalities are common.

Central disorders   **CNS-hypothalamic-pituitary disorders** can be distinguished from gonadal failure by the presence of **low** gonadotropin levels. A common cause of hypogonadotropic hypogonadism is severe physical or emotional stress. Young, usually extremely fit athletes (such as

Olympic marathoners) or high-pressure professionals can have high enough levels of their own endogenous opiates to inhibit gonadotropin secretion. Other causes include pituitary adenomas (e.g., prolactinoma) or other CNS tumors, congenital CNS lesions such as empty Sella syndrome, and Kallmann's syndrome, a genetically inherited syndrome of amenorrhea and anosmia. A less common but important defect is Sheehan's syndrome, or acute pituitary necrosis due to postpartum hemorrhagic hypotension.

Androgen insensitivity

If the patient presents with phenotypically normal breasts but the uterus is absent, **androgen insensitivity (testicular feminization)** may be present. These patients have an XY karyotype and testosterone-producing gonads, but no functioning target organ receptors. Consequently, although genetically male, masculine differentiation of the external and internal genitalia does not occur, and patients are phenotypically female. They usually have normal appearing feminine external genitalia, a short or absent vagina, scanty pubic and axillary hair, and female breast development; there are neither female nor male internal genitalia. There is a high risk of malignant transformation of the ovaries in this situation, and removal should be offered. **Congenital absence of the uterus** is another cause of primary amenorrhea. Patients with Müllerian agenesis look the same as do those with androgen insensitivity, but have normally functioning ovaries and an XX karyotype. Renal abnormalities are seen in up to a third of these patients.

Introgenic amenorrhea

Amenorrhea is unusual after oral contraception (OCP) discontinuation, but because OCPs can mask an underlying menstrual abnormality, problems can first present after discontinuation and thus appear to be "caused by" the pill itself. During use, amenorrhea is present in approximately 5% of patients without physiologic consequences; reassurance is the only treatment needed.

Because of persistently elevated levels of progesterone, Depo-Provera is associated with prolonged amenorrhea (up to 9 months after discontinuation). Many other drugs with anti-dopaminergic effects, including tricyclic antidepressants and antiemetics, can cause amenorrhea by elevating prolactin levels. Exposure to certain chemotherapeutic agents or radiation can also result in gonadal failure and amenorrhea.

Anatomic problems

A common **anatomic defect** is Ascherman's syndrome, or adhesions caused by uterine inflammation. Inflammation can be caused by postpartum curettage, endometritis, or other uterine trauma. Congenital Müllerian anomalies include an interrupted vaginal canal, uterine anomalies, lack of a vaginal orifice, and complete Müllerian agenesis. The Mayer-Rokitansky-Kuster-Hauser syndrome consists of an absent or hypoplastic vagina and an abnormal or absent uterus.

Workup

Laboratory testing is very useful. Both hyper- and hypothyroidism can result in hypogonadotropic hypogonadism. Prolactin levels should be measured; if greater than 100ng/mL, a pituitary microadenoma might be present. LH and FSH assays will distinguish between ovarian (high, due to loss of feedback) and hypothalamic-pituitary (low, the primary problem) disorders as discussed above. If a patient with ovarian failure is younger than 30, a chromosomal abnormality may be present; if older, an autoimmune syndrome such as autoimmune thyroiditis or adrenal insufficiency may coexist with ovarian failure. A progesterone challenge, done to confirm the presence of circulating estrogens, is useful. A progestin is given in an attempt to induce withdrawal bleeding. If normal bleeding occurs, the diagnosis of anovulation is made, because endogenous progesterone production is dependent on normal ovulation. If there is no bleeding following the progestin, sequential estrogen followed by progesterone administration should result in uterine bleeding unless there is an anatomical obstruction.

Hyperandrogenism

Hyperandrogenism is an endocrinologic disorder that can cause significant emotional distress. Often the most troublesome aspect is the presence of hypertrichosis (excess hair in a normal distribution), hirsutism (excess hair in atypical locations) or other signs of virilization. The final common denominator is an excess end-organ response to a functional hyperandrogenic state.

Normally the ovaries and adrenal gland make moderate amounts of androgens. Testosterone is primarily produced by the ovaries. Testosterone is converted to dihydrotestosterone (DHT), its biologically active product, at the end-organ by 5-alpha-reductase; hyperandrogenism is better correlated with DHT and reductase reductase activity than with testosterone levels. Since reductase activity cannot easily be measured, its metabolite, 3-alpha-diol glucuronide, is used instead.

The most common cause of hirsutism is **increased reductase activity**, a normal variant common in certain ethnic groups. **Polycystic ovarian syndrome** (PCO) is also associated with hyperandrogenism. Abnormal gonadotropin releasing hormone (GnRH) function results in chronically elevated LH levels, in turn leading to elevated circulating androgens. Affected women have elevated estrone levels due to peripheral conversion of the excess androgens.

Ovarian neoplasms, most commonly Sertoli-Leydig cell and Hilus cell tumors (see Chapter 66, "Gynecologic Malignancies"), can produce androgens and lead to virilization. Affected patients typically develop rapid-onset virilization with elevation of serum testosterone to more than twice normal; imaging of the ovaries followed by operative removal of any masses found should follow. **Luteoma of pregnancy** is a benign mass responsible for virilization during gestation. **Adrenal carcinomas** can also cause virilization because the excess steroids are converted to androgens in the peripheral tissues.

CAH

Congenital adrenal hyperplasia is a disorder due to a deficiency in one of the enzymes, usually 21-OH hydroxylase, involved in steroid synthesis. The hydroxylase deficiency leads to decreased cortisol production which causes release of adrenocortotropic hormone (ACTH) due to a lack of negative feedback. This excess ACTH further stimulates the adrenal gland; in the face of the enzymatic defect cortisol precursors build up which are converted to androgens. By a similar pathway, Cushing's syndrome can also cause hyperandrogenism.

Treatment

Treatment of hyperandrogenism is directed at excluding the presence of an androgen-secreting tumor, which can be accomplished with a high degree of accuracy by means of pelvic ultrasound and abdominal CT scan. Any mass found in this clinical setting should be removed as soon as possible. If no masses are identified, symptom relief is the primary concern.

OCPs are effective in reducing free circulating testosterone by raising levels of its carrier protein, sex hormone binding globulin, and by suppressing LH secretion, thereby decreasing androgen production. Because testosterone levels are high in many of these disorders, OCPs are effective in most patients with virilization who do not desire pregnancy. Spironolactone may be the most effective available inhibitor of reductase activity. GnRH antagonists have also been used to reduce ovarian androgen production, but their use is limited by significant menopausal side effects. Electrolysis, shaving, bleaching, and depilatories provide cosmetic relief. If the primary abnormality is excess adrenal androgen precursor production, suppression with steroids may be helpful.

Infertility

Infertility is defined as the inability to conceive after 1 year of sexual intercourse without contraception, while **fecundity** is the possibility of achieving a pregnancy with 1 menstrual cycle. Infertility affects 10%-15% of couples in the reproductive age group; 1 out of every 5 couples ever married has sought treatment for the inability to conceive. Age is an important factor; the prevalence of infertility approaches 90% in nulliparous women at age 40. Fecundity is approximately 20% in healthy couples not using contraception, thus, half of normal couples will conceive within 3 months, 75% within 6 months, and 90% within a year. Caffeine, tobacco, and certain drugs adversely affect fertility. Before performing any invasive procedure on the female, evaluation of the male should be completed and his willingness to father a child confirmed.

Male

Problems causing infertility in the **male** usually involve sperm abnormalities. Infertility should be clearly differentiated from **impotence**, the inability to achieve and maintain an erection. Information regarding exposure to toxins, drugs, mumps, tobacco, alcohol, antihypertensives (a classic cause of impotence), and sulfa drugs should be sought, as well as the presence of buttock and thigh claudication suggesting aortoiliac and pelvic atherosclerosis (see Chapter 37, "Vascular Surgery"). Libido and sexual function, including frequency, should be specifically addressed. If impotence is ruled out, the primary test is semen analysis to evaluate ejaculate quantity and viscosity, and sperm motility, morphology, and count.

Female

Two-thirds of infertile couples have an identifiable abnormality of the **female** partner. Female infertility factors can be broken down into **ovulatory dysfunction** (affecting about 30% of patients), **tubal and pelvic pathology** (affecting 60%), and **unexplained** infertility (accounting for the remaining 10%).

Ovulatory dysfuction

Anovulation, associated with hyperprolactinemia, thyroid abnormalities, gonadal agenesis, or polycystic ovaries, for example, is an obvious cause of infertility. Anovulatory cycles become more common as a female approaches the menopause. A history of irregular menses or absence of usual premenstrual symptoms can indicate anovulation. Findings such as a body habitus consistent with Turner's or Klinefelter's syndromes, the presence of a male-shaped escutcheon or other signs of virilization, or galactorrhea, goiter, or striae all suggest conditions that can be associated with anovulation. A consistent, biphasic half degree Celsius increase in basal body temperature (BBT) provides evidence of ovulation, as does the finding of a progesterone level greater than 5ng/mL.

Once ovulation has been confirmed, its adequacy is addressed. An endometrial biopsy, when performed 2-3 days before menses, should reveal a secretory endometrium responding to ovulation and subsequent progesterone production. If the histology is not appropriate for the day of the cycle, a **luteal phase defect** may be present. A hysterosalpingogram (HSG), a transcervical contrast study of the uterus and tubes, will radiographically demonstrate any abnormal filling contours of the uterine cavity. No "spill" bilaterally on HSG does not necessarily indicate tubal blockage because the tubes may spasm. Interestingly, HSG alone have been shown on occasion to mechanically open blocked tubes and restore fertility. A similar test, hysteroscopy, allows direct visualization of the uterine cavity and even treatment of anatomic abnormalities such as endometrial polyps, fibroids and intrauterine adhesions (Ascherman's syndrome).
(continued)

OB-Gyn
Reproductive Endocrinology and
Infertility *continued*

Cervical mucous is best assessed at mid-cycle. Due to the elevated estrogen levels, the mucous should be clear, abundant, and stretchable ("spinnbarkeit"), and should "fern" when dried. The postcoital test (PCT) evaluates both the ovulatory cervical mucus as well as the sperm-mucous interaction. Precise timing is necessary for proper interpretation; mucous should be examined as soon as possible after intercourse at the time of suspected ovulation. The usefulness of this test has recently been questioned. Lubricants can be spermicidal and produce a picture similar to that of poor mucus.

Tubal problems

Tubal patency can be demonstrated either by HSG or by chromopertubation, which consists of transcervical instillation of indigo carmine while the fimbria are observed during laparoscopy. Because of its invasive nature, chromopertubation is usually only done when other intra-abdominal pathology is suspected. In the US, nonpatent fallopian tubes most often are the result of pelvic inflammatory disease (PID). Tubal blockage can also result from endometriosis, appendicitis, or previous pelvic surgery, all of which are associated with inflammation and adhesion formation. A history of previous pelvic infection, pelvic surgery, multiple sexual partners, previous sexually transmitted disease, ectopic pregnancy, or dyspareunia (which can be a sign of endometriosis) should be sought. Because tubal factors and PID are both relatively common, most initial infertility evaluations include cervical cultures for gonorrhea and chlamydia. **Anti-sperm antibody** testing should be considered.

Treatment

Treatment depends on the abnormality present. Male factor causes such as varicocele or infection should be treated. A significant number of male patients, however, will not regain normal semen function. In these patients, assisted reproductive technologies can be of benefit. **Intrauterine insemination (IUI)** with washed sperm can be used as long as some normal sperm are present; washing allows the separation and concentration of the most promising sperm. Intracytoplasmic sperm injection is also useful for low sperm conditions. If these fail, or if azoospermia, severe oligospermia, or asthenospermia refractory to treatment are present, **therapeutic donor insemination (TDI)** can be effective. Treatment of cervical factors such as poor mucus historically has involved estrogen and mucolytic therapy. The most successful method for treating cervical factor infertility is to bypass it entirely with IUI timed to follow the LH surge. **Surgery** is required, if possible, to correct uterine abnormalities. Intrauterine polyps or submucosal leiomyomata can be resected using hysteroscopic techniques. Hysteroscopy can also be used for lysis of intrauterine synechiae or resection of a uterine septum. Except for complete bilateral tubal occlusion, the relationship between a particular uterine anatomic anomaly and infertility may not be precise. Fallopian tube obstruction can be treated by transcervical balloon tuboplasty or by conventional laparotomy or laparoscopy. Tubal surgery includes salpingolysis, neosaplingostomy and tubal reanastomoses. Unfortunately, success rates are not promising, and bypassing tubal function completely by means of **in vitro fertilization (IVF)** may be a better option in many situations.

If known, the underlying causes of anovulation should be treated. If not, there are effective means of dealing with either idiopathic anovulation or ovulatory dysfunction. Many drugs are useful. Clomiphene citrate is a synthetic drug that exerts a very weak biologic estrogenic effect, falsely lowering the true estrogen signal to the hypothalamus. The net effect is an increase in GnRH, FSH, and LH, making it useful in PCO and many other anovulatory conditions, and probably also for luteal phase defects. It is relatively safe and fairly inexpensive, but should be used for no more than 4-6 cycles.

Exogenous gonadotropins are also useful. Human menopausal gonadotropin is an extract from the urine of postmenopausal women composed of equal amounts of LH and FSH. It is expensive and has a higher complication rate than clomiphene, and induces superovulation, often being combined with IUI. It is injected daily in conjunction with close monitoring of ovarian follicles by ultrasound and estrogen levels. When follicles appear mature and estrogen levels are adequate, HCG, which mimics LH and stimulates ovulation, is injected. When combined with IUI, fecundity rates are approximately 15%. The major side effect is ovarian hyperstimulation that can develop into a life-threatening syndrome consisting of ovarian enlargement, ascites, pleural effusion, electrolyte imbalances, and hypovolemia; torsion can also occur due to the tremendous ovarian enlargement. All

OB-Gyn
Reproductive Endocrinology and Infertility *continued*

ovulation-inducing drugs increase the chances of multiple gestations. Endogenous FSH and LH can be stimulated by the pulsatile administration of GnRH. Luteal phase defects are usually treated with exogenous progesterone until the end of the first trimester when the placenta takes over progesterone production from the corpus luteum.

Bromocriptine is a dopamine agonist that directly inhibits pituitary prolactin secretion. It is useful in patients with a prolactinoma and those hyperprolactinemic from other causes to remove the prolactin-mediated inhibition of ovulation. Ovarian wedge resection can help patients with PCO by removing a significant amount of androgen-producing stromal tissue. Patients in whom ovulation cannot be induced due to decreased ovarian reserve, donor egg IVF, where both the sperm and the oocyte are donated, fertilized in vitro, and implanted into the patient's uterus, is an option. ■

Psychiatry

Hassen Al-Amin
and
Anton P Porsteinsson
Section Editors

68   DSM-IV Orientation

In psychiatry, **classification** attempts to bring order to the great diversity of phenomena encountered in clinical practice, in order to identify groups of patients that share similar clinical features so that treatment planning and prediction of outcome can be simplified. Such a system allows health professionals caring for these patients to communicate with one another with the confidence that they are indeed studying the same problem. The **Diagnostic and Statistical Manual, 4th edition (DSM-IV)** is the "bible" of psychiatry; it is the systemic classification system for psychiatric problems that all psychiatrists use throughout the world.

History

The various classification systems in psychiatry date back to the days of Hippocrates, who introduced the terms "mania" and "hysteria." Official classification of mental disorders in the United States was first attempted as part of the census of 1840 as a means to collect statistical information. Various systems were adopted over the early part of the 20th century, the most detailed developed by the Army and Veterans Administration following World War II. This classification strongly influenced the International Classification of Diseases, the sixth edition of which included mental disorders for the first time.

In 1952, the American Psychiatric Association's Committee on Nomenclature and Statistics published the first edition of the **Diagnostic and Statistical Manual of Mental Disorders (DSM-I)**. The major significance of this book was that for the first time it described the categories it listed. It was revised and published as **DSM-II** in 1968. Publication of **DSM-III** occurred in 1980, coinciding with publication of the ninth edition of the International Classification of Diseases (ICD-9). DSM-III included, for the first time, explicit diagnostic criteria, a multiaxial system (see below), and a descriptive approach that was supposed to be neutral regarding theories of causation, enabling clinicians of varying theoretic orientations to use it without difficulty. It was revised (**DSM-III-R**) in 1987.

Due to the explosive growth of the field and to the publication of ICD-10 in 1992, work started on the fourth version of the Diagnostic and Statistical Manual of Mental Disorders (**DSM-IV**). The revision process included an extensive literature review, a re-analysis and re-examination of the data, and field trials. It was published in 1994 and currently represents the definitive classification of mental disorders. It is based on a descriptive approach to diagnosis, the definition of a disorder consisting of a description of the clinical features that must be present for the diagnosis to be made. The DSM-IV reflects the current consensus of a group of experts on the classification and diagnosis of mental disorders; the criteria will require further revision as knowledge increases.

DSM-IV

The DSM-IV splits the description of the various psychiatric diagnoses into five categories, or **axes**, in an attempt to ensure that attention is given to the biological, psychological, and social aspects of a person's condition.

Axis I consists of the clinical psychiatric syndromes and other selected conditions that are usually the primary focus of attention (so-called "V codes").

Axis II consists of the personality disorders and mental retardation. The habitual use of a particular defense mechanism can be listed on Axis II.

Axis III is for listing physical conditions that are present, whether related to Axis I disorders or not.

Axis IV codes psychosocial or environmental stressors, whether positive or negative.

Axis V is the Global Assessment of Functioning Scale that quantifies the patient's overall level of functioning during a particular period.

The severity of an Axis I syndrome can be described as mild, moderate, or severe, and as being in partial or full remission. Diagnosis can be provisional or documented by prior history. The DSM-IV contains decision trees for diagnoses based on many specific signs or symptoms.
(continued)

Psychiatry
DSM-IV Orientation *continued*

Although it appears complex at first, exploration of the DSM-IV allows medical students and other trainees insight into diagnostics and decision making in the field of psychiatry. A primary care version will be published in the near future. ■

Psychiatric illness usually develops over time, and is viewed as the result of interactions between the genetic and physiologic make-up of an individual (biologic factors), the patterns of behavior and thinking that the individual acquires during development (psychologic factors), and the dynamic processes created as the result of familial and cultural interaction (social factors). Such a biopsychosocial perspective is essential when gathering the **history** and performing the **mental status exam** (**MSE**) in a patient with psychiatric illness.

The psychiatric evaluation starts with an assessment of the patient's mental status, understanding of the problem, and reactions to stressors. Overall goals include estimation of the severity of symptoms, making the diagnosis and a biopsychosocial formulation of the problem based on the DSM-IV, providing an explanation of the problem and the treatment options to the patient, and initiation of treatment by engaging the patient in psychotherapy. A common strategy is to first try to develop a rapport with the patient, next, to start to collect data using open-ended questions, and finally, to end the interview with structured, closed-ended questions and formal testing.

Psychiatric History

It is often valuable to obtain and describe the results of the psychiatric history in a relatively fixed, stylized format. **Identifying data** include the name, age, marital status, race, and reason for referral of the patient, as well as the source(s) of your information (patient, family, friends, and old records). The **chief complaint** is described, as usual, in the patient's words. **History of the present illness** should focus on current symptoms, onset, and precipitating factors. If the patient has had previous major medical or psychiatric illnesses, treatment received and the patient's compliance should be ascertained. Symptoms are often best described in chronologic order; anything that worsens or improves symptomatology can provide clues. If the patient uses technical terms, figure out what the patient believes he means. Presence or absence of suicidal or homicidal ideation is important to elicit, as is

Psychiatry
Psychiatric Evaluation and the MSE
continued

judgment of severity, and a history of drug and/or alcohol use and its relation to the patient's current condition is always important. Finally, the **past medical history**, including the patient's primary care physician, should be noted. List current medications, their dosages, and any recent changes; many medications can induce psychiatric symptoms.

Next, the **past psychiatric history** is elicited. Document dates and duration of previous psychiatric treatment, both inpatient and outpatient. Highlight precipitating factors and level of function before the onset of symptoms (deterioration of function is a major criterion in most DSM-IV diagnoses, and is used as a reference when monitoring response to treatment), type of treatment the patient has received (including psychosocial intervention and medications and their dosages, effects, and side effects), and compliance with medications and psychotherapy (including relationships with therapists). Document the major signs and symptoms present at admission and discharge, and plans for followup. Finally, because it is so pervasive and important, elaborate fully any history of drug and alcohol use, including onset, progression, effects on family and overall functioning, and any history of treatment or rehabilitation efforts.

Developmental and Social History

The developmental and social history is designed to elicit the effects of such issues on the present problem. **Peri- and postnatal complications**, if any, and a description of **developmental milestones** and **major childhood illnesses** should be documented. Describe relevant issues relating to **childhood play** and **relationships**, focusing on problematic behavioral patterns and anything suggestive of sexual or physical abuse. Elaborate on **major childhood stressors** or losses such as divorce or death in the family. Describe the patient's **education** and school performance, including relationships with peers and teachers.

Family and **sexual histories** are important. Names and ages of parents and siblings should be documented. Elaborate on the patient's relationships with them, their expectations for the patient, and their reaction to the patient's illness. A history of psychiatric illnesses in the family is particularly significant, including medications received and responses. Ask the patient about sexual orientation, satisfaction, and history of deviant behavior such as cross-dressing, fetishism, or pedophilia. If the patient is **married**, check the timing and circumstances of the marriage and relationships with the spouse and children. Describe the patient's **employment history** and level of job satisfaction, and highlight any recent changes or financial problems.

Mental Status Exam

The **mental status exam (MSE)**, although somewhat variable in description, is a relatively formal way of assessing the mental status and overall condition of the patient **at the time of the interview**. It helps to narrow the differential diagnosis, delineate the target signs and symptoms, and formulate the treatment plan. Most of the information in the MSE is obtained during the informal part of the interview, but some direct questions may be needed. Save highly structured questions and tests for the end of the interview, and prepare the patient for them by emphasizing their routine, screening nature to minimize negative reactions to such direct questioning.

The MSE is classically divided into several, discrete parts:

General appearance: Describe the patient **as you see him or her**, including clothing, grooming, and appropriateness in relation to the setting. Describe gait, posture, gestures, mannerisms, psychomotor activity, abnormal behaviors, eye contact, and any unusual motor movements. Note the presence or absence of self-injury, signs of IV substance abuse, and evidence of physical trauma.

Attitude toward the interviewer: Is the patient spontaneous and cooperative in relating information, or defensive, hostile, or guarded (and so on)?

Speech: Describe speed, tone, volume, and quantity; document dysarthria or aphasia, if present.

Mood and affect: **Mood** is the emotional state expressed by the patient, while **affect** is the state **observed** by the interviewer; decide whether the two are **congruent** with each other and **appropriate** for the thought content. *(continued)*

Psychiatry
Psychiatric Evaluation and the MSE

continued

Blunt affect refers to inadequate expression of emotional state, while **flat affect** refers to the complete absence of emotional expression.

Thought content: Describe **what** the patient is thinking. Indicate the presence of hopeless/helpless/worthless themes or thoughts of guilt or shame. Note the presence of extreme suspiciousness or paranoid ideation, and identify and elaborate on **delusions** (incorrect thoughts). It is particularly important in this section to try to use the patient's direct quotes rather than your interpretation of the words you hear so that as much objectivity as possible can be preserved. Describe obsessive or phobic ideation, and the presence or absence of suicidal or homicidal thoughts.

Thought process: Describe **how** the patient is thinking. Is the flow of thoughts organized and coherent, or does the patient jump from one idea to another with or without reasonable association (**flight of ideas** and **loosening of associations**, respectively)? Are answers not related to questions asked (**tangentiality**) or are unnecessary details included (**circumstantiality**)? Does the patient stop talking suddenly or lose track of previous thoughts for no clear reason (**thought blocking**)? Check for **thought insertion** or **broadcasting** and for **ideas of reference** (typified by statements that TV, radio, or newspapers are giving the patient special messages). Does the patient repeat the same sentence several times (**perseveration**) or repeat your questions (**echolalia**)?

Perceptions: An **illusion** is a misinterpretation of actual sensory stimuli, while a **hallucination** is a sensory experience without sensory stimulation (both common during delirium, intoxication, and withdrawal). Describe the type of experience: tactile, visual, olfactory, gustatory, or auditory. Look for **command hallucinations** and whether the patient controls the voices or acts on these commands.

Insight and judgment: Such assessment is difficult, and whether an accurate judgment can be made after one 30-minute interview can be controversial. It is sometimes easy to identify such problems, however, in severely impaired patients. Comment should always be made about patients' awareness of their illness, problems (**insight**) with how they are dealing with them, and willingness to accept treatment (**judgment**).

Level of consciousness: Is the patient alert or lethargic, or easily distractible? A level of consciousness that alternates between alert and sleepy is often seen in delirium (see Chapters 20, "Neurology," and 74, "Cognitive Disorders" for further discussion of delirium and dementia).

Orientation: Is the patient oriented to time (day, date, month, year, or season), person (family and familiar people) and place (home address, city, county, and state)?

Cognitive function: When performing tests to evaluate cognitive function, take into consideration the patient's baseline intellectual functioning and educational level. Such testing (often called the **mini-MSE; MMSE**) is especially helpful in the identification of neuropsychiatric disorders that present as impairment in one or more cognitive functions. For example, patients with dementia can present with memory loss first, before global cognitive abilities are affected. In depression, attention and concentration are significantly impaired, while schizophrenic patients usually show deficits in abstract thinking and problem solving tasks.

Test **language** by testing naming, repetition, and reading. The specific type of deficits can help differentiate Broca's from Wernicke's aphasia and identify paraphasic errors, sometimes seen in patients with dementia. Test for **attention and concentration** by asking the patient to count upward and/or downward by a specific number ("serial 7s") and repeat digits; such tasks are usually impaired in patients with delirium. Tests of **memory** include assessment of the patient's ability to register, retain, and retrieve information. Check **immediate recall** by seeing if the patient is able to remember 3 items after 5 minutes (giving clues, if needed), **recent memory** (events from the same day), and **remote recall** (significant events and dates from the past). Patients with dementia first exhibit deficits in short term memory and in learning new material, but may remember significant memories from their childhood. **Visuo-spatial and motor performance** are checked by asking the patient to copy figures such as crossed pentagons or by asking them to draw a clock face. Patients with a right parietal lobe lesion may draw half the clock only (left **neglect**) and/or have problems with tasks that require coordination of the visual and motor systems in space.

Physical Exam and Laboratory Testing

All patients should have a complete physical exam during their evaluation; timing, however, depends on presentation, medical history, and level of suspicion that an organic problem exists. In other words, the higher the suspicion that a general medical condition is causing symptoms, the higher the priority the physical exam assumes.

Laboratory testing should be individualized depending on the differential diagnosis after the initial assessment. Some purely screening labs, however, can be helpful, both to determine the patients' baseline and to ensure their well-being, because certain conditions are so prevalent. Such tests include a complete blood count (CBC) and differential, blood urea nitrogen (BUN), creatinine, electrolytes, liver function tests, urinalysis, free T4 and thyroid-stimulating hormone (TSH) to rule out thyroid disease, rapid plasma reagent (RPR) test to rule out neurosyphilis, a pregnancy test in women at childbearing age, and a urine toxicology screen. Vitamin B12 and folate levels should be measured in patients with dementia, and a baseline EKG performed before administering phenothiazines or tricyclic antidepressants (see Chapter 71, "Psychopharmacology"). Serum levels of nortriptyline, desipramine, tegretol, lithium, and valproate should be checked in appropriate patients, both to ensure a therapeutic level and to rule out toxicity (and to ensure compliance, if appropriate).

An electroencephalograph (EEG) is helpful if seizure activity is suspected, while a head CT or MRI are needed if an organic neurologic problem is suspected. These are also useful in patients with a first psychotic episode or the acute onset of psychiatric symptoms.

Finally **psychologic testing** should be done to answer a specific question. Examples include neuropsychologic testing to confirm frontal lobe dysfunction, the Minnesota

Multiphasic Personality Inventory (MMPI) to assess the personality profile of the patient, and intelligence testing to measure the patient's IQ.

Formulation

This is the part of the chart that summarizes all the relevant information obtained above, and forms the basis upon which the differential diagnosis is formulated. The problem at hand, possible causes, and precipitating factors should be discussed in terms of the biopsychosocial model. Prognostic factors obtained from the history and MSE should be discussed, and their impact on pathogenesis and prognosis evaluated. A comment should be made about the psychodynamic conflicts involved and major defense mechanisms, and how they relate to the symptomatology and behavioral patterns seen.

Diagnosis

Psychiatric diagnoses are made according to the **Diagnostic and Statistical Manual, 4th edition (DSM-IV**; see Chapter 68, "DSM-IV Orientation"), a multiaxial diagnosis scheme compatible with the biopsychosocial model. **Axis I** covers most of the psychiatric diagnoses themselves, while **Axis II** usually allows recording of developmental and personality disorders, the latter characterized by rigid patterns of maladaptive behavior and attitudes that start early in development (see Chapter 77, "Personality Disorders"); personality disorders are recorded on a different axis because they are usually chronic and resistant to treatment. **Axis III** covers any medical conditions present relevant to the diagnosis, course, and treatment of the Axis I psychiatric disorder. Stressors are recorded on **Axis IV**, including severity, type, and chronicity, to act as a reminder that psychosocial factors can precipitate or contribute to the mental disorder. **Axis V** is used to describe the level of functional impairment and consists of current and past scores on the **Global Assessment of Functioning (GAF)** scale. It serves as a baseline to monitor progression of disease and response to treatment.
(continued)

Psychiatry
Psychiatric Evaluation and the MSE
continued

Treatment Plan

The **treatment plan** includes goals and objectives of the proposed treatment based on the diagnosis and overall assessment.

If additional information is needed for the final diagnosis and plan, that should be so indicated, as should any pending laboratory tests, why they are indicated, and what information you are trying to gain from them. Medication choices should be clearly documented and justified, including dosage and any monitoring required. Specify targeted symptoms and when improvement can be expected, and document discussion with the patient about side effects.

The type of **psychotherapy** recommended should be indicated (see Chapter 72, "Psychotherapy"), and again, goals should be specific. **Referrals** (social services, medical consultation, psychological testing, and so on) should be clearly documented, including the reason for referral and the objectives. Finally, the frequency of **followup** and an estimate of the duration of treatment should be discussed. ∎

70   Psychiatric Emergencies

Psychiatric emergencies obviously abound. Very often the single most critical decision to be made in the psychiatric emergency department is whether the patient needs acute inpatient care. Most often the need for acute, sometimes involuntary, hospitalization is because of the risk of harm to patients themselves (**suicide**) or to others (**violent behavior**). The decision whether to admit or discharge a patient is one that requires considerable judgment, and thus can only be acquired through experience.

Suicide

Suicide, defined as intentional, self-inflicted death, is commonly precipitated by frustrated psychologic needs and feelings of hopelessness and helplessness resulting in intolerable psychologic pain. Suicidal patients usually have troubles problem solving and view suicide as the only way to escape unbearable stress. Suicide is the eighth most common cause of death in the US; incidence is estimated between 10-12 per 100,000 persons yearly, leading to 30,000 deaths per year; the number of attempted suicides is 8-10 times higher.

Demographics   **Men commit** suicide three times more often than women; **women attempt** suicide three to four times more often than men. Men tend to use more lethal methods, explaining their higher "success" rate. Suicide rates in women **increase with age**, peaking between 55-70, and follow a bimodal distribution in men, peaking between 15-24 and after 45. The suicide rate is rising rapidly in adolescents and young adults and is currently the third leading cause of death in males aged 15-24 (after accidents and homicides). Suicide rate is highest among **whites** but is also high among inner city blacks and native Americans. Suicide rate is lowest for married persons, twice as high for single, never-married persons; and 4-5 times higher for **divorced** or **widowed** persons. Rates are highest among **unemployed** persons and those with **low socioeconomic status**; among professionals, **physicians** are at greatest risk for suicide. Approximately 90%-95% of patients who commit or attempt suicide have a **diagnosed**

Psychiatry
Psychiatric Emergencies *continued*

major psychiatric disorder; psychiatric patients have a risk for suicide 3-12 times higher than the population at large.

Risk factors

About half the patients who commit suicide have **depression** as their primary diagnosis. The risk for suicide is highest if depression is associated with psychotic symptoms (e.g., command hallucinations) and within the first 6 months after hospital discharge. Risk is also high early after the initiation of treatment, when depression is still present but the patient's energy level is rising. About a quarter of completed suicides are related to **alcoholism**, especially in patients with overlapping mood disorder symptoms or antisocial personality disorder. Alcohol and other substances worsen depressive or psychotic symptoms and increase the risk for suicide secondary to disinhibition and impaired reality testing. Ten percent of deaths in **schizophrenic** patients are due to suicide. Risk factors associated with suicide among schizophrenics include young age, male sex, single marital status, depressive symptoms, and demoralization. **Personality disorders**, particularly borderline and antisocial types, are associated with increased risk; suicide gestures are also very frequent in these patients. A **history of previous suicide attempts** is associated with a high risk for later, successful suicide. About 40% of suicide victims have a history of a prior attempt; risk is highest within 3 months of the first attempt. Risk is increased in patients with a **family history** of suicide. Finally, **terminal illness**, **chronic pain**, **chronic disease**, and **recent surgery** are all associated with increased risk.

Suicide assessment

Suicide assessment is the process of formulating an opinion of the risk that the patient will attempt or commit suicide in the near future, and carries with it obvious implications about the need for hospitalization and treatment. Assessment in some form is indicated in all patients presenting to a psychiatric emergency room and in all patients with a major psychiatric disorder. Obviously, patients complaining of or admitting to suicidal ideation and those who have just survived a suicide attempt require careful, complete assessment, as do patients with major medical problems who show signs of depression, demoralization, or hopelessness. Finally, patients who deny suicidal intent but whose behavior suggests suicide potential (e.g., accidental overdose or single-vehicle automobile accidents) deserve assessment.

Several generalizations are helpful. Suicidal patients commonly communicate their intentions to others. **All suicide threats should be taken seriously**, even those in chronic manipulative patients who make frequent suicide gestures. Establish a rapport with patient before asking direct questions about suicide, and ask about suicidal ideation in an empathic way. "It seems you have been feeling sad for a while, have thoughts of suicide crossed your mind?" is better than "are you thinking about killing yourself?" Don't be afraid to ask about suicide. **Questioning patients about suicide does not put the idea in their heads**; patients, in fact, are often relieved that the subject has been raised for them.

Any suicide evaluation should include assessment of risk factors, mental status, and social support. Specific questions about suicidal ideation, intent, and plans should be asked to establish the potential for immediate risk.

All patients who present to a psychiatric emergency room or have pertinent risk factors should be questioned about suicide (assuming suicidal ideation is not present). As with most psychiatric problems, collateral information from family or friends is very important. If there is no evidence of suicidal ideation or intent, the patient is considered to be at low risk. Be cautious with patients who are guarded, hesitant, or show sudden improvement.

Patients often present to the psychiatric emergency room with **suicidal ideation** or admit to suicidal ideation during evaluation. In such a situation, detailed inquiry is needed. Ask about suicidal ideation itself. Is it of recent onset or chronically present? Are there any precipitating factors, such as problems with a relationship or command hallucinations? Are suicidal thoughts sporadic or continuous, and mild or severe, intrusive, and distressing? Does the patient have a sense of control over suicidal thoughts, and does the patient want to die or get treatment? Ask specifically about plans for suicide, using specific questions, and try to formulate an opinion as to the patient's intent to carry it out. Does the patient have access to the means or materials needed, and are such means potentially lethal? Has the patient taken any steps to carry out

the plan, such as making a will or hoarding pills? Does
the patient have any realistic future plans, or feel hopeless
and/or fantasize about life after suicide ("I'll join a lost
lover—no pain")? Finally, are there any deterrents to suicide such as family or religious support?

It is not unusual for patients to present to the emergency
room **after an unsuccessful suicide attempt**. Once medically stabilized, an assessment of their immediate risk for
suicide should be done. Such assessment should address
the medical seriousness of the attempt (a self-inflicted
gunshot that happened to miss the heart is more serious
than superficial scratches on the wrist, for example), as
well as both **stated** (did the patient communicate a wish
to die to others, and did the patient believe that the
method used would be lethal?) and **implied** (was the
attempt planned or impulsive, and could it realistically
cause death?) **intents**. Assess the patient's reaction to the
attempt. Is the patient relieved to be rescued or does the
patient regret that the attempt failed? Finally, the patient's
mental status, level of intoxication, degree of depression,
psychosis, or emotional turmoil, degree of cooperation
with the interviewer, and future orientation will all influence the judgment of immediate risk.

Treatment

Treatment of suicidal patients consists of **treatment of
the underlying problem** and **protecting the patient
from self-harm while risk is present**. Once the initial
evaluation and medical stabilization is complete, the decision of whether the patient needs hospitalization or treatment on an outpatient basis must be made. The decision
to hospitalize a patient in a locked, monitored inpatient
psychiatric unit should be based on the perception of the
patient's risk for suicide now and in the near future, any
underlying psychiatric diagnosis, the patient's motivation
for treatment, presence of support systems, and the availability of outpatient treatment. Patients who are believed
to be at high risk for suicide but refuse inpatient treatment can be hospitalized against their will.

Violent Behavior

Violence is common in today's society. Homicide is the
tenth leading cause of death in the US, and the second
leading cause of death among adolescent boys. Certain
psychiatric disorders are associated with increased risk

for violent behavior, but psychiatric patients as a whole do not commit violent crimes more often than does the general population. Approximately 10% of psychiatric emergency room visits are related to violence, making it important for mental health professionals to be able to assess, predict, and control violent behavior in their patients.

Males are nine times more likely to commit violent crimes than females, and violence is more common among teenagers and young adults. **Poverty** is highly associated with violence, and violence is common in persons with history of childhood abuse or among those whose parents were divorced or criminals.

Risk factors

Several unique situations increase the risk for violent behavior. Patients with **serious mental illness** (schizophrenia and mania, for example) have varying potential for violent behavior, especially when acutely psychotic, at times related to severe paranoia or command hallucinations. **Noncompliance** with treatment increases the risk for violence in severely mentally ill patients. Alcohol and drug use and **intoxication** are frequently associated with agitation, psychosis, disinhibition, and impaired judgment; drugs other than alcohol that are associated with violence include sedative-hypnotics, hallucinogens, phencyclidine (PCP), cocaine, and amphetamines. Patients who are **mentally retarded** are at increased risk for self-abusive and violent behavior; such patients have limited coping and interpersonal skills and easily get frustrated with the demands of everyday living. **Dementia and delirium** are frequently associated with assaultive and aggressive behavior, related to factors such as disorientation, perceptual disturbances, and psychotic symptoms. Violence and criminal behavior is common in **antisocial personality disorder**. In such patients, violent acts are usually planned and goal-directed. **Complex partial seizures** are occasionally associated with non-goal-directed violence. **Past violent or criminal behavior** is the best predictor of potential or future violence. Patients are usually not forthcoming with such information, which should be obtained from family members, medical records, or law enforcement sources. Finally, biologic factors such as low levels of 5-HIAA, the major metabolite of serotonin, have been associated with aggressive and suicidal behavior.

Assessment

Objectives of the initial assessment are to determine the presence of a psychiatric illness, to identify risk factors associated with violence, and to implement a treatment plan. Assessment includes a complete psychiatric history and mental status evaluation. It is important to **ensure that the working milieu is a safe environment for you, other patients, other staff, and the patient**. Potentially violent patients should be always searched by security or police officers to remove any weapons. Conduct the interview in the presence of other staff members, and keep the door open, if needed. Pay attention to your "gut feelings" about threats or threatening situations, and discuss the situation with other staff and get their input. Be aware of the patient's nonverbal language; patients usually exhibit certain signs suggestive of a potentially threatening situation. Monitor psychomotor activity (relaxed or agitated, clenching fists, pacing, pointing at interviewer), manner (cooperative or threatening), voice (normal or loud), and any psychotic signs (normal or responding to internal stimuli).

Approach the patient in calm, nonjudgmental manner. Speak softly and avoid intense eye contact. Ask questions in an empathic way, but be clear and direct. Always ask patients about homicidal ideation, intent, and plans. Vital signs should be checked on all patients. Blood alcohol level and urine drug screen should be obtained, and a screening physical exam should be performed, if possible. There are, in general, three steps in the management of violent patients: management of the acute problem, treatment of the underlying condition, and disposition.

Management

If the patient exhibits ongoing threatening or aggressive behavior and verbal strategies such as empathy or limit-setting do not work, several options for **acute management** are available. Medications can be useful for some, notably violent, psychotic patients. Get additional help; patients are more likely to follow directions or take medications after a "show of force." Seclusion can help; patients often calm down in a quiet room with decreased stimulation. Restraints should be used when patients pose a severe threat to themselves or others. Patients should be told that they are being restrained because of uncontrolled behavior. Four or five persons are needed to safely restrain a patient; each person should take a limb **in a plan agreed to beforehand**. Finally, if all of the above measures do not control the patient, medications can be administered involuntarily. Haloperidol or benzodiazepines, alone or in combination, are safe and useful.

Once the aggressive behavior is controlled, **the underlying condition must be determined and treated**. A psychotic patient is likely to respond to antipsychotics, while an intoxicated patient needs to sober up before the substance abuse problem can be addressed. A patient with antisocial personality disorder is unlikely to benefit from treatment and needs to be handled by the legal system.

Finally, the patient needs **definitive disposition**. Hospitalization is necessary for patients with violent behavior related to a psychiatric illness (e.g., a manic episode); involuntary hospitalization can be necessary. Intoxicated patients are usually discharged after referral to outpatient or inpatient rehabilitation programs unless there is a coexisting psychiatric or medical condition that necessitates hospitalization. Outpatient support systems such as family and friends should be mobilized and intensified if patients are sent home. Finally, some patients are discharged to the custody of law enforcement agencies, especially those with antisocial personality disorder associated with violent and criminal behavior. ■

| 71 | Psychopharmacology |

Psychopharmacology is a relatively young discipline. The psychotropic effects of lithium were discovered in 1949, and, soon thereafter, chlorpromazine, imipramine, and chlordiazepoxide came into use. These (and other) drugs transformed the practice of psychiatry and made independent living in the community ("mainstreaming") possible for millions of patients. This chapter provides an overview of psychopharmacologic decision-making and describes the major groups of psychotropic agents. Electroconvulsive therapy is also briefly described.

Pharmacologic Decision-Making

Psychiatric medications seldom cure the illness, but provide **palliation**. Before prescribing a psychotropic agent, the **diagnosis** and/or **target symptoms** should both be clear, and the past medical history, list of current medications, history of alcohol or drug use, and history of previous psychotropic medication use should all be known. Once a medication is prescribed, it should be given a full trial (ensuring compliance and therapeutic dosing) before discontinuing it or adding another agent. Patients should be educated about possible side effects, and regimens should be kept simple to maximize compliance. A good technique (whatever your specialty) is to choose a few medications from each group and become comfortable with their use, pharmacologic actions, and adverse effects.

Pharmacology   Most psychoactive medications are given by mouth, and most are lipophilic weak bases absorbed in the small bowel. Most have a large volume of distribution, are protein bound, and have long half-lives. Most (with the notable exception of lithium) are metabolized in the liver; bile, feces, and urine are the major sites of excretion. Psychotropic drugs are typically receptor or enzyme antagonists or agonists or neurotransmitter precursors. The **therapeutic window** is the dose or concentration within which the drug is most effective, while the **therapeutic index** (TI) is the ratio between the toxic and effective doses; the lower the TI, the more careful the dosing must be. Many psychotropic drugs have narrow TIs. Medications that produce tolerance and withdrawal should be used with close observation in a time-limited fashion, if possible, and all psychotropic medications are best withdrawn slowly unless adverse effects dictate otherwise.

Antidepressants

The drugs most commonly used to treat depression (see Chapter 76, "Mood Disorders") are the **heterocyclic antidepressants**, **monoamine oxidase inhibitors**, **serotonin specific reuptake inhibitors**, and **atypical agents**. All act to increase the amount or effects of catecholamines and/or serotonin at the synapse, deficiencies of which are the major biologic abnormality associated with depression.

Heterocyclic antidepressants

The **heterocyclic antidepressants** include the tetra-, tri-, bi-, and unicyclic antidepressants, named for and distinguished by the number of rings in their chemical structure. They all share similar efficacy and toxicity profiles, but their pharmacokinetics vary. Most are given orally and experience significant first pass metabolism. Absorption and metabolism vary widely among individuals, and because of their narrow TIs, serum drug levels often need to be measured. Cardiac conduction defects are the major medical contraindication to heterocyclic use.

Their short-term effects are **to reduce serotonin and norepinephrine (NE) reuptake at the synapse, potentiating the effects of both neurotransmitters**. Long-term administration is associated with **decreased sensitivity (downregulation)** of the beta-adrenergic and perhaps serotonin receptors, which correlates with the 2 week delay typically seen before therapeutic effect is seen, suggesting that factors other than simple catecholamine deficiency are involved in depression. Because they are all equally efficacious, side effects, which vary depending on the cholinergic, histaminic, and alpha-adrenergic receptor antagonist affinity, often are the major factors influencing selection. **Desipramine** and **nortriptyline** are the least anticholinergic, **amitriptyline** the most. Desipramine has potent norepinephrine reuptake inhibition while **clomipramine** is the strongest serotonin reuptake inhibitor. Anticholinergic effects include dry mouth, blurred vision, constipation, urinary retention, and occasional exacerbation of narrow angle glaucoma or anti-cholinergic delirium. Sedation is the most common anti-histaminic effect and orthostatic hypotension is the most common problem caused by alpha-adrenergic blockade. Weight gain and sexual dysfunction are two significant problems also encountered with many of these drugs. Tricyclics should be avoided during pregnancy and lactation.

MAO-Is

Monoamine oxidase inhibitors (MAO-I) are as effective but used less frequently than the other antidepressants because of the need to adhere to a tyramine-free diet. Monoamine oxidase is the enzyme primarily responsible for the metabolism of biogenic amines; ingested tyra-mine, if not metabolized, leads to a catecholamine excess and can precipitate a hypertensive crisis. The MAO-Is act to **inhibit the metabolism of catecholamines, thereby prolonging their effect at the synapse**. The currently available MAO-Is are **phenelzine, tranylcypromine**, and **isocarboxazid**. **Selegine** is a MAO-type B inhibitor approved for use in Parkinson's disease, and reversible MAO inhibitors are available outside the US. MAO-Is are as efficacious as the other antidepressants for the treat-ment of major depression, and may be more helpful for atypical depression. Careful patient education about dietary restrictions is mandatory, and symptoms of hyper-tensive crisis should be discussed and patients instructed to seek medical help if they arise. Other side effects include orthostatic hypotension, sleep disturbances, and sexual dysfunction.

SSRIs

Serotonin-specific reuptake inhibitors (SSRIs), as their name implies, are specific **inhibitors of presynaptic serotonin reuptake, potentiating the synaptic effects of serotonin**. They are as effective as the other antidepres-sants and are generally better tolerated than are either the heterocyclics or MAO-Is. **Fluoxetine, fluvoxamine, paroxetine**, and **sertraline** are the four agents available in the US (while clomipramine is a SSRI, it has a hetero-cyclic structure and is thus classified with the hetero-cyclics). SSRIs are only available in oral form, and differ in terms of active metabolites and half-lives. SSRIs are also helpful in panic and obsessive-compulsive disorders, bulimia, social phobia, and possibly obesity. The most common side effects are nausea and diarrhea, headache, nervousness, insomnia, and drowsiness; if patients are able to tolerate these for a few weeks, tolerance will often develop. Sexual dysfunction is not uncommon. Birth defects do not appear to be more frequent with fluoxetine, but pregnancy is still a relative contraindication for their use. Serotonergic agents should not be used with MAO-Is.

Atypical anti- depressants

There are several so-called "**atypical**" **antidepressants** that do not fall into one of the classes above. **Bupruprion** is a useful drug for depression, but its dose should be limited to less than 450mg per day and the drug not be given to patients with bulimia or electrolyte disturbances to avoid precipitating seizures. The mechanism of action is unknown, although it is suspected to involve the noradrenergic system. It is effective, generally safe and well tolerated, and produces few sexual side effects.

Nefazodone, recently approved by the FDA, is a weak serotonin reuptake inhibitor and receptor antagonist and a mild norepinephrine reuptake inhibitor. It produces few sexual or other side effects, and may be especially effective in depression with prominent anxiety symptoms.

Trazodone, a relatively specific serotonin reuptake inhibitor and serotonin agonist, is useful as much for its potent sedative effects as for its antidepressant qualities. A rare but significant side effect in males is priapism; more frequent or prolonged erections are an indication to stop the medication. Trazodone is also frequently used in low dosages to control agitation in demented patients.

Venlafaxine is a nonselective biogenic amine, serotonin, norepinephrine, and dopamine reuptake inhibitor, and does not possess anticholinergic, antihistaminic, or alpha-1-adrenergic antagonist activity. Venlafaxine may have a faster onset of action than the other antidepressants; patients resistant to other antidepressants respond to venlafaxine about a third of the time. Venlafaxine is generally well tolerated, but dose-related diastolic hypertension can occur.

Antipsychotics

Schizophrenia and other psychotic conditions (see Chapter 73, "Psychotic Disorders") are associated with increased dopaminergic activity; the **classic antipsychotics** are thus all **dopamine receptor antagonists**. **Clozapine** and **risperidone** are two novel antipsychotics with features that offer several therapeutic advantages. *(continued)*

Psychiatry
Psychopharmacology *continued*

Dopamine antagonists

The **dopamine receptor antagonists** include **chlorpromazine** (used since the 1950s), **haloperidol**, and **fluphenazine**. While all are postsynaptic dopamine receptor antagonists, they vary considerably in chemical structure and potency—all are equally efficacious, but the dose needed to reach the desired effect varies widely. Low potency drugs, in general, are more sedating, cause more orthostasis, are more likely to have anticholinergic side effects, and probably lower the seizure threshold to a greater extent. High potency agents, in contrast, are more likely to be associated with extrapyramidal symptoms and neuroleptic malignant syndrome (discussed below). While the therapeutic action of these drugs is believed to be due mainly to blockade of the dopaminergic receptors, it appears that other factors are involved, because while the receptor blockade occurs immediately, the antipsychotic effects take more time to develop.

Side effects

Side effects of the classic antipsychotics are critically important and can largely be explained by the varying antagonist effects on a variety of receptor systems, including dopaminergic, muscarinic cholinergic, alpha-1-adrenergic, and histamine receptors. Lower potency agents generally have greater affinity for the cholinergic (cardiac conduction delays, dry mouth, blurred vision, constipation, and urinary retention), alpha-adrenergic (orthostatic hypotension), and histamine (weight gain and sedation) receptors. Various hematologic and problems can occur, as can sexual problems such as impotence, anorgasmia, and decreased libido.

High potency antipsychotics have a higher affinity for the dopaminergic D1 receptor and are thus most likely to cause so-called "**extrapyramidal**" **symptoms** (**EPS**). Several dopaminergic side effects are seen early after medication is started. **Acute dystonia** classically occurs within 1-5 days after initiation of treatment (or increase in dose), and presents with ophisthotonus, torticollis, oculogyric crisis, and, rarely, laryngeal involvement. Diphenhydramine or benzotropine can be used for treatment. Drug-induced **Parkinsonism** (from dopaminergic blockade) is common, presenting with masked facies, cogwheeling, resting tremors, festinant gait, stiffness, and drooling; lowering the dose of the responsible antipsychotic, switching to a lower potency agent, or administering anticholinergic agents are all treatment options.

Akathisia refers to a distressing, subjective feeling of restlessness in the legs often causing pacing; lowering the dose of the antipsychotic, switching to a lower potency agent, or administering propranolol can all help.

Neuroleptic malignant syndrome, a rare, potentially lethal reaction to these drugs, is characterized by muscular rigidity, fluctuation in the level of consciousness, autonomic dysfunction (hyperthermia, unstable blood pressure, diaphoresis, and tachycardia), leukocytosis, and elevated creatinine phosphokinase levels. This is a medical emergency and mandates hospitalization, discontinuation of the responsible drug, and treatment with bromocriptine, amantadine, or dantrolene. The most concerning late side effect is **tardive dyskinesia (TD)**, which rarely occurs before 6 months of treatment have passed. It consists of involuntary, abnormal, irregular choreoathetoid movements of any muscle (most often mouth and tongue), varying from minimal to grossly incapacitating; movements can initially worsen when the antipsychotic is withdrawn. There is no consistently effective treatment. If the antipsychotic can be withdrawn, improvement occurs about half the time. Patients who must continue medication are generally switched to clozapine or risperidone.

Indications

Therapeutic indications for the classic antipsychotics include all psychotic disorders, whether "functional" or secondary to a general medical condition or substance use. Schizophrenia is the best known indication, but idiopathic psychoses arising, for example, in mania or depression are often improved by antipsychotics. Antipsychotics are also helpful in patients with severe agitation, violent behavior, and movement disorders. Selection depends on the underlying disorder and risk of side effects. Noncompliance is very common in these patients, making the use of long-term depot formulations very attractive.

Other antipsychotics

Clozapine, a dopaminergic D1 and D4 and serotonin antagonist, is an effective antipsychotic that is associated with significantly fewer EPS. It appears to be more effective for the treatment of the negative symptoms (see Chapter 73, "Psychotic Disorders") of schizophrenia, and has been successful in patients resistant to traditional antipsychotics. Agranulocytosis occurs in 1%-2% of patients making weekly monitoring of the white blood cell count necessary. Seizures, hypertension, tachycardia, and sialorrhea can occur. **Risperidone** has significant D2 and serotonin antagonist activity. It also seems to improve negative symptoms, but does not have the hematologic side effects of clozapine. It also has fewer neurologic side effects than traditional antipsychotics.

Antianxiety Agents and Hypnotics

This group consists mainly of the **benzodiazepines** and **buspirone** (**barbiturates** are rarely prescribed today). The **benzodiazepines** enhance GABAminergic activity via activation of a benzodiazepine receptor. They have anxiolytic, sedative, anti-convulsant, and muscle-relaxant properties, and are among the most prescribed medications in the world. The main differences between the various benzodiazepines are rates of absorption and half-lives; most are metabolized in the liver, and many have active metabolites. Benzodiazepines interact in an additive fashion with all sedating medications, including alcohol, and have significant abuse potential. They are very useful for short-term sedation, but can produce respiratory depression, particularly when used with narcotics or in the elderly.

Benzodiazepines are useful in most disorders where anxiety is prominent. Insomnia and alcohol withdrawal are other common indications, and they have been used with success in panic disorders and mania. Treatment should be specific, brief, and predetermined in duration, and should probably be avoided altogether in patients with a history of abuse. Tolerance develops readily. The most commonly used agents are **diazepam**, **lorazepam**, **chlordiazepoxide**, **alprazolam** and **clonazepam**. **Flumazenil** is a specific benzodiazepine receptor **antagonist**, useful for benzodiazepine overdose.

Buspirone, a relatively nonsedating anxiolytic, is a serotonin type 1A receptor agonist. Efficacy is delayed, but it has few side effects and no abuse potential. It is effective in generalized anxiety disorder, major depression, and, possibly, in agitation and impulsivity.

577

Agents for Bipolar Disorder

Cade discovered the psychotherapeutic effects of **lithium** in Australia in 1949. Lithium is the most commonly used agent for treatment of acute mania and the prophylaxis of patients with unipolar and bipolar disorders (see Chapter 76, "Mood Disorders"). The therapeutic mechanism of action is not known, although lithium affects the serotonergic and several second messenger systems.

The most common side effects associated with lithium are gastric upset, mild cognitive impairment, weight gain, tremor, fatigue, polydipsia and polyuria, hypothyroidism, and "lithium acne." Lithium has a narrow therapeutic range and toxicity is frequent. Mild toxicity typically occurs with levels above 1.5meq/L and severe toxicity, requiring hospitalization, can be seen with levels as low as 2meq/L. Toxicity causes progressively worsening gastrointestinal (diarrhea and vomiting) and neurologic (drowsiness, weakness, ataxia, delirium, hyperreflexia, focal neurologic signs, seizures, and even coma) symptoms.

Lithium is useful in the treatment of acute mania, prophylaxis of bipolar disorder and other mood disorders, augmentation of antidepressant treatment, schizophrenia, and explosive and violent behaviors. Careful monitoring of serum levels is recommended, and lithium should be avoided during pregnancy due to mild teratogenic effects.

Others

Carbamazepine is an anticonvulsant that has been found to be effective both as prophylaxis for and in the treatment of acute mania. It may be especially effective in rapidly-cycling bipolar disorder. Its mechanism of action is unclear. Carbamazepine is associated with both transient leukopenia and, rarely, aplastic anemia, mandating hematologic monitoring. **Valproate** and **divalproex sodium** are also anticonvulsants that have been found to be effective in psychiatric disorders. Although generally well-tolerated, they can occasionally cause pancreatitis and severe hepatotoxicity. Indications for the use of these drugs include acute mania, prophylaxis of both bipolar disorder and other depressive disorders, antidepressant augmentation, agitation, and intermittent explosive disorder.
(continued)

Psychostimulants

The three psychostimulants available in the US are **dextroamphetamine**, **methylphenidate**, and **pemoline**, all useful in the treatment of depressive disorders, attention deficit hyperactivity disorder (see Chapter 79, "Child Psychiatry"), and narcolepsy. Dextroamphetamine and methylphenidate stimulate catecholamine release from presynaptic neurons and inhibit catecholamine reuptake and monoamine oxidase-mediated metabolism; actions of pemoline (which has a delayed onset relative to the other two) are less well understood. Psychostimulants are generally well-tolerated. While dextroamphetamine and methylphenidate are highly addictive, abuse is infrequent if patient selection is optimal.

Electroconvulsant Therapy

Electroconvulsant therapy (ECT) is a safe and effective treatment for major depression, mania, and schizophrenia, but is currently underutilized because of its historic "black eye." ECT acts by inducing generalized seizures in a controlled environment and by other, unknown mechanisms, causing downregulation of postsynaptic beta-adrenergic receptors.

Modern ECT is performed while the patient is anesthetized and undergoing careful physiologic monitoring with an anesthesiologist present (see Chapter 12, "Anesthesiology and Pain Management"). Electricity is administered via electrode(s) placed in either a bitemporal or unilateral (over the nondominant hemisphere) fashion. Unilateral treatment is thought to be associated with fewer adverse effects while bilateral treatment appears to be more effective; most clinicians start with unilateral treatment and switch to bilateral if response is not adequate. Seizure activity is monitored by electroencephalography or tonic-clonic movements in an extremity temporarily "protected" from pharmacologic paralysis; the shortest effective duration of seizure activity during ECT is believed to be 25 seconds. Treatments are most commonly administered 2-3 times a week, typically (for treatment of depression) for 6-12 sessions.

The mortality associated with ECT (.004%) is very low, and contraindications are anything contraindicating general anesthesia. Space-occupying lesions of the central nervous system, elevated intercranial pressure, and severely compromised cardiac status are relative contraindications. Common side effects include postictal confusion, headaches, and delirium, and, most importantly, impaired short-term memory. Memory impairment is especially prominent during the course of ECT itself, and usually resolves over several weeks with complete return to baseline 6 months after treatment is finished. Mild, transient cardiac arrhythmias and hypertension can occur during therapy.

While ECT is very effective in treating indicated disorders, it does nothing to prevent their recurrence. Therefore, after successful treatment, prophylactic medications or intermittent maintenance ECT treatments are usually needed. ∎

72　Psychotherapy

Psychotherapy is the systematic use of a human relationship for therapeutic purposes—to effect enduring changes in the patient's feelings and behavior. Along with psychopharmacologic treatment, discussed in the previous chapter, psychotherapy is the fundamental means of treating patients with psychiatric illnesses.

Features common to all forms of psychotherapy include a confiding relationship between the patient and the clinician, an effort to understand the cause of the patient's distress and to develop a method for relieving it, an attempt to obtain new information about the nature and sources of the patient's problems and ways of dealing with them, facilitation of emotional arousal (which seems to be a prerequisite for attitudinal and behavioral changes), the enhancement of a sense of mastery through successful experiences in order to increase hope, and the critical importance of the personal qualities of the therapist to help strengthen patient's expectations.

Psychoanalysis

Classic "Freudian" **psychoanalysis** is the technique whereby Freudian concepts are used to understand and treat psychiatric problems. It is the most intensive form of psychotherapy—the patient is seen at least 3-4 times a week for several years. The patient reclines, and the analyst sits behind the couch, out of the patient's visual range, to minimize the effects of the therapist's presence. The concept of **transference** is fundamental to psychotherapy, and is generally defined as the set of feelings, beliefs, fantasies, and reactions that a patient brings to the doctor-patient relationship and may project onto the therapist. **Countertransference** refers to the expectations and emotions the therapist may have toward the patient.

The patient is encouraged to free-associate and speak without hesitation about anything that comes to mind. Patients undergoing psychoanalysis need to be psychologically minded, highly motivated, verbal, and be able to tolerate the stress generated by analysis. The clinician uses interpretation and clarification to understand and help patients resolve conflicts. Although controversial, adjuvant psychotropic drugs are sometimes used. Psychoanalysis works particularly well for neuroses, personality disorders, paraphilias, and sexual disorders.

Psychoanalytically-oriented Psychotherapy

Psychoanalytically-oriented psychotherapy is based on the same principles as is psychoanalysis, but is less intensive. There are two types: insight-oriented and supportive psychotherapy.

Interpretation is the hallmark of **insight-oriented psychotherapy**. Interpretation attempts to bring unconscious processes to conscious awareness. Other useful techniques include informative comments, which help the patient understand social or educational issues, and summaries and recapitulation to help maintain therapeutic focus. There is less emphasis on free association, but more on interpersonal and day-to-day reality issues, and it seems to work for many of the same problems that are treated with classic psychotherapy.

In **supportive psychotherapy** the goal is to understand the patient's psychodynamic structure. Goals are to strengthen defenses, reduce anxiety, and restore psychologic homeostasis; psychotropic drugs and family or group therapy are used on an "as-needed" basis. Patients are seen at frequencies ranging from daily to once every few months, and more emphasis is paid to external and interpersonal events. Indications for this type of therapy are adjustment disorders, impulse disorders, psychosomatic disorders, and psychoses.

Brief Psychotherapy

Types of brief psychotherapy

Brief dynamic psychotherapy is based on Freudian psychoanalytic concepts. This short-term treatment generally consists of 10-40 sessions over a year or less. The goal is to develop insight into underlying problems, leading to psychologic and behavioral changes. Because of the increasing emphasis on primary care and cost containment, interest in this treatment modality is increasing.

Suitable patients must be highly motivated, psychologically minded, able to define a specific problem to be addressed, and able to tolerate the temporary increase in

Psychiatry
Psychotherapy *continued*

anxiety or sadness that this type of therapy can evoke. Patients must also be able to develop a therapeutic alliance and work with the therapist. Patients with fragile ego structures (suicidal or psychotic, for example) or poor impulse control (such as substance abusers, those with antisocial personalities, and borderline patients) are poor candidates.

There are several types of brief psychotherapy. In **brief focal psychotherapy** (Tavistock-Malan), a definite focus of treatment is identified and the termination date is set in advance. The goal is to clarify the nature of defenses, anxieties, and impulses. Malan emphasized the identification and interpretation of transference (including negative transference), often linked to relationships with parents.

Time-limited psychotherapy (Boston University-Mann) is strictly limited to 12 sessions, and termination is a major focus. The general focus is on identification of central conflict-causing present and past pain, emphasis on self-image, and, in young people, treatment of maturational crisis.

Short-term dynamic psychotherapy (Davanloo) emphasizes the evaluation of the patient's ego function. Criteria for success include psychological mindedness, high motivation, good response to trial transference interpretation, flexible defenses, and the ability to tolerate anxiety, guilt, and depression. Important to this approach is flexibility of the therapist to adapt the technique to suit the patient's needs, control of patient's regressive tendencies, active intervention to prevent overdependence on the therapists, and fostering intellectual insight. No specific termination date is given to the patient, although duration of therapy is short.

In **short-term anxiety-provoking psychotherapy** the focus is on Oedipal (triangular) conflict. Treatment is divided into four major phases. First is the patient-therapist encounter, in which a working alliance is established and an outline for the focus of treatment is obtained. During early therapy, transference is clarified as soon as it appears, leading to the establishment of a true therapeutic alliance. During the height of treatment, active concentration on Oedipal conflicts is chosen as the therapeutic focus occur. The repeated use of anxiety-provoking questions and confrontation about the avoidance of pregenital characterologic issues the patient uses to avoid dealing with the therapist are important. Encouragement and support is provided as the patient becomes anxious while struggling to understand conflicts. The final phase is evidence of change and termination of psychotherapy, which emphasizes demonstration of a change in the patient's behavior outside therapy and evidence that adaptive patterns of behavior are being used.

Interpersonal psychotherapy (Weissman and Klerman) is designed to improve interpersonal skills. The ideal patient is an outpatient with a non-bipolar, non-psychotic depressive disorder; interpersonal behavior is emphasized as a cause of the disorder and as a method of cure. The therapist attempts to be supportive, empathic, and flexible, with minimal attention paid to transference.

Cognitive Therapy

Cognitive therapy is a short-term, structured therapy that requires active participation by the patient and collaboration with the therapist to achieve treatment goals. Cognitive therapy is based on the theory that behavior is secondary to the way in which individuals think about themselves and their roles in the world. Maladaptive behavior is secondary to ingrained, stereotyped thoughts that lead to **cognitive distortion**, errors in thinking based on erroneous assumptions developed from previous experiences. Therapy is aimed at correcting these cognitive distortions and self-defeating behaviors that result.

Cognitive therapy can be done on an individual or group basis, with or without medication. Therapy is time-limited, generally consisting of 15-25 weekly sessions. Patients are assigned readings and homework, are asked to record what they are thinking in certain stressful situations (such as "I am no good," or "she doesn't like me"), and to ascertain the underlying, often relatively unconscious assumptions that add to negative thoughts. This is called "recognizing and correcting automatic thoughts," and functions to make the patient aware of distorted thinking and the assumptions on which the problems are based.
(continued)

The cognitive model of depression includes Beck's **cognitive triad**, a description of the thought distortion that occurs when an individual is depressed. The triad includes a negative view of self, a negative interpretation of present and past experiences, and a negative expectation of the future. Cognitive therapy is primarily useful in dysthymic disorder, nonendogenous depressive disorders, and symptoms not sustained by a pathologic family.

Behavior Therapy

Types of behavior therapy

Behavior therapy is based on the principles of learning theory. **Operant conditioning** is based on the observation that behavior is shaped by its consequences. In other words, if behavior is positively reinforced it will increase, if punished, it will decrease, and if it elicits no response, it will be extinguished. **Classical conditioning** is based on the observation that behavior is shaped by its association with anxiety-provoking stimuli. For example, a person can be conditioned to feel fear in an otherwise neutral situation paired with a noxious stimulus.

The goal of behavior therapy is to modify learned, maladaptive behavior patterns. It is most effective for specific, well-delineated, circumscribed maladaptive behavior such as phobias, overeating, or sexual dysfunction, and for psychophysiologic disorders such as asthma, hypertension, pain, or insomnia, in which symptom occurrence is coupled with or worsened by stress.

Behavior therapy techniques include **token economy**; a form of positive reinforcement where a patient is rewarded for desired behavior with various tokens such as food. **Systematic desensitization** (Wolpe), used with or without medication, is based on counterconditioning: a person can overcome anxiety by approaching the feared situation or object gradually in a pharmacologically relaxed state. **Graded exposure** is similar to systematic desensitization, except that relaxation training is not involved and treatment is usually carried out in real-life situations. In **flooding**, the patient is exposed immediately to the most anxiety-provoking stimulus; if applied in an imaginary sense (as opposed to real-life) it is called **implosion**. Flooding is felt to be the most effective behavioral treatment if the patient can tolerate the anxiety. **Aversion therapy**, most effective with alcohol abuse, paraphilias, and behaviors associated with impulsive or compulsive qualities, is a form of classical conditioning in which an aversive stimulus such as an electric shock, a substance that induces vomiting (e.g., Antabuse), or social disapproval is coupled with the undesired behavior. Finally, in **participant modeling**, the patient learns a new behavior primarily by observation and imitation. Irrational fears can be unlearned by observing a fearless model confront the feared object. A variant of this technique, in which real-life problems are acted out under the therapist's observation or direction, is called **behavior rehearsal**.

Group Therapy

In **group therapy**, carefully selected patients are placed into a group to help each other. The advantages of group therapy include the opportunity for feedback from the patient's peers and the opportunity for both patient and therapist to observe the patient's psychologic, emotional, and behavioral responses to a diversified group of people.

Goals of group therapy are diverse, including support, improved social skills, specific symptomatic relief, and resolution of intrapsychic conflicts. Groups usually meet once or twice a week, and can be homogeneous or heterogeneous depending on the diagnosis. The primary indications for group therapy include patients with psychotic and anxiety disorders, phobias, sexual problems, and personality disorders. Families and couples where the overall "system" needs change are also ideal. Contraindicated are patients at risk for suicide and those with sadomasochistic tendencies. Duration of treatment varies from weeks to years, and can be time-limited or open-ended.

Marital Therapy

Marital therapy is a form of psychotherapy used to modify the interaction of two people who are in conflict with each other over one or several areas—social, emotional, sexual, or economic. The therapist establishes a therapeutic contract with the patient couple and attempts to reverse or change maladaptive patterns of behavior and encourage personality growth and development. *(continued)*

Psychiatry
Psychotherapy *continued*

Indications for initiating marital therapy include failure of individual therapy to resolve marital difficulties, onset of distress in one or both partners that is clearly related to marital events, and request by a couple in conflict. Contraindications include patients with psychoses, one or both partners who seriously want a divorce, a spouse who refuses to participate, and usually active domestic violence.

Crisis Intervention

A psychologic crisis refers to an individual's inability to solve a problem. **Crisis intervention** is designed to offer the immediate help that a person in crisis needs to re-establish emotional homeostasis. It is based on crisis theory, which emphasizes the immediate response to the immediate situation and the longterm development of psychologic adaptation aimed at preventing future problems.

Caplan emphasized that crisis is characteristically self-limited. Crisis is characterized by an initial phase in which anxiety and tension rise, followed by a later phase in which problem solving mechanisms alleviate the initial crisis. The patient and therapist work together at resolving the crisis, and the goal is to arrive at a clear understanding of the psychodynamics involved and an awareness of how they are responsible for the current problem. Techniques include reassurance, suggestion, environmental manipulation, and medication, and it is essential to end therapy as soon as the crisis has been resolved.

Highly motivated patients with a history of specific stressful situations of recent origin that produced anxiety are ideal candidates. Crisis intervention is both therapeutic and preventive because it enables many patients to attain a level of emotional functioning superior to before onset of the crisis.

Biofeedback

According to the concept of biofeedback, autonomic responses can be controlled by operant or instrumental conditioning. Biofeedback provides the ability to gain some degree of voluntary control over bodily functions that normally operate outside consciousness. Physiologic manifestations of anxiety and tension (e.g., headache, pain, or tachycardia) can be alleviated by teaching the patient to be aware of the physiologic differences between tension and relaxation, helping the patient to be aware of which state is present and how to control it. ■

73   Psychotic Disorders

A **psychosis** is the inability to distinguish what is real from what is not. Psychotic disorders can exist as independent problems (the subject of this chapter), but many other psychiatric disorders can include psychotic symptoms as part of their presentation or later course. **Schizophrenia** is, by far, the most common and important psychotic disorder. **Schizoaffective disorder, delusional disorder, schizophreniform disorder, brief psychosis**, and **postpartum psychosis** also fall within the category of psychotic disorders.

Schizophrenia

Schizophrenia is a common and chronic mental illness, characterized by continued, episodic recurrence and progressive deterioration of cognitive, social, and overall functioning. It is associated with higher suicide, mortality, and morbidity rates than the general population. Although equally prevalent between genders (lifetime prevalence of about 1%), age of onset peaks between 15-25 years in men and 25-35 years in women.

There are three major classes of symptoms: "**positive**" symptoms that **respond** to treatment (delusions, hallucinations, loose associations, and bizarre speech and behavior); "**negative**" symptoms that **often do not** (social withdrawal, anhedonia, lack of drive, attention deficits, poverty of speech content, and alogia), and **prodromal** (apparent, often in hindsight, before the onset of illness) or **residual** (those that remain after active symptoms are controlled) symptoms. DSM-IV criteria require that the prodromal or residual symptoms persist for 6 months or more, and that significant positive symptoms be present for at least 1 month (less, with treatment); significant decline from baseline social, personal, and occupational functioning since the onset of symptoms must be present.

Etiology

Both biologic and psychosocial factors have been "blamed" for schizophrenia. **Genetics** and **biologic abnormalities** are present in affected patients, but it is clear that **environmental factors** contribute significantly to phenotypic expression. Abnormalities of the limbic system, frontal lobes, basal ganglia, and brainstem have been found in schizophrenic patients; imaging often reveals cerebral atrophy, enlarged ventricles, decreased volume of the hippocampal-amygdala complex and parahippocampal gyrus, and decreased blood flow to the dorsolateral prefrontal cortex. Patients with schizophrenia commonly have abnormal smooth visual pursuit and saccadic eye movements, immune responses (e.g., decreased interleukin production), and abnormal hormonal response (e.g., decreased prolactin and growth hormone production). Several neurotransmitter systems are abnormal in schizophrenia. While no one system alone accounts for all problems, abnormalities of dopamine, serotonin, norepinephrine, and various amino acids (such as GABA and glutamine) have generated the most interest.

Psychosocial factors usually act to precipitate acute deterioration, but can affect the chronic course of the illness. Psychoanalytic theories explain schizophrenia in terms of "ego defects" and intrapsychic conflicts that result in regression, consequently manifest as psychotic symptoms. Defense mechanisms in patients with schizophrenia include denial, projection, and regression. Social and learning theories focus on interpersonal difficulties during childhood that hinder normal development in susceptible individuals—extreme suppression or expression of emotional responses in the families of patients with schizophrenia increases the relapse rate and can precipitate an acute episode.

Presentation

Patients with schizophrenia usually look odd, disheveled, and unkempt, reflecting poor grooming and self-neglect. They can be extremely agitated and screaming, immobile and completely silent, or frankly **catatonic**. Affect is usually inappropriate, with patients commonly displaying extreme happiness, unprovoked anxiety, or anger, but is sometimes flat or blunted, reflective of anhedonia and depression. Bizarre **delusions** (religious, persecutory, erotomanic, somatic, or grandiose, for example) are very common, and patients can talk about being controlled by outside forces such as the devil or a spiritual power. **Ideas of reference** (TV and radio giving special, individual messages) are common. Although suicidal thoughts are common, homicidal ideation is rare. Patients can have a prominent **formal thought disorder**, manifest by disorganized, incoherent speech, loose associations, thought blocking, flight of ideas, neologisms, word salad, tangentiality, and circumstantiality; others can be completely mute and unresponsive. Auditory **hallucinations** are common; patients describe hearing voices that comment on their behavior, give them commands, or are threatening or hostile. Sometimes patients deny hearing voices but are seen talking or laughing to themselves as if they are responding to internal stimuli. Olfactory and tactile hallucinations can also occur; visual hallucinations are rarer and should prompt consideration of other causes (such as alcohol withdrawal). **Illusions**, (misinterpretation of actual sensory stimuli) can occur during the active phases of the illness. Judgment and insight are frequently poor, affecting compliance.

Although schizophrenic patients can look confused and bizarre, they are usually alert and oriented; short-term memory and long-term recall are mostly intact. Cognitive impairment is evident by neuropsychologic testing. Schizophrenic patients usually demonstrate poor abstract thinking, difficulty in problem solving, and frontal lobe dysfunction; on average, these patients have lower IQs than do those in the general population, and measured IQ usually deteriorates as the disease progresses.

DSM-IV describes five subtypes, based on the predominant symptomatology:

Subtypes

Paranoid type: Prominent features in these patients are delusional ideation and/or hallucinations, and problems are usually of late onset, without severe exacerbations. Patients are typically suspicious, tense, guarded, and sometimes even hostile and aggressive. Patients usually have good premorbid function, and prognosis is better than other types.

Disorganized type: The characteristic feature of this subtype is a significant formal thought disorder, and problems are usually of early and insidious onset. Patients show inappropriate emotions such as outbursts of laughing, and demonstrate unusual facial grimacing. Behavior is disorganized and unproductive. Patients usually have poor premorbid function and a poor prognosis.

Catatonic type: Presentation varies, and includes stupor, negativism, motor excitement, posturing, rigidity, or mutism. Patients can shift from one state to another.

Stereotypes, mannerisms, and waxy flexibility are also seen. Onset is usually sudden, and prognosis is better than the other types.

Residual type: Negative symptoms such as eccentric behavior, asociality, and illogical thinking predominate; patients do not have prominent delusions, hallucinations, or catatonic behavior, but can have mild loosening of associations. Prognosis is poor, and patients are often resistant to treatment.

Undifferentiated type: Patients who do not fall into one of the subtypes above are classified here.

Related disorders

Many disorders can produce problems suggestive of schizophrenia. Schizophrenia, however, has a unique pathogenesis and characteristic clinical course. Patients with **schizoaffective disorder** (see below) fulfill criteria of both schizophrenia and an affective disorder; affective symptoms exist in conjunction with psychotic symptoms and usually persist beyond the active phase of the psychotic presentation. The diagnosis of **delusional disorder** (see below) requires the presence of non-bizarre delusions without hallucinations or negative or residual symptoms of schizophrenia. **Schizophreniform disorder** and **brief psychotic disorder** (see below) are differentiated from schizophrenia by the short duration of symptoms. Patients with schizophrenia can have **depressive symptoms** or irritability and agitation that look like **mania** (see Chapter 76, "Mood Disorders"); such symptoms, however, are brief in relation to the rest of the illness. Patients with schizoid, schizotypal, or borderline **personality disorders** (see Chapter 77, "Personality Disorders") can have odd beliefs, eccentric behavior, inappropriate affect, and, occasionally, psychotic symptoms. Such symptoms, however, have no clear onset and persist throughout life in a very mild form with no spontaneous exacerbation. An unusual degree of control over symptoms and the presence of primary or secondary gains suggest the diagnosis of **factitious** or **malingering disorder** (see Chapter 78, "Somatoform Disorders"). Finally, if the psychotic symptoms can be attributed to a specific mental condition or substance use, then the diagnosis is **psychotic disorder due to general medical condition** or **substance-induced psychotic disorder**, respectively.
(continued)

Psychiatry
Psychotic Disorders *continued*

In addition to the symptoms themselves, treatment should address factors that continue to encourage relapse, such as problems with employment, family, and social relationships. Individual, group, and family psychotherapy as well as cognitive and behavioral approaches are all useful. Education for both the patient and family is essential to ensure proper compliance and followup.

Treatment

Almost every patient with schizophrenia should be on medication and receive followup throughout life. **Conventional medications treat the positive symptoms only and do not cure the disease** (although some novel antipsychotics such as Clozapine can improve negative symptoms, also). Maintenance therapy can improve prognosis and decrease the number and severity of relapses; 30%-50% of patients with schizophrenia, however, are not adequately compliant with treatment. This can be related to poor insight, denial, and social or financial factors, but **is usually due to dissatisfaction with the effects of the medication itself**. It is thus crucial to prepare patients for the side effects, reassuring them that there are always alternative treatment options, should side effects develop; such alternatives, of course, are preferable to no therapy at all. So-called "**extrapyramidal symptoms**" (**EPS**) can be related to acute (dystonia and akathisia) or chronic (tardive dyskinesia; TD) antipsychotic use.

Antipsychotics

Antipsychotics such as haloperidol, Prolixin, Mellaril, and Trilafon minimize agitation, irritability, and aggression within hours, but improvements in delusional and hallucinatory symptoms are not apparent for 1-2 weeks. Hallucinations can disappear or become mild enough that they no longer affect daily activities. Delusions rarely disappear completely, but patients can gain insight and stop acting on them. Patients can stop talking about their delusions spontaneously or talk about them as something that happened in the past only; occasionally patients gain enough insight to dismiss the delusions as unreal. **Benzodiazepines** are useful to control agitation during an acute psychotic episode. About a third of patients, especially those with predominant negative symptoms, are resistant to treatment with typical antipsychotics. Some such patients can respond to treatment with **atypical neuroleptics** such as Clozapine or Risperidone. Clozapine is not associated with EPS or TD, but can cause marrow suppression. Risperidone is as effective as the typical neuroleptics with fewer side effects, but its effect on patients with refractory symptoms is not yet clear.

Thymoleptics such as lithium, Tegretol, or valproic acid have several useful functions. In addition to alleviating affective symptoms, they can reduce persistent agitation and aggression in some patients, and may augment the beneficial effects of the antipsychotics on psychotic symptoms in others (although efficacy in this regard is still controversial). **Antidepressants** have been used to treat negative symptoms resistant to conventional treatment, and **electroconvulsive therapy (ECT)** has been used in refractory cases with success. ECT seems to be most helpful in patients with prominent affective and positive psychotic symptoms.

Reasons for hospitalization include the need for observation and confirmation of the diagnosis, initiation of treatment, and management of acute exacerbations. Patients can be committed involuntarily when their suicidal or homicidal ideations are significant enough that they are considered dangerous to themselves or others.

Schizoaffective Disorders

Schizoaffective disorders are seen in those patients with prominent psychotic **and** affective symptoms. Patients should have **both** the diagnosis of schizophrenia, **and** enough affective symptomatology (see Chapter 76, "Mood Disorders") to meet diagnostic criteria for a major mood disorder (bipolar, depression or mixed); the affective symptoms should last a significant portion of the total duration of the psychotic illness, including both the active and residual periods. In addition, positive symptoms (delusions or hallucinations) should be present for at least 2 weeks without prominent mood symptoms. The course of the illness resembles that of schizophrenia, but, in general, prognosis is better (although worse than that of mood disorder). Poor prognostic factors include prominent negative symptoms, early onset, poor premorbid function, and progressively deteriorating course. Treatment approach is generally similar to that of schizophrenia, with the addition of antidepressants or mood stabilizers frequently helpful.
(continued)

Psychiatry
Psychotic Disorders *continued*

Delusional Disorder

Delusional disorder is a relatively uncommon problem characterized mainly by prominent, **non-bizarre** delusions **without** the positive, negative, or residual symptoms typical of schizophrenia. "Non-bizarre" means that the subject of the delusion can actually happen in real life; the belief is **delusional**, however, if it is **not** really happening to the patient. For example, stomach cancer is real. A patient with the delusion of having such a cancer, despite evidence otherwise, has a non-bizarre delusion. Interestingly, limbic system and basal ganglia dysfunction commonly presents as delusional disorder. No formal thought disorder, mood symptoms (affect is usually congruent with their delusion), or cognitive deficits are seen. Such patients do not usually have hallucinations, but tactile or olfactory hallucinations are "allowed" if they are part of the delusional theme (e.g., itching and numbness due to the delusion of a skin cancer). DSM-IV criteria require the presence of the delusion for one month before making the diagnosis.

Six types of delusions are recognized, in some ways similar to several of the personality disorders (see Chapter 77). Patients with the **erotomanic** type believe that a famous person is in love with them, and those with the **grandiose** type talk about discovering an important invention, or being the friend of an important figure. The **jealousy** type is seen more in men than women. Patients insist that their spouse is having an affair with someone else, and interpret minor incidents as supportive of their belief. Patients with the **persecutory** type believe that there is a person or agency trying to inflict harm on them, and are usually angry and/or hostile because of their paranoia. The **somatic** type is rare. Patients usually present with a delusion related to their body, typically insisting they have a brain tumor in spite of negative results. Patients can become frustrated and visit many physicians before seeing a psychiatrist. This disorder is differentiated from a somatoform disorder (see Chapter 78, "Somatoform Disorders") by the fact that patients with the latter accept the fact that they might not have an illness, while those with delusional disorder do not. Finally, patients with the **mixed** type present with more than one delusion of the above types. Patients with this diagnosis can also develop delusions that do not fit with any of the types discussed above.

Treatment approach is similar to that for schizophrenia. Most patients improve; in about half, delusions disappear completely. Delusions persist, however, in about 30% of patients.

Schizophreniform Disorder

Schizophreniform disorder is very similar to schizophrenia. By definition, however, symptoms last **less than 6 months**. Patients usually recover completely and do not show a decline in function. The course of the illness is short, and patients with schizophreniform disorder have a better prognosis than do those with schizophrenia. Favorable prognostic factors include absence of blunted or flat affect, presence of confusion at the peak of the psychotic episode, acute onset of psychotic symptoms, and good premorbid functioning. Short duration of illness and presence of affective symptoms are also associated with better prognosis. Treatment approach is similar to that of schizophrenia, although long-term medication is not needed.

Brief Psychotic Disorder

Patients with **brief psychotic disorder** have one or more of the major positive psychotic symptoms lasting **less than a month**; affective symptoms and attention deficits are frequently seen. DSM-IV requires that schizophrenia, schizoaffective disorder, and psychotic disorder due to general medical condition be ruled out; a complete workup to rule out medical problems is essential before making this diagnosis. By definition, patients improve in a short period of time and usually return to their baseline of functioning. Again, favorable prognostic factors include good premorbid functioning, the presence of precipitating factors (that presumably can be corrected), acute onset and short duration of symptoms, few negative symptoms, and presence of affective symptoms. Treatment approach is similar to that of schizophrenia, except that a short duration of medication use is adequate. *(continued)*

Psychiatry
Psychotic Disorders *continued*

Postpartum Psychosis

Patients with psychotic symptoms in the postpartum period, usually beginning within days to weeks of the delivery, are given the diagnosis of **postpartum psychosis**. Prodromal symptoms include decreased energy and sleep, restlessness, changes in mood, and emotional exhaustion. Such symptoms, often referred to as the "postpartum blues," are common and self-limited. Patients with true postpartum psychosis, however, become irritable, suspicious, and delusional about the baby. They may describe the baby as being defective, and can have thoughts of harming the baby or not wanting to take care of it; significant affective symptoms are often present. Always rule out medical problems or substance use in this situation. Patients may need to be hospitalized, especially if they have delusions of harming the baby or themselves, and can have recurrent episodes. Such patients usually benefit from a supportive network of family and friends. ■

74   Cognitive Disorders

Cognitive Disorders and Disorders due to Medical Conditions

DSM-IV has provided major changes in conceptualization and terminology of many psychiatric illnesses. The old categorization of mental disorders as **organic or functional** is not valid anymore, because it is clear that all psychiatric disorders are related in some way to biologic abnormalities at some level. This chapter deals with the disorders generally referred to as **organic mental disorders** in DSM-III-R: **cognitive disorders** and **psychiatric disorders due to medical conditions**.

Cognitive Disorders

These disorders include **delirium, dementia,** and **amnestic disorders**. In each, the prominent clinical manifestation is a deficit in cognitive function (memory, language, or attention). These disorders can be caused by a specific problem, a general medical condition, or substance abuse, alone or in combination. If the type of impairment is not clear, then the diagnosis is **cognitive disorder not otherwise specified (NOS)**. Delirium and dementia are also covered in Chapter 20, "Neurology").

Delirium

Delirium, defined as an **altered level of consciousness** and/or **a state of global cognitive impairment**, is a syndrome with both psychiatric (mood, perception, and behavior) and neurologic (tremor, asterixis, incoordination, and urinary incontinence) manifestations. It is common in hospitalized patients, especially those elderly and stressed, and independently worsens prognosis.

Causes are multiple. In hospitalized patients, medication use or misuse, withdrawal, and systemic illness and major stress are especially common; complete sensory deprivation and lack of sleep (common in ICUs) can worsen symptoms. Delirium usually resolves a few days after treatment of the causative factor. It can, however, last for weeks, depending on the cause, severity, duration, and concomitant problems.

(continued)

Psychiatry
Cognitive Disorders *continued*

The most important treatment for delirium is to identify and treat the underlying cause. Take precautions to avoid injury in agitated patients, and use physical restraints if necessary. Make the patient's environment as familiar and constant as possible. Visual aids such as a clock and calendar and gentle and regular reorientation to time, place, and person (including opening the shades and turning on the lights during the day) can decrease discomfort and agitation. Chemical "restraints" (medication) can be helpful to treat agitation and insomnia, but should be used with caution. Haloperidol (Haldol), an antipsychotic, is very useful, and short-acting benzodiazepines can help patients sleep.

Dementia

Dementia is the syndrome of **loss of previously acquired cognitive function with a normal level of consciousness**. Dementia usually occurs in the elderly; about 5% of Americans over 65 years and 20% of those over 80 are demented. DSM-IV classifies dementia into subtypes according to identified problems such as Alzheimer's disease, Picks disease, cerebrovascular disease, hypothyroidism, or substance use. Dementia is not inevitable with advancing age, but often no cause is found in elderly, demented patients.

Dementia typically results in personality change and a significant decline in social and occupational functioning, eventually interfering with basic activities of daily living (ADL). Patients eventually become disoriented to time and place, forget their addresses, and forget where objects are left. They usually maintain orientation to person until late stages of the illness. Problems with memory are an early and prominent feature of dementia. Short-term memory is obviously impaired, but long-term memory is usually also present, although more difficult to detect. All patients with dementia exhibit difficulties in planning and organizing their activities (executive functioning). Patients (especially those with Alzheimer's or vascular dementia) can develop aphasia, and complaints of insomnia, headache, dizziness, and generalized weakness are common.

Alzheimer's dementia is a histologic diagnosis, but the clinical diagnosis can be made antemortem if other possible causes are excluded. Pathologic findings include generalized atrophy of the brain, enlargement of the ventricles, widened cortical sulci, pathognomonic senile plaques (amyloid deposits), neurofibrillary tangles, neuronal loss, and neuronal degeneration. Decreased norepinephrine and cholinergic activity have been found to occur in these patients. Symptoms usually arise after 65, and include memory impairment, aphasia, agnosia, and abnormal executive functioning. Affected patients steadily decline, late in the course of the disease becoming bedridden, incoherent, completely amnestic, and incontinent.

Vascular dementia (formerly termed multi-infarct dementia in DSM-III-R) is present in patients who have significant cerebrovascular atherosclerosis or infarcts in many areas of the brain due to thrombotic or embolic vascular occlusion. Occasionally, it can be differentiated from Alzheimer's dementia by sudden onset and stepwise deterioration. Focal neurologic findings are common.

Dementia can be due to **HIV disease** (see Chapter 19, "HIV and AIDS"). Most patients with AIDS have central nervous system involvement with visible parenchymal abnormalities seen on MRI. Dementia usually occurs late in the disease.

The diagnosis of **substance-induced persisting dementia** is made when symptoms of dementia persist beyond the normal course of intoxication or withdrawal. Many substances can cause dementia after chronic use, including alcohol, inhalants, and heavy metals.

Parkinson's disease is caused by low levels of dopamine in the basal ganglia, and is associated with resting tremor, masked facies, shuffling gait, bradykinesia, limb stiffness, and slow thinking (bradyphenia). **Huntington's disease**, transmitted in an autosomal dominant fashion, is characterized by choreoathetoid movements (**chorea**). Patients commonly have dementia of the subcortical type, with more psychomotor retardation, depressive, and psychotic

Psychiatry
Cognitive Disorders *continued*

symptoms, and less impairment in memory, language, and insight. **Pick's disease** affects mainly the frontal and temporal lobes, and is associated with neuronal loss, gliosis, and neuronal Pick's bodies. Behavior and personality changes occur before cognitive impairments; hypersexuality, placidity, and hyperorality are characteristic.
Creutzfeldt-Jakob disease is a rare infectious disease caused by a prion (proteinaceous substance with no DNA or RNA). It causes tremor, ataxia, and myoclonus, and is rapidly progressive, causing death in 6-12 months.
Binswanger's disease refers to the situation where multiple subcortical infarcts leading to dementia is present.

Other causes

Many other conditions can be associated with dementia, including head trauma, tumors, hydrocephalus, neurosyphilis, renal failure, Wilson's disease, B12 or folate deficiency, and autoimmune disorders such as lupus erythematosis and multiple sclerosis. When the diagnosis of **dementia due to general medical condition** is made, the underlying disease should be recorded on axis III.

Dementia is usually progressive and irreversible. A major focus of the initial evaluation of these patients, therefore, is trying to identify the few reversible causes of dementia (nutritional deficiencies, tumors, and so on), present only about 10%-15% of the time. Patients with irreversible dementia have many needs, such as maximization of physical health and attention to diet, exercise, and recreation. Tacrine, a cholinesterase inhibitor, can improve cognitive deficits in about a quarter of patients with Alzheimer's dementia. Short-acting benzodiazepines can be used to treat insomnia and agitation; antipsychotics and antidepressants can also be useful. "Start low and go slow" when prescribing medications for the elderly, and avoid long-acting benzodiazepines and medications with anticholinergic activity.

Individual supportive **psychotherapy** can help with coping mechanisms and provide strategies to compensate for memory loss such as taking notes, keeping calendars, and maintaining visual clues in the environment. Families and caretakers also need counseling to help them deal with grief, frustration, and, occasionally, guilt that surfaces when taking care of patients with dementia.

Amnestic disorders

Amnestic disorders are those problems that solely affect memory; other cognitive abilities such as attention and concentration remain intact. Many areas of the brain are involved in memory, including the thalamic dorsomedial nucleus, hippocampus, mammillary bodies, and amygdala; any damage to these areas, especially if bilateral or left-sided, can result in memory dysfunction. DSM-IV requires a causative factor (either identified or presumed) for diagnosis (if none is identified, amnestic disorder NOS is present); this specificity helps differentiate them from amnestic states seen with dissociative disorders. If the duration of the memory deficit is less than a month, it is termed **transient**. Amnesia can be **anterograde** (inability to learn new information) or **retrograde** (inability to remember old information). **Immediate recall** (memory at three minutes or so) and memory of remote childhood experiences are often unaffected. Onset can be sudden (amnesia caused by trauma or a cerebrovascular accident; CVA) or gradual (brain tumor or thiamine deficiency).

Many problems occurring in the central nervous system (CNS) can cause amnestic disorders, whether acutely or after resolution of the active phase of the illness. In addition to the usual focal neurologic findings, **tumors** can present with psychiatric symptoms or syndromes. Tumors in the temporal or parietal lobes are usually associated with memory deficits, while those arising in the frontal lobes or limbic system can present with psychiatric symptoms such as abnormal perceptions, delusions, mood changes, language deficits, or delirium caused by increased intracranial pressure. Memory deficits can persist after removal of the tumor. **CVAs** that involve the bilateral medial thalamus or hippocampus usually result in memory deficits. Such infarcts almost always involve larger areas of the brain, so focal neurologic findings are prominent. **Herpes simplex encephalitis** usually affects the frontal and temporal lobes, and thus can cause memory deficits. Associated neurologic findings include seizures, disorientation, changes in the level of consciousness, and anosmia (loss of taste or smell); common psychiatric symptoms include olfactory and gustatory hallucinations, bizarre delusional ideations, and personality changes secondary to involvement of the frontal lobes. Amnestic disorders due to herpes simplex encephalitis are usually chronic.
(continued)

MS

Multiple sclerosis (MS), a demyelinating disease that affects the white matter in many areas of the brain, can cause an amnestic disorder due to involvement of the temporal lobes and diencephalon. About half of patients have memory problems that usually produce problems with both immediate and delayed recall. Some improvement can occur with steroids. Both open and closed **head injuries** can cause amnesia. Memory problems often involve the time directly surrounding the accident, and a decreased attention span, difficulty in problem solving, aggressiveness, irritability, changes in personality, and depression can all be seen. Severity of memory loss usually correlates with severity of trauma and the degree of improvement in the first week after injury. Patients who receive **electroconvulsive therapy** (ECT; see Chapter 71, "Psychopharmacology") develop retrograde amnesia for events surrounding the treatment, and, commonly, anterograde amnesia for the few hours following. Memory deficits are transient, lasting 6 months, at most, after finishing therapy. **Korsakoff's syndrome** is caused by thiamine deficiency due to poor nutrition, and is usually seen in persons with chronic alcoholism. Commonly, patients cannot remember things from the recent past or learn new tasks, but memory for remote events is intact. Confabulation is prominent. The syndrome is usually preceded by **Wernicke's encephalopathy** (confusion, ataxia, and nystagmus) which is treatable with thiamine. **Transient global amnesia** is characterized by very short (up to 24 hours), transient amnesia. Patients are usually alert, somewhat confused, and cannot describe their problem, and invariably recover completely in few hours.

Many other disorders present with various types of memory loss. Dementia is always associated with other cognitive deficits that progress over many years, and delirium causes characteristic changes in the level of consciousness. Patients with **dissociative disorders** have selective memory deficits associated with disorientation to self, and, usually, a history of a stressful life event. **Factitious disorder** should be considered if primary or secondary gains are identified and a clear cause for amnesia is not identified.

Primary goals are to identify and treat the underlying cause of the amnestic disorder and to slow deterioration. Frequent orientation to date and place can help decrease anxiety. Individual supportive psychotherapy is indicated to help patients deal with the denial and frustration associated with the disorder, and to help them deal with the experience after recovery.

Mental Disorders due to General Medical Condition

Psychiatric symptoms can be part of the presentation of many medical conditions. When symptoms meet criteria for a specific psychiatric disorder, DSM-IV allows the diagnosis of a **disorder secondary to a specific medical condition** or **due to substance use**. Such mental disorders previously (DSM-III-R) were classified as organic mental disorders, but now are classified with the "parent" psychiatric disorder itself. This approach has two advantages: assurance that medical illness will always be part of the differential diagnosis, and elimination of the misleading absolute separation of organic and functional mental disorders.

There are three specific diagnoses in this area that do not meet criteria for a known psychiatric disorder. **Catatonia** is a state of immobility, mutism, and extreme negativism, often associated with echolalia (repeating others' words), echopraxia (repeating others' actions), or purposeless and unprovoked hyperactivity. If such symptoms can be attributed to a physical condition and mania or delirium are not present, the diagnosis of **catatonic disorder due to general medical condition** is made. The diagnosis of **personality change due to general medical condition** is made when a medical condition exists that is clearly causing uncharacteristic (for the patient) behavior and attitudes; such changes cannot be explained by another mental disorder, delirium, or dementia. Such personality changes are classified as labile, disinhibited, aggressive, apathetic, paranoid, or combined subtypes. A classic example is a patient with a frontal lobe lesion who becomes indifferent to social norms, disinhibited in

Psychiatry
Cognitive Disorders *continued*

regard to sexual behavior, and emotionally labile (**frontal lobe syndrome**), who might be given the diagnosis of "personality change due to frontal lobe tumor, combined type." Finally, the diagnosis of **mental disorder NOS due to general medical condition** is given to a patient with a combination of symptoms that do not fit in any major DSM-IV category and a possible causative medical condition; an examples is a patient with dissociative symptoms associated with complex partial seizures.

Because of their relative frequency, certain medical conditions should usually be specifically kept in mind when evaluating a patient with new or recently changed psychiatric symptoms. **Complex partial seizures** (see Chapter 20, "Neurology"), formerly known as **temporal lobe epilepsy**, are commonly associated with behavioral abnormalities and an altered level of consciousness. Aura symptoms include changes in mood, fear, and anxiety. Patients can report unusual sensations such as "being in a dream," tunnel vision, jamais vu, or deja vu, and somatic complaints such as blushing, hyperventilation, or strange sensations in the stomach. Others can exhibit uncontrolled automatic movements such as lip smacking, chewing, or facial grimacing, and some develop delusions, hallucinations, or, rarely, violent behavior. Chronic, behavioral changes, together referred to as the epileptoid personality, can develop during the interictal phase. Hyperorality with slow and circumstantial speech, heightened experience of emotions, hyperreligiosity with increased concern about philosophical and ethical issues, and hyposexuality or occasionally hypersexuality are characteristic.

All psychiatric patients should be screened for **thyroid disease** by checking free T4 and thyroid-stimulating hormone (TSH) levels; even subclinical disease can cause behavioral changes or worsen a preexisting psychiatric condition. Patients with hypothyroidism can become depressed, apathetic, and slow, or can present with a manic-like psychosis, including paranoid delusions and hallucinations. Patients taking lithium are at risk to develop thyroid disease and should be monitored regularly. Patients with hyperthyroidism can present with panic-like symptoms such as hyperventilation, tachycardia, sweating, nervousness, and fear of impending death, or symptoms of mania, including tremors, hyperactivity, pressured speech, intrusive behavior, cognitive impairment, insomnia, and psychotic symptoms.

Acute intermittent porphyria is an autosomal dominant disorder producing enzymatic defects that result in the accumulation of porphyrins. Most common in women, it causes abdominal pain, motor neuropathies, mood swings, angry outbursts, extreme anxiety, depression, and psychosis. Barbiturates are contraindicated in these patients because they can precipitate attacks. ■

75   Anxiety Disorders

Anxiety disorders are among the most common psychiatric problems. A reasonable amount of anxiety is a normal human emotion; what constitutes pathologic anxiety varies. In general, anxiety that is persistent, interferes with normal functioning, or is perceived by the patient as troublesome, merits treatment. Discussed here are **panic disorder** and **agoraphobia**, **specific** and **social phobia**, **obsessive compulsive disorder**, **post-traumatic stress disorder** and **acute stress disorder**, **generalized anxiety disorder**, **anxiety disorders due to a general medical condition** or **substance induced anxiety disorder**, and **anxiety disorder NOS**.

Panic Disorder and Agoraphobia

The essential feature of **panic disorder** is the presence of recurrent **panic attacks**, which are discrete periods of intense fear accompanied by somatic symptoms such as palpitations, tachypnea, sweating, trembling, chest pain, nausea, dizziness, paresthesias, and chills or hot flashes. Panic attacks can also be accompanied by feelings of losing control, impending doom, or derealization. Panic attacks can occur in any anxiety disorder, but in panic disorder they occur repeatedly, unexpectedly, and lead to anticipatory anxiety. Panic disorder is often accompanied by **agoraphobia**, anxiety about being in places or situations from which escape might be difficult or embarrassing or help unavailable; this anxiety leads to pervasive avoidance of or significant duress during such situations. Due to the prominence of somatic symptoms, these patients need a full workup to exclude organic medical problems.

Age of onset varies considerably, but is typically in late adolescence or early adulthood; if agoraphobia develops, it usually happens within the first few years. Other psychiatric conditions such as major depression, other anxiety disorders, and substance use disorders frequently coexist, and a third to half of patients have agoraphobia with their panic disorder; the rest, panic disorder alone (isolated agoraphobia without panic disorder is uncommon). Panic disorders are 2-3 times more common in women, and some evidence of a genetic predis position exists.

Causes

Biologic abnormalities exist in patients with panic disorder. Patients display an increased sympathetic tone, and the autonomic nervous system seems to adapt more slowly and respond excessively to stimuli in contrast to unaffected patients. Abnormalities of GABA, serotonin, and norepinephrine have also been identified. Behavior theory postulates that agoraphobia is caused by paired association of events (anxiety and social situations) through classical conditioning; stimulus generalization can then occur. Psychoanalytic theory theorizes that panic attacks result from unsuccessful repression against anxiety-provoking impulses. Freud conceptualized anxiety as a signal to the ego that a dangerous situation exists. Neurosis then forms, to reduce the anxiety and avoid danger.

Treatment

Heterocyclic antidepressants, monoamine oxidase inhibitors (MAOIs), selective serotonin reuptake inhibitors (SSRIs), and benzodiazepines are all effective in the treatment of panic disorder (see Chapter 71, "Psychopharmacology"). A common approach is to start with a low dose of a heterocyclic antidepressant; because some patients initially experience a stimulant-like reaction, the dose should be slowly increased. Like depression, therapeutic effects are delayed, and patients need support, education, and encouragement during this "lag" period. If heterocyclics fail or are not tolerated, benzodiazepines, SSRIs and MAOIs are second line drugs. Medications can eventually be stopped in this situation, but should be tapered slowly to reduce the risk of relapse. It is very important to combine pharmacotherapy with psychotherapy. Cognitive and behavior therapy have been proved effective in panic disorders and agoraphobia. The focus in cognitive therapy is on the patient's tendency to misinterpret mild bodily sensations as life-threatening. Behavior therapies focus on relaxation techniques, respiratory training, and desensitization through exposure to the feared stimulus. Psychodynamically oriented psychotherapy (see Chapter 72, "Psychotherapy") may be of benefit for some patients.

(continued)

Psychiatry
Anxiety Disorders *continued*

Specific Phobia and Social Phobia

Phobias are the single most common mental disorder in the United States, but only a very small percentage of patients seek treatment. A phobia is an irrational fear of an object, situation, or activity, resulting in avoidance, marked distress, or impairment in functioning or relationships. In **specific phobia** the feared object is concrete and focal, and in **social phobia** there is fear of scrutiny or embarrassment. Specific phobia is divided into animal, natural environment, blood-injections-injury, situational, and other types, while social phobia is generalized as a fear that involves most social situations.

Causes

Age of onset appears to be bimodal, with peaks occurring in childhood and the mid-20s; if traumatic in origin, age at onset is more variable. Approximately 1 in 10 persons develop specific or social phobias during their lifetimes. Phobias appear to be more common in females, and there appear to be familial patterns for both disorders. Biologic theories focus on a state of heightened autonomic arousal, but behavior theories are most often used to explain pathogenesis. Classical conditioning (see Chapter 72, "Psychotherapy") with generalization creating a specific phobia is illustrated by a patient experiencing a sudden, loud noise while playing with a white rat during childhood, then becoming fearful of rats or objects resembling them. Social phobia is explained by lack of social skills, faulty evaluation of one's own performance, hypersensitivity to criticism, or early, unpleasant social experiences. Psychoanalytic theories do not differ between phobias and explain them in the same manner as other neuroses.

Treatment

The most successful treatments are behavioral, usually using relaxation techniques combined with gradual exposure (**systematic desensitization**). **Flooding** involves putting someone immediately into the feared situation to teach them they can survive. Medications such as low dose beta-blockers before anxiety-provoking situations can help in specific situations, and MAOIs and SSRIs appear to be useful in social phobia.

Obsessive Compulsive Disorder

The cardinal feature of **obsessive compulsive disorder** (**OCD**) is the presence of recurrent obsessions or compulsions that the person recognizes as excessive or unreasonable, are severe enough to cause marked distress, are time consuming, or cause significant impairment. **Obsessions** are recurrent, intrusive thoughts, feelings, ideas, or sensations, while **compulsions** are recurrent, purposeful, intentional behaviors. If obsessions or compulsions are resisted, anxiety occurs. Most commonly, both coexist, but in a small minority of patients an obsession or compulsion can exist alone. The most common obsessions are fear of contamination, pathologic doubt, somatic obsessions, the need for symmetry, aggressive obsessions, and sexual obsessions, while the most common compulsions are checking, washing, counting, a need to ask, a need for symmetry, and precision. Severity typically waxes and wanes. People may scrub their hands, be unable to leave the home, or, because of rituals, take hours to finish a simple task such as eating a meal. Onset is usually gradual, but can be sudden, typically following a stressful event. OCD usually begins in adolescence or early adulthood, but can occur in children. Treatment is efficacious, with a 60%-80% response rate.

Causes

There appears to be a biologic component to these disorders; dysfunction of the serotonergic system has been implicated. Increased activity in the caudate nucleus and orbital gyri, areas of concentrated serotonin and dopamine activity, that normalize after successful treatment with serotonin reuptake inhibitors, can be seen by PET scanning. Dysfunction of dopaminergic neurons is further supported by the fact that obsessions and compulsions sometimes develop in postencephalitic Parkinsonism. There is high concordance rate in twins; 35% of first degree relatives of afflicted individuals have OCD. Behaviorists believe obsessions are conditioned stimuli—previously neutral stimuli become associated with noxious or anxiety-provoking events, and thus become capable of producing noxious emotions on later exposure. Compulsions are established secondary to their anxiety-relieving qualities. Psychoanalytic explanations focus on three defense mechanisms: isolation, undoing, and reaction formation. An impulse is **isolated** from its accompanying affect. Due to a constant threat that the affect may escape the defense of isolation, a compensatory mechanism is formed whereby a compulsive act is initiated that aims to **undo** the consequences the patient

Psychiatry
Anxiety Disorders *continued*

fears the obsessional thoughts may have. Through **reaction formation**, abnormal character traits are formed.

Treatment

Both pharmacologic and behavior treatment are helpful. Serotonin-specific drugs have been shown to be effective in OCD, but take 3-4 weeks to work, have a response rate of only 40%-60%, and have a high relapse rate after discontinuation. MAOIs and lithium are also used. Behavior therapy is as effective as pharmacotherapy but more durable. The principal approaches are exposure and response prevention; the combination of pharmacotherapy and behavior therapy potentiate each other. Psychosurgical treatment can be used as a last resort.

Post-Traumatic Stress Disorder and Acute Distress Disorder

Post-traumatic stress disorder (PTSD) wasn't recognized as an independent diagnosis until 1980, although descriptions of stress-related syndromes date back to the Civil War. Post-traumatic stress disorder is characterized by symptoms developing after an exposure to an extreme, traumatic stressor. The stressor involves the possibility of death or serious injury, and the person's response involves intense fear, helplessness, or horror. The trauma is reexperienced through recurrent and intrusive recollections, including dreams, flashbacks, intrusive thoughts, and physiologic or psychologic distress on exposure to reminders of the trauma. There is persistent avoidance of reminders of the trauma with decreased responsiveness to such reminders, and, frequently, persistent hyperarousal. The minimum duration of symptoms is one month. If onset is more than 6 months after the trauma, it is specified as delayed onset. If symptoms last less than 3 months the disorder is specified as acute, and if more than 3, chronic. **Acute stress disorder** is a new diagnosis first introduced in the DSM-IV (1994), applying to patients in whom symptoms occur within 4 weeks of trauma and last for 2 days to 4 weeks.

Post-traumatic stress disorder can occur at any age. Symptoms usually begin within 3 months after trauma, and duration varies widely. The course often waxes and wanes, and comorbidities, especially substance use and depressive disorders, are very common. Community-based studies reveal a lifetime prevalence of 1%-14%; up to 58% of high-risk individuals (such as combat veterans) develop the disorder, and there is a relationship between level of combat and risk of PTSD. Victims of sexual assault are at especially high risk for subsequent mental health problems, including suicide.

Causes

Psychodynamic theories focus on the inability of the victim to process or rationalize the trauma that precipitated the disorder. Psychoanalytic models postulate that the trauma reactivates latent conflicts originating in infancy. Behavior models postulate that the trauma becomes paired, through classical conditioning, with physical or mental reminders of the trauma. Through instrumental learning, the patient avoids both the trauma and the reminders. Psychobiologic explanations focus on abnormalities of certain neurotransmitters, including norepinephrine, dopamine and endogenous opiates. The hypothalamic-pituitary-adrenal axis has been found to be hyperactive in some patients; hyperreactivity of the autonomic nervous system is also a common finding.

Treatment

Initiating assessment and treatment as close to the traumatic event as is possible is believed to prevent or minimize the disorder. Support, discussion of the event, and instruction and education about coping mechanisms are the major therapeutic approaches. Sedatives and hypnotics can help. When faced with a patient who already has PTSD, a multifaceted approach is imperative. Psychoeducation, family therapy, and group therapy with others who have experienced similar trauma have proved helpful. Pharmacotherapy for PTSD is mostly empiric. Some heterocyclics and MAOIs have been shown to reduce intrusive recollections; as have SSRIs in anecdotal reports. Clonidine, beta-blockers, lithium, and carbamazepine decrease hyperarousal and intrusive recollections in some patients. Short-term antipsychotic use can help if poor impulse control or psychotic features are prominent, but benzodiazepines should generally be avoided.

Generalized Anxiety Disorder

Causes & treatment

Generalized anxiety disorder is characterized by excessive anxiety and worry about a number of events and activities occurring with high frequency for a period of at least 6 months. These worries are difficult to control and are accompanied by a variety of symptoms, including muscle tension, restlessness, fatigue, problems concentrating, irritability, and sleep disturbance. The course is chronic and fluctuating, and coexistence with other psychiatric disorders, especially panic and major depressive disorders, is common. Lifetime prevalence is around 5%, and females are more commonly affected. In contrast to many of the anxiety disorders, there is minimal evidence for genetic transmission.

Psychodynamic theories, previously described, focus on neuroses. Behavior theories emphasize the disorder as a conditioned response, while biologic theories implicate abnormalities in the function of various neurotransmitters, especially the serotonergic system. The major psychotherapeutic approaches are cognitive-behavioral, supportive, and insight oriented. Various relaxation techniques, systematic desensitization, and cognitive therapy are helpful. Marked reduction in the level of anxiety commonly occurs after discussing the problem with a sympathetic therapist. Pharmacologic therapy utilizes anxiolytics such as the benzodiazepines and Buspirone; benzodiazepines should only be used for short periods of time while psychotherapy begins. Heterocyclics, beta-blockers, and SSRIs can also be used.

Other Anxiety Disorders

Other anxiety disorders categorized in the DSM-IV include **anxiety disorder due to a general medical condition**, **substance-induced anxiety disorder**, and **anxiety disorder NOS**. General medical conditions such as hyperthyroidism, pheochromocytoma, hypoglycemia, congestive heart failure, pulmonary embolism, chronic obstructive pulmonary disease, pneumonia, vitamin B12 deficiency, vestibular disorders, and encephalitis can cause anxiety or symptoms mimicking a panic attack. Various substances can do the same, such as caffeine, cocaine, alcohol, amphetamines, bronchodilators, anticholinergics, insulin, oral contraceptives, antihistamines, antiparkinsonian medications, corticosteroids, and various psychotropics. Anxiety disorder NOS encompasses disorders with prominent anxiety symptoms that do not meet criteria for other anxiety disorders. ■

76 Mood Disorders

The mood disorders are characterized by a disturbance in mood as their cardinal feature. **Mood** is sustained emotional tone, while affect is the external expression of present emotional context. The presence of altered mood itself, be it depression, elation, or irritability is not sufficient to warrant a diagnosis of a mood disorder. Specific signs and symptoms that produce functional impairment need to be present for the required period of time. According to DSM-IV, mood disorders are divided into **depressive disorders, bipolar disorders**, and two disorders based on etiology: **mood disorders due to a general medical condition**, and **substance-induced mood disorders**. The bipolar disorders (bipolar I disorder, bipolar II disorder, cyclothymia, and bipolar disorder NOS) differ from the depressive disorders (major depressive disorder, dysthymia, and depressive disorder NOS) by the presence of manic, hypomanic, or mixed episodes.

Theories of Mood Disorders

Biologic

The **biologic** school postulates that mood disorders are associated with organic derangements. The **neurotransmitters** norepinephrine and serotonin, both biogenic amines, are believed to be reduced in amount or effect in depression and increased in mania. Drugs that are highly effective in these conditions have relatively specific neurochemical effects on these neurotransmitter systems (see Chapter 71, "Psychopharmacology"), and nearly all effective treatments for depression lead to an increase in the amount of norepinephrine and serotonin at the synapse. With time there is a decrease in the sensitivity of the postsynaptic beta-adrenergic and 5-hydroxitryptamine type 2 ($5-HT_2$) receptors, which is consistent with the delayed therapeutic efficacy of the antidepressants. Abnormalities of dopamine, acetylcholine, GABA, and neuroactive peptides have also been implicated. **Neuroendocrine hormone abnormalities** are another possible factor. Hypercortisolemia is the most common endocrine abnormality seen with depression, and blunted TSH release and decreased growth hormone activity have also been reported. **Sleep abnormalities** in mood disorders are present more than half the time. There is decreased REM latency (time until beginning of first

REM period), increased REM density in the first half of sleep, and increased overall REM sleep, as well as initial and terminal insomnia and multiple awakenings.

Genetic

There is strong evidence for **genetic transmission**, in whole or in part, for most or all of the mood disorders. Proponents of this school stress that the problems arise from the individual's intrinsic DNA rather than environmentally-induced or acquired biologic changes.

Psychosocial

The third major school implicates **psychosocial issues**. **Environmental stressors** are believed critical. The risk of suffering an episode of depression rises several-fold in the first 6 months after stressful life events. These events are less likely to play a role in recurrent episodes, and overall are believed more to "tip the scales" in a person with an underlying predisposition toward a mood disorder rather than be the cause per se. **Psychoanalytic theory** postulates that following real or perceived loss of a loved object, anger is turned inward instead of toward the lost object (Freud). This happens as part of the loved object having been internalized and ambivalently held. Others argue that instability in parent-child interactions leads to vulnerability to separation and loss that extends into adulthood. Mania has been seen as a defense against depression through reaction formation. According to **cognitive theory**, learned negative views lead to feelings of depression. The cognitive triad of Beck is a negative view of self, a negative interpretation of personal experiences, and negative expectations of the future; this triad fuels depression.

Depressive Disorders

Major depression

Depressive disorders are divided into **major depressive disorder**, **dysthymia**, and **depressive disorder not otherwise specified** (**NOS**).

The essential feature of a **major depressive disorder** is either **depressed mood** or **loss of interest or pleasure in nearly all activities**. Signs and symptoms include social withdrawal, loss of libido, changes in appetite or weight, sleep disturbances, low energy levels, and changes in psychomotor activity. Symptoms tend to be worse in the morning, and feelings of worthlessness or guilt, difficulty thinking or concentrating, and difficulty making decisions are often present. Recurrent thoughts of death or suicidal ideation or frankly delusional or psychotic thought processes are seen in severe cases. Symptoms must be present for at least two weeks and cause significant impairment or distress to warrant the diagnosis.

Depression can present differently in children and adolescents. Somatic complaints, agitation, and single voice auditory hallucinations are seen relatively more often in prepubertal children, while substance abuse, school difficulties, rejection sensitivity, promiscuity, and antisocial behavior can be symptoms of depression in a formerly well-behaved adolescent. Depression is a common but under-diagnosed condition in the elderly, where it commonly causes somatic complaints, apathy, memory loss, disorientation, and sometimes confusion severe enough to masquerade as dementia (**pseudodementia**). About half the patients with true depression have significant depressive symptoms prior to the diagnosis of their first episode.

The natural history of depression is surprisingly poor. Studies conducted in the pre-drug era show that "untreated" depression recurs in 50%-80% percent of cases. Treatment works; an untreated episode lasts 6-13 months, while treatment, on the average, shortens this to 3 months. Those receiving antidepressants for less than 3 months almost always suffer recurrent symptoms. About two-thirds of treated patients recover within a year, and nearly 80% within 2 years; most of the rest have chronic illness. Multiple recurrences are common, but those who remain on prophylactic psychopharmacologic treatment appear to suffer fewer relapses.

Major depressive disorder is common, with an overall lifetime prevalence of about 15% (25% in women). It is more common in rural areas and nursing home populations. Mean age at onset is 40, but depressive disorder can occur at any age. Depression has a strong genetic component. Race and socioeconomic status are not risk factors, but family history is—first degree relatives of depressed patients are 2-10 times as likely to have major depression and 1.5-2.5 times as likely to have a bipolar disorder as are controls. Concordance rates for monozygotic twins are 50%.
(continued)

DSM-IV divides major depressive disorder into **single episode** or **recurring**. Single episodes carry more uncertainty about the future course, both whether recurrence will occur and whether the next episode will be depressive or manic (at which point it becomes a bipolar disorder); depression manifest as a single episode may even be later reclassified as another psychiatric or medical condition. Specifiers rate the most recent episode by **severity**, **presence of psychotic features**, and **remission**. Severity can be mild, moderate, or severe; psychotic features, if present, mood congruent or incongruent, and the episode can be in partial or full remission. If the most recent episode is of unknown severity, it is labeled unspecified.

Certain **subtypes** of major depressive disorders are recognized based on the syndromic picture of the last episode. "With melancholic features" identifies a subgroup of patients who seem to be particularly responsive to somatic therapy. These patients exhibit loss of pleasure or lack of reactivity with depressed mood, diurnal variation, early morning awakening, marked psychomotor retardation or agitation, loss of appetite or weight loss, or excessive or inappropriate guilt. "With atypical features" identifies a subgroup whose biologic symptoms (oversleeping, overeating) are opposite those usually seen. These patients have prominent anxiety and often complain of a heavy, leaden feelings in the arms and legs. This subgroup may respond better to monoamine oxidase inhibitors or selective serotonin reuptake inhibitors. "With catatonic features" implies that electroconvulsive therapy (ECT) may be particularly effective; catatonia is most often seen in mood disorders (particularly bipolar I disorder) and schizophrenia. "With postpartum onset" specifies that the onset was within 4 weeks of delivery, and "chronic course" requires that full syndromic criteria are present for at least 2 years. Longitudinal course specifiers describe the course of recurrent episodes and include seasonal patterns, rapid cycling in bipolar disorders, and a recurrent course with or without full interepisodic recovery.

Dysthymic disorder

By definition, **dysthymic disorder** is a chronic condition. It is characterized by a depressed mood present for most of the day on more days than not for a minimum of 2 years. Patients exhibit appetite and sleep disturbances, fatigue, low self esteem, poor concentration, impaired decision making, and hopelessness.

Dysthymic disorder often has an early and insidious onset and a chronic course. Patients with dysthymic disorder commonly develop major depression ("double depression"); such individuals are less likely to have a full recovery from the depressive episode, and are more likely to suffer recurrence. Dysthymic disorder often coexists with personality disorders, substance use disorders, and anxiety disorders, and is more common in women and among first degree relatives of people with major depressive disorder. Dysthymic disorder is specified as of early or late onset (before or after age 21, respectively) and can have the same atypical features as major depressive disorder.

Depressive disorders NOS

Depressive disorder NOS is a residual category that includes disorders with depressive symptomatology that does not meet criteria for another depressive disorder or adjustment disorder. Examples include premenstrual dysphoric disorder, minor depressive disorder, and recurrent brief depressive disorder, all of which are being studied for consideration as separate diagnostic entities. This diagnosis can also be used where a depressive disorder is present but further diagnostic clarification is not possible at the time.

Bipolar Disorders

The presence of manic, hypomanic, or mixed manic depressive episodes define bipolar disorders. **Hypomanic** symptomatology is characterized by elated, irritable, or expansive mood, as well as other signs and symptoms such as rapid and pressured speech, hyperactivity, diminished sleep, grandiosity, racing thoughts and flights of ideas, impaired concentration, hypersexuality, excessive partying or excessive work, and impulsive acts such as overspending or making foolish business investments. Full-blown **mania** requires the existence of psychotic features, marked social or vocational impairment, hospitalization, or a history of a previous manic episode.

Bipolar I disorder

Bipolar I Disorder requires the presence of at least one full-blown **manic episode**. Episodes can be manic only or a mixture of manic episodes with hypomania, depressive,

Psychiatry
Mood Disorders *continued*

and mixed episodes; mixed episodes have the simultaneous presence of depressed and manic features nearly every day for at least a week. Psychotic features are present about half the time and tend to be grandiose and mood congruent. Insight is frequently lost, and patients often get into severe financial and social trouble.

Bipolar I Disorder is a recurrent problem; over 90% of individuals with one manic episode have more, and often manic and depressive episodes follow each other in succession. The number of episodes tends to be more frequent than in major depression, and, with advancing age, the interepisodic period tends to become shorter ("kindling"). Most patients return to their previous level of function between episodes, although 20%-30% retain partial symptomatology.

Bipolar I Disorder is equally common between genders, races, and ethnic groups. Mean age at onset is the early 20s; if much later, a medical cause should be diligently sought for. There is a strong familial pattern. Of first degree relatives of an affected patient, 4%-24% have Bipolar I Disorder, 1%-5% Bipolar II Disorder, and 4%-24% major depressive disorder; concordance for monozygotic twins is 79%.

DSM-IV specifies whether the last episode was manic, mixed, or depressive, and specifies severity by the same criteria as a major depressive episode. If the last episode was depressed, it can have melancholic features, atypical features, or be chronic. The course of Bipolar I Disorder can be with or without full interepisodic recovery, with a seasonal pattern, or with rapid cycling (4 or more distinct episodes in 1 year), all of which have specific implications for treatment.

Bipolar II disorder   Hypomania is the major trait of Bipolar II Disorder; manic or mixed episodes preclude the diagnosis but otherwise diagnostics and subtypes are the same. The course is very similar to Bipolar I Disorder, except a smaller percentage of patients have partial interepisodic recovery. Five to 15% of patients with Bipolar II Disorder develop a manic episode within 5 years and are reclassified as Bipolar I Disorder.

Cyclothymia

Cyclothymia, defined as a chronic mood disturbance of at least 2 years duration involving frequent hypomanic and mild depressive episodes that do not meet the full criteria or major depression, is perceived as a chronic but less severe variant of Bipolar Disorder. To be present, there should be no periods of euthymia longer than 2 months, and impairment cannot be severe. It usually has an insidious onset and chronic course, and there is a 15%-50% risk that the person will eventually develop Bipolar I or II Disorder. Onset is usually early in life; first degree relatives have a higher incidence of mood and substance related disorders.

Bipolar Disorder NOS is a residual diagnostic category for disorders with bipolar features that do not meet the criteria for other bipolar disorders.

Other Mood Disorders

The essential feature of **mood disorders due to a general medical condition** is that the mood disturbance is felt to be due to an organic medical problem. It can meet criteria for one of the mood disorder episodes, and must impair social or vocational functioning. The temporal relationship with the medical disorder may be diagnostic, and there may also be a previously established relationship in the literature. Some of the most common medical conditions where a concomitant mood disorder can be seen are Cushing's syndrome, hypoadrenalism, hypo- and hyperthyroidism, Parkinsonism, Huntington's disease, stroke, dementia, vitamin B12 deficiency, systemic lupus erythematosis, hepatitis, HIV, and pancreatic cancer.

The course is very variable, and depends on the underlying medical condition. According to the DSM-IV, the disorder can be divided into the subtypes of "with depressive features," "with major depressive-like episodes," "with manic features," and "with mixed features."

Substance-Induced Mood Disorders exist when there is a prominent and persistent disturbance in mood that is presumed to be causally related to the use of a substance. The substance may be a drug of abuse, a medication, or a toxin, and the mood disturbance can occur in the context of intoxication or withdrawal. To be present, it must cause a significant disturbance in functioning that is in excess of the usual symptoms or problems occurring in connection with intoxication or withdrawal.

Treatment

Treatment for mood disorders focuses both on immediate and long term needs of the patient. Hospitalization may be needed or the patient can be treated as an outpatient, depending on the degree of immediate impairment. Treatment is often divided into **somatic** and **psychosocial** treatments; a combination of the two is probably most effective. Diagnostic clarity is very important, and contributory problems such as a medical disorders or substance abuse need to be corrected.

**Psycho-
pharmacology**

Three-quarters of major depressive episodes respond to **medication**. The **antidepressants** include selective serotonin reuptake inhibitors (SSRIs), heterocyclic antidepressants, monoamine oxidase inhibitors (MAO-I), venlafaxine, nefazodone, buproprion, and lithium (see Chapter 71, "Psychopharmacology"). No single medication can be recommended as optimal for every patient. The heterocyclics have traditionally been the first line of treatment for depression, but lately many clinicians are using the SSRIs in this role, although their long-term efficacy and safety are not well established. Some circumstances call for different approaches. The addition of an antipsychotic or ECT is needed in psychotic depression. If the depression has atypical features, MAO-I may work better, and if the depressive episode is part of a bipolar disorder, a mood stabilizer such as lithium or an anticonvulsant must be used. The lag time between starting medication and clinical improvement is commonly at least 2-3 weeks, longer in geriatric patients. Duration of treatment should probably be at least 9-12 months, longer (or lifelong) if depression is recurrent, is of late onset, or is particularly severe.

Pharmacologic treatment of manic episodes differs. Acute hospitalization, sometimes involuntary, is often needed. Antipsychotics and/or benzodiazepines are introduced to quickly bring the excitation and agitation under control. **Mood stabilizers** are used for definitive treatment; lithium, carbamazepine, and valproic acid are most frequently used. They all have significant side effects and require careful monitoring of serum levels. Much data support anticonvulsants over lithium for patients with rapid cycling varieties of bipolar disorder or those who consistently have mania following depression.

ECT

Electroconvulsive therapy (ECT) is the treatment of choice for psychotic depression, when the depression is extremely severe or includes catatonia, and when antidepressants are not tolerated. Relative indications include treatment-resistant depression, and sometimes acute mania. Despite a historic "black eye," ECT is safe and is the most effective treatment for depression.

Psychotherapy

Psychotherapeutic therapy is useful for many of these patients, especially those with significant depression (see Chapter 72, "Psychotherapy"). Individual, group, and family therapy are all effective, but are often deferred until after the most serious symptoms are under control. **Interpersonal therapy** was developed for the outpatient treatment of depression. Emphasis is on ongoing current personal issues such as interactions with spouse, family members, boss, and coworkers. Patterns are observed, feelings clarified, and alternate courses of action are explored with the goal of an improvement in interpersonal skills; treatment is usually highly focused and short term. **Cognitive therapy** is based on the premise that a depressed person has errors in thinking that result in unrealistic thoughts about self and the world. The patient is taught to reverse these faulty conclusions and eliminate or replace negativity, with the desired result being a change in thinking, behavior, and mood. The therapist takes a very active role and treatment is highly structured and short term. **Psychodynamic psychotherapy** is generally longer-term, and focuses on the premise that unresolved conflicts or painful experiences in one's childhood persist into adult life, creating problems. By understanding and resolving childhood conflicts, the patient is freed from repeating patterns and able to meet life's demands more successfully.

Education of the patient and family should be an integral part of any treatment, with the goals being improved compliance, understanding of the illness, and adaptation in society. Education and support are considered by many the cornerstones of successful treatment of these disorders. ■

77   Personality Disorders

Personality refers to the enduring qualities of a person manifest by ways of behaving in a wide variety of circumstances. **Personality disorders** are patterns of inflexible, maladaptive personality traits that cause significant impairment in social or occupational functioning, subjective distress, or both. By definition, personality disorders are long-standing and deeply ingrained; onset is usually in adolescence or early adulthood.

General Overview

Many theories of causality exist. Twin studies support the existence of a genetic contribution to personality disorders—concordance is higher among monozygotic twins, and monozygotic twins raised apart have concordance rates similar to those raised together. A child's temperament may predict the future development of a personality disorder, especially if there is not "goodness of fit" between parents and the child. Freud suggested that personality disorders represent a fixation at an early developmental stage, while Reich believed that characteristic defensive styles persons use largely determine personality. Cognitive and behavioral therapists view personality disorders as learned behaviors.

A useful generalization is to view personality disorders as patterns of behavior that patients somehow learn to use in order to cope with their problems. In psychodynamic terms, these patterns are referred to as **defenses**, unconscious mental processes that the ego uses to resolve internal conflicts; effective defenses reduce internal anxiety. Even if such patterns of behavior are seen as maladaptive by other people (a "personality disorder"), **patients themselves often feel no distress because their anxiety is controlled**. Individuals with a personality disorder are often very reluctant to engage in therapy and give up their defensive styles, because, in doing so, anxiety is temporarily worsened.

DSM-IV groups personality disorders into three clusters. Those in cluster A can be described as "**odd and eccentric**," and include schizotypal, schizoid, and paranoid disorders. Those in cluster B, the "**dramatic, emotional,**

and erratic," include histrionic, narcissistic, antisocial, and borderline personality disorders, while those in cluster C, the **"anxious and fearful,"** include avoidant, dependent, and obsessive/compulsive personality disorders (as well as personality disorders NOS).

Cluster A: "Odd and Eccentric"

Schizotypal

Patients with **schizotypal personality disorder** exhibit **strikingly peculiar behavior**, speech, thinking, and perception. Patients are withdrawn and avoidant, display "magical thinking," peculiar ideas, mild paranoid tendencies, delusions, and derealization. Relatives of schizophrenic patients are at higher risk to develop the disorder, and some patients with schizotypal personality disorder go on to develop full-blown schizophrenia (see Chapter 73, "Psychotic Disorders"). Psychotherapy should be supportive and structured; free association and unstructured reflection is often poorly tolerated. Social skills training can be advantageous, but antipsychotic medications are not particularly helpful.

Schizoid

Schizoid personality disorder is characterized by a lifelong pattern of **social withdrawal**. Affected persons are detached and indifferent to others, have bland, constricted affect, are typically anhedonic, and seem eccentric, isolated, or lonely. They often find living situations and jobs that involve little or no contact with others. Such individuals rarely seek help or initiate treatment.

Psychotherapeutic emphasis is on being warm and caring; as trust develops, patients can open up to the therapist, often revealing deep fears of closeness and unbearable dependency. Pharmacotherapy is not strongly indicated unless concomitant disorders develop.

Paranoid

Persons with **paranoid personality disorder** are typically **suspicious**, mistrustful, and perceive themselves to be exploited by others. They typically refuse to take responsibility for their own feelings, instead projecting them onto others. They are often hostile, irritable, and intense. People who are litigious, bigoted, or pathologically jealous often have "real" paranoid personality disorders. Patients rarely seek treatment on their own. Supportive psychotherapy may be the optimal approach. Straightforwardness, honesty, respect, and clear specific communications are encouraged. Once trust has devel-

oped, the patient may be able to tolerate alternative explanations and perceptions. Social skills training and behavior therapy such as role playing are successful at times.
Pharmacotherapy is generally viewed with suspicion by
the patient, but if severely agitated, anxiolytics or antipsychotics can help.

Cluster B: "Dramatic, Emotional, and Erratic"

Histrionic

Individuals with **histrionic personality disorder** are dramatic, extroverted, **attention-seeking**, shallow, exhibition-
istic, and seductive; underneath this "front" can be nag-
ging self-doubt and inability to enter into long-lasting
interpersonal relationships. These patients are often eager
for the attention that therapy brings; once the flamboy-
ance is peeled away, however, an inability to recognize
their own feelings or explain their motivations often surfaces. The therapist should show concerned professional-
ism and a high degree of constancy and reliability.
Encouraging patients to look at their behavior and clarify
their emotions can be helpful. Patients can do well in
group therapy, but pharmacotherapy is of limited use
unless concomitant disorders are present.

Narcissistic

Narcissistic personality disorder is characterized by
grandiosity, feelings of entitlement, low empathy, and a
heightened sense of self-importance. Patients are hypersensitive to evaluation by others and handle rejections
very poorly. Treatment of narcissistic personality disorder
is difficult. If progress is to be made, patients usually
have to take a self-critical look at their own thinking and
behavior. There is some disagreement on how this is best
achieved. Some psychotherapeutic schools encourage
strict limit-setting and confrontation, while others recommend a more supportive approach. Medications are of
very limited use.

Antisocial

Individuals with **antisocial personality disorder** show a
pattern of behavior (usually starting before age 18)
marked by the **inability to conform to social norms**;
such patients act irresponsibly, exploitatively, and without
guilt. Affected patients manipulate others for personal
gain and have little concern about the effect of their
actions, and frequently get in trouble with the law. There
is a strong familial pattern, and concomitant substance
use disorders are common. These patients almost never

seek treatment on their own unless the goal is to avoid responsibility, punishment, or some other secondary gain, and are often seen in the forensic or emergency room setting. They can be charming and manipulative and often are able to fool even experienced professionals; access to background information and past history is thus invaluable. Patients with antisocial personality disorder are recognized as among the most difficult to treat in all of psychiatry. Some success has been achieved in settings where the patients are forced to participate in therapy (such as in jail). Firm limits are essential, and early termination of therapy by the patient is very common.

Psychopharmacology is not helpful for the disorder itself.

Borderline

Borderline personality disorder is characterized by a pervasive pattern of **instability** in interpersonal relationships, affect, mood, behavior, and self-image. Patients are classically self-mutilating and indirectly self-destructive and their relationships typically chaotic. Patients can display chronic suicidality and may make multiple suicide attempts. These patients almost always appear to be in a state of crisis, and "micropsychotic" episodes can occur during periods of more intense stress. Psychotherapy is intense with problematic transference (see Chapter 72, "Psychotherapy")—patients are inclined to see others as either all good or all bad and can quickly switch from one camp to the other. Patients are demanding and manipulative; countertransference can also be problematic. Regression is frequent. Such patients display characteristic maladaptive defenses, including primitive idealization and devaluation, splitting, and projective identification (whereby the patient unconsciously tries to coerce the therapist to act out a particular type of behavior). Constancy on the part of the therapist, limit-setting, and genuine interest can lead to development of trust with subsequent stabilization of mood. Consistency is very important, because these patients try to fulfill their pathologic beliefs that everyone ultimately fails them. Borderline patients frequently require hospitalization for self-injurious and impulsive behaviors. Hospitalization should be minimized in order to minimize regression and the perceived "break" from intensive outpatient therapy. Medications are beneficial in some patients. Antipsychotics can reduce impulsivity and irritability and treat micropsychotic episodes, and antidepressants can improve the dysphoria present in most patients. There is increasing evidence of the usefulness of serotonergic agents in this disorder. Antiepileptics and lithium can be helpful if mood instability is prominent and impulsive behavior problematic.

Cluster C: "Anxious and Fearful"

Avoidant

Individuals with **avoidant personality disorder** are **hypersensitive to rejection**, leading to an avoidant, introverted life. While there is **desire** for social interaction (differentiating it from schizoid personality disorder), patients are too fearful of rejection to allow themselves to actually enter into relationships. Because these patients enter into relationships only if they perceive there is a high likelihood of their being liked, psychotherapeutic goals are to build trust through acceptance and benevolent concern. Once trust is established, the therapist can encourage the patient to take on bigger tasks and focus on assertiveness and social skills training. Encouragement and praise is important. Group therapy can be quite helpful as well as social skills training. When anxiety is prominent antianxiety agents can be useful.

Dependent

Dependent personality disorder is characterized by **excessive reliance on others for emotional support**. Such patients get others to assume responsibility for major areas in their lives, feel helpless when alone, and demean themselves to gain acceptance or tolerate mistreatment by others. Psychotherapy can be effective, but the therapist must be able to control excessive, dependent transference. The therapist must also be able to tolerate the patient's pathological relationships, because patients can become too anxious and terminate therapy if they perceive a strong push from the therapist to end a relationship based on dependency. Patients can do well in group therapy and assertiveness training. Anxiety and depression are common among these patients and can be treated appropriately with medications.

Obsessive/ compulsive

Obsessive/compulsive personality disorder is characterized by perfectionism, **behavioral rigidity**, formality, intellectualizing, affective constriction, and indecisiveness. Patients often have strong self-doubts that they overcome with excessive devotion to certain actions, causes, or work, ignoring other areas of their lives. Freud theorized that this disorder represents arrest at the anal stage of development. Such patients have a reputation for being difficult to treat, but often seek treatment on their own because they appear to know that they are suffering. Patients are often superficial, intellectualizing, and unable to get to the point, and the therapist can become bored or risk getting into a "power struggle" because of the urge to move the therapy along. Encouraging free association is initially frustrating, but can reveal the deep emotions that these patients are defending against. Excessive interpretation may not be useful. Group therapy can be quite useful.

NOS

Personality disorder not otherwise specified (NOS) is reserved for personality disorders that cannot be classified as one of the subtypes above. Passive/aggressive, depressive, sadomasochistic, and sadistic personality disorders can be placed under this heading, as can patients who share features from various subtypes but fall into no single category. ■

The somatoform disorders make up a group of problems that present with physical symptoms for which no sufficient medical explanation can be found. The symptoms or complaints are either not consistent with any medical disorder or the magnitude of disability suffered by the patient is not fully explained by any organic problem present. These patients often undergo numerous diagnostic procedures and therapeutic regimes. Patients suffer significant disability in social, occupational, and other realms secondary to their symptoms or the resulting unnecessary treatments.

Diagnosis

Differentiating a somatoform disorder from an organic medical problem can often be difficult, but obviously is the primary goal. Usually, the psychiatrist does not see these patients until this has been done. Somatoform disorders are distinguished from malingering and factitious disorders (also discussed below) by the unconscious nature of the motives behind symptoms and their perpetuation. Somatic complaints can also be seen in delusional or major depressive patients, but in these patients, the diagnosis differs based on the intensity of the belief in the symptom, the presence of other neurovegetative symptoms, or the presence of a clear psychosocial stressor with a time limited course. There are 7 diagnostic categories of somatoform disorders outlined in the DSM-IV: **somatization disorder**, **conversion disorder**, **hypochondriasis**, **body dysmorphic disorder**, **pain disorder**, **undifferentiated somatoform disorder**, and **somatoform disorder not otherwise specified (NOS)**.

There are many theories for the existence of somatoform disorders. Both abnormalities in the immune system and malfunction of certain areas of the brain causing misinterpretation of sensory information have been postulated as causes. Psychodynamic theories suggest that the patient uses somatic symptoms to express stress, emotional conflicts, or as a means to get unconscious needs met. The classic concepts of primary and secondary gains often nicely apply to these patients.

In general, women are afflicted more than men, and these disorders are more common in lower socioeconomic strata. They often coexist with medical disorders, and a thorough medical workup of all patients with somatic complaints is initially required. The diagnosis of somatoform disorder is one of exclusion: one must first rule out any medical or other psychiatric condition that might be responsible for the complaints. The course and prognosis of the various somatoform disorders differ, but the longer they persist, the poorer the prognosis. Treatment also differs, but once medical or psychiatric disorders are ruled out, further diagnostic and therapeutic medical procedures should be limited. Psychiatric interventions can be of significant benefit in these disorders, and can limit the overall extent of medical expenditures.

Somatization Disorder

This disorder is defined by a **multiplicity of somatic complaints involving many organ systems**. It was previously called **Briquet's Syndrome**, after Paul Briquet, the French physician who initially described these symptoms. Afflicted patients are often vague historians with multifocal complaints who seek care from multiple caregivers. They are at increased risk of morbidity from their diagnostic workup, and often hold the belief that they have been sickly most of their lives. Many of these patients have additional mental disorders such as major depression or personality disorders or traits. Women are more commonly affected, and symptoms are noted early, often during adolescence.

It is particularly important to rule out general medical conditions that have a fluctuating course and multiple symptoms (for example, multiple sclerosis, systemic lupus erythematosis, AIDS, hyperparathyroidism, or hyperthyroidism). Over half of these patients have a coexisting medical disorder, but somatization disorder is also present if the extent of the patient's symptoms or disability cannot be explained by the medical disorder. These patients experience fluctuations in the severity and nature of their symptoms that are increased by psychologic or physical stress. It is imperative to consolidate the patient's care to a single primary physician. Sustained and intense communication between the primary physician and all specialists, including the psychiatrist, is essential for successful treatment. Frequent, regularly scheduled visits (not based on symptoms) can reduce the number of "crises." Once a thorough medical work up is complete, further diagnostic procedures or therapeutic treatments should be avoided, except when clearly indicated. While classic analytic psychotherapy can often worsen symptoms, cognitive, behavioral, and group therapies can be quite successful.

Conversion Disorder

This disorder is defined by the involvement of **"pseudoneurologic" symptoms**, or those that involve impairment in sensory and/or motor systems, leading to seizures, paralysis, paresthesia, blindness, deafness, and so on. There is an involuntary loss or limitation of physical function that does not follow well-established neurologic distributions. Freud described the psychological basis of this disorder as a result of an unconscious conflict that causes anxiety in the patient. He believed that the patient developed the symptom as a way of reducing the anxiety (**primary gain**), then received increased emotional and physical attention as a result of being sick (**secondary gain**). These patients often present with "la belle indifference," a seeming lack of concern about their physical symptoms. The patient's symptoms are usually based on a "role model" such as a family member or friend, or the patient's own previous neurological disorder.

This is the most common of the somatoform disorders, and again is most common in women. Symptomatology is often fairly short, but occasionally can be chronic and unremitting. As with all somatoform disorders, a primary medical or neurologic illness causing the symptoms of concern must be excluded, keeping in mind that many of these patients do have coexisting medical disease. Common medical and neurologic disorders that coexist or mimic conversion disorder include seizure disorders, multiple sclerosis, polymyositis, myasthenia gravis, and optic neuritis.

Patients with the best prognosis have good pre-morbid function, have a shorter duration of symptoms before treatment, and receive timely psychiatric intervention (i.e., psychotherapy). Many of these patients are suggestible and may thus respond symptomatically to powerful reassurance and encouragement. A majority remit spontaneously even without formal intervention. Those who do not remit spontaneously carry an increased risk for significant morbidity and disability.

Hypochondriasis

Patients with hypochondriasis are described as being **preoccupied with somatic symptoms**. These symptoms become exaggerated and are the major focus of the patient's energies. The time and energy they expend seeking diagnoses and treatments for their symptoms often result in significant impairment in social and occupational function. Medical workup again fails to explain the symptoms or the extent of impairment due to the symptoms. The incidence of hypochondriasis is roughly equal in males and females. It is commonly seen in 20- to 30-year olds, and commonly results in chronic symptoms and disability. There is often a ruminative, obsessive, anxious quality to the presentation of these patients, contrasting sharply with la belle indifference.

In patients suspected of hypochondriasis, it is important to rule out delusional perceptions of somatic symptoms. While true delusions cannot be altered, the preoccupation with symptoms in hypochondriasis can be swayed when the patient is confronted. Symptoms can focus on one organ or system or can be multifocal. Again, patients engage in "doctor shopping" and receive excessive treatment and long workup, and again it is important for the patient to have frequent, regularly scheduled medical visits to avoid acute care visits. The course of this disorder is chronic with episodic exacerbations associated with stressors, but some patients eventually improve. These patients often have coexistent depressive and/or anxiety disorders, for which pharmacotherapy can be useful. Many patients are resistant to individual psychotherapy, but group therapy can be quite effective.

Body Dysmorphic Disorder

Body dysmorphic disorder is described as a **preoccupation with an imagined bodily flaw or an exaggerated distortion of a real defect**. This preoccupation causes significant distress in the patient's self perception and affects social and occupational functioning. These people are frequently seen by dermatologists, plastic surgeons, and dentists. It is most common in young women, especially in teenagers, and is often a chronic problem. Symptoms usually remain constant over time with variations occurring in the intensity of anxiety and in which body part is the area of focus. The most common preoccupation is with facial flaws. Some patients become housebound, and many engage in frequent mirror checking behavior. They typically undergo multiple procedures without relief of their anxieties, and can be at high risk of suicide secondary to depression, anxiety, and impaired social and occupational functioning. Patients can have delusions of reference (for example, if people are laughing as the patient enters the room, the patient may think that people are laughing at his or her flaw), but no other delusional symptoms are present. Frequently coexistent are major depression, anxiety disorders such as obsessive-compulsive disorder, or schizoid and narcissistic personality disorders.

Body dysmorphic disorder must be distinguished from a normal concern with one's physical appearance, anorexia nervosa, and psychotic distortions of body parts. Surgical, dermatological, or dental treatments do not lessen the severity of the symptoms, and often make them worse because actual scars and defects develop. Selective serotonin reuptake inhibitors have been found to be helpful in the pharmacotherapy of this disorder. Psychotherapy is also helpful.

Pain Disorder

Pain disorder is defined as the presence of symptoms of **pain that are not in accord with medical or neurologic evidence**, or to an extent that is **not fully accounted for by an existing medical or neurologic disorder**. There must be psychological factors involved that can account for the symptoms. Persons with pain disorders often are found to have difficulty verbally expressing their emotional feelings (alexithymia) and thus are thought to express their feelings through the exhibition of somatic distress.

Pain disorders are very commonly seen in general medical practice. There is considerable variation in their prevalence, and they are commonly seen in blue collar workers, often attributed to job-related injuries (low back pain is one of the most common complaints). Patients have increased rates of benzodiazepine and opioid dependence, engage in doctor shopping, and again often receive many unwarranted medical and surgical interventions. They may have associated mood and anxiety disorders.

True physical pain generally has a waxing and waning course with good response to analgesics. Psychogenic pain, however, begins abruptly and increases in intensity. This pain is constant, and its intensity varies little with change in attention levels or treatment with analgesics. The poorest prognosis is found in patients with character pathology, those who are involved in litigation or who may benefit financially from their illness, those who are addicted to analgesics, and those who have a long history of the disorder. Analgesics and surgery (including nerve blocks and ablative procedures) are generally not helpful. Treatment with antidepressants and serotonin reuptake inhibitors has been successful in some cases. Behavior treatment and individual psychotherapy have also been effective.

Undifferentiated Somatoform Disorder

This disorder is described by **symptoms or physical complaints for which no medical or neurologic condition can be found or can explain the extent of disability suffered by the patient** and do not correspond to any of the above categories. The symptoms must persist for at least 6 months and cause the patient significant distress or dysfunction. Typically, patients complain of symptoms involving the autonomic nervous, gastrointestinal, or genitourinary systems, fatigue, or weakness. The symptoms of this disorder can also overlap with those seen in chronic fatigue syndrome.

Somatoform Disorder (Not Otherwise Specified)

This is a diagnosis that is usually made when **symptoms consistent with a somatoform disorder are found**, but **the criteria for the specific disorders described above, and outlined in the DSM-IV are not met**.
"Pseudocyesis," or false pregnancy, is one example.
(continued)

Psychiatry
Somatoform Disorders *continued*

Related Disorders

Factitious disorders

Factitious disorder, malingering, and other related psychiatric illnesses, not classified as somatoform disorders, can present with similar symptoms. **Factitious disorder** (also called **Munchausen's Syndrome**, after the Baron von Munchausen who was infamous for his fantastic story telling) is present when symptoms are **consciously** produced, but with an **unconscious** benefit: the symptoms are produced to allow the patient to remain in the sick role. Patients will often subject themselves to significant harm in order to remain "sick." They may inject foreign substances into their blood to cause infections or electrolyte abnormalities, or may misuse medications such as insulin or anticoagulants to feign endocrine or coagulation abnormalities. A variant of this disorder exists called factitious disorder with psychologic symptoms, in which patients feign psychiatric symptoms to obtain hospital care. Interestingly, the disorder is most common in health care workers. "Munchausen's by proxy" means that the patient's symptoms are induced by the caregiver (most commonly, mother to child), and serve to keep the caregiver linked with the sick role.

Malingering

A **deliberate** production of symptoms for a **conscious goal** (such as disability benefits, workman's compensation, or to avoid jail) is referred to as **malingering**. These patients generally give a vague history, often refuse a complete physical or medical workup, and engage in doctor shopping. Risk taking can be considerable in these patients, and is seen mostly in males

Other disorders

Patients with **delusional disorder with somatic complaints** hold fast to their beliefs in the delusion. The somatic complaints in this type of delusional disorder are monosymptomatic, and often focus on organ dysfunction, infection, or abnormally shaped body parts. In young children and the elderly, somatic complaints are often the primary presenting complaints in **major depression**, because it is uncommon for patients in either of these age groups to present with the complaint of feeling sad or having a depressed mood. Somatic complaints in major depression will clear as the other symptoms of depression clear with typical antidepressant medications.
Adjustment disorder, unspecified can present with somatic complaints. It is defined as a **maladaptive**

response to a clear psychosocial stressor; the response to the stressor is in excess of what would be normally expected. The course of the somatic symptoms is time limited, usually resolving within six months after the stressful situation is resolved. Finally, **anxiety disorders** often present with physical symptoms (palpitations, sweating, shortness of breath). Thorough interviewing usually permits the identification of panic disorder or generalized anxiety disorder. These conditions are quite amenable to pharmacologic therapy and psychotherapy, but often run a chronic course. ■

79   Child Psychiatry

Child psychiatrists specialize in the treatment of children with psychiatric illnesses, including problems relating to development or problems in which communication with the child may be different than in adults. Child psychiatrists need to be creative and imaginative, and be able to effectively work with non-medical people such as parents, school teachers, social workers, nurses, and art and recreational therapists who can provide a better understanding of patients and their lives. Specific diagnostic and theoretic issues for the various disorders are discussed in their respective chapters. This chapter focuses specifically on the issues surrounding causality, diagnosis, and treatment of psychiatric disorders in children.

General Concepts

Troubled children usually present with a constellation of problems that makes it hard to adapt to life's stressors in a healthy way; such children may lack coping skills or the cognitive ability to understand the world. Difficulties can be divided into internalizing and externalizing disorders.

Internalizing disorders are seen in children who are unable to outwardly manifest their difficulties, and absorb their pain and misinterpretations. These children are depressed or anxious, may be "quietly psychotic," or suffer from overwhelming fear. Such children have a poor sense of identity and sometimes starve themselves or throw up because they believe the only control they have over their own lives is what they put in their mouths. Internalizing disorders are usually manifest as poor self esteem, declining school performance, withdrawal from others, and even suicide attempts. Depression can be considered an internalizing disorder if the major symptoms are social withdrawal, apathy, and lack of motivation.

Externalizing disorders manifest by outwardly disruptive behavior. Children with externalizing disorders are typified by those with aggression toward others, who set fires, are disruptive, steal, lie, and cheat, or have periods of severe rage. Some children with conduct disorder or opposition defiant disorder may be externalizers, and anxiety can present this way.

Confidentiality is a significant issue in therapeutic relationships with children and adolescents; psychotherapy is likely to be effective only if a mutual, trusting relationship is established. The (verbal) contract usually agreed upon is that anything the child tells the therapist will be kept in strict confidence; parents, school, siblings, or anyone else will not be told what is said unless the child gives permission to do so. **This excludes issues relating to safety, however: if the therapist believes that the safety of the child (or others) is compromised, confidentiality will be violated** (see Chapter 47, "Adolescent Medicine" for a discussion of emancipation and consent).

One way of establishing rapport with children is to allow them to know about and defend or rebut comments made about them by others. Information from school, parents, friends, siblings, or any other source usually should be discussed with the child. In this context, parents are told that their comments will likely be shared with the child, and that the child may say things that will not be shared with the parents. In so doing, the therapist automatically aligns with the child (the patient), enabling an empathic and trustworthy atmosphere to be established, in the hope of improving the quantity and quality of information imparted to the therapist.

Mood Disorders

Major depression is common (see Chapter 76, "Mood Disorders") and can begin in childhood. The signs to look for can be remembered by the mnemonic **SIG E CAPS**: **suicidal thoughts**, **loss of interest** in usual activities (**anhedonia**), **guilt**, **lack of energy**, **lack of concentration**, **loss or gain in appetite**, **psychomotor restlessness** or **depression**, and **sleep difficulties**.

If the "SIG E CAPS" signs and symptoms are present for two weeks or more, the diagnosis of major depression can be made. Prior to planning therapy, non-psychiatric causes of depression should be ruled out; particularly common in children and adolescents are substance abuse, thyroid disease, electrolyte abnormalities, infections, head trauma, and **child abuse or neglect** (see Chapter 58, "Child Abuse").
(continued)

Therapy begins the moment you interact with the child. By presenting yourself in an empathetic way, you may be lucky enough to create an environment whereby the child feels at ease and feels understood. Empathy, in this context, is the ability to place yourself in someone else's position; by doing so you can learn what children think and begin to hypothesize why they act the way they do, and, from there, begin to develop a treatment plan. If you suspect that the child might be suicidal, you need to ensure the child's safety through inpatient hospitalization or a "family watch" system, where somebody is in constant contact with the child. Treatment plans often have to be individualized; an example is children who are depressed over the loss of a parent who have not had the chance to mourn. In a similar fashion, children depressed because of poor school performance may require testing to rule out a specific learning disability.

Medication

As of August, 1994, no study has shown an overall benefit to **antidepressant medication** use in childhood depression. Despite this, many psychiatrists believe that some children do better with medication. As the child ages, too (especially into adolescence), the chances of responding to psychopharmacotherapy are greater. Medication prescribed depends on a combination of factors, including what medications have been tried in the past, whether family members have found certain antidepressants effective, and side effects. The use of psychotropic medications in children raises important ethical and personal questions, including the potential for interfering with growth and development, thinking processes, creativity, or learning. What is the "meaning" of taking medicine to this child, and what does having to take a medicine daily for "psychiatric reasons" mean to the family?

As is the case with any therapeutic intervention, antidepressants should be used for a specific reason. Symptoms to target include sleep difficulties, poor appetite and weight loss, poor concentration, lack of energy, and loss of interest. Sleep disorders often improve first, followed by concentration and appetite. It may take several weeks of therapy before improvement is seen (see Chapter 76, "Mood Disorders"). Blood pressure (including orthostatic changes), weight, and anticholinergic side effects such as dry mouth, headaches or dizziness, or difficulties urinating need to be followed. Of great importance is an ongoing assessment of the patient's suicidal tendencies. Because there is an increase in energy levels **before** improvement in mood, **the period just after initiation of treatment may represent the highest risk for suicide**.

The most widely used medication is probably imipramine (see Chapter 71, "Psychopharmacology"). Desipramine, also a tricyclic antidepressant and the major metabolite of imipramine, is seldom used today because of evidence linking it to the sudden death of several children. Prozac and Zoloft (selective serotonin reuptake inhibitors; SSRIs) are also of value. Some believe that these drugs provide more energy than imipramine, thus, they may be of special benefit if significant amotivation is present.

Psychotherapy

Psychosocial intervention should be initiated along with psychopharmacotherapy. Many techniques are useful, including **individual** and **family therapy** and **peer group involvement** such as participation in after-school organizations or summer youth camps. A major part of treatment in child psychiatry is family therapy, including discussion of parenting techniques, strategies, and communication styles, and the use of role playing. The alliance developed with the patient sometimes makes family therapy tricky, occasionally to the point of needing to defer this part of treatment to another therapist.

Attention Deficit Hyperactivity Disorder

Attention deficit hyperactivity disorder (**ADHD**) probably accounts for the most number of referrals to a child psychiatrist other than major depression. The hallmarks of this diagnosis include problems with **attention**, **impulsiveness**, and **overactivity**. These symptoms, however, may in fact represent the final common pathway of many disorders other than ADHD, such as depression, severe trauma, or child abuse. Therefore, prior to making the diagnosis, a careful and detailed history is mandatory; the diagnosis should also await observation over time rather than being applied after one parent/child interview, and should be made using information from all aspects of the child's life, including home, school, and daycare settings.

Connor's scale is a very simple questionnaire designed to indicate the possibility of ADHD; it is not, however, sufficient to make the diagnosis. Many similar question-naires exist, but, again, the presence of symptoms can be due to a variety of disorders.

Treatment

Treatment for ADHD needs to be multimodal; although medication is unquestionably of value, concomitant behavior- or psychotherapy is required. Typical medications used to treat attentional problems include methylphenidate (Ritalin), dextroamphetamine, clonidine, and tricyclic antidepressants; occasionally lithium or an SSRI such as Prozac are used. Ritalin, however, can "help" almost anyone, even if they don't have problems with tasks requiring prolonged attention. Ritalin and dex-troamphetamine are fairly safe, although they inhibit appetite and thus can cause weight loss. These effects typ-ically occur during initiation of treatment; patients are usually able to develop tolerance. When used in excess, however, psychostimulants can cause insomnia, weight loss, motor restlessness (akathisia) or tics, and headaches, as well as high blood pressure and growth retardation.

There must also be an ongoing therapeutic relationship with patient and family. Family therapy focuses on sup-porting the parents and their attempts to set limits, as well as with children who may view themselves as different than their peers and need a great deal of support around this issue. Group therapy for children with attentional problems is also helpful.

Post Traumatic Stress Disorder

Post traumatic stress disorder (PTSD) is also common in childhood. Although classified as an anxiety disorder (see Chapter 75, "Anxiety Disorders"), it can also be viewed as a dissociative phenomenon. The diagnosis is dependent on experiencing an extreme, traumatic event or events, out of line with ordinary life (typically, in chil-dren, sexual or physical abuse by a family member). PTSD is categorized as type I or II based on whether the problem resulted from one overwhelming experience (such as a rape or plane crash) or from a pattern of ongo-ing trauma (such as sexual abuse within the family), respectively; treatment between the two differs. Affected patients who suffer recurrent trauma can develop a defense mechanism whereby they are able to dissociate themselves from the situation; in effect, "disconnect" from what is going on. Such children will often report feelings of watching the trauma happen to them and feeling sorry for the person experiencing the trauma, but not actually of being caught up in it themselves. They believe that they are able to leave their bodies and watch the trauma occurring to them. Physiologic studies suggest a hyper-aroused state; children may have elevated cortisol levels, an exaggerated startle response, and seem to be constantly "on guard," as if they are unable to settle themselves and are constantly in fear of being retraumatized.

Treatment for PTSD is multimodal. Psychopharmacologic support can sometimes help, especially antidepressants if symptoms of depression are present. The main psychotherapeutic goal is to allow children to recall their stories in narrative without having the associated affect of "breaking down"; this can take years to accomplish. Helping patients develop defense mechanisms whereby they are able to gain mastery over the experience and feel less of a victim can help. The use of narrative through journals or creating stories or artwork with the child can also help. Once the child is able to talk about the experience, help with the management of emotions surrounding the experience is often the final part of therapy. ■

80 Substance Abuse

A **psychoactive substance** is anything that, when taken into the body, alters mental status or level of consciousness. **Addiction** and **abuse** are terms that have acquired different meanings in both lay and medical settings. The former has been discarded by the World Health Organization for the more appropriate term, **dependence**, which can be physiologic or psychologic. Physiologic dependence implies a need to use a psychoactive substance to prevent withdrawal symptoms, while psychologic dependence implies persistent craving to prevent going into a dysphoric state. Abuse of a substance is defined as excessive or improper use.

Diagnosis

Diagnostic criteria outlined in DSM–IV for substance dependence require a maladaptive pattern of substance use, leading to clinically significant impairment or distress. Specific criteria include **tolerance**, defined by a need for increased amounts of the substance to achieve intoxication or desired effect, or markedly diminished efficacy with continued use of the same amount, **withdrawal** (or need for the same or closely related substance to avoid withdrawal symptoms), an **increase in amount** or duration of use of the substance, persistent desire or **unsuccessful efforts to cut down** or control substance use, **excessive time spent** in activities necessary to obtain the substance or recover from its effects, **interference** with social, occupational, or recreational activities, or **continued use** despite knowledge of physical or psychologic ill effects. Three or more of these items over the past year are necessary to define the diagnosis.

It is most convenient to divide commonly abused substances into **stimulants**, that generally cause excitation, **depressants**, that generally produce somnolence or relaxation, **psychedelics** and **hallucinogens**, that lead to perceptual changes and euphoria, and **miscellaneous** or less commonly abused drugs.

Stimulants

Caffeine

Caffeine is the most popular stimulant drug used in the United States. Sources are widespread. Natural sources include the coffee bean, tea leaves, the cacao tree, and the cola nut, yielding respectively coffee, tea, chocolate, and soft drinks (often with "cola" in their name). Other sources of caffeine are guaraná from the seeds of a South American jungle shrub, available in the United States as tablets marketed in health food stores as "Zoom" and "Zing," and maté, made from leaves of the holly plant, that is an ingredient in herbal teas with names like "Morning Thunder." The caffeine addict can drink up to 16 cups of coffee per day. Cessation of intake leads to real withdrawal symptoms within 24-36 hours, including irritability, headache, nausea, and vomiting. Caffeine has physical effects, causing tremulousness and increased gastric acidity. At present, there is no firm link between reasonable coffee intake and carcinogenesis.

Nicotine

Nicotine, obtained from the tobacco plant, was brought to Europe from North and South America during the age of exploration. Tobacco can lead to altered states of consciousness, and nicotine tolerance can develop in hours (rather than in days or weeks as is the case for most other drugs). This shortened period of adaptation puts the casual experimenter in danger of becoming addicted. Cigarettes, because they are less harsh and are filtered, are more likely to be inhaled deeply relative to cigars or pipes. Chewing or taking tobacco as snuff deliver a relatively higher dose of nicotine but these forms of use are less addictive because delivery to the brain is less efficient than from inhalation. Nicotine addicts who also abuse other substances describe quitting nicotine use as much more difficult than curtailing the use of other substances. Physicians have tried chewing gum containing nicotine and skin patches with nicotine but these do little to curb the psychologic craving for nicotine.

The recent occupation of Somalia brought another novel natural stimulant to light: **khat** (also known as Qat, Chat, and Miraa). The leaves and twigs of the East African plant are chewed for their stimulating effect, the active ingredients resembling amphetamines. **Betel nut** is popular in Asia, and, when chewed, imparts a black color to the teeth. Betel nut contains acrolein, a stimulant that behaves like caffeine. Yohimbe is the source of **yohim-bine**, an alpha-2 antagonist that can be brewed into a stimulating tea. It is used medically to treat impotence, and is regarded by some as an aphrodisiac. Ephedra, the source of **ephedrine**, grows in arid areas. It is used to brew "Mormon tea," because the religion prohibits ingestion of caffeine.

Cocaine

Cocaine is a natural stimulant derived from the coca plant; South Americans chew the leaves for increased energy for day-to-day tasks. Cocaine was first utilized by physicians at the turn of the century for treatment of illnesses such as alcohol dependence. Cocaine was used by the wealthy and famous (even Sherlock Holmes). When its abuse potential became apparent, steps were taken to curb its availability. The Coca Cola Company, which previously had included cocaine as an ingredient of its drinks eliminated the drug, but still includes a drug-free extract of coca leaves in the soda. Cocaine is a widely used and highly potent mucous membrane topical local anesthetic in the medical setting.

Cocaine exerts varying effects depending on the mode of use. Inhaled and injected cocaine are much more potent than are ingested or topical. The more efficient delivery results in a euphoric and hyperstimulated state, and users can behave overtly psychotic, experiencing hallucinations and paranoid delusions, and can become violent. Physical effects include tremors, tachycardia, mydriasis, hypertension, and cardiac damage. Toxic doses can result in seizures, and withdrawal can cause extreme depression. Cocaine hydrochloride and its free base form, **crack**, have short half-lives. This makes management easier; if intervention is necessary, IV barbiturates or benzodiazepines can be used. Respiratory depression may occur with cocaine overdose. In the emergency department the cocaine metabolite, mercoyl ecognine, is often found in the urine of recent users.

Amphetamines

Amphetamines are synthetic stimulants, first developed in Germany in the 1930s. First suggested for use in improving the productivity of workers and soldiers during World War II, amphetamines later became widely used in diet pills. Amphetamines also became favored by truck drivers and athletes. Currently amphetamines have been restricted for use in only a few situations. The effects are similar to those of cocaine, but display a much longer duration of action. Hepatic metabolism of amphetamines is much slower than that of cocaine, thus their toxicity is greater. Withdrawal symptoms parallel those of cocaine, and suicidal attempts and extreme depression can be seen after use. Psychoses will respond to haloperidol or phenothiazines, and acidification of the urine with ammonium chloride will aid in amphetamine excretion.

Depressants

Alcohol intoxication

Alcohol is the most widely used and oldest known psychoactive substance. What began as the ingestion of crudely fermented brews centuries ago has evolved into a problem affecting millions. Alcohol use is assessed from two perspectives: the toxic effects due to acute ingestion, and the syndrome of chronic alcoholism.

Acute intoxication is due to absorption into the blood. Absorption occurs at a higher rate than does oxidation and elimination; thus, levels rise. Serum levels are accurate indicators of intoxication, although significant individual variations in the ability to metabolize alcohol exist. The legal limit for intoxication is 100mg/dL, although some individuals will be incapacitated at much lower levels. Levels between 100-400mg/dL produce symptoms ranging from lack of coordination to delirium, and levels in excess of 500mg/dL may be fatal. Most people will clear alcohol at a rate ranging between 20 and 30mg/dL per hour; this often provides a rough guideline for estimating time of recovery from alcohol's effects. Roughly, the better the function at higher serum levels, the greater the tolerance. The chronic alcoholic has a long-standing history of dependence on alcohol, needs to drink to prevent withdrawal, has poor work and family relationships, drinks alone, often may have a legal record, and often needs medical intervention because of alcohol use.

Patients seen for alcohol related problems generally fit into one of 3 categories: those **acutely intoxicated**, those **withdrawing** from alcohol, and those with medical complications from **longstanding alcohol abuse**. The intoxicated patient will have slurred speech, and impaired judgment, and can be violent or euphoric. Poor motor coordination, orthostatic hypotension, and dizziness can be present. Severely intoxicated patients may have decreased

Psychiatry
Substance Abuse *continued*

respiratory rate, hypothermia, and may become comatose. Idiosyncratic intoxication refers to the development of aggression and antegrade amnesia following ingestion of minuscule amount of alcohol. The behavioral changes usually subside within several hours or days and the patient typically ends the episode after prolonged sleep.

Withdrawal

Alcohol withdrawal peaks 2-48 hours after the last drink. Symptoms include irritability, depression and anxiety, with auditory, tactile, or visual hallucinations (true visual hallucinations are rare and strongly suggest alcohol withdrawal). Tachycardia, sweating, hypertension, tremors, nausea and vomiting can be present. This syndrome, **delirium tremens** ("DTs"), when occurring in hospitalized patients can be highly morbid or even fatal. Benzodiazepines are used to treat withdrawal, as are clonidine and atenolol. Phenothiazines are not recommended because of the chance that they might lower seizure thresholds and lead to further complications. Alcohol itself, when administered under medical supervision, is safe and may be the best overall treatment for acute withdrawal.

Wernicke–Korsakoff syndrome is actually two separate disorders. **Wernicke's encephalopathy** is an acute disorder, consisting of cerebellar ataxia, oculomotor disturbances such as nystagmus, and impaired mentation. This can be fatal if untreated. **Korsakoff's psychosis** is chronic, and typically follows an acute episode of Wernicke's encephalopathy. It is characterized by severe memory impairment usually manifested as retrograde amnesia and inability of the patient to remember anything: he or she literally lives only in the present.

Opiates

Drugs derived from morphine and other constituents of opium are called **opiates**. The analgesic properties of these compounds have been known for hundreds of years, being utilized in crude form until a German pharmacist isolated morphine (named for Morpheus, the Greek god of dreams) in the early 1800s. Since then, dozens of synthetic derivatives have been made. Heroin is semisynthetic derivative while Demerol is purely synthetic. All opiates essentially produce the same effects, but differ in onset and duration of action. The opiates that are injectable are more easily abused.

Tolerance and physical dependence develop rapidly over 2-3 days and the user will have withdrawal symptoms upon discontinuation of the drug. Opiate intoxication is characterized as euphoria, flushing, miosis, drowsiness, bradycardia, hypothermia, and decreased respiratory rate. Withdrawal symptoms and signs are typically opposite to the pharmacological effects seen with opiates. The severity of the withdrawal syndrome varies with the size of the opioid dose and the duration of dependence. Symptoms can appear 4-6 hours after the last dose and peak within 36-72 hours, and include nausea, vomiting, dilated pupils, insomnia, lacrimation, hyperpyrexia, and abdominal pain. Clonidine can reduce the autonomic symptoms of withdrawal. Methadone is used for chronic support, although, being an opiate also, it obviously merely substitutes one drug for another. Its benefits include reduced mental status effects and legality.

Sedative-hypnotics

Sedative-hypnotics, also known as downers or sleeping pills, are divided into barbiturate sedatives, non-barbiturate sedatives, and minor tranquilizers. These share many characteristics with alcohol, and elicit many of the moods and cognitive effects seen with acute alcohol ingestion. Tolerance to the mood-related effects of these drugs develops at a more rapid rate than physiological tolerance. People who take the drug, therefore, are at increased risk of overdose. The shared properties make this group of drugs acceptable treatment for withdrawal from alcohol, but thus they also are extremely dangerous when used in combination.

Barbiturates

The first **barbiturate** drug, barbital, was introduced in 1903. Since then, numerous derivatives have appeared. Barbiturates are useful clinically. Long-acting barbiturates like phenobarbital can be used as daytime sedatives. Intermediate-acting barbiturates like amobarbital and secobarbital have the most alcohol-like behavior and end up being abused. Short-acting barbiturates, such as thiopental, are useful as anesthetics.

Non-barbiturate sedatives include methaqualene (Quaaludes) and chloral hydrate. A "Mickey Finn" (watch an old movie) refers to chloral hydrate added to alcohol to sedate an unsuspecting victim. Chloral hydrate is sometimes used to sedate children for procedures.
(continued)

Minor tranquilizers

Minor tranquilizers refer to the benzodiazepines (and seldom used meprobamate). Meprobamate was the first of this class to be released (1954), but has since been replaced by the benzodiazepines. Benzodiazepines are widely used in the inpatient and outpatient setting as anxiolytics and sleeping pills, but are illegally abused due to their mood-altering properties. Benzodiazepines are metabolized by oxidation in the liver to active metabolites, many of which are also benzodiazepines. Caution must thus be used in alcoholics or in anyone with impaired hepatic function.

Psychedelics or Hallucinogens

These substances, despite their name, rarely produce true hallucinations, rather euphoria and perceptual changes. Patients may be in panic states and appear extremely apprehensive due to their lack of ability to effectively deal with the perceptual distortions. Symptoms subside in hours but may recur periodically years after last use (flashbacks).

LSD

Lysergic acid diethylamide (LSD) is the most famous psychedelic. It was synthesized from ergot (a plant fungus that attacks cereal grains) by Albert Hoffman in 1938. It became popular in the 1960s, then saw a decline in use that has since reversed. Other drugs in this class include **peyote**, **mescaline**, and **mushrooms** (psylocybin is the active ingredient). **Ibogaine**, derived from the African plant, iboga, produces effects comparable to LSD and has recently been proposed as a treatment for opiate addiction.

PCP

Phencyclidine (PCP) is not easily classified because of the bewildering effect on the CNS. First proposed as an anesthetic, the drug produces severe delusional and psychotic states in the user. Now approved as a veterinary anesthetic, the drug appears in crudely synthesized form and is either injected or smoked after being sprinkled on marijuana or tobacco. Users are often psychotic and extremely violent, and often cannot feel (or disregard) pain — not a good combination. Management of these patients includes physical restraint and benzodiazepines to counteract the anxiety the patient experiences because of delusions. For the violent patient on PCP, haloperidol may be useful in combination with urine acidification to enhance excretion.

Marijuana

Known as ganja, kaya, herb, and weed, **marijuana** (cannabis) has been used for centuries. It produces a dreamy state of well-being referred to as a "high." Symptoms associated with the drug are dependent on the setting in which it is used and pre-existing psychiatric function. There seems to be no physical dependence associated with the drug. The metabolic products from the drug are fat soluble; metabolites are detectable up to 7 days after last use in the occasional user and up to 30 days in the chronic user. Debate continues as to potential medical uses and legality of the drug — it seems to be no more intrinsically harmful than alcohol.

Miscellaneous

Certain unusual sources of psychoactive substances are easily obtained, such as **glue**, **solvents**, and **aerosol propellants**. The effects are similar to mild anesthesia. **Nitrous oxide** (laughing gas) is obtainable from spray cans of whipped cream ("whip-its") or sold in balloons at rock concerts. **Benzotropine** (cogentin) can be misused for its "buzz." Finally, street chemists will experiment with unusual combinations of drugs and chemicals with disastrous results. Notable are adulterations added to "cut" pure heroin or cocaine or to enhance effects. A recent example of the latter is "Crazy Eddie," a mixture of embalming fluid (formaldehyde) and crack. ■